T0142184

Essentials in Ophthalmology

Series Editor
Arun D. Singh

More information about this series at http://www.springer.com/series/5332

Jorge L. Alió
Editor

Keratoconus

Recent Advances in Diagnosis and Treatment

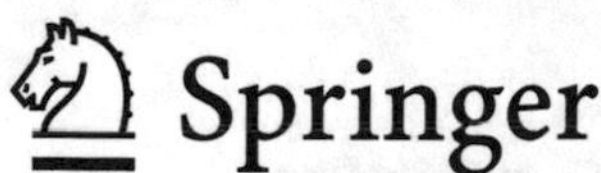

Editor
Jorge L. Alió, MD, PhD, FEBO
Keratoconus Unit
Department of Refractive Surgery
Vissum Alicante, Alicante, Spain

Division of Ophthalmology
Miguel Hernández University
Alicante, Spain

ISSN 1612-3212 ISSN 2196-890X (electronic)
Essentials in Ophthalmology
ISBN 978-3-319-82933-3 ISBN 978-3-319-43881-8 (eBook)
DOI 10.1007/978-3-319-43881-8

Softcover reprint of the hardcover 1st edition 2016

Printed on acid-free paper

This Springer imprint is published by Springer Nature
The registered company is Springer International Publishing AG
The registered company address is: Gewerbestrasse 11, 6330 Cham, Switzerland

Foreword

When Jorge Alió invited me to write the introduction to this fascinating book, I was both honoured and delighted. The task brought together three components which have made a significant impact upon the world of corneal disease and refractive surgery, namely a better understanding of keratoconus and corneal biomechanics together with the lifelong contributions of Jorge Alió.

For science to better understand the nature of any given problem, it is often best to investigate extremes of that problem. Fortunately most of the world's population possess corneas whose biological and biomechanical properties fall within defined limits; however, there are a significant number within the pathological group defined as keratoconus whereby the mechanical properties are well outside the normal range. This book gathers together our knowledge of keratoconus and in doing so allows a far more comprehensive appreciation of deviation from the norm and how that comes about.

The volume starts with a detailed review of the magnitude of the problem in terms of both genetics and epidemiology and immediately follows by relating structural changes observed by histopathology. Corneal genetics is a rapidly moving field with genetic screening for granular dystrophies already a reality. Major advances are now being made in the field of keratoconus, and it will not be too long before we see genetic screening for individuals within this group. Today ever-evolving diagnostic techniques allow earlier diagnosis with the implications that in future early diagnosis in children and early intervention will limit if not prevent severe visual problems associated with keratoconus.

The section on diagnostic tools is a comprehensive survey of what is currently available and gives useful reviews of the advantages and disadvantages of specific techniques. Great emphasis is placed on topography and tomography together with various theories as to the usefulness of each of these techniques. It should be specially mentioned that one chapter addresses the topic of the new and important role of corneal epithelial thickness study in the diagnosis of keratoconus assisted by very high frequency ultrasound devices, an issue that probably will deserve further attention due to its relevance in the coming years.

While biomechanics are discussed, it is unfortunate that to date we do not have any reliable clinical devices to measure changes in biomechanical properties. Laboratory studies have concentrated on extensiometry whereby strips of cornea are cut from donor eyes and then loaded with weights whilst measuring changes in length, Hooke's law. These studies are of limited if any value because they destroy the integrity of the hemisphere of the cornea and ignore the stress-strain relationships that are thereby lost. This is of particular importance in the evaluation of a patchy differential elasticity in keratoconus. More recent studies using interferometry have given useful values for corneal biomechanics but have not yet reached the clinical forum. The promise of Brillouin scatter for making such measurements is also confounded by problems because these measurements are totally dependent upon water content which varies as a function of corneal depth and therefore water concentration should be monitored simultaneously by perhaps the use of Raman scatter, but this in turn is dependent upon detailed knowledge of temperature at the point of measurement.

Descriptions of therapeutic interventions form a significant part of this volume and the advent of cross-linking is emphasised. It has always been of some concern that removing or cutting into corneas with excessive elasticities may lead to exacerbation of the problem over time. The use of intra-corneal rings and segments is reported to have some success, but we should be aware of the experience of retinal surgeons when they report their findings of silicon compression rings in detachment surgery. Over a 20–30-year period erosion has been reported because of the differential rigidity between these devices and the underlying sclera, and sometimes these devices have worked their way through the entire sclera and have been found in the choroid. Collagen does not react well to prolonged positive or negative stress. In a similar fashion Excimer ablation may well correct a degree of the refractive error in the short term, but in removing tissue will certainly weaken the globe and may exacerbate the process over a patient's lifetime.

The section on cross-linking is comprehensive, and the introduction of this technique may well herald a new era in the treatment of keratoconus; as for the first time we have a potential treatment regime which is targeting one of the underlying elements of the disease process, i.e. loss of rigidity, by inducing cross-linking between the glycoprotein elements associated with the collagen helixes and increasing rigidity results. While the nature of the process is not fully understood and the relative contributions from fibres associated with collagen and elements in the surrounding matrix have not been defined, the clinical results are clearly significant. The initial clinical regime with a 30 min soaking riboflavin followed by 30 min of ultraviolet irradiation has been modified by many groups, and now much faster procedures have been developed. As the understanding of the photochemistry becomes apparent, further modifications may be made to improve the outcome of the procedure including riboflavin with various additives together with additional oxygen being made available and pulsing the ultraviolet radiation. A useful discussion is presented concerning the presence or absence of the epithelium prior to the commencement of the cross-linking procedure. This is extremely important as the epithelium presents a barrier to the diffusion of riboflavin and at the same time absorbs around 20 % of the incident UV radiation. Treatments with the epithelium on must first defeat the barrier properties and then have sufficient power in the radiating source to compensate for the loss of energy absorbed by the epithelium. Even if these two elements are rectified, there is a further component in ensuring adequate cross-linking and that is the presence of sufficient oxygen. Currently as reported most groups treat with the epithelium off, but the obvious goal is to treat with epithelium on using suitably modified protocols and components.

This is an excellent compendium of our current knowledge of keratoconus and will become a handbook for those in the field. I have no hesitation whatsoever in commending it to you and congratulate all the authors of the various chapters in doing a fantastic job and in particular Jorge Alió for bringing it together and making it possible.

London, UK John Marshall

Preface

During recent years, especially in the last 10 years, an increasing interest in the diagnosis and treatment of keratoconus has arisen.

Over these years, the topic has been in continuous evolution with noteworthy improvements that have transformed keratoconus into a completely different entity in terms of clinical understanding and potential treatment. The progress of the knowledge about the subject has been so great and in depth that the practical clinician has observed it with eyes wide open and astonished at the changes in the paradigms on keratoconus diagnosis and treatment modalities. Publications in peer-reviewed journals and tabloids have increased enormously as well.

This is why we believe that, in this moment, there is a need to summarise the most updated knowledge in keratoconus management and treatment in a book like the one that you, the reader, have now in your hands. Even though a book when published may never be complete and updated, the reader will find along the different chapters a considerable amount of new information on the diagnosis and different modern therapeutic modalities of keratoconus that can be used practically to assist the medical management of keratoconus patients.

We would like to thank all the co-authors of this book and all those who have supported this endeavour, especially Springer, for their kindness in publishing this book, for the contribution that this may provide to those interested in using better treatment alternatives for keratoconus patients.

I would like to thank especially my colleagues and most especially my family for the time, dedication and understanding in the many weeks, days and hours that have been taken to build up this book. I would like to thank also my truly loyal secretary, Ruth Waterhouse, for the coordination that she has made during the edition of this book and for her quiet support in putting it altogether.

Miguel Hernández University
Alicante, Spain

Jorge L. Alió

Contents

Contributors

Jorge L. Alió, MD, PhD, FEBO Keratoconus Unit, Department of Refractive Surgery, Vissum Alicante, Alicante, Spain

Division of Ophthalmology, Miguel Hernández University, Alicante, Spain

Jorge L. Alió del Barrio, MD, PhD Keratoconus Unit, Department of Refractive Surgery, Vissum Alicante, Alicante, Spain

Division of Ophthalmology, Miguel Hernández University, Alicante, Spain

Renato Ambrósio Jr., MD, PhD Department of Ophthalmology, Instituto de Olhos Renato Ambrósio, Rio de Janeiro, RJ, Brazil

VisareRio, Rio de Janeiro, Brazil

Universidade Federal de São Paulo, São Paulo, Brazil

Rio de Janeiro Corneal Tomography and Biomechanics Study Group, Rio de Janeiro, Brazil

David F. Anderson, MBChB, FRCOphth, PhD Southampton Eye Unit, University Hospital Southampton, Southampton, UK

University of Southampton, Southampton, UK

Timothy J. Archer, MA(Oxon), DipCompSci(Cantab) London Vision Clinic, London, UK

Francisco Arnalich Montiel, MD, PhD Ophthalmology Department, IRYCIS, Ramón y Cajal University Hospital, Madrid, Spain

Cornea Unit, Hospital Vissum Madrid, Madrid, Spain

FangJun Bao, PhD, MD Eye Hospital, Wenzhou Medical University, Wenzhou, Zhejiang, China

The Institution of Ocular Biomechanics, Wenzhou Medical University, Wenzhou, Zhejiang, China

Adel Barbara, MD, FRCOphth IVision Medical Center, Keratoconus and Refractive Surgery Centre, Haifa, Israel

Ramez Barbara, MBChB Southampton Eye Unit, University Hospital Southampton, Southampton, UK

Michael W. Belin, MD Department of Ophthalmology and Vision Science, Southern Arizona VA Healthcare System, University of Arizona, Tucson, AZ, USA

Luca Buzzonetti, MD Ophthalmology Department, Bambino Gesù IRCCS Children's Hospital, Rome, Italy

Institute of Ophthalmology, Catholic University, Rome, Italy

Annalisa Canovetti, MD U.O. Oculistica, Nuovo Ospedale S. Stefano, Prato, Italy

Francisco Cavas-Martínez, PhD Department of Graphical Expression, Technical University of Cartagena, Cartagena, Murcia, Spain

Kathryn Colby, MD, PhD Department of Ophthalmology and Visual Science, University of Chicago, Chicago, IL, USA

Ernesto De la Cruz Sánchez, PhD Faculty of Sports Science, University of Murcia, Santiago de la Ribera, Murcia, Spain

Ahmed Elsheikh, PhD School of Engineering, University of Liverpool, Liverpool, UK

NIHR Biomedical Research Centre for Ophthalmology, Moorfields Eye Hospital NHS Foundation Trust and UCL Institute of Ophthalmology, Liverpool, UK

Fernando Faria Correia, MD Rio de Janeiro Corneal Tomography and Biomechanics Study Group, Rio de Janeiro, Brazil

Cornea and Refractive Surgery Department, Hospital de Braga, Braga, Portugal

Cornea and Refractive Surgery Department, Instituto CUF, Porto, Portugal

Life and Health Sciences Research Institute (ICVS), School of Health Sciences, University of Minho, Braga, Portugal

ICVS/3B's-PT Government Associate Laboratory, Braga/Guimarães, Portugal

Roberto Fernández Buenaga, MD, PhD Keratoconus Unit, Department of Refractive Surgery, Vissum Corporation, Edificio Vissum, Alicante, Spain

Francisco J. Fernández Cañavate, PhD Department of Graphical Expression, Technical University of Cartagena, Cartagena, Murcia, Spain

Daniel García Fernández-Pacheco, PhD Department of Graphical Expression, Technical University of Cartagena, Cartagena, Murcia, Spain

Pierre Fournié, MD, PhD Department of Ophthalmology, CRNK, CHU Toulouse, Hôpital Pierre-Paul Riquet, Toulouse, France

Stéphane D. Galiacy, PhD CRNK, CHU Toulouse, Hôpital Pierre-Paul Riquet, Toulouse, France

Brendan Geraghty, PhD School of Engineering, University of Liverpool, Liverpool, UK

NIHR Biomedical Research Centre for Ophthalmology, Moorfields Eye Hospital NHS Foundation Trust and UCL Institute of Ophthalmology, Liverpool, UK

Marine Gobbe, MST(Optom), PhD London Vision Clinic, London, UK

Farhad Hafezi, MD, PhD Center for Applied Biotechnology and Molecular Medicine (CABMM), University of Zurich, Zurich, Switzerland

ELZA Institute, Dietikon, Zurich, Switzerland

University of Southern California, Los Angeles, CA, USA

University of Geneva, Geneva, Switzerland

Parwez Hossain, MBChB, FRCOphth, PhD Southampton Eye Unit, University Hospital Southampton, Southampton, UK

University of Southampton, Southampton, UK

Salim Ismail, BSc, MSc (Hons) Department of Ophthalmology, New Zealand National Eye Centre, Faculty of Medical and Health Sciences, University of Auckland, Auckland, New Zealand

Aylin Kılıç, MD Department of Cataract and Refractive Surgery, Istanbul Göz Hastanesi, Istanbul, Turkey

Sabine Kling, PhD Center for Applied Biotechnology and Molecular Medicine (CABMM), University of Zurich, Zürich, Switzerland

Ivo Lenzetti, MD U.O. Oculistica, Nuovo Ospedale S. Stefano, Prato, Italy

I-Ping Loh, MSc Department of Ophthalmology, New Zealand National Eye Centre, Faculty of Medical and Health Sciences, University of Auckland, Auckland, New Zealand

Alex Malandrini, MD U.O. Oculistica, Nuovo Ospedale S. Stefano, Prato, Italy

François Malecaze, MD, PhD Department of Ophthalmology, CRNK, CHU Toulouse, Hôpital Pierre-Paul Riquet, Toulouse, France

Jennifer Jane McGhee, BSc Department of Ophthalmology, New Zealand National Eye Centre, Faculty of Medical and Health Sciences, University of Auckland, Auckland, New Zealand

Luca Menabuoni, MD U.O. Oculistica, Nuovo Ospedale S. Stefano, Prato, Italy

José Nieto Martínez, PhD Department of Graphical Expression, Technical University of Cartagena, Cartagena, Murcia, Spain

David O'Brart Department of Ophthalmology, Guy's and St. Thomas' Hospital, London, UK

King's College London, London, UK

Gianni Petrocelli, MD Ophthalmology Department, Bambino Gesù IRCCS Children's Hospital, Rome, Italy

Roberto Pini, PhD Institute of Applied Physics, Italian National Research Council, Sesto Florence, Italy

Ana Belén Plaza Puche, PhD Keratoconus Unit, Vissum Alicante, Alicante, Spain

Dan Z. Reinstein, MD, MA(Cantab), FRCSC, FRC, Ophth London Vision Clinic, London, UK

Columbia University Medical Center, New York, NY, USA

Centre Hospitalier National d'Ophtalmologie, Paris, France

School of Biomedical Sciences, University of Ulster, Coleraine, UK

Francesca Rossi, PhD Institute of Applied Physics, Italian National Research Council, Sesto Florence, Italy

Pablo Sanz Díez, OD, MSc Keratoconus Unit, Department of Refractive Surgery, Vissum Alicante, Alicante, Spain

Division of Ophthalmology, Miguel Hernández University, Alicante, Spain

Giuliano Scarcelli, PhD Fischell Department of Bioengineering, University of Maryland, College Park, MD, USA

Mohamed Shafik Shaheen, MD, PhD Department of Ophthalmology, University of Alexandria, Alexandria, Egypt

Ahmed Shalaby, MD Department of Ophthalmology, University of Alexandria University Main Hospital, Alexandria, Egypt

Trevor Sherwin, BSc (Hons), PhD Department of Ophthalmology, New Zealand National Eye Centre, Faculty of Medical and Health Sciences, University of Auckland, Auckland, New Zealand

Ronald H. Silverman, MS, PhD Department of Ophthalmology, Columbia University Medical Center, New York, NY, USA

F.L. Lizzi Center for Biomedical Engineering, Riverside Research, New York, NY, USA

Joaquin Silvestre-Albero Inorganic Chemistry Department, University de Alicante, Alicante, Spain

Andrew M.J. Turnbull, MBChB Southampton Eye Unit, University Hospital Southampton, Southampton, UK

Raksha Urs, PhD Department of Ophthalmology, Columbia University Medical Center, New York, NY, USA

Paola Valente, MD Ophthalmology Department, Bambino Gesù IRCCS Children's Hospital, Rome, Italy

Alfredo Vega Estrada, PhD Keratoconus Unit, Vissum Alicante, Alicante, Spain

Francesco Versaci, MSE CSO srl, Florence, Italy

Gabriele Vestri, MSE CSO srl, Florence, Italy

QinMei Wang, MD Eye Hospital, Wenzhou Medical University, Wenzhou, Zhejiang, China

The Institution of Ocular Biomechanics, Wenzhou University, Wenzhou, Zhejiang, China

Amy Watts, OD, FAAO Department of Ophthalmology, Massachusetts Eye and Ear Hospital, Boston, MA, USA

Seok Hyun Yun, PhD Wellman Center for Photomedicine, Massachusetts General Hospital, Cambridge, MA, USA

Department of Dermatology, Harvard Medical School, Boston, MA, USA

Hussam Zaghloul, MD Department of Ophthalmology, Alexandria Armed Forces Hospital, Alexandria, Egypt

Part I

Introduction

1 What Is Keratoconus? A New Approach to a Not So Rare Disease

Jorge L. Alió

Keratoconus is today a classic topic in ophthalmology. Its history is associated to a background of a corneal disease with a blinding potential and no hope for treatment. It is only since the late 1950s that contact lenses have become a partial solution for the visual loss for some cases of keratoconus while other approaches were nonexisting. Those patients diagnosed with keratoconus had the same category as any corneal dystrophy with no potential treatment and no therapeutic recommendations to perform. The patients had no hope for the future and could not do anything about preventing its progress or being informed about the potential long-term complications or any consistent and reliable therapeutic approach.

Since those historical and recent "black days" until now there has been a tremendous evolution. At this moment in 2016, there is a completely different approach for the diagnosis and treatment of keratoconus.

The study and diagnosis of keratoconus has radically changed since the early seventeenth century when the Jesuit Priest Christoph Scheiner [1] experienced and reported that glasses of different shapes reflect light in different ways, until nowadays, corneal diagnostic technology has taken a huge step forward. Scheiner used the optical phenomenon he described to assess the curvature of the human cornea. In doing it, he was able to compare the light reflections of different shapes and he even described some pathologies that were evident cases of keratoconus. Since those early days and later on when the sophistications for the measurement of corneal curvature were introduced in the late nineteenth century by Javal until almost recently with the development of modern corneal topographics, a new diagnostic universe has appeared [2]. A universe of precise diagnosis, developing early indicators of the disease [3] and indeed creating grading in categories of the disease according to severity [4].

In parallel to that, new corneal surgical approaches have been developed. Most probably, the first corneal grafts performed by Edward Zirm in Prague were advanced keratoconus cases [5]. It is unclear in the literature, but most probably, those cases really were as hopeless as to deserve a new surgery with a huge potential of unknown complications and a lack of the adequate technology to perform them. For sure all of them failed.

Today, an array of surgical approaches exists for corneal grafting in keratoconus [6]. The development of anterior lamellar graft and more recently, the potential to peel off the Descemet membrane from the innermost layers of the cornea (DALK) has completely changed the biological perspective of these patients in which corneal

J.L. Alió, M.D., Ph.D., F.E.B.O. (✉)
Keratoconus Unit, Department of Refractive Surgery, Vissum Alicante, Alicante, Spain

Division of Ophthalmology, Miguel Hernández University, Alicante, Spain
e-mail: jlalio@vissum.com

J.L. Alió (ed.), *Keratoconus*, Essentials in Ophthalmology, DOI 10.1007/978-3-319-43881-8_1

biological failure rejection was one of the main problems. Even though deep anterior lamellar graft has not demonstrated superior outcomes to penetrating graft in terms of visual and refractive outcome, its biological benefits are clear [6].

However, it is not only about the anatomical exchange of corneal tissue but rather about improving it in a different shape with better optical performance and with a better biological stability. This last issue has been precisely approached by the new invasive pharmacology of the cornea, based on the use of riboflavin and ultraviolet activation has revolutionized the therapy of corneal disease starting with keratoconus. These invasive pharmacological methods have just started and even though today they are widely and successfully used, it is probably just the beginning of a new era in the treatment of corneal disease and particularly in the treatment of keratoconus.

What are the consequences of all these improvements happening in diagnosis, technology, surgical capabilities, and emerging innovative therapies? The first is that keratoconus has become today a pandemic disorder. Those of us today who dedicate our professional time to cornea diseases have never seen so many cases, so many presentations in meetings, and so many publications about keratoconus as in the last 10 years. The reason for this is clear: there were many more cases than expected. The definition of keratoconus as a rare disease is no longer sustainable: some areas of the world, due to genetic and environmental factors, are suffering an epidemic outbreak of keratoconus, which is really based on the improved and more accessible diagnostic capabilities we have and the diagnostic precision that we have achieved. This increase in the number of cases has led to the development of keratoconus experts, specialized units, and even a new journal (*International Journal of Keratoconus and Corneal Ectatic Diseases*), solely dedicated to what has been until now a rare disease. In Cornea and Comprehensive Ophthalmological meetings, discussions on keratoconus are vivid. Databases of keratoconus have been created worldwide such as the one that we created in Spain 8 years ago called the Iberia Keratoconus Database which, in a few years, has collected over 3000 cases of keratoconus of the Iberian peninsula with cases from all areas of Spain and Portugal (Red Tematica de Investigacion Oftalmologica OFTARED, Ministerio de Ciencia y Tecnologia, Spain). All these patients represent at this moment a huge amount of information. Patients today have hope for the treatment of a disease that was formerly hopeless. They not only hope to achieve vision but also better vision. As an example, refractive surgery, formerly forbidden might have a role in keratoconus in certain special conditions and it is today demanded by these patients (see Chaps. 12–15).

All these improvements, all this progress, all this newly developed knowledge, in our opinion, have led to the need for the development of this new book. In this book, the reader will see how modern approaches to keratoconus from different perspectives are improving our understanding about its etiology and pathogenesis, its evolution, its classification, its diagnosis, the application of technology to therapy, the use of surgical and invasive pharmacological tools and, finally the future perspectives that we have for those patients who, unfortunately, have keratoconus.

Patients suffering from keratoconus, even though unfortunate, are lucky enough to live in an era in which keratoconus, a disease that was formerly untreatable, is now starting to be treated successfully and can lead to good visual outcomes. A better future is available already and further improvements are coming soon for these patients.

Compliance with Ethical Requirements Jorge L. Alió declares that he has no conflict of interest. No human or animal studies were carried out by the author for this chapter.

References

1. Christof S. Oculus hoc est: fundamentum opticum. Innsbruck: Daniel Agricola; 1619.
2. Wilson S, Klyce S. Advances in the analysis of corneal topography. Surv Ophthalmol. 1991;35:269–77.
3. Barbara A. Textbook on keratoconus. New insights. Section 2. Diagnosis of keratoconus and diagnostic tools. 1st ed. New Delhi: Jaypee Brothers

Medical Publishers Ltd; 2012. p. 35–96. ISBN 978-93-5025-404-2.
4. Alio J, Vega-Estrada A, Sanz-Diez P, Peña-Garcia P, Duran-Garcia ML, Maldonado M. Titulo: keratoconus management guidelines. Int J Kerat Ect Cor Dis. 2015;4:1–39.
5. Zirm E. Eine erfolgreiche totale Keratoplastik. Albrecht von Graefes Arch Ophthal. 1906;64:580–93.
6. Arnalich F, Barrio J, Alio JL. Corneal surgery in keratoconus: which type, which technique, which outcomes? Eye Vis. 2016;3:2.

Modern Pathogenesis of Keratoconus: Genomics and Proteomics

2

Pierre Fournié, Stéphane D. Galiacy, and François Malecaze

2.1 Introduction

Despite numerous intensive studies, the pathogenesis of keratoconus remains unknown. Eye rubbing and the presence of allergies seem to be the only commonly identified factors.

The majority of keratoconus cases are temporally sporadic and some forms are defined by the existence of several clinically affected patients within the same family. Autosomal dominant (with reduced penetrance) and autosomal recessive transmission modes have been described [1]. Several studies suggest the existence of subclinical forms within the relatives of an affected patient with keratoconus [2, 3]. Identical twins show strong concordance of keratoconus with a high degree of phenotypic similarities, suggesting a key role for a genetic component [4].

Extreme variations in the prevalence of keratoconus are observed in relation to ethnicity. One study investigating its prevalence in Asian and Caucasian individuals living in similar geographic zones demonstrated an unequal distribution of the disease. Its incidence is four times higher among Asian individuals compared to Caucasians [5]. Others studies report differences in the severity and evolution of the disease in relation to ethnicity, which provides another strong argument in favour of a genetic component [6, 7]. While the multifactorial origin is accepted, the genetic component undoubtedly has a major role [8, 9].

Two pathophysiological mechanisms, probably interrelated, have been proposed: a biomechanical change or a biological origin. The biological origin of the disease can be investigated based on either a candidate hypothesis or a comparative analysis without candidate.

2.2 Candidate-Driven Approach

2.2.1 Candidate Gene Approach

The candidate gene approach is based on the knowledge of the disease biochemistry and pathology and consists of identifying mutations in encoding genes for the proteins of the affected tissue. Several studies found enzymatic and biochemical anomalies in affected corneas [9, 10]. The association of keratoconus with osteogenesis imperfecta [11] and mitral valve disease [12, 13] indicates a potential role for collagen anomalies in its occurrence. Studies investigating the pathogenesis of

P. Fournié, M.D., Ph.D. (✉) • F. Malecaze, M.D., Ph.D.
Department of Ophthalmology, CRNK, CHU Toulouse, Hôpital Pierre-Paul Riquet, Toulouse, France
e-mail: fournie.p@chu-toulouse.fr; malecaze.fr@chu-toulouse.fr

S.D. Galiacy, Ph.D.
CRNK, CHU Toulouse, Hôpital Pierre-Paul Riquet, Toulouse, France
e-mail: galiacy.s@chu-toulouse.fr

J.L. Alió (ed.), *Keratoconus*, Essentials in Ophthalmology, DOI 10.1007/978-3-319-43881-8_2

keratoconus have attempted to identify mutations in genes coding for components of interleukin-I [14], proteases [15, 16], protease inhibitors [17, 18], and collagens. Type I, III, IV, V, VI, VII, and VIII collagens are present in the cornea. The first collagen-encoding gene tested was COL6A1, but no significant relationship with keratoconus was detected [19]. Similarly, other collagen-encoding genes of the cornea were tested and eliminated [10]. Negative results obtained from linkage analyses do not exclude the role of these encoding genes in certain types of keratoconus. Indeed, the degree of genetic heterogeneity of this disease is unknown and mutations of several encoding genes from families that have not been tested may yet play a role in the emergence of keratoconus. One candidate gene study led to the identification of related mutations among patients affected by keratoconus. Mutations affecting the gene VSX1 were identified. This gene codes for a putative transcription factor and is also involved in posterior polymorphous dystrophy [20]. VSX1, however, has a role in only 0.1–0.4 % of familial keratoconus and thus its importance in the pathogenesis of keratoconus remains low.

2.2.2 Syndromic Keratoconus

Keratoconus is occasionally associated with other genetic or ophthalmologic diseases such as Down's syndrome, Leber congenital amaurosis, atopic diseases, conjunctivitis, some pigmentary retinopathies, mitral valve prolapse, collagen vascular diseases, and Marfan's syndrome [9, 10, 21]. It remains difficult, however, to establish a direct relationship between these diseases and keratoconus. Interpretations of these relationships are indeed challenging because of the relatively high prevalence of keratoconus, which remains probably underestimated. As a result, it is difficult to determine if these diseases are associated as co-factors triggering a keratoconus genetic susceptibility or if they are directly involved in the disease pathogenesis. This is an issue of particular significance when considering associated genetic diseases that are the results of the alteration of known genes and where a genetic analysis would help identify the gene responsible for keratoconus.

Down's syndrome is strongly related with keratoconus, with an estimated prevalence of 0.5–15 %, which is 10–300 times higher than the general population [10, 22, 23]. This suggests a link between keratoconus and chromosome 21. Numerous genetic studies have targeted this chromosome and some of them suggest its involvement in the pathogenesis of the disease [19]. This relationship, however, has also been attributed to some environmental factors such as eye rubbing, which may play a co-factor role, resulting in a strong prevalence of keratoconus [23].

Among all associated diseases, the direct cause of keratoconus is largely unknown and remains a matter of continued debate. This is predominantly due to the lack of basic information regarding the real prevalence of keratoconus and the impact of environmental factors.

2.2.3 Non-candidate-Driven Approach

An interesting global approach using 'omic' techniques aims to identify the origin of keratoconus without taking into account any preconceived ideas of the pathogenesis of the disease. In this approach, corneas affected by keratoconus are compared with healthy corneas during a particular cell machinery stage: the DNA (genomics), the RNA (transcriptomics), or the protein (proteomics). Transcriptomics is used to analyse, at the mRNA level, which genes are being expressed and in what ratios, whereas proteomics looks at the proteins that are subsequently translated.

2.2.4 Linkage Analysis

Unlike studies investigating candidate genes, genetic linkage analyses do not rely on any knowledge of the pathogenesis or biochemistry of the disease. Linkage analyses highlight genetic regions that contain genetic variants bound to a phenotype.

To date, 17 distinctive genetic regions have been identified [8], indicating the existence of a strong genetic heterogeneity in the development of keratoconus. Among these regions, only three have been independently verified (5q21, 5q32, and 14q11). These studies implicate two genes as potential minor candidates (*MIR184* and DOCK9). More recently, global sequencing of the genome and/or exome has replaced linkage analyses.

2.2.5 Genome-wide Association Studies

The relative failure of previous approaches and the recent advancements in molecular biology have promoted new studies. Using the state-of-the-art technologies of high-throughput genotyping, recent studies have compared the frequency of hundreds of thousands of genetic variants distributed among chromosomes. The most convincing studies detected linkage with variants of the gene *LOX* (lysyl oxidase, involved in the cross-linking of stromal collagen) [24, 25]. Other authors have concentrated on comparing intermediary phenotypes rather than groups of individuals (case–control study). Lu et al., for example, identified a region associating keratoconus with central corneal thinning [26]. Complementary meta-analyses have identified several variants in or near this region (*FOXO1*, *FNDC3B*, *RXRA-COL5A1*, *MPDZ-NFIB*, *COL5A1*, and *BANP-ZNF469*). One of these variants, *BANP-ZNF469*, was also found in an independent Australian cohort [27]. The role played by variants of this particular gene was confirmed in a study by Lechner et al. [28]. *ZNF469* is a gene that is also involved in another corneal syndrome (brittle cornea syndrome) and is linked to a thin and fragile cornea. This gene is currently the most important identified genetic factor in the pathogenesis of keratoconus.

2.2.6 Transcriptomics–Proteomics

Several studies have compared proteomes between patients affected by keratoconus and control patients. Comparability of results is difficult, due to differences in tissue type (tear fluid, corneal tissue: epithelium and/or stroma), age, disease severity, and development stage of keratoconus. A number of studies provide evidence that keratoconus is characterized by a cytokine imbalance in tear fluid and that these inflammatory mediators operate actively at the ocular surface. More than 1500 proteins have been identified in the analysis of the tear film. Higher levels of proteolytic activity and increased levels of proinflammatory cytokines, cell adhesion molecules, matrix metalloproteinases (MMP), glycoproteins, and transporter proteins have been observed compared to controls [29 32]. In particular, studies have shown a strong concordance of elevated Interleukin 6 (IL6), tumour necrosis factor α (TNFα), and MMP9 in tears from keratoconus patients [29, 33–35]. MMP9 is one of the matrix-degrading enzymes produced by the human corneal epithelium and regulated by cytokine IL6. In addition to IL6, TNFα is considered a major pathogenic factor in systemic and corneal inflammation. TNFα induces the expression of MMP9. Balasubramanian et al. [29] found higher levels of MMP9 in tears from keratoconic eyes, but the difference was not statistically significant. They indicated that the observed discrepancy might be explained because they used antibodies to the active MMP9. Shetty et al. [35] observed that MMP9, IL6, and TNFα were strongly upregulated at the mRNA level in keratoconus patient epithelia. However, whereas tears of keratoconus patients demonstrated an acute increase in MMP9 and IL6 levels over controls, TNFα levels did not show any significant associations with different grades of keratoconus. They demonstrated that the administration of cyclosporine A strongly reduced the inflammatory stimulation and expression of MMP9 in tears of keratoconus patients and decreased the production of IL6, TNFα, and MMP9 by corneal epithelial cells, while follow-up of 20 keratoconus patients over 6 months demonstrated significant local topographical changes in the cornea measured by keratometry. Although overall change in keratometry may not be very significant in the study, the authors suggest that cyclosporine A may be a promising new treatment modality for keratoconus [35].

We should take into account that the reported changes in tear film cytokine profile may not necessarily reflect intracorneal processes in keratoconus.

It is however becoming clear that mediators of inflammation are present in the keratoconus cornea. Keratoconus could be an inflammatory disorder as many studies are indicating elevated levels of inflammatory markers but with contradictory findings. Differences in the expression of some proteins (matrix components, cytokeratin, etc.) have also been observed at both the epithelial and stromal levels [35–37]. Findings overlap only partially, however, bringing into question not only the different pathophysiological routes involved but also the sampling procedures. Although keratoconus is not caused by corneal inflammation itself—clinical and histological findings show little evidence of this inflammation—data strongly substantiate the emerging concept of underlying inflammatory pathways in the pathogenesis of keratoconus. We must also bear in mind that there is the possibility that the changes in these inflammatory mediators may be an epiphenomenon of change in corneal structure.

Overall, it cannot be ruled out that keratoconus originates in events which take place outside the cornea but which are ultimately responsible for the induction of its ectasia. Numerous proteases, immunoglobulins, and cytokines have been found in tear fluid of patients but could reflect changes in lacrimal gland and conjunctiva.

Are these changes cause or effect and are they genetic or environmental in origin? The source of these proteins remains unknown. Atopy, eye rubbing, contact lens wear, oxidative stress [33, 38, 39], and genetic factors have been suggested to cause the disease. Balasubramanian et al. [40] made an interesting observation that eye rubbing increased inflammatory cytokines and MMP levels in tears in normal eyes and in keratoconus.

In addition to local activation of inflammatory pathways, there is accumulating evidence that systemic inflammatory changes [41] and systemic oxidative stress [33, 38, 39] may affect the corneal microenvironment in keratoconus. The interaction of corneal and systemic cellular inflammatory mediators that contribute to development of keratoconus is poorly understood.

Apoptosis of keratocytes is found as well [42, 43]. Based on an RNA study, Mace et al. demonstrated that keratoconus might be related to a deregulation of the proliferation pathways and cellular differentiation [43]. Inadequate balance between cytokines (pro- and anti-inflammatory) may lead to an altered corneal structure and function, triggering an increase in metalloproteinases and keratocytes apoptosis. The exact underlying molecular mechanisms remain to be elucidated.

These studies have shown that keratoconus demonstrates a corneal structural imbalance, associated with a metabolic stress, and an imbalance between apoptosis and proliferation. To date, however, these studies have failed to identify a clinically usable biomarker to screen keratoconus or assess its degree of severity.

2.3 Conclusion

The pathogenesis of keratoconus remains a mystery. Global analyses are beginning to highlight important affected pathways, but considerably more effort is required to understand the development of this disease. Scientific evidence has shown that keratoconus is a multifactorial disease involving complex interaction of both genetic and environmental factors.

Genetic susceptibility is now considered a key factor in the occurrence of keratoconus, but despite extensive studies, no contributing gene has yet been identified. Finding a gene responsible for keratoconus is crucial, as it would allow for the characterization of diagnostic criteria by comparing phenotypes and genotypes. This would aid surgeons as keratoconus is a contraindication to corneal refractive surgery, but it would also help to elucidate the pathogenesis of this disease.

Compliance with Ethical Requirements Pierre Fournié, Stéphane D. Galiacy, and François Malecaze declare that they have no conflict of interest. No human or animal studies were carried out by the authors for this chapter.

References

1. Wang Y, Rabinowitz YS, Rotter JI, Yang H. Genetic epidemiological study of keratoconus: evidence for major gene determination. Am J Med Genet. 2000;93:403–9.
2. Rabinowitz YS, Garbus J, McDonnell PJ. Computer-assisted corneal topography in family members of patients with keratoconus. Arch Ophthalmol. 1990;108:365–71.
3. Salabert D, Cochener B, Mage F, Colin J. Keratoconus and familial topographic corneal anomalies. J Fr Ophtalmol. 1994;17:646–56.
4. Tuft SJ, Hassan H, George S, et al. Keratoconus in 18 pairs of twins. Acta Ophthalmol. 2012;90:e482–6.
5. Pearson AR, Soneji B, Sarvananthan N, Sandford-Smith JH. Does ethnic origin influence the incidence or severity of keratoconus? Eye. 2000;14:625–8.
6. Tay KH, Chan WK. Penetrating keratoplasty for keratoconus. Ann Acad Med Singapore. 1997;26:132–7.
7. Tuft SJ, Moodaley LC, Gregory WM, et al. Prognostic factors for the progression of keratoconus. Ophthalmology. 1994;101:439–47.
8. Abu-Amero KK, Al-Muammar AM, Kondkar AA. Genetics of keratoconus: where do we stand? J Ophthalmol. 2014;2014:641708. doi:10.1155/2014/641708.
9. Edwards M, McGhee CN, Dean S. The genetics of keratoconus. Clin Exp Ophthalmol. 2001;29:345–51.
10. Rabinowitz YS. Keratoconus. Surv Ophthalmol. 1998;42:297–319.
11. Beckh U, Schonherr U, Naumann GO. Autosomal dominant keratoconus as the chief ocular symptom in Lobsteinosteogenesisimperfectatarda. Klin Monatsbl Augenheilkd. 1995;206:268 72.
12. Sharif KW, Casey TA, Coltart J. Prevalence of mitral valve prolapse in keratoconus patients. J R Soc Med. 1992;85:446–8.
13. Street DA, Vinokur ET, Waring 3rd GO, et al. Lack of association between keratoconus, mitral valve prolapse, and joint hypermobility. Ophthalmology. 1991;98:170–6.
14. Wilson SE, He YG, Weng J, et al. Epithelial injury induces keratocyte apoptosis: hypothesized role for the interleukin-1 system in the modulation of corneal tissue organization and wound healing. Exp Eye Res. 1996;62:325–7.
15. Kenney MC, Chwa M, Opbroek AJ, Brown DJ. Increased gelatinolytic activity in keratoconus keratocyte cultures. A correlation to an altered matrix metalloproteinase-2/tissue inhibitor of metalloproteinase ratio. Cornea. 1994;13:114–24.
16. Sawaguchi S, Yue BY, Sugar J, Gilboy JE. Lysosomal enzyme abnormalities in keratoconus. Arch Ophthalmol. 1989;107:1507–10.
17. Sawaguchi S, Twining SS, Yue BY, et al. Alpha-1 proteinase inhibitor levels in keratoconus. Exp Eye Res. 1990;50:549–54.
18. Sawaguchi S, Twining SS, Yue BY, et al. Alpha 2-macroglobulin levels in normal human and keratoconus corneas. Invest Ophthalmol Vis Sci. 1994;35:4008–14.
19. Rabinowitz YS, Maumenee IH, Lundergan MK, et al. Molecular genetic analysis in autosomal dominant keratoconus. Cornea. 1992;11:302–8.
20. Héon E, Greenberg A, Kopp KK, et al. VSX1: a gene for posterior polymorphous dystrophy and keratoconus. Hum Mol Genet. 2002;11:1029–36.
21. Bawazeer AM, Hodge WG, Lorimer B. Atopy and keratoconus: a multivariate analysis. Br J Ophthalmol. 2000;84:834–6.
22. Cullen JF, Butler HG. Mogolism (Down's syndrome) and keratoconus. Br J Ophtalmol. 1963;47:321–30.
23. Shapiro MB, France TD. The ocular features of Down's syndrome. Am J Ophthalmol. 1985;99:659–63.
24. Bykhovskaya Y, Li X, Epifantseva I, et al. Variation in the lysyl oxidase (LOX) gene is associated with keratoconus in family-based and case-control studies. Invest Ophthalmol Vis Sci. 2012;53:4152–7.
25. Dudakova L, Liskova P, Trojek T, et al. Changes in lysyl oxidase (LOX) distribution and its decreased activity in keratoconus corneas. Exp Eye Res. 2012;104:74–81.
26. Lu Y, Vitart V, Burdon KP, et al. Genome-wide association analyses identify multiple loci associated with central corneal thickness and keratoconus. Nat Genet. 2013;45:155–63.
27. Sahebjada S, Schache M, Richardson AJ, et al. Evaluating the association between keratoconus and the corneal thickness genes in an independent Australian population. Invest Ophthalmol Vis Sci. 2013;54:8224–8.
28. Lechner J, Porter LF, Rice A, et al. Enrichment of pathogenic alleles in the brittle cornea gene, ZNF469, in keratoconus. Hum Mol Genet. 2014;23:5527–35.
29. Balasubramanian SA, Mohan S, Pye DC, Willcox MD. Proteases, proteolysis and inflammatory molecules in the tears of people with keratoconus. Acta Ophthalmol. 2012;90:e303–9.
30. Jun AS, Cope L, Speck C, et al. Subnormal cytokine profile in the tear fluid of keratoconus patients. PLoS One. 2011;6:e16437.
31. Lema I, Brea D, Rodriguez-Gonzalez R, et al. Proteomics analysis of the tear film in patients with keratoconus. Mol Vis. 2010;16:2055–61.
32. Pannebaker C, Chandler HL, Nichols JJ. Tear proteomics in keratoconus. Mol Vis. 2010;16:1949–57.
33. Lema I, Duran JA. Inflammatory molecules in the tears of patients with keratoconus. Ophthalmology. 2005;112:654–9.
34. Lema I, Sobrino T, Duran JA, et al. Subclinical keratoconus and inflammatory molecules from tears. Br J Ophthalmol. 2009;93:820–4.
35. Shetty R, Ghosh A, Lim RR, et al. Elevated expression of matrix metalloproteinase-9 and inflammatory cytokines in keratoconus patients is inhibited by

cyclosporine A. Invest Ophthalmol Vis Sci. 2015;56:738–50.
36. ChaerkadyR SH, Scott SG, et al. The keratoconus corneal proteome: loss of epithelial integrity and stromal degeneration. J Proteomics. 2013;87:122–31.
37. Joseph R, Srivastava OP, Pfister RR. Differential epithelial and stromal protein profiles in keratoconus and normal human corneas. Exp Eye Res. 2011;92:282–98.
38. Kenney MC, Brown DJ. The cascade hypothesis of keratoconus. Cont Lens Anterior Eye. 2003;26: 139–46.
39. Lema I, Duran JA, Ruiz C, et al. Inflammatory response to contact lenses in patients with keratoconus compared with myopic subjects. Cornea. 2008;27:758–63.
40. Balasubramanian SA, Pye DC, Willcox MD. Effects of eye rubbing on the levels of protease, protease activity and cytokines in tears: relevance in keratoconus. Clin Exp Optom. 2013;96:214–8.
41. Karaca EE, Ozmen MC, Ekici F, et al. Neutrophil-to-lymphocyte ratio may predict progression in patients with keratoconus. Cornea. 2014;33:1168–73.
42. Kim WJ, Rabinowitz YS, Meisler DM, et al. Keratocyte apoptosis associated with keratoconus. Exp Eye Res. 1999;69:475–81.
43. Mace M, Galiacy SD, Erraud A, et al. Comparative transcriptome and network biology analyses demonstrate antiproliferative and hyperapoptotic phenotypes in human keratoconus corneas. Invest Ophthalmol Vis Sci. 2011;52:6181–91.

3 Epidemiology of Keratoconus

Ramez Barbara, Andrew M.J. Turnbull, Parwez Hossain, David F. Anderson, and Adel Barbara

3.1 Introduction

The burden of a disease is determined by its incidence and prevalence, which in turn inform the provision of relevant healthcare services including screening programmes, primary and specialist medical care. Genetic and environmental factors affect the incidence and prevalence of keratoconus and it has become apparent that previous estimates of prevalence have been overly conservative, as new diagnostic modalities have enabled earlier detection of corneal changes and also the diagnosis of sub-clinical, or 'forme fruste' disease. This latter classification has proved important in the field of keratorefractive surgery, where preoperative assessment has identified previously undiagnosed, sub-clinical keratoconus and thus protected patients from iatrogenic worsening of ectasia. Furthermore, cases previously thought to be unilateral have frequently been shown with modern imaging to be bilateral, with one eye at an earlier sub-clinical stage. It is now accepted that truly unilateral keratoconus does not exist [1], although it may present unilaterally in the context of asymmetric environmental factors, such as eye rubbing [2, 3]. Improved knowledge of the epidemiology of keratoconus has increased our understanding of the underlying pathogenesis, and earlier recognition of subclinical keratoconus has contributed to a surge in new management strategies designed to ameliorate the long-term burden of disease.

3.2 Incidence and Prevalence

The epidemiological burden of a disease informs the provision of healthcare services. A review of early studies of the prevalence of keratoconus between 1936 and 1966 found a range of 50–230 cases per 100,000 (0.05–0.23 %) [4]. A review of later studies (1959–2011) [5] found prevalence estimates ranging from 0.3 per 100,000 (0.0003 %) in Russia to 2340 per 100,000 (2.3 %) in Maharashtra, India [6]. Taken in isolation however, figures for either prevalence or incidence fail to illustrate important regional and ethnic variations. These will be discussed in more detail in the following sections.

R. Barbara, M.B.Ch.B. (✉) • A.M.J. Turnbull, M.B.Ch.B.
Southampton Eye Unit, University Hospital
Southampton, Southampton, UK
e-mail: Ramezborbara@gmail.com

P. Hossain, M.B.Ch.B., F.R.C.Ophth., Ph.D.
D.F. Anderson, M.B.Ch.B., F.R.C.Ophth., Ph.D.
Southampton Eye Unit, University Hospital
Southampton, Southampton, UK

University of Southampton, Southampton, UK
e-mail: parwez@soton.ac.uk

A. Barbara, M.D., F.R.C.Ophth.
IVision Medical Centre, Keratoconus and Refractive
Surgery Centre, Haifa, Israel
e-mail: adelbarbara@yahoo.com

J.L. Alió (ed.), *Keratoconus*, Essentials in Ophthalmology, DOI 10.1007/978-3-319-43881-8_3

Many early studies were limited by their reliance on older imaging modalities. This includes Kennedy's oft-cited paper from 1986, in which keratometry and keratoscopy were used to estimate the prevalence in Minnesota, USA as 54.5/100,000 (0.0545 %) [7]. More recent studies using videokeratography (topography) provide more sensitive estimates [8]. For example, a prevalence of 3.18 % was recorded in a population-based study of Israeli Arabs [9], consistent with other studies from Israel, Iran and Lebanon [10–13]. Furthermore, cases previously thought to be unilateral have frequently been shown with modern imaging to be bilateral, with one eye at an earlier sub-clinical stage. It is now accepted that truly unilateral keratoconus does not exist [14], although it may present unilaterally in the context of asymmetric environmental factors, such as eye rubbing [2, 3, 14].

In 2015, Gordon-Shaag et al [8] provided an excellent summary of published prevalence studies and emphasized the important methodological differences between hospital- or clinic-based reports and population-based studies [8]. Hospital-based studies tend to underestimate true prevalence because they fail to include asymptomatic patients, those with early disease and those being managed in a non-hospital setting. Population-based studies are considered the gold standard for measuring prevalence, but they too can be hampered by certain selection biases [10]. Tables 3.1 and 3.2, reproduced from Gordon-Shaag et al [8], summarize the key hospital- and population-based studies of keratoconus prevalence to date. They highlight important geographic variations in prevalence, as well as the increased estimates that have resulted from newer imaging modalities.

Whilst the heterogeneous methodology of prevalence studies limits the accuracy of direct comparisons between studies, it is clear that estimates of prevalence have increased dramatically over the last few decades. This was highlighted in a review by McMonnies, discussing screening for keratoconus prior to refractive surgery [15]; in this review, the author highlighted several studies, including one from 2003 [16] employing Atlas anterior corneal topography, biomicroscopy and ultrasound pachymetry that found a keratoconus prevalence of 0.9 % in refractive surgery candidates, i.e. four times the upper range of estimate of prevalence prior to 1966 [15]. A 2010 study in Yemen [17] using TMS-2 topography, biomicroscopy and pachymetry found a combined keratoconus/forme-fruste keratoconus prevalence in LASIK/PRK candidates of 5.8 %, i.e. 25 times greater than the mean prior to 1966 [15]. In these studies however, sampled patients were candidates for keratorefractive surgery and as KC is strongly associated with myopia the data is exposed to self-selection bias [15].

Middle Eastern and central Asian ethnicity is considered a risk factor for keratoconus [1]. Studies have reported prevalence of 2.3 % in India [6], 2.34 % among Arab students in Israel [10] and 2.5 % in Iran [13]. Although these studies had some methodological flaws, the concordance of results supports a true prevalence in some Asiatic countries of similar magnitude [13]. A lower prevalence of keratoconus in Japanese compared with Caucasian populations has been reported [5].

Estimates of annual incidence of keratoconus range from 1.4 to 600 cases per 100,000 population [18]. However, there is a paucity of recent studies of incidence that have benefited from modern imaging technology and diagnostic sensitivity. Assiri et al reported an incidence of 20 per 100,000 per year in one Saudi Arabian province [18], although this was likely to have been an underestimate given that the figure was based on referrals to a tertiary clinic. Elsewhere, incidence has been estimated at 1.3/100,000/year in Denmark [19]. Ethnic differences are influential, with an incidence of 25/100,000/year for Asians compared with 3.3/100,000/year for Caucasians ($p<0.001$) having been demonstrated in a single catchment area [20]. In a similar UK study, Pearson et al [21], demonstrated annual incidence of keratoconus of 19.6/100,000 and 4.5/100,000 in Asian and Caucasian communities, respectively.

Table 3.1 Hospital/clinic-based epidemiological studies of KC (Gordon-Shaag et al BioMed Research International 2015—reproduced with kind permission from authors)

Author	Location	Age in years	Sample size	Incidence/100,000	Prevalence/100,000	Method
Tanabe et al. (1985) [105]	Muroran, Japan	10–60	2601-P		9	Keratometry
Kennedy et al. (1986) [7]	Minnesota, USA	12–77	64-P	2	54.5	Keratometry + retinoscopy
Ihalainen (1986) [67]	Finland	15–70	294-P	1.5	30	Keratometry + retinoscopy
Gorskova and Sevost'ianov (1998) [106]	Urals, Russia				0.2–0.4	Keratometry
Pearson et al. (2000) [21]	Midlands, UK	10–44	382-P	4.5-W 19.6-A	57 229	Keratometry + retinoscopy
Ota et al. (2002) [107]	Tokyo, Japan		325-P	9		Keratometry?
Georgiou et al. (2004) [20]	Yorkshire, UK		74-P	3.3-W 25-A		Clinical examination
Assiri et al. (2005) [18]	Asir, Saudi Arabia	8–28	125-P	20		Keratometry
Nielsen et al. (2007) [19]	Denmark		NA	1.3	86	Clinical indices + topography
Ljubic (2009) [108]	Skopje, Macedonia		2254		6.8	Keratometry
Ziaei et al. (2012) [109]	Yazd, Iran	25.7 ± 9	536	22.3 (221)		Topography

A Asian (Indian, Pakistani and Bangladeshi), *W* white, *P* patient, *NA* not available

Table 3.2 Population-based epidemiological studies of KC (Gordon-Shaag et al BioMed Research International 2015—reproduced with kind permission from authors)

Author	Location	Age in years (mean)	Sample size	Prevalence/ 100,000 (cases)	Method	Sampling method
Hofstetter (1959) [110]	Indianapolis, USA	1–79	13345	120 (16) Placido disc[a]	Rural volunteers	
Santiago et al. (1995) [111]	France	18–22	670	1190	Topography	Army recruits
Jonas et al. (2009) [6]	Maharashtra, India	>30 (49.4 ± 13.4)	4667	2300 (128)	Keratometry[a]	Rural volunteers (8 villages)
Millodot et al. (2011) [10] Jerusalem, Israel	18–54 (24.4 ± 5.7)	981	2340 (23)	Topography	Urban volunteers (1 college)	
Waked et al. (2012) [11]	Beirut, Lebanon	22–26	92	3300 (3)	Topography	Urban volunteers (1 college)
Xu et al. (2012) [112]	Beijing, China	50–93 (64.2 ± 9.8)	3166	900 (27) Optical low coherence reflectometry[a]	Rural + urban volunteers	
Hashemi et al. (2013) [13]	Sharud, Iran	50.83 ± 0.12	4592	760 (35)	Topography	Urban volunteers from random cluster
Hashemi et al. (2013) [31]	Tehran, Iran	14–81 (40.8 ± 17.1)	426	3300 (14)	Topography Urban volunteers (stratified cluster)	
Shneor et al. (2014) [9]	Haifa, Israel	18–60 (25.05 ± 8.83)	314	3180 (10)	Topography	Urban volunteers (1 college)
Hashemi et al. (2014) [12]	Mashhad, Iran	20–34 (26.1 ± 2.3)	1073	2500 (26)	Topography	Urban volunteers (stratified cluster in 1 university)

[a]The methods for detecting KC used in these studies are now considered inadequate and the results should be interpreted with caution

3.3 Environmental and Genetic Factors: Separate or Synergistic?

While increasing estimates of prevalence have largely been attributed to advances in imaging and detection, partly driven by the boom in refractive surgery, we may be witnessing a true increase in the incidence of keratoconus for other reasons. Keratoconus is thought to be caused by a complex interplay of environmental and genetic factors, as well as biomechanical and biochemical disorders [14, 22–24]. Whilst their exact nature remains unclear, the relevance of environment and genetic factors explains the wide variation in prevalence across geographic areas. Varying prevalence among groups of different ethnicity living in the same geographic location suggests a genetic basis for disease. For example, higher prevalence than the British average has been found in Indian, Pakistani and Bangladeshi communities living in the United Kingdom [20, 21]. Further evidence of a genetic basis to the disease includes a significant association with consanguinity [25], autosomal dominant patterns of familial inheritance [26], higher concordance between monozygotic than dizygotic twins [27] and an association with other genetic disorders [28]. In one study, 10 % of patients with keratoconus had a family history of the disease, compared with just 0.05 % of the age-matched control group [29]. While both dominant and recessive patterns of autosomal inheritance have been proposed [9, 26], most cases of keratoconus to date have been deemed sporadic [28].

Current thinking is that geographic variations in prevalence can be explained by specific environmental factors promoting the expression of genetic factors related to ethnicity [15]. This may occur through epigenetic modifications including DNA methylation, which alters gene expression and subsequent phenotype [30]. Epigenetic modifications may result from environmental stressors including toxins and microbial exposure [30], but the most widely discussed are ultraviolet light exposure and eye rubbing [15].

3.4 Ultraviolet Light Exposure

Higher prevalence of keratoconus has been identified in Saudi Arabia [18], Iran [31], New Zealand [32], Israel [9] and some Pacific Island populations [5]. One explanation for this distribution is that these are areas with high ultraviolet (UV) light exposure—an environmental factor widely implicated in keratoconus [15]. Excess UV exposure may be geographical in origin (latitudinal or altitudinal), or related to outdoor pursuits including work and leisure activities. It is proposed that UV light increases the production of reactive oxygen species within the cornea [33] and that keratoconic corneas lack the ability to process excess reactive oxygen species [34] which leads to oxidative stress, cytotoxicity and corneal thinning [35].

While UV exposure and other environmental factors may play a role in determining the prevalence of keratoconus, the observation that Asians living in the United Kingdom have a prevalence of KC 7.6 times that of Caucasians suggests that non-environmental (i.e. genetic) factors are predominant [20]. Similarly, the prevalence of keratoconus is much higher in non-Persians (Arabs, Turks and Kurds) living in Tehran (7.9 %) than Persians (2.5 %) [31]. An argument against the role of excess UV exposure is that natural corneal collagen cross-linking is induced by UV light, which might be expected to reduce the prevalence and rate of progression of keratectasia in these areas [36].

3.5 Eye Rubbing and Allergy

Another environmental stressor widely studied in the context of keratoconus is eye rubbing and its relation to atopic or allergic disease. The association between eye rubbing and keratoconus was first described in 1956 [37]. While some studies have found similar rates of eye rubbing among patients with keratoconus and normal controls [10, 38], the association with eye rubbing is now widely accepted [8].

Recurrent epithelial trauma, similar to that caused by contact lens wear, results in the release of matrix metalloproteinases 1 and 13, interleukin-1 and tumour necrosis factor-alpha that lead to stromal remodelling and keratocyte apoptosis [39–41]. In turn, this may cause epigenetic modifications that facilitate the gene expression required for development of keratoconus [15]. Raised intraocular pressure caused by eye rubbing has also been cited as a contributory factor [42]. Interestingly, the duration of eye rubbing in patients with keratoconus appears longer than that associated with allergic eye disease not associated with keratoconus [43], possibly explaining why the majority of atopic patients do not go on to develop keratectasia. In hot and dry climates, high levels of dust may induce frequent eye rubbing, providing another potential explanation for the higher prevalence in these areas [8].

Some of the most compelling evidence to support a role for eye rubbing comes from reports of asymmetric keratoconus attributed to asymmetric eye rubbing [44, 45]. In 1984, Coyle described an 11-year-old boy who could stop his paroxysmal atrial tachycardia by rubbing his left eye, thus eliciting the oculo-cardiac reflex—a manoeuvre he performed up to 20 times a day. Although initially he had a normal ocular examination, when examined four years later he was found to have unilateral keratoconus [3]. It is possible that if this patient had been assessed with modern topography, he would have been found to have bilateral, albeit highly asymmetrical involvement.

The prevalence of atopic/allergic disease in developed countries has risen in recent years [46], and similar increases in keratoconus could be related to this [47]. Similar to keratoconus, the aetiology of atopy is thought to be a combination of genetic and environmental factors, linked via epigenetic modifications [15]. There is controversy as to whether there is a true association between atopy and keratoconus, and if there is, to what extent this might be. Whilst allergic eye disease causes itch that leads to the urge for patients to rub their eyes, atopy is common in the general population as well as the population of keratoconics. Some studies have recorded low correlations between atopy and keratoconus in large series [48–50] but others have reported strong associations [51–53].

More recently, using univariate analysis, Bawazeer et al found that keratoconus was associated with eye rubbing, atopy and family history [54]. However, multivariate analysis of the same data by the same group revealed eye rubbing as the only significant predictor of disease [54]. So, while atopy may contribute to keratoconus, it is thought to be more through the promotion of eye rubbing than the atopic process itself [54]. Evidence supporting this theory also comes from other conditions in which eye rubbing of a non-atopic origin is a feature. For example, both Leber's congenital amaurosis and Down syndrome are associated with repeated eye rubbing and keratoconus [55]. However, whether keratoconus arises in these patients due to eye rubbing, or a genetic link, is yet to be elucidated.

3.6 Gender

Results concerning gender preponderance vary between studies. Jonas [6], Laqua [56], Amsler [57] and Hammerstein [58] demonstrated female preponderance of 53 %, 57 %, 65 % and 66 % female dominance, respectively. Ertan [59], Street [60], Fatima [61], Pouliquen [62] and Owens [32] demonstrated male preponderance of 62 %, 62 %, 53 %, 57 % and 59 %, respectively. Others have demonstrated no significant gender differences [7] and overall keratoconus is not considered to favour one gender over the other. In the Collaborative Longitudinal Evaluation of Keratoconus (CLEK) study [63], the progression rates of keratoconus were found to be equivalent in both men and women.

3.7 Age

Keratoconus is a disease of adolescence and young adulthood typically presenting between the ages of 20 and 30 years [64], and diagnosis uncommon after the age of 35 years [4]. An exception to this is the diagnosis of older patients when presenting for other reasons, e.g. as candidates for cataract or keratorefractive surgery, where ectasia went undetected in earlier life due to either mild symptoms or less sophisticated imaging. Younger age of diagnosis may imply different aetiological factors. In a Japanese study, HLA antigen association was found to be higher in keratoconics diagnosed under the age of 20 years, in particular HLA-A26, B40 and DR9 antigens [65].

It should be noted that age of diagnosis is quite different from age of onset, and the latency between the two remains unclear. Younger age of onset predicts greater severity [66], faster progression and/or shorter time to penetrating keratoplasty [66]. Early diagnosis of keratoconus is crucial, as treatment including corneal collagen cross-linking can now be offered to arrest disease progression, and this has been facilitated by recent advances in imaging. In a Finnish cohort, Ihalainen (1986) reported that 73 % of patients were aged 24 years or below at the first onset of symptoms, with a mean age of 18 years [67]. Olivares Jimenez et al [68] reported a mean age of symptom onset of 15.39 years in a Spanish cohort. Again, ethnic differences are apparent, with Asians having a significantly lower age (4–5 years less) of first presentation compared with Caucasians [20, 21, 69]. As estimates of prevalence increase, estimates of age of onset decrease for the same reasons of earlier and more sensitive diagnosis [8].

Low numbers of patients reported as diagnosed with keratoconus aged over 50 years are somewhat surprising given the chronic nature of the disease [8] and several explanations have been proposed for this. Some have pointed to associations with conditions that reduce life expectancy, including mitral valve prolapse [70], obesity [71] obstructive sleep apnoea [71, 72] and Down syndrome, although the mortality rate in keratoconics has not been found to differ from that of the general population [73]. A genuine increase in prevalence due to rising rates of allergy in young people could be the explanation, although it could simply be that more young patients are being diagnosed due to technological advances [8].

3.8 Associations with Other Diseases

Keratoconus has been associated with several other syndromic conditions. This has helped understand both the epidemiology and pathophysiology of the disease.

3.8.1 Down Syndrome

Patients with Down syndrome tend to have a higher than average prevalence of keratoconus [74] varying between 0 and 30 % across several studies [75–78]. Cullen et al found 5.5 % prevalence of keratoconus among 143 Down syndrome patients who were mainly Caucasian [79]. Shapiro et al found an incidence of 15 % among 53 patients [77]. Hestnes et al found an incidence of 30 % [76]. In contrast, an Italian study found no keratoconus among 157 children with Down syndrome aged 1 month—18 years [80], and a similar finding was reported in separate studies of Malaysian and Chinese children [80–82]. It is unclear whether the higher prevalence of keratoconus in some populations of Down syndrome is related to eye rubbing and atopy, or some other phenotypic consequence of the chromosomal abnormality.

While patients with Down syndrome and keratoconus are at risk of acute corneal hydrops and secondary corneal opacification [83–85], keratoplasty is generally reserved for patients with minimal intellectual disability and eye rubbing tendency as higher post-operative complications are reported for this group [81]. Early diagnosis and subsequent treatment with corneal collagen cross linking would be expected to halt the progression of keratoconus in this population and reduce the requirement for corneal transplant [82].

3.8.2 Leber's Congenital Amaurosis

Keratoconus is more commonly found with Leber's congenital amaurosis (LCA) than other hereditary blinding diseases [83], possibly due to a connection with the CRB1 gene [84, 85]. Keratoconus was identified in 26 % (5/19 patients) of LCA patients with mutations in aryl hydrocarbon receptor interacting protein-like 1 protein (AIPL1) [86]. While some hypothesize that eye rubbing due to poor vision (the 'oculo-digital sign') is the associating factor, it is now considered more likely to be genetic factors that link keratoconus with LCA [83].

3.8.3 Connective Tissue Disorders

Connective tissue disorders encompass a wide range of conditions characterized by defective collagen or elastin. Several of these syndromes have been associated with keratoconus.

- Mitral Valve Prolapse
- Mitral valve prolapse is one of the most commonly associated connective tissue diseases with keratoconus, and is in turn associated with Ehlers–Danlos syndrome. Prevalence of mitral valve prolapse in patients with keratoconus varies between 5.7 % and 58 % [87–89], while the prevalence of mitral valve prolapse in the general population is between 0.36 % and 7 % [90, 91].
- Recently, it was found that the distribution of the cross-linking enzyme lysyl oxidase (LOX) is markedly decreased in keratoconus patients

[92]. This causes changes in the extracellular matrix which could help explain the association with mitral valve prolapse [93].

- Ehlers–Danlos Syndrome
- Ehlers–Danlos syndrome (EDS) is thought to be associated with keratoconus due to defective collagen synthesis and processing [94]. The association was first described by Kuming and Joffe in 1977 [95]. A study by Woodward et al found that keratoconus patients are five times more likely to have hypermobility of the metacarpophalyngeal and wrist joints [96]. Of the six subtypes of EDS, vascular and kyphoscoliotic EDS (previously known as types IV and VI, respectively) have ocular manifestations including myopia and blue sclera [94], but keratoconus remains rare with this syndrome [97]. McDermott et al found just one keratoconus patient when examining the corneal topography of 72 patients with various EDS subtypes [98]. In 1975, Robertson found 50 % of 44 keratoconus patients to have features of classical EDS (previously types I and II) [99]. Recent studies have found no evidence of keratoconus in EDS patients; however, there was some evidence of corneal thinning [100, 101] and steepening [101, 102].
- Osteogenesis Imperfecta
  Osteogenesis imperfecta is a rare autosomal dominant inherited disease with collagen type I abnormality. It is classically known for its ophthalmic manifestation of blue sclera, but an association with keratoconus in some families with osteogenesis imperfecta has also been found [92, 103].
- Marfan syndrome
  Marfan syndrome is an autosomal dominant connective tissue disease with multiple ocular manifestations including ectopia lentis, axial myopia, retinal detachment and glaucoma. However, an association with keratoconus has only been rarely reported [104].

3.9 Discussion

It is clear that the prevalence of keratoconus has been underestimated until fairly recently. Studies have also highlighted significant geographic variations in disease, helping to shed light on the underlying pathophysiology and risk factors. Improved understanding of the epidemiology of keratoconus and earlier recognition of subclinical disease has contributed to a surge in new management strategies, as the true burden of the disease is realized. Rather than disease management being supportive through refractive correction and contact lenses, with full-thickness penetrating keratoplasty advocated for advanced disease, keratoconus can now be addressed at a much earlier stage with efforts to slow or prevent progression. Consequently, there is a potential role for national screening programmes at schools or universities to enable the early detection of keratoconus in certain high-risk groups. Early detection through the use of new technologies should lead to earlier treatment, promising to reduce the demand for corneal transplantation, improve the quality of life for patients and reduce the economic strain on already stretched healthcare services worldwide.

Compliance with Ethical Requirements The authors declare that they have no financial interest in the material published. No human or animal studies were carried out by the authors for this chapter.

No human or animal studies were carried out by the authors for this article.

References

1. Gomes JA, Rapuano CJ, Belin MW, Ambrósio Jr R, Group of Panelists for the Global Delphi Panel of Keratoconus and Ectatic Diseases. Global consensus on keratoconus diagnosis. Cornea. 2015;34(12):e38–9.
2. Ioannidis AS, Speedwell L, Nischal KK. Unilateral keratoconus in a child with chronic and persistent eye rubbing. Am J Ophthalmol. 2005;139(2):356–7.
3. Coyle JT. Keratoconus and eye rubbing. Am J Ophthalmol. 1984;97:527–8.
4. Krachmer JH, Feder RS, Belin MW. Keratoconus and related noninflammatory corneal thinning disorders. Surv Ophthalmol. 1984;28(4):293–322.
5. Gordon-Shaag A, Millodot M, Shneor E. The epidemiology and etiology of keratoconus. Int J Kerat Ect Cor Dis. 2012;1:7–15.
6. Jonas JB, Nangia V, Matin A, Kulkarni M, Bhojwani K. Prevalence and associations of keratoconus in rural maharashtra in central India: the central India eye and medical study. Am J Ophthalmol. 2009;148:760–5.
7. Kennedy RH, Bourne WM, Dyer JA. A 48-year clinical and epidemiologic study of keratoconus. Am J Ophthalmol. 1986;101(3):267–73.

8. Gordon-Shaag A, Millodot M, Shneor E, Liu Y. The genetic and environmental factors for keratoconus. Biomed Res Int. 2015;2015:795738.
9. Shneor E, Millodot M, Gordon-Shaag A, Essa M, Anton M, Barbara R, Barbara A. Prevalence of keratoconus among young arab students in israel. Int J Kerat Ect Cor Dis. 2014;3(1):9–14.
10. Millodot M, Shneor E, Albou S, Atlani E, Gordon-Shaag A. Prevalence and associated factors of keratoconus in Jerusalem: a cross-sectional study. Ophthalmic Epidemiol. 2011;560747.
11. Waked N, Fayad AM, Fadlallah A, El Rami H. Keratoconus screening in a lebanese students' population. J Fr Ophtalmol. 2011;35(1):23–9.
12. Hashemi H, Khabazkhoob M, Yazdani N, Ostadimoghaddam H, Norouzirad R, Amanzadeh K, et al. The prevalence of keratoconus in a young population in Mashhad. Iran Ophthalmic Physiol Opt. 2014;34(5):519–27.
13. Hashemi H, Beiranvand A, Khabazkhoob M, Asgari S, Emamian MH, Shariati M, et al. Prevalence of keratoconus in a population-based study in Shahroud. Cornea. 2013;32(11):1441–5.
14. Gomes JAP, Tan D, Rapuano CJ, Belin MW, Ambrósio R, Guell JL, et al. Global consensus on keratoconus and ectatic diseases. Cornea. 2015;34(4): 359–69.
15. Cw M. Screening for keratoconus suspects among candidates for refractive surgery. Clin Exp Optom. 2014;97(6):492–8.
16. Ambrosio R, Klyce S, Wilson SE. Corneal topographic and pachymetric screening of keratorefractive patients. J Refract Surg. 2003;19:24–9.
17. Bamashmus MA, Saleh MF, Awadalla MA. Reasons for not performing keratorefractive surgery in patients seeking refractive surgery in a hospital-based cohort in "yemen". Middle East Afr J Ophthalmol. 2010;17(4):349–53.
18. Assiri AA, Yousuf BI, Quantock AJ, Murphy PJ. Incidence and severity of keratoconus in Asir province Saudi Arabia. Br J Ophthalmol. 2005;89: 1403–6.
19. Nielsen K, Hjortdal J, Aagaard Nohr E, Ehlers N. Incidence and prevalence of keratoconus in Denmark. Acta Ophthalmol Scand. 2007;85(8):890–2.
20. Georgiou T, Funnell CL, Cassels-Brown A, O'Conor R. Influence of ethnic origin on the incidence of keratoconus and associated atopic disease in Asians and white patients. Eye. 2004;8:379–83.
21. Pearson AR, Soneji B, Sarvananthan N, Sandford-Smith JH. Does ethnic origin influence the incidence or severity of keratoconus? Eye. 2000;4(4):625–8.
22. Sugar J, Macsai MS. What causes keratoconus? Cornea. 2012;31(6):716–9.
23. Edwards M, McGhee CN, Dean S. The genetics of keratoconus. Clin Exp Ophthalmol. 2001;29(6): 345–51.
24. Barbara A. Textbook on Keratoconus: New Insights. In: F. Malecaze, N. Chassaing, P Calvas. Genetic of Keratoconus. 1st edition. New Delhi, India. Jaypee Brothers Medical Publishers (P). Ltd. 2012. Chapter 2.
25. Gordon-Shaag A, Millodot M, Essa M, Garth J, Ghara M, Shneor E. Is consanguinity a risk factor for keratoconus? Optom Vis Sci. 2013;90(5):448–54.
26. Burdon KP, Coster DJ, Charlesworth JC, Mills RA, Laurie KJ, Giunta C, et al. Apparent autosomal dominant keratoconus in a large Australian pedigree accounted for by digenic inheritance of two novel loci. Hum Genet. 2011;124(4):379–86.
27. Tuft SJ, Hassan H, George S, Frazer DG, Willoughby CE, Liskova P. Keratoconus in 18 pairs of twins. Acta Ophthalmol. 2012;90(6):e482–6.
28. Nowak DM, Gajecka M. The genetics of keratoconus. Middle East Afr J Ophthalmol. 2011;18(1):2–6.
29. Rabinowitz YS. The genetics of keratoconus. Ophthalmol Clin North Am. 2003;16(4):607–20.
30. Barros SP, Offenbacher S. Epigenetics: connecting environment and genotype to phenotype and disease. J Dent Res. 2011;88(5):400–8.
31. Hashemi H, Khabazkhoob M, Fotouhi A. Topographic Keratoconus is not Rare in an Iranian population: the Tehran Eye Study. Ophthalmic Epidemiol. 2013;20(6):385–91.
32. Owens H, Gamble G. A profile of keratoconus in New Zealand. Cornea. 2003;22:122–5.
33. Marchitti SA, Chen Y, Thompson DC, Vasiliou V. Ultraviolet radiation: cellular antioxidant response and the role of ocular aldehyde dehydrogenase enzymes. Eye Contact Lens. 2011;37(4):206–13.
34. Kenney MC, Brown DJ, Rajeev B. Everett Kinsey lecture. The elusive causes of keratoconus: a working hypothesis. CLAO J. 2000;26(1):10–3.
35. Cristina Kenney M, Brown DJ. The cascade hypothesis of keratoconus. Cont Lens Anterior Eye. 2003;26(3):139–46.
36. Chan E, Snibson GR. Current status of corneal collagen cross-linking for keratoconus: a review. Clin Exp Optom. 2013;96(2):155–64.
37. Frederick R. Contact lenses in treatment of keratoconus. Br J Ophthalmol. 1956;40(5):295–304.
38. Weed KH, MacEwen CJ, Giles T, Low J, McGhee CNJ. The dundee university scottish keratoconus study: demographics, corneal signs, associated diseases, and eye rubbing. Eye (Lond). 2008;22(4):534–41.
39. Mackiewicz Z, Määttä M, Stenman M, Konttinen L, Tervo T, Konttinen YT. Collagenolytic proteinases in keratoconus. Cornea. 2006;25(5):603–10.
40. Zhou L, Zhao SZ, Koh SK, Chen L, Vaz C, Tanavde V, et al. In-depth analysis of the human tear proteome. J Proteomics. 2012;75(13):3877–85.
41. Wilson SE, He YG, Weng J, Li Q, McDowall AW, Vital M, et al. Epithelial injury induces keratocyte apoptosis: hypothesized role for the interleukin-1 system in the modulation of corneal tissue organization and wound healing. Exp Eye Res. 1996;62(4):325–7.
42. McMonnies CW. Mechanisms of rubbing-related corneal trauma in keratoconus. Cornea. 2009;28(6): 607–15.
43. Krachmer JH. Eye rubbing can cause keratoconus. Cornea LWW. 2004;23(6):539–40.
44. Jafri B, Lichter H, Stulting RD. Asymmetric keratoconus attributed to eye rubbing. Cornea. 2004;23(6):560–4.

45. Zadnik K, Steger-May K, Fink BA, Joslin CE, Nichols JJ, Rosenstiel CE, et al. Between-eye asymmetry in keratoconus. Cornea. 2002;21(7):671–9.
46. Romagnani S. The increased prevalence of allergy and the hygiene hypothesis: missing immune deviation, reduced immune suppression, or both? Immunology. 2004;112(3):352–63.
47. Cw M. Keratoconus fittings: apical clearance or apical support? Eye Contact Lens. 2004;27(1):15–20.
48. Spencer WH, Fisher JJ. The association of keratoconus with atopic dermatitis. Am J Ophthalmol. 1959;47:332–44.
49. Galin MA, Berger R. Atopy and keratoconus. Am J Ophthalmol. 1958;45:904–6.
50. Roth HL, Kierland RR. The natural history of atopic dermatitis. A 20-year follow-up study. Arch Dermatol. 1964;89:209–14.
51. Davies PD, Lobascher D, Menon JA, Rahi AH, Ruben M. Immunological studies in keratoconus. Trans Ophthalmol Soc U K. 1976;96(1):173–8.
52. Rahi A, Davies P, Ruben M, Lobascher D, Menon J. Keratoconus and coexisting atopic disease. Br J Ophthalmol. 1977;61(12):761–4.
53. Gasset AR, Hinson WA, Frias JL. Keratoconus and atopic diseases. Ann Ophthalmol. 1978;10:991–4.
54. Bawazeer AM, Hodge WG, Lorimer B. Atopy and keratoconus: a multivariate analysis. Br J Ophthalmol. 2000;84(8):834–6.
55. McMonnies CW, Boneham GC. Keratoconus, allergy, itch, eye-rubbing and hand-dominance. Clin Exp Optom. 2003;86:376–84.
56. Laqua H. Hereditary diseases in keratoconus. Klin Monbl Augenheilkd. 1971;159:609–18.
57. Amsler M. The "forme fruste" of keratoconus. Wien Klin Wochenschr. 1961;73:842–3.
58. Hammerstein W. Keratoconus concurrent in identical twins. Ophthalmology. 1972;165:449–52.
59. Ertan A, Muftuoglu O. Keratoconus clinical findings according to different age and gender groups. Cornea. 2008;27:1109–13.
60. Street DA, Vinokur ET, Waring 3rd GO, Pollak SJ, Clements SD, Perkins JV. Ack of association between keratoconus, mitral valve prolapse, and joint hypermobility. Ophthalmology. 1991;98:170–6.
61. Fatima T, Acharya MC, Mathur U, Barua P. Demographic profile and visual rehabilitation of patients with keratoconus attending contact lens clinic at a tertiary eye care centre. Cont Lens Anterior Eye. 2010;33(1):19–22.
62. Pouliquen Y, Forman MR, Giraud JP. Evaluation of the rapidity of progression of keratoconus by a study of the relationship between age when first detected and age at operation. J Fr Ophtalmol. 1981;4(3): 219–21.
63. Fink BA, Sinnott LT, Wagner H, Friedman C, Zadnik K, CLEK Study Group. ZKCSG. The influence of gender and hormone status on the severity and progression of keratoconus. Cornea. 2010;29(1):65–72.
64. Galvis V, Sherwin T, Tello A, Merayo J, Barrera R, Acera A. Keratoconus: an inflammatory disorder? Eye (Lond). 2015;29(7):843–59.
65. Adachi W, Mitsuishi Y, Terai K, Nakayama C, Hyakutake Y, Yokoyama J, Mochida C, Kinoshita S. The association of HLA with young-onset keratoconus in Japan. Am J Ophthalmol. 2002;133(4):557–9.
66. Caroline P, Andre M, Kinoshita B, and Choo J. Etiology, Diagnosis, and Management of Keratoconus: New Thoughts and New Understandings. Pacific Univ Coll Optom. 2008
67. Ihalainen A. Clinical and epidemiological features of keratoconus genetic and external factors in the pathogenesis of the disease. Acta Ophthalmol Suppl. 1986;178:1–64.
68. Caroline P, Andre M, Kinoshita B, and Choo J. Etiology, Diagnosis, and Management of Keratoconus: New Thoughts and New Understandings. Pacific Univ Coll Optom. 2008. 12–15.
69. Cozma I, Atherley C, James NJ. Influence of ethnic origin on the incidence of keratoconus and associated atopic disease in Asian and white patients. Eye (Lond). 2005;19(8):924–6.
70. Beardsley TL, Foulks GN. An association of keratoconus and mitral valve prolapse. Ophthalmology. 1982;89(1):35–7.
71. Pihlblad MS, Schaefer DP. Eyelid laxity, obesity, and obstructive sleep apnea in keratoconus. Cornea. 2013;32(9):1232–6.
72. Arora R, Gupta D, Goyal JL, Jain P. Results of corneal collagen cross-linking in pediatric patients. J Refract Surg. 2012;28(11):759–62.
73. Moodaley LC, Woodward EG, Liu CS, Buckley RJ. Life expectancy in keratoconus. Br J Ophthalmol. 1992;76(10):590–1.
74. Van Splunder J, Stilma JS, Bernsen RM, Evenhuis HM. Prevalence of ocular diagnoses found on screening 1539 adults with intellectual disabilities. Ophthalmology. 2004;111(8):1457–63.
75. Rabinowitz YS. Keratoconus. Surv Ophthalmol. 1998;42(4):297–319.
76. Hestnes A, Sand T, Fostad K. Ocular findings in Down's syndrome. J Ment Defic Res. 1991;35(3): 194–203.
77. Shapiro MB, France TD. The ocular features of Down's syndrome. Am J Ophthalmol. 1985;99(6): 659–63.
78. Walsh SZ. Keratoconus and blindness in 469 institutionalised subjects with Down syndrome and other causes of mental retardation. J Ment Defic Res. 1981;25(4):243–51.
79. Cullen JF, Butler HG. Mongolism (Down's Syndrome) and Keratoconus. Br J Ophthalmol. 1963;47:321–30.
80. Fimiani F, Iovine A, Carelli R, Pansini M, Sebastio G, Magli A. Incidence of ocular pathologies in Italian children with Down syndrome. Eur J Ophthalmol. 2007;17(5):817–22.
81. García García GP, Martínez JB. Outcomes of penetrating keratoplasty in mentally retarded patients with keratoconus. Cornea. 2008;27(9):980–7.
82. Koppen C, Leysen I, Tassignon MJ. Riboflavin/UVA cross-linking for keratoconus in Down syndrome. J Refract Surg. 2010;26(9):623–4.

83. Elder MJ. Leber congenital amaurosis and its association with keratoconus and keratoglobus. J Pediatr Ophthalmol Strabismus. 1994;31(1):38–40.
84. Ehrenberg M, Pierce EA, Cox GF, Fulton AB. CRB1: one gene, many phenotypes. Semin Ophthalmol. 2013;28(5–6):397–405.
85. McMahon TT, Kim LS, Fishman GA, Stone EM, Zhao XC, Yee RW, Malicki J. CRB1 gene mutations are associated with keratoconus in patients with leber congenital amaurosis. Invest Ophthalmol Vis Sci. 2009;50(7):3185–7.
86. Dharmaraj S, Leroy BP, Sohocki MM, Koenekoop RK, Perrault I, Anwar K, et al. The phenotype of Leber congenital amaurosis in patients with AIPL1 mutations. Arch Ophthalmol. 2004;122(7):1029–37.
87. Kalkan Akcay E, Akcay M, Uysal BS, Kosekahya P, Aslan AN, Caglayan M, Koseoglu C, Yulek F, Cagil N. Impaired corneal biomechanical properties and the prevalence of keratoconus in mitral valve prolapse. J Ophthalmol. 2014;2014:402193.
88. Lichter H, Loya N, Sagie A, Cohen N, Muzmacher L, Yassur Y, et al. Keratoconus and mitral valve prolapse. Am J Ophthalmol. 2000;129(5):667–8.
89. Sharif KW, Casey TA, Coltart J. Prevalence of mitral valve prolapse in keratoconus patients. J R Soc Med. 1992;85(8):446–8.
90. Turker Y, Turker Y, Baltaci D, Basar C, Akkaya M, Ozhan H, Melen Investigators. OHMI. The prevalence and clinical characteristics of mitral valve prolapse in a large population-based epidemiologic study: the MELEN study. Eur Rev Med Pharmacol Sci. 2015;19(12):2208–12.
91. Savage DD, Garrison RJ, Devereux RB, Castelli WP, Anderson SJ, Levy D, McNamara PM, Stokes 3rd J, Kannel WB, Feinleib M. Mitral valve prolapse in the general population. 1. Epidemiologic features: the Framingham Study. Am Heart J. 1983;106(3):571–6.
92. Greenfield G, Stein R, Romano A, Goodman RM. Blue sclerae and keratoconus: key features of a distinct heritable disorder of connective tissue. Clin Genet. 1973;4(1):8–16.
93. Dudakova L, Jirsova K. JK. The impairment of lysyl oxidase in keratoconus and in keratoconus-associated disorders. J Neural Transm. 2013;120(6):977–82.
94. Castori M. Ehlers-danlos syndrome, hypermobility type: an underdiagnosed hereditary connective tissue disorder with mucocutaneous, articular, and systemic manifestations. ISRN Dermatol. 2012;2012:751768.
95. Kuming BS, Joffe L. Ehlers-Danlos syndrome associated with keratoconus. A case report. S Afr Med J. 1977;52(10):403–5.
96. Woodward EG, Morris MT. Joint hypermobility in keratoconus. Ophthalmic Physiol Opt. 1990;10:360–2.
97. Ja C. Corneal abnormalities in Ehlers-Danlos syndrome type VI. Cornea. 1993;12(1):54–9.
98. McDermott ML, Holladay J, Liu D, Puklin JE, Shin DH, Cowden JW. Corneal topography in Ehlers-Danlos syndrome. J Cataract Refract Surg. 1998;24(9):1212–5.
99. Robertson I. Keratoconus, the Ehlers-Danlos syndrome: a new aspect of keratoconus. Med J Aust. 1975;1:571–3.
100. Pesudovs K. Orbscan mapping in Ehlers-Danlos syndrome. J Cataract Refract Surg. 2004;30(8):1795–8.
101. Villani E, Garoli E, Bassotti A, Magnani F, Tresoldi L, Nucci P, et al. The cornea in classic type ehlers-danlos syndrome: Macro- and microstructural changes. Invest Ophthalmol Vis Sci. 2013;54:8062–8.
102. Gharbiya M, Moramarco A, Castori M, Parisi F, Celletti C, Marenco M, et al. Ocular features in joint hypermobility syndrome/ehlers-danlos syndrome hypermobility type: a clinical and in vivo confocal microscopy study. Am J Ophthalmol. 2012;154(3):593–600.
103. Beckh U, Schönherr U, Naumann GO. Autosomal dominant keratoconus as the chief ocular symptom in Lobstein osteogenesis imperfecta tarda. Klin Monbl Augenheilkd. 1995;206(4):268–72.
104. Maumenee IH. The eye in the Marfan syndrome. Trans Am Ophthalmol Soc. 1981;79:684–733.
105. Tanabe U, Fujiki K, Ogawa A, Ueda S, Kanai A. Prevalence of keratoconus patients in Japan. Nihon Ganka Gakkai Zasshi. 1985;89(3):407–11.
106. Gorskova EN, Sevost'ianov EN. Epidemiology of keratoconus in the Urals. Vestn Oftalmol. 1998;114(4):38–40.
107. Ota R, Fujiki K, Nakayasu K. Estimation of patient visit rate and incidence of keratoconus in the 23 wards of Tokyo. Nihon Ganka Gakkai Zasshi. 2002;106(6):365–72.
108. Ljubic AD. Keratoconus and its prevalence in Macedonia. Macedonian J Medical Sci. 2009;2(1):58–62.
109. Ziaei H, Jafarinasab MR, Javadi MA, et al. Epidemiology of keratoconus in an Iranian population. Cornea. 2012;31(9):1044–7.
110. Hofstetter HW. A keratoscopic survey of 13,395 eyes. Am J Optometry. 1959;36(1):3–11.
111. Santiago PY, Assouline M, Ducoussau F, et al. Epidemiology of keratoconus and corneal topography in normal young male subjects. Invest Ophthalmol Vis Sci. 1995;36:S307.
112. Xu L, Wang YX, Guo Y, You QS, Jonas JB. Prevalence and associations of steep cornea/keratoconus in greater Beijing. The Beijing Eye Study. PLoS One. 2012;7(7):e39313.

Histopathology (from Keratoconus Pathology to Pathogenesis)

4

Trevor Sherwin, Salim Ismail, I-Ping Loh, and Jennifer Jane McGhee

Histopathology (compound of three Greek words: ἱστός histos "tissue", πάθος pathos "suffering", and -λογία -logia "study of") refers to the microscopic examination of tissue in order to study the manifestations of disease. Specifically, in clinical medicine, histopathology refers to the examination of a biopsy or surgical specimen by a pathologist, after the specimen has been processed and histological sections have been placed onto glass slides. In contrast, cytopathology examines free cells or tissue fragments (From https://en.wikipedia.org/wiki/Histopathology, released under the Creative Commons Attribution-Share-Alike License).

4.1 Introduction

In keratoconus, the study of disease manifestation in tissue biopsies has provided a large portion of the investigations into the pathogenesis of this enigmatic disease. The lack of an animal model has led to the view that this is largely a human disease and the success of corneal transplantation for end-stage disease has enabled the availability of tissue for histopathologic study. This chapter aims to summarise the major findings from the published literature on the histopathology of keratoconus. The chapter will further draw upon the authors' own insights into this field and draw some conclusions as to how pathological findings can inform the underlying pathogenesis and will also lead to an hypothesis as to how keratoconus may progress as informed by the histopathology.

Histopathology is necessarily difficult to interpret by definition. The study always involves the examination of biopsied/excised tissue, and as such, the examination of diseased tissue that has been removed as part of a corneal transplant operation. Keratoconic tissue removed for corneal transplant is deemed to be untreatable by other means and thus can be considered end-stage disease. Therefore, the pathogenic processes that researchers are trying to understand by examining this tissue are probably not active anymore and therefore are difficult to decipher but not impossible. Liken it, for instance, to a post-mortem examination where the pathologists job is to use the information present in the now deceased tissues to decipher what caused the current condition (the condition of being deceased)—this is a very similar process to the histologist examining dystrophic tissues to decide what cellular processes have led to the current presentation of the tissue.

T. Sherwin, B.Sc. (Hons), Ph.D. (✉) • S. Ismail, B.Sc., M.Sc. (Hons) • I-Ping Loh, M.Sc. • J.J. McGhee, B.Sc.
Department of Ophthalmology, New Zealand National Eye Centre, Faculty of Medical and Health Sciences, University of Auckland, Auckland, New Zealand
e-mail: t.sherwin@auckland.ac.nz

J.L. Alió (ed.), *Keratoconus*, Essentials in Ophthalmology, DOI 10.1007/978-3-319-43881-8_4

Furthermore, the nature of histological tissue processing, preparation and examination means that sections of tissue are analysed with a view to extrapolating findings to interpret the pathology of the whole sample. Given that the extent of the pathology may vary widely within the sample, many sections of tissue need to be observed in order to attribute how much the pathology within each section equates to the disease of the whole sample. However, the range of pathology across the sample can be of potential use, especially in a highly organised and symmetrical tissue like the cornea.

For instance, the authors have, in previous work, used the range of degradation across keratoconic cones to delineate early and later signs of keratoconic progression. Accordingly the complete absence of Bowman's layer in the central cone was hypothesised to be preceded by the more subtle breaks in Bowman's that occurred in the periphery of the same tissue. Subsequent investigation of the cellular incursion across this normally acellular barrier was believed to be an active process as cellular invasion coincided with an upregulation of cathepsin enzymes in those cells immediately adjacent to the matrix breaches.

Thus, using careful observation and marrying those observations with recurring themes allows the researcher to piece together previous occurrences within tissue using histological examination. Of course the traditional histological stains that were used for centuries are now supplemented by the more modern technique of immunohistochemistry that now allows very precise labelling and localisation of proteins, peptides and even amino acids within the tissue sections.

In order to define the limitations of this chapter, the authors will discuss the published literature that describes examination of corneal tissue by electron and light microscopical examination utilising histological and immunological labelling methods. This chapter will be limited to these techniques and will not evolve into cytological or molecular methods as this would impinge upon other chapters within this book.

4.2 Signs of Keratoconus: Clinical vs. Pathological

Clinical observations of morphological changes in keratoconus have been well documented since Nottingham first described keratoconus as a distinct condition amongst the corneal ectatic conditions in his treatise "Practical observations on conical cornea: and on the short sight, and other defects of vision connected with it" [1]; however, since then significant advances have been made in the recognition of this condition.

Indeed, computerised corneal topographical assessment now facilitates the diagnosis of keratoconus, which prior to the development of this technology was extremely difficult due to the absence of clinical signs in the early stages of the disease, the highly variable nature of the signs once apparent and the subsequent lack of alignment with disease progression.

In 1965 Duke Elder's 'System of Ophthalmology' [2] established the clinical signs of keratoconus:

"1. A thinning of the cornea at the apex of the cone from one-half to one-fifth of its normal dimensions.
2. An endothelial reflex appears in the central portion of the cornea at the peak of the cone
3. Vertical lines are seen in the deeper layers of the stroma
4. An increased visibility of the nerve fibres which form a network of grey lines interspersed with small dots
5. Fleischer's ring, a line running round the base of the cone
6. Ruptures of Descemet's membrane of characteristic appearance
7. Ruptures in Bowman's membrane in advanced cases producing superficial linear scars."

However in that same seminal text, Duke-Elder noted that:

> … pathological investigations have provided little to add to the biomicroscopic appearance.

This chapter aims to address some of the advances made in pathological investigations since Duke Elder's observation that have indeed enabled some insights into the pathogenesis behind the biomicroscopic signs. In particular, we highlight the advances made since the advent of immunohistochemistry and the insights that this technique has brought.

4.3 Structural Changes in Keratoconus

The characteristic thinning and other biomicroscopical signs of disease progression in keratoconus would be predicted to correlate with the alteration of structural elements and this has indeed been shown to be the case.

4.3.1 Bowman's Layer

Structural abnormalities and defects in Bowman's membrane in the central part of keratoconic cornea have been well documented. Examination of the collagen organisation in keratoconic tissue by scanning electron microscopy found sharply edged defects and ruptures of varying degrees in Bowman's layer in all keratoconic corneas examined [3]. Two further studies reported discontinuities in Bowman's layer and distorted stroma beneath these defects, including fibrotic regions where the epithelium was in direct contact with the stroma [3, 4]. The latter study also suggested localised areas of disease progression as abnormalities of the extracellular matrix (ECM) were not uniform within an individual keratoconic cornea.

Analyses of keratoconus mostly target the central cone of the cornea for analysis, since this is the area of greatest disease involvement. Our studies have targeted the peripheral keratoconic cone in the hope of identifying early pathological features [5]. We showed that discrete incursion of fine cellular processes into Bowman's membrane was decipherable in the periphery of keratoconic corneas. These cell processes were keratocytic in origin and were often observed in conjunction with a defined indentation from the basal epithelium.

4.3.2 Stroma–Collagen Lamellae

Transmission electron microscopy (TEM) studies of diseased tissue have revealed that the thickness of collagen lamellae in keratoconus is unaltered, but the number of lamellae appears to be significantly less than in normal tissue [6]. Synchrotron X-ray diffraction studies have indicated no difference in interfibrillar spacing between collagens in keratoconus and control corneas unambiguously demonstrating that thinning of the corneal stroma in keratoconus is not a result of closer packing of the fibrils in the corneal stroma. However, some evidence is presented for a reduction in the volume of proteoglycan along the collagen fibrils in keratoconic cornea [7]. These data suggest a progressive loss of lamellae within the stroma in keratoconus but the role of the keratocytes and the fate of the collagen are not known. Low angle X-ray scattering has shown that the orientation of collagen fibrils within the lamellae is altered in keratoconus [8], suggesting that loss of structural integrity, degradation and/or insufficient repair mechanisms may all be important in the disease process. The variability of the histopathology data is not unique as biochemical analyses of the stromal matrix components within the keratoconic stroma have been inconclusive: One study described decreased collagen and total protein levels in keratoconic tissue by western blotting [9]. A second found a 5% increase in type I collagen in keratoconus [10]; while a third study described no differences in collagen composition of biochemical extracts from keratoconus [11].

4.3.3 Descemet's Membrane

Ruptures and folds in Descemet's membrane are a common feature in keratoconus [12]. The structural changes behind these ruptures are unclear as several studies of extracellular matrix proteins reveal no differences in detection of types I, III, IV, V, VI or VIII collagen between keratoconic and normal tissue. The same was true of laminin, entactin and perlecan [3, 13] with one study noting that while the immunoreactivity was identical in normal scarred and keratoconic corneas, the reaction was discontinuous within the defects in the keratoconic cones [14]. One argument for the lack of matrix changes surrounding the defects in Descemet's membrane suggests that environmental factors such as eye rubbing and UV exposure are responsible rather than matrix degradation.

4.3.4 Matrix Deposition and Scar Formation

Keratoconus proteomic data shows widespread decreases in many extracellular matrix proteoglycan core proteins, type I, III, V, VI and XII collagen, as well as lumican and keratocan proteins [15–17]. The expression of TGF-β, IL-1, vimentin and tenascin (scar associated matrix protein) was increased in keratoconic corneas [18]. An increase in type IX collagen and an altered pattern in endostatin (anti-angiogenic and induces endothelial cell apoptosis [19]) was found in patients with keratoconus [20].

As the important components for wound healing response and scar formation [21], fibronectin, type III, laminin and tenascin were localised most intensively in areas of defects in keratoconic corneas [21–23]. In keratoconus-associated hydrops, deposition of small amounts of fibronectin in Descemet's membrane and punctate staining of collagen III throughout the stroma with the most intense labelling in the posterior stroma, immediately adjacent to Descemet's membrane, was observed. Similarly, staining for laminin in hydrops-associated keratoconic corneas was observed in stroma immediately adjacent to Bowman's layer and Descemet's membrane [22]. ECM deposition was found to be uniquely in localised areas of the stroma, corresponding to the site of hydrops involvement [22].

4.4 Cellular Changes in Keratoconus

There are a number of key cellular aberrations to the cornea that are commonly observed in keratoconus. Although keratoconus is primarily considered to be an anterior corneal disease, histopathological observations have been reported to affect each layer of the cornea albeit to varying degrees.

4.4.1 Epithelium

The often thinned keratoconic corneal epithelium shows normal cellular morphology at the periphery with highly elongated cells present at the cone apex of the superficial epithelium. These superficial cells appear in a concentric arrangement and further down are accompanied by highly reflective structures and fold-like changes in the basal epithelial layer [24]. Recent methods for analysing epithelial thickness include spectral domain optical coherence tomography (OCT) and ultrahigh resolution OCT which have confirmed older histopathological reports of pronounced deviation in epithelial thickness in keratoconic corneas [25, 26]. It has been reported that where the epithelium is of a higher thickness in keratoconic corneas, the cells are relatively taller suggesting the thickness is due to abnormally large sized cells rather than increased cell proliferation [27]. TUNEL staining, an indicator of the presence of apoptotic cells, appears to show much more variation in staining patterns across the epithelium with a general pattern of apoptosis deeper within the epithelium continuing all the way down to the basal epithelium, a pattern not usually observed in normal corneas [28, 29]. Loss of epithelial cell density is reported as a likely possible cause for the epithelial thinning observed in keratoconus [30] with remaining cells showing a marked increase in cell area [31, 32]. It has been suggested that loss of desmoglein 3 (DSG3), a desmosomal protein, reduces the cells ability to adhere to each other and this may be responsible for epithelial cell loss in keratoconus; however, a study of 10 keratoconic corneas found that half of these corneas stained very positively for DSG3 while all reference corneas showed no or low expression [33]. Variable immunohistochemistry results like these are not uncommon in keratoconus and this has resulted in a lack of a reliable diagnostic marker for the dystrophy. Exacerbating this observed variation in histopathological results, there would appear to be distinct stages of disease progression with cellular differences notable in early, intermediate and advanced stages of keratoconus. Tsubota et al. [32] analysed such cellular differences at each stage of disease progression in a total of 20 keratoconic corneas and reported cells that were slightly elongated in early keratoconic epithelia to highly elongated, sharp spindle-like epithelial cells that increased in frequency from intermediate to advanced stages of keratoconus.

Beyond the basal epithelium, the basement membrane appears irregular and contains localised breaks in keratoconus, showing an erratic pattern of laminin 1 and 5 staining with type VII collagen variably localised to the basement membrane anomalies. Similarly, Integrin ß4 which is uniformly positive in the basement membrane and in the lateral and apical membranes of epithelial cells of normal corneas is much more variable in keratoconic corneas [34]. Type XII collagen staining is reported to be reduced in the basal epithelium/basement membrane region which may play an important role in changing the cell–matrix interactions that would be observed within normal corneas [35]. Although immunohistochemical (IHC) studies have been largely superceded by gene expression assays, a recent report showed a reduction in the collagen fibril-maturing enzyme lysyl oxidase (LOX) in epithelial cells and a reduction in collagen IV in the basement membrane of keratoconus patients. The IHC results in this study correlated positively with concurrent gene expression data and the authors indicate that the reduced expression of collagen IV by basal epithelial cells may be responsible for the thinning of the basement membrane which contributes to the pathology of keratoconus [12]. Similar to superficial epithelial cells, the cells of the basal epithelium also appear larger in terms of surface area and show a much more irregular arrangement in keratoconic corneas [14]. In advanced cases of keratoconus, there are cell membrane ruptures that lead to a significant reduction in basal epithelial cell numbers which in turn leads to only a few layers of flattened superficial epithelium lying on an abnormal basement membrane [36, 37].

Although current evidence provides convincing data that the epithelium is heavily involved in keratoconus pathogenesis it is still unclear whether it is epithelial abnormalities that drive the disease process or are a consequence of disease initiation of alternative aetiology (such as from within the stroma) [27, 38].

4.4.2 Cellular Incursion into Bowman's Layer

Although this is a normally acellular layer, ruptures in the membrane characteristically seen to varying levels in keratoconic corneas [3] facilitates abnormal cellular interactions allowing epithelial cells to come into direct contact with the stroma [4]. Our own studies have revealed indentation of the basal epithelium and infiltration by fine cellular processes of keratocytic origin into the Bowman's layer [5]. These cellular processes have been observed to extend through the Bowman's layer, effectively linking the stroma and epithelium [5]. Staining for vimentin confirms these invading cells to be of mesenchymal origin and therefore have migrated up from the stroma below [5]. Particularly evident at the peripheral regions of keratoconic corneas, is the additional movement of integrin a3ß1-positive basal epithelial cells down into the Bowman's layer at regions of stromal cell incursion which indicates a clear disease phenotype of abnormal cellular interaction. Immunolabelling for cathepsin B reveals distinct variation in staining localisation in keratoconic corneas with increased distribution of cathepsin B within keratocytic cells in association with the damaged Bowman's membrane [5]. This increase in cathepsin B staining differs not only in the staining patterns observed in normal corneas but also between adjacent keratocytes not linked to breaks in the Bowman's layer in keratoconic corneas.

It would appear that defects in the Bowman's layer facilitate an increase in nerve fibres that are observed to be thickened and closely associated with stromal cells moving up into the Bowman's layer [39]. The direct interaction of epithelial cells and keratocytes in keratoconic corneas may in part be mediated by the appearance of these nerve fibres. However, the prominent nerve fibres observed microscopically in the clinic are not present in all keratoconic corneas [27] and new techniques such as in vivo confocal microscopy has not been able to fully elucidate their presence [31, 40, 41]. It is clear though, that nerve fibres in keratoconic corneas show an abnormal pattern [13, 31, 40] of association with Schwann cells which may result in the reduced corneal sensitivity reported by some affected patients [27].

4.4.3 Stroma

The resident keratocytes of the corneal stroma appear to have alterations in both morphology and number in keratoconus. It has been reported that overall keratocyte density is lower in keratoconic corneas [28, 29, 42]. Similar to epithelial cells, keratocyte apoptosis seems to be increased in keratoconus and this has been offered as an explanation for the general reduction in keratocyte numbers observed in keratoconic corneas [29]. When keratocytic density across the width of the stroma is compared from anterior to posterior there appears to be a distinct difference with keratocyte densities being lower in the anterior-most portion of the stroma compared to the more posterior regions. These observations have given strength to suggestions that keratoconus is primarily an anterior corneal disease. Although a recent report of histochemical analysis of the keratoconic stroma showed a general reduction of keratocytes at the anterior stroma, there was an overall increase in the number of cells present within this region when compared to normal corneas. These non-keratocytic cells were observed to show lighter staining of the cytoplasm (agranular) with a higher organelle count (lysosomes, endoplasmic reticulum and mitochondria) and likely to represent differentiated cells or cells of a non-keratocyte lineage [27]. It has been observed that the anterior-most stromal cells (whether they be activated keratocytes or non-keratocyte origin cells) send cellular processes (pseudopodia) into the Bowman's layer towards the basal epithelial lamina [43]. It has been hypothesised that this cellular activity is responsible for breakdown of corneal tissue in the anterior stroma and which may contribute to the collapse of epithelial cells in towards the Bowman's layer [5, 27, 44]. The invasion of cells that are not normally resident in the anterior stroma may be intrinsically involved in this structural breakdown of the anterior corneal layers and determining their true nature would provide significant insight into this enigmatic disease.

4.4.4 Endothelium

Similar to the Descemet's membrane (see section 4.3.3), the endothelium may become detached from the layers anterior although in many cases it maintains a normal appearance. Despite this, some cellular abnormalities such as elongated pleomorphic cells containing dark intracellular structures and endothelial cell loss have been reported [45, 46]. This cell loss can be associated with apoptosis [28] but in general it is the accompanying Descemet's membrane rupture that would appear to be responsible for significant endothelial cell degradation [45] in keratoconic corneas.

4.5 Keratoconic Changes in Secreted Enzymatic Factors

The cells of the various layers of the cornea secrete an abundance of factors that influence the milieu in which the cells are housed. In keratoconus, the levels of these secreted molecules are altered and this could produce an altered proteolytic or inflammatory cascade in response to localised trauma.

4.5.1 Matrix metalloproteinases

One of the largest groups of secreted molecules are the enzymes—the metalloproteinases and the lysyl oxidases, both being associated with collagen degradation and oxidative stress [47, 48].

These can be broken down into groups based on their target structural molecules. The metalloproteinases (MMPs) number upwards of 25, are tissue specific and calcium and zinc dependant. These molecules are responsible for the remodelling of the cornea by cleaving collagen, gelatin and elastin. These MMPs are believed to contribute to corneal thinning through a reduction in collagen volume in keratoconus [49, 50].

The family of metalloproteinases consist of collagenases being MMP1, 8 and 13; stromelysins being MMP3 and 10; matrilysins being MMP7 and 26 and gelatinases being MMP2 (previously Gelatinase A) and 9, and membrane-bound MMPs, being MMPs 14 through 17 and MMP24 [51].

Mackiewicz et al. utilising keratoconus tissue removed during penetrating keratoplasty vs. cadaver tissue determined the localisation of seven such enzymes [52]. MMP1 staining was increased and extended in the keratoconic tissue, being identified not only in the epithelium but also in the stroma. Such findings are supported by other research [53]. MMP1 has the ability to degrade corneal collagens Types I and II and is upregulated by EMMPRIN (extracellular matrix metalloproteinase inducer, CD147). EMMPRIN is a member of the immunoglobulin superfamily of adhesion molecules and has been shown to be upregulated in tumour cells and may be responsible for inducing MMP secretion by fibroblasts closely associated with cancer cells, thus allowing for invasion and metastasis [54]. Seppala et al. identified increased levels of both EMMPRIN and MMP1 in the epithelium and stroma; however, the correlation between areas of pathology and MMP1 staining was not as strong as between EMMPRIN and these damaged areas, whilst MMP1 was also localised to undamaged areas, leading to the conclusion that EMMPRIN may also upregulate the other members of the MMP family thus inducing destruction of the collagen fibrils. EMMPRIN could be considered as "a regulator of keratoconus associated structural, MMP-mediated destruction" [53].

Likewise, MMP13 staining was increased in the epithelium and very posterior stroma and it has been postulated that this molecule could also be involved in corneal thinning. [52]. Initially it was shown through IHC that MMP2 (Gelatinase A) and MMP14 levels were unchanged and identified only in keratocytes [55] though Makiewicz et al. found staining of these molecules further afield in keratoconus, having being detected in Bowman's and Descemet's membranes and the endothelium [52]. Increased expression of MMP14 in the basal epithclial cells as well as in keratocytes points to the potential for increased degradation of Bowman's membrane and decreased volume of the stroma due to the gelatinase and protease activity of this molecule [50].

Other authors have detected no elevation in the expression of MMPs 3 and 10 in comparing normal with keratoconic tissue [56].

MMP8 levels were reduced in comparison to controls and it was suggested that this may lead to impairment of corneal remodelling in the disease state [52].

The levels of MMP9 expression are elevated in the tear film and in culture supernatants of primary keratoconic epithelial cell lines. Expression is promoted by IL-1β and TNF-α, two pro-inflammatory cytokines [57]. However, this increase of MMP9 has not been detected by IHC methods [58–60].

Again, the results of staining for the expression of MMP14 have varied with no change detected by one group [52] while elevated levels in the corneal stroma were detected by other researchers [50]

4.5.2 Matrix metalloproteinases Tissue Inhibitors

Much research has been aimed at elucidating the relationship of the MMPs to their native tissue inhibitors, the TIMPs. These molecules belong to a family of four and are involved in corneal remodelling and scar development [59].

TIMP1 is an inducible inhibitor normally limited to the corneal epithelium but increased staining was observed in the stroma and keratocytes in keratoconus, particularly in areas associated with scar tissue [59]. TIMP1 inhibits the activation of MMP9. TIMP2 staining was somewhat increased with scattered staining of the ECM whereas in normal tissue it is limited to epithelial cells, keratocytes and endothelial cells.

TIMP3 was located throughout the cornea in normal tissue, being a matrix-associated protein; however, in 50 % of the keratoconic tissue studied, there was a loss of expression in areas of loosened epithelium and thinning. The authors postulated that this loss of expression may occur in areas of increased enzymatic activity [59]. Others, using TUNEL staining, found localisation of TIMP3 to the basal epithelium and the anterior stroma of keratoconic tissue. The increased levels of TIMP1 and 3 were found in scarred keratoconic tissue as was an increase in the number of cells found to be TUNEL positive, a marker for apoptosis [61]. The authors considered that an imbalance in the ratio of TIMP1:TIMP3 could induce cell death as TIMP1 inhibits the apoptotic effect of TIMP3.

4.5.3 Cathepsins

There are approximately a dozen members of the cathepsin protease family, which are distinguished by their structure, catalytic mechanism and which proteins they cleave. Most of the members become activated at the low pH found in lysosomes but there are exceptions such as cathepsin K, which works extracellularly after secretion by osteoclasts in bone resorption. They have an important role in the cellular turnover.

Cathepsin B, a cysteine protease, is normally expressed in the epithelial layer but it has been shown to have increased labelling of the epithelial cells in keratoconus in 90 % of tissue studied with further staining of stroma. However, no definite relationship between the levels of staining and the clinical features of the tissue could be identified [60]. The authors also noted a similar increase of staining for cathepsin G, a neutral serine proteinase. They suggested that these enzymes could contribute to an increase in gelatin- and casein-digestion, inducing the tissue abnormalities seen in keratoconus. Brookes et al. detected increased staining for both cathepsins B and G not only in the epithelium but also in anterior keratocytes, in particular those in close association with nerves passing through the stroma and into Bowman's membrane. They noted a marked increase in staining in areas of disruption in this layer [39].

Cathepsin K, a cysteine protease, is found to have increased levels of expression in the epithelium and Descemet's membrane and through the anterior stroma of keratoconic tissue in comparison to normal tissue. Its presence in both normal and diseased corneas points to a potential role in tissue remodelling, given its ability to cleave collagen Type I [52]. The members of the cathepsin family have been strongly implicated in cell turnover through the mechanism of apoptosis with their release into the intracellular space [62]. Staining for apoptotic cells in both normal and keratoconic tissue, utilising TUNEL and ssDNA stain, found much greater levels of apoptotic cells in all layers of the cornea in the diseased tissue with a reduction in the numbers of ssDNA positive cells (a marker of early stages of apoptosis) but with a good correlation between the localisation of both markers [28].

4.6 Recurrence of Pathology

Once the corneal integrity has deteriorated significantly due to advanced keratoconus, surgical intervention is inevitable. Penetrating keratoplasty (PK) utilises a full thickness corneal replacement and has been a well-accepted clinical choice for decades. However, it can be complicated by endothelial rejection which leads to graft failure. In recent years, deep anterior lamellar keratoplasty (DALK) has gained popularity as it leaves the recipient Descemet's membrane and endothelium in place, thereby maintaining tissue integrity and eliminating the risk of endothelial graft rejection [63, 64].

Since the 1970s [65, 66], there have been case reports of corneal grafts exhibiting characteristics of keratoconus several years after initial success of the transplantation. Clinically, the refractive stability of those grafts was found to have deteriorated with increased astigmatism, sub-epithelial and anterior stromal scarring, corneal thinning, Vogt's striae, Munson sign, increased endothelial reflex and visibility of the nerve fibres in the cornea [67]. Corneal topography showed irregular or asymmetric patterns with localised corneal steeping [68]. Histopathologically, various features (Fig. 4.1) such as epithelial oedema, breaks in Bowman's layer, stromal thinning and folds, folded stromal lamellae, stromal ectasia, thinning in central cornea, thickening of Descemet's membrane and endothelial atrophy have been observed [67–70]. All of these characteristics are reminiscent of the pathology of keratoconus, indicating the possibility of recurrent keratoconus post-transplantation.

The incidence of recurrence of keratoconus is reported to be rare, occurring at a rate of 5.4–11.7 % and with a latency of 17.9–21.0 years post-PK [71, 72], and at 1.6 % with a dramatic shorter latency period of 5 years for post-DALK eyes [73, 74]. Such reported incidences of recurrence of keratoconus in grafted corneal tissue may provide important clues as to the pathogenesis of keratoconus.

There are three speculated mechanisms for the recurrence of keratoconus:

(a) The host route: Recurrence of the host's disease in the graft, such that the cells from the remaining host cornea induce the grafted tissue to develop keratoconic pathology. This seems to be the most accepted mechanism due to the slow progression of recurrence post-PK, as the initial appearance of keratoconus takes decades to develop and similarly the recurrence of the disease in the grafted tissue takes two decades to resurface. It is speculated that the remaining abnormal keratocytes from the host continue to migrate and infiltrate the donor cornea [75, 76] gradually replacing the donor keratocytes and producing abnormal collagen. Or alternatively, the residual basal epithelial cells may secrete proteolytic or autolytic enzymes that lead to loss of collagen fibres [73, 77, 78]. The speculated host route was further supported by the dramatic shorter time frame of recurrence (3–4 years) for post-DALK [74, 79]. DALK

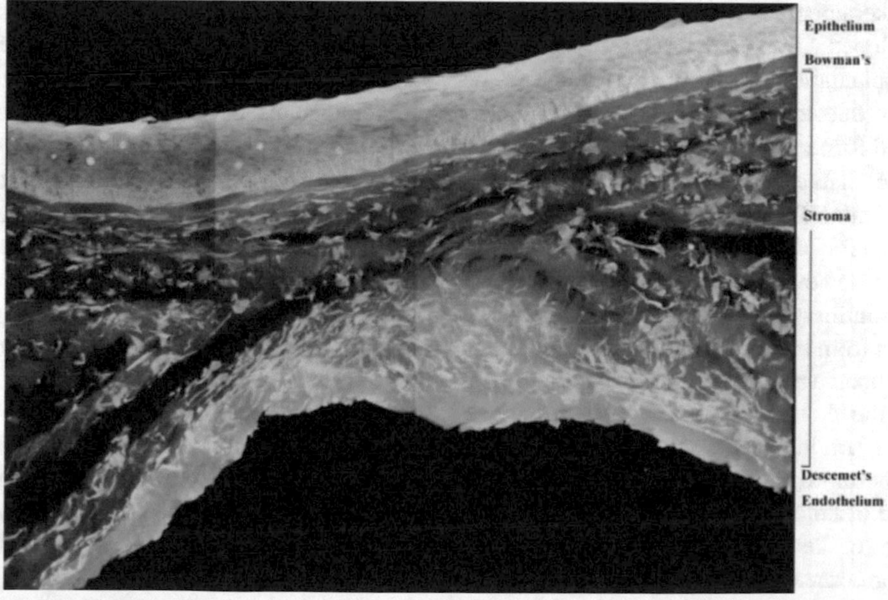

Fig. 4.1 Anteroposterior section of keratoconic corneal button obtained after transplant surgery. The section has been stained using Celltracker green which stains the cytoplasm of all living cells green and counter immunolabelled with an antibody to Integrin α3β1, which labels the basal epithelium. Many of the histopathological features of keratoconus are visible in this tissue section including epithelial hypertrophy, epithelial basement membrane irregularities, breaks in Bowman's layer, stromal fibrosis and central corneal thinning. Bar = 100 μm

is thought to provide less possibility of graft rejection by retaining the recipient stromal bed; however, the earlier onset of recurrence could be the result of either increased host keratocyte invasion in to the donor tissue and/or donor tissue weakening due to the excision of the donor Descemet's membrane prior to transplant [73]. In opposition to this theory however, is the fact that recurrence has been reported when a corneal button size of greater than 8 mm was used to minimise the volume of host cornea that remained in the tissue bed that could effectively lead to recurrence [71]. Also, the ability of significant numbers of abnormal host keratocytes to infiltrate the donor tissue and lead to keratoconus manifestation is debateable. Thus, there might be other mechanisms that lead to the recurrence.

(b) The donor route: Transmission of undiagnosed keratoconus from the donor cornea [80]. One case [81] report described using the two corneas of a donor which were grafted on an advanced keratoconic eye and a corneal leukoma eye. Both keratoconic and non-keratoconic recipient eyes eventually developed reported keratoconus post-transplantation. This was assumed to be likely due to the presence of as yet undetected forme fruste keratoconus in the donor tissue that eventuated once grafted to the recipients. This report could serve as evidence for a possible donor transmission route; however, there are no studies known that routinely follow the fate of contralateral grafts from the same donor to establish if this occurs on a regular basis. Also, presumption that the donor tissue must have had forme fruste keratoconus is completely unproven. Furthermore, one case [69] reported recurrence of keratoconus 7 years after the initial graft for keratoconus; however, the fellow donor cornea appears to be normal 12 years post-transplantation. It is speculated that this could still occur due to donor transmission if the donor exhibited unilateral keratoconus [75] or the second graft is yet to develop keratoconus. Certainly long-term follow-up analysis will be needed in order to determine the likelihood of this mechanism in majority of cases of recurrent keratoconus. It does seem to be clear though that the recurrence of keratoconus via donor transmission is not the sole mechanism responsible.

(c) Mechanical trauma such as contact lens wearing or eye rubbing can cause damage to the sutured cornea and failure of the wound healing process leading to apoptosis and a weakened graft cornea [82, 83]. However, it is difficult to isolate mechanical trauma as the major route [79] for the recurrence during latency period as there are plenty of reported recurrences with no evidence of eye rubbing or contact lens wearing. Nevertheless, mechanical trauma is most likely to at least play the role of 'second-hit' [83].

No doubt each of the three speculated mechanisms of recurrence of keratoconus in grafted corneal tissue can explain the development of disease in certain isolated cases, but none appear to be the major underlying mechanism for the recurrence, especially when the recurrence is rare.

Interestingly, the classical signs of keratoconus such as corneal thinning and epithelial incursion are not unique only for post-transplantation for keratoconus but also for other indications [84]. This has raised doubt whether the observation of recurrence has sometimes been confused with failed graft due to decompensation. Perhaps the clues lie away from the central graft and towards the peripheral region where the graft–host junction is sited. At the graft–host junction, lamellar disruption and thinning were observed [85–87], and stress test studies show that the graft–host junction remains weak even after the wound appears to have healed [77]. Adding to that, the epithelium at graft–host junction is much thickened (Fig. 4.2). Thus, corneal decompensation may be due to the increased physical stress at the graft–host junction during wound healing between the weakened keratoconus host and the normal thickness graft [84].

In addition to wound healing, impaired nerve innervation post-transplantation will likely lead to epithelial complications later on [88]. Being a primarily central corneal disease, the peripheral

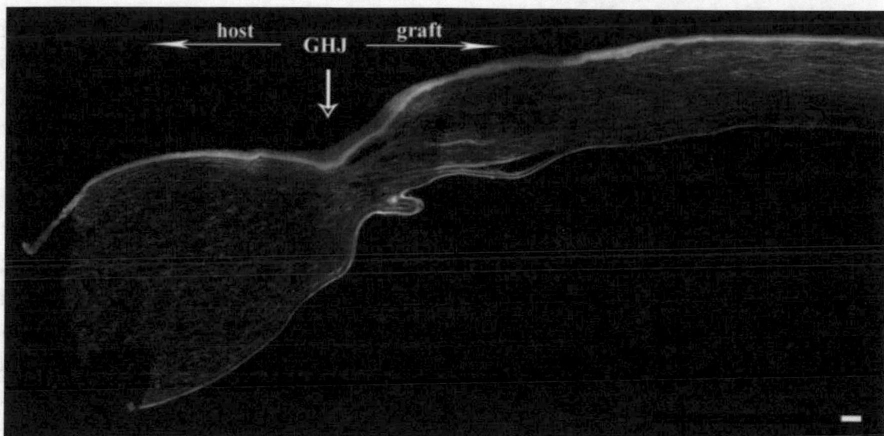

Fig. 4.2 An anteroposterior section of the junction between the host tissue and a corneal graft (GHJ) many years after the original operation. The graft tissue including some of the host tissue was removed during a regraft operation and processed for immunohistochemistry. Many of the histological features which may represent the recurrence of keratoconus are present in the graft material including epithelial oedema, breaks in Bowman's layer, stromal thinning and folds, folded stromal lamellae, stromal ectasia, thinning in central cornea, lipid thickening of Descemet's membrane and endothelial atrophy are visible. Bar = 100 μm

innervation in keratoconic corneas appears to be intact [13]. In terms of nerve re-innervation post-PK, despite the sub-basal nerve fibre density being significantly reduced [89], patients had higher nerve fibre density and greater nerve branch density than patients who underwent PK for other indications. This might partially explain the lower rate of recurrence after PK for keratoconus at around 11.7 % [72] than other stromal dystrophies at 21 % [90]. Taken together, the weakened graft–host junction, impairment in nerve re-innervation and mechanical insults such as eye rubbing and contact lens wearing can all cause damage which might lead to apoptosis indicating a fourth speculated mechanism of abnormal wound healing [85].

4.7 A Role for Inflammation in Keratoconus

Keratoconus has long been categorised as a non-inflammatory corneal dystrophy due to the lack of neovascularisation and cellular infiltration [91, 92]. However, there has been increasing evidence that may refute this concept [17, 93]. In keratoconus with acute corneal hydrops, dendritic cells (presumed leukocytes) [94] were observed clinically with in vivo confocal microscopy. Recently, studies using tear fluids of keratoconic patients revealed elevated levels of interleukin-6 (IL-6), tumour necrosis factor-α (TNF-α) and matrix metalloproteinase (MMP)-9 [95–100]. The expression of other factors such as MMP-1, -3, -7, -13, IL-4, -5, -6, -8, TNF-β [97] and tissue plasminogen activator (t-PA) [17] was also elevated, whereas lactoferrin and IgA [101, 102] were reduced in keratoconus. Tears from keratoconic patients associated with eye rubbing and contact lens wearing showed an increase not only in MMP13, IL-6, -10 and TNF-α, but also in the intercellular adhesion molecule (ICAM)-1 and vascular cell adhesion molecule (VCAM)-1 that are known to be important for inflammatory response [95, 103, 104]. Tear fluid of pseudokeratoconus caused by ocular rosacea [105] showed significantly elevated levels of IL1 and MMP9 [106, 107].

4.7.1 Immunohistochemical Evidence of Inflammation

The central cornea has a resident population of epithelial and stromal dendritic cells (DC), which function as antigen-presenting cells (APCs).

Although the corneal periphery contains mature and immature resident bone marrow-derived CD11c⁺DC, the central cornea is endowed exclusively with immature and precursor DC, both in the epithelium and the stroma, wherein Langerhans cells and monocytic DC reside, respectively [108–111]. In addition to the DC, macrophages are present in the posterior corneal stroma [108, 109].

Immunohistochemical labelling in central cornea of keratoconus showed $CD11b^+$ macrophages, $CD45^+$ leucocytes and HLA-DR MHC-II receptor on APCs localised in increasing number in epithelium and stroma (Fig. 4.3) [22, 112]. The density of APCs decreased from the paracentral towards the central part of the cornea [111]. Dendritic cells in keratoconus had the appearance of brighter bodies and shorter dendrites than those found in inflamed corneas [111]. Another macrophage marker, CD68, seemed to provide conflicting findings given its presence in epithelial basement membrane [17, 112, 113].

In hydrops-associated keratoconus, extensive presence of $CD11b^+$ macrophages have been observed. Though the number of leukocytes and APCs appeared reduced when associated with hydrops, $langerin^+$ DC numbers were similar with and without hydrops [22]. A huge elevation of numbers of leucocytes were noticed in the stroma, epithelium and even the endothelium in hydrops-associated keratoconus with subsequent neovascularisation [22]. (The authors find that neovascularisation in sections of keratoconic tissue is best identified using antibodies to Von Willebrand Factor (Fig. 4.4))

This suggested a chronic inflammatory process with recruitment of inflammatory cells [22]; however, the signs of inflammation appeared to attenuate in hydrops-associated keratoconus indicating that inflammation is not specifically associated with the occurrence of hydrops [22]. Thus, we believe inflammation in keratoconus is likely to be a chronic process rather than an acute occurrence.

4.8 Pathology Informing Pathogenesis

Modern histological techniques can be effectively used to determine pathological changes occurring within the matrix and cells in keratoconic corneal tissue. However, the real question to be answered is whether investigation of pathological changes within the tissue can add to the analysis of the pathogenesis of the disease or are we simply looking at the effect of disease progression. Many of the pathological phenomena that occur in keratoconus (described earlier)

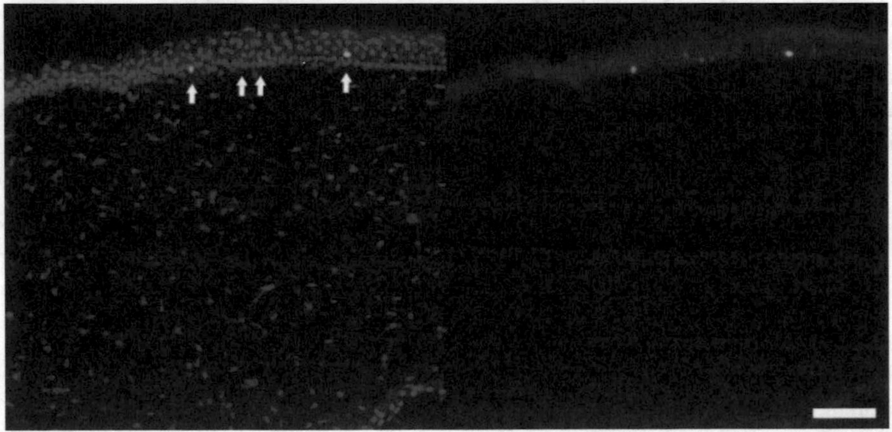

Fig. 4.3 A section of keratoconic tissue labelled with CD11b (*green*) shows macrophages present in the basal layers of the epithelium. The same section is also shown counterstained with DAPI (*blue*) which stains the nuclei of all the cells of epithelium and keratocytes within the stroma and CD11b highlighted with arrows to show the localisation of the macrophages within the epithelium. Bar = 100 μm

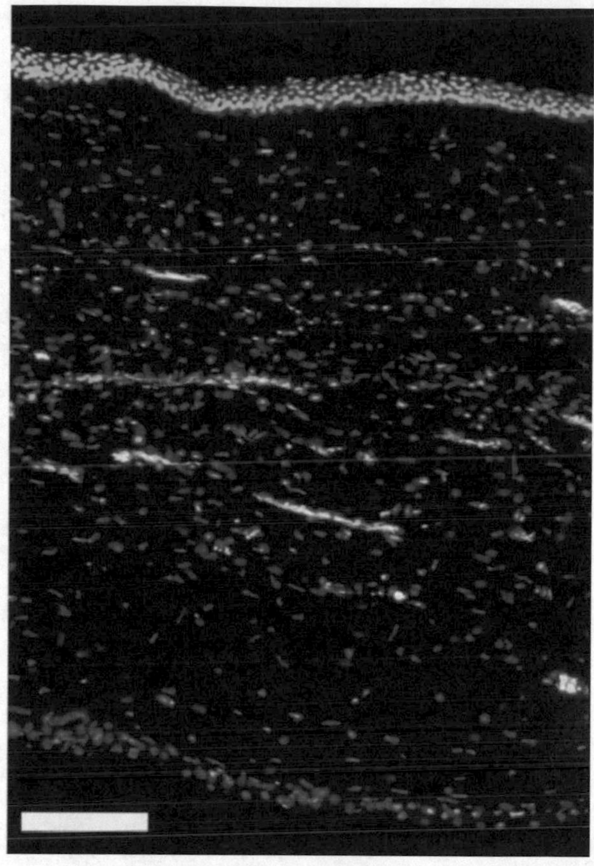

Fig. 4.4 A section of keratoconic tissue is shown with extensive neovascularisation as revealed by labelling using antibodies to Von Willebrand Factor. Bar = 100 μm

mirror tissue remodelling processes in that changes in cell activation, enzyme secretion matrix removal, deposition and remodelling are all involved in corneal repair. This has led to the proposal that progression of keratoconus is in fact due to aberrant repair mechanisms which continuously try to repair the matrix loss in keratoconus but instead compound that loss further. The beginning of this destructive cycle may begin with an external environmental trigger and afterwards be fuelled by aberrant internal processes. This is further supported when we combine molecular studies with the histological data. Recently, in our laboratory we were able to show that cells isolated from keratoconic corneas expressed the main repair modulating molecules at levels higher than normal corneas and equated to the levels found in a normal wounded cornea. However when the keratoconic corneas were supplied with a secondary insult they were unable to mount an adequate repair response [114].

In summary, modern histopathology can successfully combine with molecular techniques to uncover the elusive pathogenesis of keratoconus.

Declaration Trevor Sherwin, Salim Ismail, I-Ping Loh and Jennifer Jane McGhee declare that they have no conflict of interest.

All procedures followed were in accordance with the ethical standards of the responsible committee on human experimentation (institutional and national) and with the Helsinki Declaration of 1975, as revised in 2000. Informed consent was obtained from all patients for being included in the study.

No animal studies were carried out by the authors for this article

References

1. Nottingham J. Practical observations on conical cornea: and on the short sight, and other defects of vision connected with it. London: John Churchill; 1854.

2. Duke-Elder S, Leigh A. System of ophthalmology, vol. III: diseases of the outer eye. St. Louis: Mosby; 1965.
3. Sawaguchi S, Fukuchi T, Abe H, Kaiya T, Sugar J, Yue BY. Three-dimensional scanning electron microscopic study of keratoconus corneas. Arch Ophthalmol. 1998;116(1):62–8.
4. Kenney MC, Nesburn AB, Burgeson RE, Butkowski RJ, Ljubimov AV. Abnormalities of the extracellular matrix in keratoconus corneas. Cornea. 1997;16(3): 345–51.
5. Sherwin T, Brookes NH, Loh IP, Poole CA, Clover GM. Cellular incursion into Bowman's membrane in the peripheral cone of the keratoconic cornea. Exp Eye Res. 2002;74(4):473–82.
6. Takahashi A, Nakayasu K, Okisaka S, Kanai A. Quantitative analysis of collagen fiber in keratoconus. Nippon Ganka Gakkai Zasshi. 1990;94(11):1068–73.
7. Fullwood NJ, Tuft SJ, Malik N, Meek KM, Ridgway A, Harrison RJ. Synchrotron X-ray diffraction studies of keratoconus corneal stroma. Invest Ophthalmol Vis Sci. 1992;33(5):1734–41.
8. Daxer A, Fratzl P. Collagen fibril orientation in the human corneal stroma and its implication in keratoconus. Invest Ophthalmol Vis Sci. 1997;38(1):121–9.
9. Critchfield JW, Calandra AJ, Nesburn AB, Kenney MC. Keratoconus: I. biochemical studies. Exp Eye Res. 1988;46(6):953–63.
10. Radda T, Menzel E, Freyler H, Gnad H. Collagen types in keratoconus. Graefes Arch Clin Exp Ophthalmol. 1982;218(5):262–4.
11. Zimmermann DR, Fischer RW, Winterhalter KH, Witmer R, Vaughan L. Comparative studies of collagens in normal and keratoconus corneas. Exp Eye Res. 1988;46(3):431–42.
12. Shetty R, Sathyanarayanamoorthy A, Ramachandra RA, Arora V, Ghosh A, Srivatsa PR, et al. Attenuation of lysyl oxidase and collagen gene expression in keratoconus patient corneal epithelium corresponds to disease severity. Mol Vis. 2015;21:12–25.
13. Patel DV, McGhee CNJ. Mapping the corneal subbasal nerve plexus in keratoconus by in vivo laser scanning confocal microscopy. Invest Ophthalmol Vis Sci. 2006;47(4):1348–51.
14. Niederer RL, Perumal D, Sherwin T, McGhee CN. Laser scanning in vivo confocal microscopy reveals reduced innervation and reduction in cell density in all layers of the keratoconic cornea. Invest Ophthalmol Vis Sci. 2008;49(7):2964–70.
15. Chaerkady R, Shao H, Scott SG, Pandey A, Jun AS, Chakravarti S. The keratoconus corneal proteome: loss of epithelial integrity and stromal degeneration. J Proteome. 2013;87:122–31. doi:10.1016/j.jprot.2013.05.023.
16. Cheung IM, McGhee CN, Sherwin T. A new perspective on the pathobiology of keratoconus: interplay of stromal wound healing and reactive species-associated processes. Clin Exp Optom. 2013;96(2):188–96. doi:10.1111/cxo.12025.
17. Galvis V, Sherwin T, Tello A, Merayo J, Barrera R, Acera A. Keratoconus: an inflammatory disorder? Eye (Lond). 2015;29(7):843–59. doi:10.1038/eye.2015.63.
18. Zhou L, Yue BY, Twining SS, Sugar J, Feder RS. Expression of wound healing and stress-related proteins in keratoconus corneas. Curr Eye Res. 1996;15(11):1124–31.
19. O'Reilly MS, Boehm T, Shing Y, Fukai N, Vasios G, Lane WS, et al. Endostatin: an endogenous inhibitor of angiogenesis and tumor growth. Cell. 1997;88(2): 277–85.
20. Maatta M, Heljasvaara R, Sormunen R, Pihlajaniemi T, Autio-Harmainen H, Tervo T. Differential expression of collagen types XVIII/endostatin and XV in normal, keratoconus, and scarred human corneas. Cornea. 2006;25(3):341–9. doi:10.1097/01.ico.0000178729.57435.96.
21. Zieske JD. Extracellular matrix and wound healing. Curr Opin Ophthalmol. 2001;12(4):237–41.
22. Fan Gaskin JC, Loh IP, McGhee CNJ, Sherwin T. An immunohistochemical study of inflammatory cell changes and matrix remodeling with and without acute hydrops in keratoconus inflammatory cell and matrix variations in keratoconus. Invest Ophthalmol Vis Sci. 2015;56(10):5831–7. doi:10.1167/iovs.14-15123.
23. Tuori A, Virtanen I, Aine E, Uusitalo H. The expression of tenascin and fibronectin in keratoconus, scarred and normal human cornea. Graefes Arch Clin Exp Ophthalmol. 1997;235(4):222–9.
24. Somodi S, Hahnel C, Slowik C, Richter A, Weiss D, Guthoff R. Confocal in vivo microscopy and confocal laser-scanning fluorescence microscopy in keratoconus. Ger J Ophthalmol. 1996;5(6):518–25.
25. Yadav R, Kottaiyan R, Ahmad K, Yoon G. Epithelium and Bowman's layer thickness and light scatter in keratoconic cornea evaluated using ultrahigh resolution optical coherence tomography. J Biomed Opt. 2012;17(11):116010. doi:10.1117/1.jbo.17.11.116010.
26. Zhou W, Stojanovic A. Comparison of corneal epithelial and stromal thickness distributions between eyes with keratoconus and healthy eyes with corneal astigmatism >/= 2.0 D. PLoS ONE. 2014;9(1), e85994. doi:10.1371/journal.pone.0085994.
27. Mathew JH, Goosey JD, Bergmanson JP. Quantified histopathology of the keratoconic cornea. Optom Vis Sci. 2011;88(8):988–97. doi:10.1097/OPX.0b013e31821ffbd4.
28. Kaldawy RM, Wagner J, Ching S, Seigel GM. Evidence of apoptotic cell death in keratoconus. Cornea. 2002;21(2):206–9.
29. Kim WJ, Rabinowitz YS, Meisler DM, Wilson SE. Keratocyte apoptosis associated with keratoconus. Exp Eye Res. 1999;69(5):475–81. doi:10.1006/exer.1999.0719.
30. Ucakhan OO, Kanpolat A, Ylmaz N, Ozkan M. In vivo confocal microscopy findings in keratoconus. Eye Contact Lens. 2006;32(4):183–91. doi:10.1097/01.icl.0000189038.74139.4a.

31. Hollingsworth JG, Efron N, Tullo AB. In vivo corneal confocal microscopy in keratoconus. Ophthalmic Physiol Opt. 2005;25(3):254–60.
32. Tsubota K, Mashima Y, Murata H, Sato N, Ogata T. Corneal epithelium in keratoconus. Cornea. 1995;14(1):77–83.
33. Nielsen K, Heegaard S, Vorum H, Birkenkamp-Demtroder K, Ehlers N, Orntoft TF. Altered expression of CLC, DSG3, EMP3, S100A2, and SLPI in corneal epithelium from keratoconus patients. Cornea. 2005;24(6):661–8.
34. Tuori AJ, Virtanen I, Aine E, Kalluri R, Miner JH, Uusitalo HM. The immunohistochemical composition of corneal basement membrane in keratoconus. Curr Eye Res. 1997;16(8):792–801.
35. Cheng EL, Maruyama I, SundarRaj N, Sugar J, Feder RS, Yue BY. Expression of type XII collagen and hemidesmosome-associated proteins in keratoconus corneas. Curr Eye Res. 2001;22(5):333–40.
36. Joseph R, Srivastava OP, Pfister RR. Differential epithelial and stromal protein profiles in keratoconus and normal human corneas. Exp Eye Res. 2011;92(4):282–98. doi:10.1016/j.exer.2011.01.008.
37. Rabinowitz YS. The genetics of keratoconus. Ophthalmol Clin. 2003;16(4):607–20.
38. Teng C. Electron microscope study of the pathology of keratoconus: part I. Am J Ophthalmol. 1963;55(1):18–47.
39. Brookes NH, Loh IP, Clover GM, Poole CA, Sherwin T. Involvement of corneal nerves in the progression of keratoconus. Exp Eye Res. 2003;77(4):515–24.
40. Efron N, Hollingsworth JG. New perspectives on keratoconus as revealed by corneal confocal microscopy. Clin Exp Optom. 2008;91(1):34–55. doi:10.1111/j.1444-0938.2007.00195.x.
41. Hollingsworth JG, Bonshek RE, Efron N. Correlation of the appearance of the keratoconic cornea in vivo by confocal microscopy and in vitro by light microscopy. Cornea. 2005;24(4):397–405.
42. Erie JC, Patel SV, McLaren JW, Nau CB, Hodge DO, Bourne WM. Keratocyte density in keratoconus. A confocal microscopy study(a). Am J Ophthalmol. 2002;134(5):689–95.
43. Rock M, Moore M, Anderson J, Binder P. 3-D computer models of human keratocytes. Eye Contact Lens. 1995;21(1):57–60.
44. Sherwin T, Brookes NH. Morphological changes in keratoconus: pathology or pathogenesis. Clinical Exp Ophthalmol. 2004;32(2):211–7. doi:10.1111/j.1442-9071.2004.00805.x.
45. Jongebloed WL, Dijk F, Worst JG. Keratoconus morphology and cell dystrophy: a SEM study. Doc Ophthalmol. 1989;72(3–4):403–9.
46. Rabinowitz YS. Keratoconus. Surv Ophthalmol. 1998;42(4):297–319.
47. Kenney MC, Brown DJ. The cascade hypothesis of keratoconus. Contact Lens Anterior Eye. 2003;26(3):139–46.
48. Sawaguchi S, Yue BY, Sugar J, Gilboy JE. Lysosomal enzyme abnormalities in keratoconus. Arch Ophthalmol. 1989;107(10):1507–10.
49. Collier SA. Is the corneal degradation in keratoconus caused by matrix-metalloproteinases? Clin Exp Ophthalmol. 2001;29(6):340–4.
50. Collier SA, Madigan MC, Penfold PT. Expression of membrane-type 1 matrix metalloproteinase (MT1-MMP) and MMP-2 in normal and keratoconus corneas. Curr Eye Res. 2000;21(2):662–8. doi:10.1076/0271-3683(200008)21:2;1-v;ft662.
51. Fournié PR, Gordon GM, Dawson DG, Edelhauser HF, Fini ME. Correlations of long-term matrix metalloproteinase localization in human corneas after successful laser-assisted in situ keratomileusis with minor complications at the flap margin. Arch Ophthalmol. 2008;126(2):162–70.
52. Mackiewicz Z, Maatta M, Stenman M, Konttinen L, Tervo T, Konttinen YT. Collagenolytic proteinases in keratoconus. Cornea. 2006;25(5):603–10. doi:10.1097/01.ico.0000208820.32614.00.
53. Seppala HP, Maatta M, Rautia M, Mackiewicz Z, Tuisku I, Tervo T, et al. EMMPRIN and MMP-1 in keratoconus. Cornea. 2006;25(3):325–30. doi:10.1097/01.ico.0000183534.22522.39.
54. Biswas C, Zhang Y, DeCastro R, Guo H, Nakamura T, Kataoka H, et al. The human tumor cell-derived collagenase stimulatory factor (renamed EMMPRIN) is a member of the immunoglobulin superfamily. Cancer Res. 1995;55(2):434–9.
55. Brown D, Chwa MM, Opbroek A, Kenney MC. Keratoconus corneas: increased gelatinolytic activity appears after modification of inhibitors. Curr Eye Res. 1993;12(6):571–81.
56. Saghizadeh M, Brown DJ, Castellon R, Chwa M, Huang GH, Ljubimova JY, et al. Overexpression of matrix metalloproteinase-10 and matrix metalloproteinase-3 in human diabetic corneas: a possible mechanism of basement membrane and integrin alterations. Am J Pathol. 2001;158(2):723–34. doi:10.1016/s0002-9440(10)64015-1.
57. Li D-Q, Lokeshwar BL, Solomon A, Monroy D, Ji Z, Pflugfelder SC. Regulation of MMP-9 production by human corneal epithelial cells. Exp Eye Res. 2001;73(4):449–59.
58. Fini ME, Yue BY, Sugar J. Collagenolytic/gelatinolytic metalloproteinases in normal and keratoconus corneas. Curr Eye Res. 1992;11(9):849–62.
59. Kenney MC, Chwa M, Alba A, Saghizadeh M, Huang ZS, Brown DJ. Localization of TIMP-1, TIMP-2, TIMP-3, gelatinase A and gelatinase B in pathological human corneas. Curr Eye Res. 1998;17(3):238–46.
60. Zhou L, Sawaguchi S, Twining SS, Sugar J, Feder RS, Yue BY. Expression of degradative enzymes and protease inhibitors in corneas with keratoconus. Invest Ophthalmol Vis Sci. 1998;39(7):1117–24.
61. Matthews FJ, Cook SD, Majid MA, Dick AD, Smith VA. Changes in the balance of the tissue inhibitor of

matrix metalloproteinases (TIMPs)-1 and -3 may promote keratocyte apoptosis in keratoconus. Exp Eye Res. 2007;84(6):1125–34. doi:10.1016/j.exer.2007.02.013.
62. Chwieralski C, Welte T, Bühling F. Cathepsin-regulated apoptosis. Apoptosis. 2006;11(2):143–9.
63. Han DC, Mehta JS, Por YM, Htoon HM, Tan DT. Comparison of outcomes of lamellar keratoplasty and penetrating keratoplasty in keratoconus. Am J Ophthalmol. 2009;148(5):744–51.
64. Sarnicola V, Toro P, Gentile D, Hannush SB. Descemetic DALK and predescemetic DALK: outcomes in 236 cases of keratoconus. Cornea. 2010;29(1):53–9.
65. Jahne M. Recurrence of keratoconus after keratoplasty. Z Arztl Fortbild. 1974;68(9):434–6.
66. Damaske E. Value of therapeutic soft contact lenses in the treatment of recurrent corneal erosions. Ophthalmologica. 1979;178(5):289–96.
67. Barbara R, Barbara A. Recurrent keratoconus. Int J Kerat Ect Cor Dis. 2013;2(2):65.
68. Bourges JL, Savoldelli M, Dighiero P, Assouline M, Pouliquen Y, BenEzra D, et al. Recurrence of keratoconus characteristics: a clinical and histologic follow-up analysis of donor grafts. Ophthalmology. 2003;110(10):1920–5. doi:10.1016/s0161-6420(03)00617-1.
69. Kremer I, Eagle RC, Rapuano CJ, Laibson PR. Histologic evidence of recurrent keratoconus seven years after keratoplasty. Am J Ophthalmol. 1995;119(4):511–2.
70. Thalasselis A, Etchepareborda J. Recurrent keratoconus 40 years after keratoplasty. Ophthalmic Physiol Opt. 2002;22(4):330–2.
71. Patel SV, Malta JB, Banitt MR, Mian SI, Sugar A, Elner VM, et al. Recurrent ectasia in corneal grafts and outcomes of repeat keratoplasty for keratoconus. Br J Ophthalmol. 2009;93(2):191–7. doi:10.1136/bjo.2008.142117.
72. Pramanik S, Musch DC, Sutphin JE, Farjo AA. Extended long-term outcomes of penetrating keratoplasty for keratoconus. Ophthalmology. 2006;113(9):1633–8. doi:10.1016/j.ophtha.2006.02.058.
73. Feizi S, Javadi M-A, Rezaei KM. Recurrent keratoconus in a corneal graft after deep anterior lamellar keratoplasty. J Ophthalmic Vis Res. 2012;7(4):328–31.
74. Javadi MA, Feizi S, Kanavi MR, Faramarzi A, Hashemian J, Mirbabaee F. Acute hydrops after deep anterior lamellar keratoplasty in a patient with keratoconus. Cornea. 2011;30(5):591–4. doi:10.1097/ICO.0b013e3181d92866.
75. Abelson MB, Collin HB, Gillette TE, Dohlman CH. Recurrent keratoconus after keratoplasty. Am J Ophthalmol. 1980;90(5):672–6.
76. Nirankari VS, Karesh J, Bastion F, Lakhanpal V, Billings E. Recurrence of keratoconus in donor cornea 22 years after successful keratoplasty. Br J Ophthalmol. 1983;67(1):23–8.
77. Cannon DJ, Foster CS. Collagen crosslinking in keratoconus. Invest Ophthalmol Vis Sci. 1978;17(1):63–5.
78. Bechrakis N, Blom ML, Stark WJ, Green WRRECURRENTKERATOCONUS. Cornea. 1994; 13(1):73–7. doi:10.1097/00003226-199401000-00012.
79. Bergmanson JP, Goosey JD, Patel CK, Mathew JH. Recurrence or re-emergence of keratoconus—what is the evidence telling us? Literature review and two case reports. Ocul Surf. 2014;12(4):267–72. doi:10.1016/j.jtos.2014.05.004.
80. Krivoy D, McCormick S, Zaidman GW. Postkeratoplasty keratoconus in a nonkeratoconus patient. Am J Ophthalmol. 2001;131(5):653–4.
81. Unal M, Yucel I, Akar Y, Akkoyunlu G, Ustunel I. Recurrence of keratoconus in two corneal grafts after penetrating keratoplasty. Cornea. 2007;26(3):362–4. doi:10.1097/ICO.0b013e31802c9e2e.
82. Yeniad B, Alparslan N, Akarcay K. Eye rubbing as an apparent cause of recurrent keratoconus. Cornea. 2009;28(4):477–9.
83. McGhee CNJ. 2008 Sir Norman McAlister Gregg lecture: 150 years of practical observations on the conical cornea–what have we learned? Clin Exp Ophthalmol. 2009;37(2):160–76.
84. Brookes NH, Niederer RL, Hickey D, McGhee CNJ, Sherwin T. Recurrence of keratoconic pathology in penetrating keratoplasty buttons originally transplanted for keratoconus. Cornea. 2009;28(6):688–93.
85. Hayes S, Young R, Boote C, Hawksworth N, Huang Y, Meek KM. A structural investigation of corneal graft failure in suspected recurrent keratoconus. Eye (Lond). 2010;24(4):728–34. doi:10.1038/eye.2009.159.
86. de Toledo JA, de la Paz MF, Barraquer RI, Barraquer J. Long-term progression of astigmatism after penetrating keratoplasty for keratoconus: evidence of late recurrence. Cornea. 2003;22(4):317–23.
87. Jhanji V, Chan E, Nambiar M, Vajpayee RB. Morphology of graft–host junction in cases with postkeratoplasty corneal ectasia. Cornea. 2013;32(7):1031–3. doi:10.1097/ICO.0b013e318281af60.
88. Feiz V, Mannis MJ, Kandavel G, McCarthy M, Izquierdo L, Eckert M, et al. Surface keratopathy after penetrating keratoplasty. Trans Am Ophthalmol Soc. 2001;99:159–70.
89. Niederer RL, Perumal D, Sherwin T, McGhee CN. Corneal innervation and cellular changes after corneal transplantation: an in vivo confocal microscopy study. Invest Ophthalmol Vis Sci. 2007;48(2):621–6. doi:10.1167/iovs.06-0538.
90. Marcon AS, Cohen EJ, Rapuano CJ, Laibson PR. Recurrence of corneal stromal dystrophies after penetrating keratoplasty. Cornea. 2003;22(1):19–21.
91. Galvis V, Tello A, Barrera R, Nino CA. Inflammation in keratoconus. Cornea. 2015;34(8):e22–3. doi:10.1097/ico.0000000000000499.
92. Krachmer JH, Feder RS, Belin MW. Keratoconus and related noninflammatory corneal thinning disorders. Surv Ophthalmol. 1984;28(4):293–322.
93. Sugar J, Macsai MS. What causes keratoconus? Cornea. 2012;31(6):716–9.doi:10.1097/ICO.0b013e31823f8c72.
94. Forrester JV, Xu H, Kuffová L, Dick AD, McMenamin PG. Dendritic cell physiology and function in the eye. Immunol Rev. 2010;234(1):282–304.
95. Balasubramanian SA, Pye DC, Willcox MD. Effects of eye rubbing on the levels of protease, protease

activity and cytokines in tears: relevance in keratoconus. Clin Exp Optom. 2013;96(2):214–8.
96. Jun AS, Cope L, Speck C, Feng X, Lee S, Meng H, et al. Subnormal cytokine profile in the tear fluid of keratoconus patients. PLoS ONE. 2011;6(1), e16437.
97. Balasubramanian SA, Mohan S, Pye DC, Willcox MD. Proteases, proteolysis and inflammatory molecules in the tears of people with keratoconus. Acta Ophthalmol. 2012;90(4):e303–9. doi:10.1111/j.1755-3768.2011.02369.x.
98. Lema I, Duran JA. Inflammatory molecules in the tears of patients with keratoconus. Ophthalmology. 2005;112(4):654–9. doi:10.1016/j.ophtha.2004.11.050.
99. Lema I, Sobrino T, Duran JA, Brea D, Diez-Feijoo E. Subclinical keratoconus and inflammatory molecules from tears. Br J Ophthalmol. 2009;93(6):820–4. doi:10.1136/bjo.2008.144253.
100. Solomon A. Inflammation in the pathogenesis of keratoconus. In: Barbara A, editor. Textbook on keratoconus: new insights. Wife Goes On; 2011.
101. Balasubramanian SA, Pye DC, Willcox MDP. Levels of lactoferrin, secretory IgA and serum albumin in the tear film of people with keratoconus. Exp Eye Res. 2012;96(1):132–7.
102. Mkaddem SB, Rossato E, Heming N, Monteiro RC. Anti-inflammatory role of the IgA Fc receptor (CD89): from autoimmunity to therapeutic perspectives. Autoimmun Rev. 2013;12(6):666–9.
103. Lema I, Durán JA, Ruiz C, Díez-Feijoo E, Acera A, Merayo J. Inflammatory response to contact lenses in patients with keratoconus compared with myopic subjects. Cornea. 2008;27(7):758–63.
104. Wojcik KA, Blasiak J, Szaflik J, Szaflik JP. Role of biochemical factors in the pathogenesis of keratoconus. Acta Biochim Pol. 2014;61(1):55–62.
105. Dursun D, Piniella AM, Pflugfelder SC. Pseudokeratoconus caused by rosacea. Cornea. 2001;20(6):668–9.
106. Afonso AA, Sobrin L, Monroy DC, Selzer M, Lokeshwar B, Pflugfelder SC. Tear fluid gelatinase B activity correlates with IL-1a concentration and fluorescein clearance in ocular rosacea. Invest Ophthalmol Vis Sci. 1999;40(11):2506–12.
107. McMonnies CW. Inflammation and keratoconus. Optom Vis Sci. 2015;92(2):e35–41. doi:10.1097/opx.0000000000000455.
108. Hamrah P, Huq SO, Liu Y, Zhang Q, Dana MR. Corneal immunity is mediated by heterogeneous population of antigen-presenting cells. J Leukoc Biol. 2003;74(2):172–8.
109. Hamrah P, Liu Y, Zhang Q, Dana MR. The corneal stroma is endowed with a significant number of resident dendritic cells. Invest Ophthalmol Vis Sci. 2003;44(2):581–9.
110. Hamrah P, Zhang Q, Liu Y, Dana MR. Novel characterization of MHC class II-negative population of resident corneal Langerhans cell-type dendritic cells. Investig Ophthalmol Vis Sci. 2002;43(3):639–46.
111. Mayer WJ, Mackert MJ, Kranebitter N, Messmer EM, Grüterich M, Kampik A, et al. Distribution of antigen presenting cells in the human cornea: correlation of in vivo confocal microscopy and immunohistochemistry in different pathologic entities. Curr Eye Res. 2012;37(11):1012–8.
112. Mathew J, Goosey J, Burns A, Bergmanson J. Immunohistochemistry and ultrastructure of anterior stromal cells in keratoconus. Invest Ophthalmol Vis Sci. 2010;51(13):6230.
113. Kenney MC, Chwa M, Lin B, Huang GH, Ljubimov AV, Brown DJ. Identification of cell types in human diseased corneas. Cornea. 2001;20(3):309–16.
114. Cheung IM, McGhee CN, Sherwin T. Deficient repair regulatory response to injury in keratoconic stromal cells. Clin Exp Optom. 2014;97(3):234–9.

Keratoconus in Children

5

Luca Buzzonetti, Paola Valente,
and Gianni Petrocelli

Keratoconus typically has its onset at puberty and progresses until the third to fourth decade of life, when it usually stabilizes [1]. Although it is a relatively rare disease at the age of 10 years, in pediatric patients keratoconus is often more advanced at diagnosis [2] and its progression may be more frequent and more rapid with a sevenfold higher risk of requiring corneal grafting [3]. Childhood onset cases have a more aggressive progression than those of later onset [4]; therefore, detection of progressive keratoconus in early stages of the disease is necessary to prevent severe visual impairment [5, 6].

Some authors report that young age is associated with more severe forms of keratoconus and faster progression, with an inverse correlation between age and severity [7, 8]. After congenital corneal opacities, keratoconus represents one of the most common causes of pediatric corneal transplantation causing about 15–20 % of all corneal transplants in children [9, 10]. A retrospective monocentric study confirms that at diagnosis keratoconus is more severe in children than in adults, and the age of the youngest child included in the study was 6 years [5]. The diagnosis of pediatric keratoconus is often made late. It depends on the scarcity of functional complaints in children, especially before the age of 8. Furthermore, it is supposed that progression of keratoconus is "explosive" in these patients (Fig. 5.1), with a short time between the onset of functional symptoms and the development of a severe form of keratoconus [11]. The late diagnosis predisposes children to serious complications including corneal perforation, microbial keratitis, glaucoma, and amblyopia.

As reported in the literature keratoconus can be associated with systemic and ocular diseases [12, 13]. In children these associations are typical and include Down's syndrome, atopy, Ehlers–Danlos syndrome, Marfan syndrome, mitral valve prolapse, Arterial Tortuosity Syndrome, Laurence–Moon–Biedl Syndrome, Costello Syndrome, Intellectual Disability. Ocular conditions include vernal keratoconjunctivitis (VKC), Leber congenital amaurosis (LCA), retinitis pigmentosa, aniridia, iridocorneal endothelial syndrome, blue sclera, corneal dystrophies such as granular and macular dystrophy, posterior polymorphous dystrophy, fleck dystrophy, Fuchs endothelial dystrophy, and lattice-granular dystrophy.

L. Buzzonetti, M.D. (✉)
Ophthalmology Department, Bambino Gesù IRCCS
Children's Hospital, Rome, Italy

Institute of Ophthalmology, Catholic University,
Rome, Italy
e-mail: luca.buzzonetti@opbg.net

P. Valente, M.D. • G. Petrocelli, M.D.
Ophthalmology Department, Bambino Gesù IRCCS
Children's Hospital, Rome, Italy
e-mail: paola.valente@opbg.net;
gianni.petrocelli@opbg.net

J.L. Alió (ed.), *Keratoconus*, Essentials in Ophthalmology, DOI 10.1007/978-3-319-43881-8_5

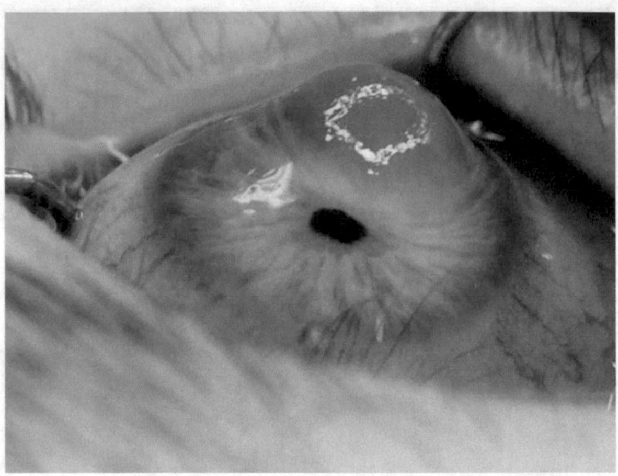

Fig. 5.1 Acute keratoconus in a 13-year-old patient

The incidence of keratoconus in patients with Down's syndrome has been reported in up to 15 % [1]. The eye rubbing, frequently observed in patients with Down's syndrome, represents one of the main pathogenetic hypothesis of keratoconus [14, 15].

Howard et al. [16] described a case of hyperthyroidism and acute hydrop secondary to underlying keratoconus in a child with trisomy 21, and they hypothesized that thyroid gland dysfunction may be associated with the development of keratoconus.

Many studies have discussed on the probably association of atopy with keratoconus [17, 18]. Copman and Gasset reported that the prevalence of eczema and asthma was higher in keratoconus patients than in control group [19, 20].

In children with keratoconus, percentage of patients with VKC ranged from 8.8 to 36 % [21]. The literature has reported that changes in corneal topography are more severe and faster in pediatric patients with keratoconus and VKC than keratoconus alone, and the progression of keratoconus in atopy takes place more rapidly [18, 22, 23]. It is of note that allergic keratoconjunctivitis with eye rubbing may increase the incidence of corneal hydrops in children with keratoconus.

In children with keratoconus the association with LCA has been documented in some reports. The incidence of keratoconus has been noted in 29 % of children with LCA and 2 % of all children with blindness. Keratoconus in patients with LCA occurred in 2 % of 0- to 14-year-olds and it is absent prior to 9 years of age and its incidence increases with increasing age [24]. There is no definitive consensus about the origin of keratoconus in patients with LCA. A working hypothesis suggests that keratoconus could result from the repetitive trauma to the cornea secondary to the characteristic extraocular sign of Franceschetti's oculodigital sign in LCA patients, comprising three components: eye poking, pressing, and rubbing [25].

5.1 Treatment

Corneal cross-linking (CXL) is actually the standard, low-invasive, safe treatment for patients affected by keratoconus [26, 27], with documented clinical progression or perceived risk of progression. Since younger patients usually show a fast progression of keratoconus [5], cross-linking in children and adolescents is actually indicated as soon as the diagnosis has been made [6].

Few authors reported clinical outcomes after CXL in pediatric patients affected by keratoconus. Caporossi et al. [4] published the largest study on pediatric CXL. This prospective study of 152 eyes of 77 patients 18 years old and under (range 10–18 years) treated by Epi-off CXL, at 36 month follow-up showed improvement in best corrected visual acuity (BCVA), *K* readings, asymmetry index values, and coma values. The authors then suggested that riboflavin-UVA-induced cross-linking stabilized the progression of keratoconus in all cases and led to functional improvement in 80% of cases, with statistically significant results.

However, some are the considerations related to Epi-off technique in children: the severe pain induced by epithelial debridement and the consequent temporary visual loss that usually make postoperative management more complicated, the risk of postoperative complications (stromal haze [28] and infections [29]), and the variable period of visual recovery (2–6 months) [26, 30, 31].

Therefore, CXL performed without epithelial removal and by shortening the surgical time could represent a great advantage in children, providing local anesthesia and making the cross-linking treatment and its follow-up management more comfortable. In fact the preservation of the epithelial layer could avoid postoperative pain and visual impairment, as well as all complications related to epithelial debridement.

Recently, it has been proposed a new transepithelial CXL technique in which a iontophoresis system provides riboflavin delivery in corneal stroma [30, 31]. Iontophoresis is a noninvasive delivery system designed to enhance the penetration of molecules as well as riboflavin into tissue using a small electric current.

We published the first clinical study on transepithelial CXL by iontophoresis of riboflavin in pediatric patients [32]. We evaluated visual acuity, and refractive and corneal aberrometric changes through 15-month follow-up in 14 eyes of 14 pediatric patients (mean age 13±2.4 [SD] years; range, 10–18 years) affected by keratoconus (stage 1 or 2 according to Amsler-Krumeich classification). In opposite to previous reports on transepithelial technique in pediatric eyes [33, 34], we did not report keratoconus progression over 15 months; furthermore, we did not observe an improvement in refractive, topographic, and aberrometric parameters, excepting for BCVA.

Our unpublished data at 24-month follow-up, recorded in 27 eyes of 17 patients (mean age 14±2.5), seem to confirm the same "trend" (Tables 5.1 and 5.2).

These early findings suggest that iontophoresis-assisted transepithelial CXL performed by means of riboflavin delivery could halt the keratoconus progression in pediatric patients up to 24 months. For sure longest follow-ups need to indicate if this technique could really become an alternative to Epi-off one, currently still considered the "gold standard."

Table 5.1 Corrected distance visual acuity, manifest spherical equivalent, and refractive astigmatism measured preoperatively and 24 months after cross-linking (27 eyes, 17 patients, mean age 14±2.5)

	Preoperative	24 months postoperative
CDVA	7.5±1.8	8.1±2.1 (P=0.1)
Spherical equivalent (D)	−1.5±1.6	−1.7±2.0 (P=0.5)
Refractive astigmatism (D)	−1.4±1.9	−1.3±1.3 (P=0.8)

CDVA corrected distance visual acuity, *D* diopters

Table 5.2 Topographic and tomographic data measured preoperatively and 24 months after cross-linking

	Preoperative	24 months postoperative
K_{max} (D)	47.9±3.2	48.6±3.6 (P=0.06)
K_{min} (D)	43.1±9.0	43.6±9.2 (P=0.07)
K_{avg} (D)	44.5±9.2	47.0±9.3 (P=0.2)
Posterior elevation map (μ)	17.96±28.5	16.81±21.5 (P=0.77)

D diopters, μ micron

Intracorneal ring segments (ICRS) have been demonstrated to be effective in improving visual acuity and reducing the refractive error and the mean keratometry in selected cases of keratoconic eyes of adult patients [35, 36]. However, up to now poor is the experience about ICRS implantation in pediatric patients. Estrada et al. [37] reported the outcomes of ICRS in the surgical correction of different levels of severity of keratoconus obtained in a large multicenter series of cases: 611 consecutive keratoconic eyes of 357 patients ranging in age from 10 to 73 years (mean age: 35.15 ± 11.62 years), but they did not separately analyze pediatric patients. Generally, ICRS are not preferred in the pediatric patients for aggressive nature of keratoconus, tendency of eye rubbing, and noncompliance. Kankariya et al. [38] observed that although the option of ICRS (less invasive) is not commonly utilized in pediatric eyes, in adolescent patients with end-stage keratoconus and imminent keratoplasty (more invasive), this option may be worth considering.

Pediatric keratoplasty still represents a very challenging surgery, generally performed when corneal opacification induces a visual deprivation [39]. The Penetrating Keratoplasty (PK), actually the "gold standard" in pediatric keratoplasty, has shown a prognosis for graft survival of approximately 50–60 % [40, 41], mainly because of endothelial rejection [42, 43]. Deep anterior lamellar keratoplasty (DALK) diffusion is currently limited in pediatric patients and few papers report outcomes after big-bubble DALK in children. Harding et al. [44] treated 13 eyes of 9 pediatric patients affected by partial thickness corneal scarring and mucopolysaccharidoses performing DALK with manual dissection, except for one eye that underwent big-bubble DALK with conversion to PK because of an intraoperative inadvertent perforation. Ashar et al. [45] observed that DALK is a feasible option in children with stromal corneal pathology. The authors evaluated 26 eyes: three underwent big-bubble procedure, while 23 layer-by-layer dissection.

Recently, the femtosecond solid-state laser was successfully used in several corneal surgical procedures and Buzzonetti et al. [46] proposed a standardized big-bubble technique in DALK assisted by femtosecond laser called Intrabubble. The laser provides a pre-Descemet's plane lamellar dissection to a predefined corneal depth and the creation of a stromal channel, 50 µm above the thinnest corneal point, into which a smooth cannula for air injection can be introduced. The Intrabubble can be considered a standardized procedure: the femtosecond laser is accurate in achieving the desired corneal depth and the big-bubble, and provides good refractive outcomes for the good alignment of donor and recipient configuration. We successfully applied this technique also to pediatric patients [47] in an attempt to decrease the rejection percentage, to improve the refractive outcome, and thus provide an anti-amblyopic effect.

We are using the IntraLase femtosecond laser (IntraLase FS Laser, Abbott Medical Optics, Inc.) that works by applying the applanation lens after obtaining a proper vacuum seal using a 10 mm diameter suction ring. However, this size can result too big to perform the treatment in smallest eyes. Thus, we experimented docking without suction ring by fixing the ocular bulb by four silk conjunctival stitches sutured over the skin (Fig. 5.2). This technique effectively provides a safe and effective applanation (Fig. 5.3).

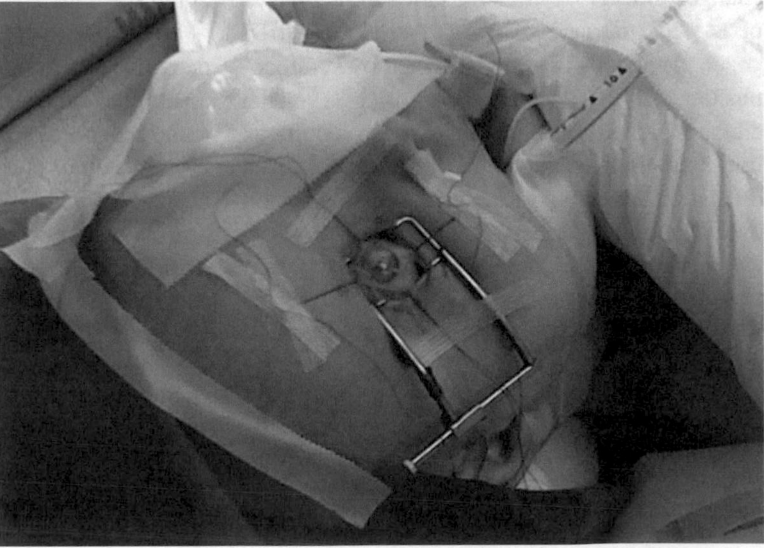

Fig. 5.2 To perform docking without suction ring we fixed the ocular bulb by four silk conjunctival stitches sutured over the skin

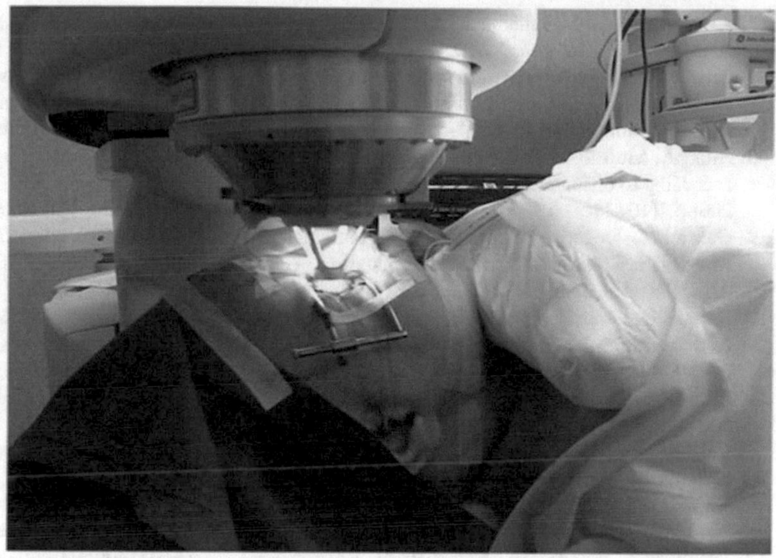

Fig. 5.3 The docking without suction ring effectively provides a safe and effective applanation

Few authors investigated the application of femtosecond laser in pediatric keratoplasty [47–49], but long-term follow-up after big-bubble DALK has not yet been reported. In a comparison between pediatric patients that underwent big-bubble DALK using mechanical trephine (seven patients, mean age 11.4±3.0; Group 1) or femtosecond laser (seven patients, mean age 11.6±4.2; Group 2), 2 year after surgery (at least 16 months after complete suture removal) we observed that (unpublished data), respectively, BCVA was 0.7±0.1D and 0.7±0.2D ($P=0.3$), spherical equivalent −4.5±0.7D and −2.4±1. ($P=0.09$), and refractive astigmatism 4.8±2.2D and 3.3±1.3D ($P=0.2$).

We did not record statistically significant differences, but our findings suggest that femtosecond laser could decrease spherical equivalent and refractive astigmatism amount. If these data will be confirmed, they will can be added to all the other typical advantages of DALK: immune rejection of corneal endothelium cannot occur, surgical procedure is extraocular, topical corticosteroids can usually be discontinued earlier, and lower is loss of endothelial cell density; compared with PK, DALK may have superior resistance to rupture of the globe after blunt trauma and sutures can be removed earlier [50].

In conclusion, keratoconus in children needs a prompt diagnosis in order to plan the most appropriate therapeutic strategy. Since the high frequency of association with systemic diseases, a best cooperation between pediatricians and ophthalmologists could improve the treatment of these young patients.

Compliance with Ethical Requirements *Conflict of Interest.* Luca Buzzonetti, Paola Valente, and Gianni Petrocelli declare that they have no conflict of interest.

Informed Consent. All procedures followed were in accordance with the ethical standards of the responsible committee on human experimentation (institutional and national) and with the Helsinki Declaration of 1975, as revised in 2000. Informed consent was obtained from all patients for being included in the study. No animal studies were performed by the authors for this chapter.

References

1. Rabinowitz YS. Keratoconus. Surv Ophthalmol. 1998;42:297–319.
2. McAnena L, O'Keefe M. Corneal collagen crosslinking in children with keratoconus. J AAPOS. 2015;19:228–32.
3. Leoni-Mesplie S, Mortemosque B, Touboul D, et al. Scalability and severity of keratoconus in children. Am J Ophthalmol. 2012;154:156–62.
4. Caporossi A, Mazzotta C, Baiocchi S, et al. Riboflavin UVA-induced corneal collagen cross-linking in pediatric patients. Cornea. 2012;31:227–31.
5. Reeves SW, Stinnett S, Adelman RA, et al. Risk factors for progression to penetrating keratoplasty in patients with keratoconus. Am J Ophthalmol. 2005;140:607–11.
6. Chatzis N, Hafezi F. Progression of keratoconus and efficacy of pediatric (corrected) corneal collagen cross-linking in children and adolescents. J Refract Surg. 2012;28:753–8.

7. Al Suhaiba Al Suhaibani AH, Al-Rajhi AA, Al-Motowa S, Wagoner MD. Inverse relationship between age and severity and sequelae of acute corneal hydrops associated with keratoconus. Br J Ophthalmol. 2007;91(7):984–5.
8. Ertan A, Muftuoglu O. Keratoconus clinical findings according to different age and gender groups. Cornea. 2008;27(10):1109–13.
9. Gabrić N, Dekaris I, Vojniković B, Karaman Z, Mravicić I, Katusić J. Corneal transplantation in children. Coll Antropol. 2001;25(Suppl):17–22.
10. Beltaief O, Farah H, Kamoun R, Ben Said A, Ouertani A. Penetrating keratoplasty in children. Tunis Med. 2003;81(7):477–81.
11. Slim EA, Jarade EF, Charanek BM, Antoun JS, Hemade AI, Awada SH, Fakhoury HW, Cherfan CG. Acute corneal hydrops mimicking infectious keratitis as initial presentation of keratoconus in a 10-year-old child. Case Rep Ophthalmol Med. 2015;2015:308348.
12. Javadi MA, Rafee'i AB, Kamalian N, Karimian F, Ja'farinasab MR, Yazdani S. Concomitant keratoconus and macular corneal dystrophy. Cornea. 2004;23(5): 508–12.
13. Cremona FA, Ghosheh FR, Rapuano CJ, Eagle Jr RC, Hammersmith KM, Laibson PR, Ayres BD, Cohen EJ. Keratoconus associated with other corneal dystrophies. Cornea. 2009;28(2):127–35.
14. Courage ML, Adams RJ, Reyno S, Kwa PG. Visual acuity in infants and children with Down syndrome. Dev Med Child Neurol. 1994;36:586–93.
15. Watt T, Robertson K, Jacobs RJ. Refractive error, binocular vision and accommodation of children with Down syndrome. Clin Exp Optom. 2015;98(1):3–11.
16. Howard S, Raine J, Dattani M. Corneal rupture in a child with Down syndrome and hyperthyroidism. BMJ Case Rep. 2009; 2009. pii: bcr08.2008.0842. doi: 10.1136/bcr.08.2008.0842. Epub 2009 Mar 5.
17. Lowell FC, Carroll JM. A study of the occurrence of atopic traits in patients with keratoconus. J Allergy Clin Immunol. 1970;46:32–9.
18. Kaya V, Karakaya M, Utine CA, Albayrak S, Oge OF, Yilmaz OF. Evaluation of the corneal topographic characteristics of keratoconus with orbscan II in patients with and without atopy. Cornea. 2007;26(8):945–8.
19. Copeman PWM. Eczema and keratoconus. BMJ. 1965;2:977–9.
20. Gasset AR, Hinson WA, Frias JL. Keratoconus and atopic disease. Ann Ophthalmol. 1978;10:991–4.
21. Kok YO, Tan GF, Loon SC. Review: keratoconus in Asia. Cornea. 2012;31(5):581–93.
22. Lapid-Gortzak R, Rosen S, Weitzman S, et al. Videokeratography findings in children with vernal keratoconjunctivitis versus those of healthy children. Ophthalmology. 2002;109:2018–23.
23. Rehany U, Rumelt S. Corneal hydrops associated with vernal conjunctivitis as a presenting sign of keratoconus in children. Ophthalmology. 1995;102(12):2046–9.
24. Dharmaraj S, Leroy BP, Sohocki MM, Koenekoop RK, Perrault I, Anwar K, Khaliq S, Devi RS, Birch DG, De Pool E, Izquierdo N, Van Maldergem L, Ismail M, Payne AM, Holder GE, Bhattacharya SS, Bird AC, Kaplan J, Maumenee IH. The phenotype of Leber congenital amaurosis in patients with AIPL1 mutations. Arch Ophthalmol. 2004;122(7):1029–37.
25. Weleber RG, Francis PJ, Trzupek KM, Beattie C.Leber Congenital Amaurosis. In: Pagon RA, Adam MP, Ardinger HH, Wallace SE, Amemiya A, Bean LJH, Bird TD, Fong CT, Mefford HC, Smith RJH, Stephens K, editors.GeneReviews®[Internet]. Seattle (WA): University of Washington, Seattle; 1993-2016. 2004 Jul 7 [updated 2013 May 2].
26. Caporossi A, Mazzotta C, Baiocchi S, Caporossi T. Long-term results of riboflavin ultraviolet a corneal collagen cross-linking for keratoconus in Italy: the Siena eye cross study. Am J Ophthalmol. 2010;149:585–93.
27. Gomes JAP, Tan D, Rapuano CJ, et al. Global consensus on keratoconus and ectatic diseases. Cornea. 2015;34:359–69.
28. Mazzotta C, Balestrazzi A, Baiocchi S, Traversi C, Caporossi A. Stromal haze after combined riboflavin-UVA corneal collagen cross-linking in keratoconus: in vivo confocal microscopic evaluation. Clin Exp Ophthalmol. 2007;35:580–2.
29. Zamora KV, Males JJ. Polymicrobial keratitis after a collagen cross-linking procedure with postoperative use of a contact lens: a case report. Cornea. 2009;28(4):474–6.
30. Bikbova G, Bikbov M. Transepithelial corneal cross-linking by iontophoresis of riboflavin. Acta Ophthalmol. 2013;92:e30–4.
31. Mastropasqua L, Nubile M, Calienno R, Mattei PA, Pedrotti E, Salgari N, Mastropasqua R, Lanzini M. Corneal cross-linking: intrastromal riboflavin concentration in iontophoresis-assisted imbibitions versus traditional and transepithelial techniques. Am J Ophthalmol. 2014;157:623–30.
32. Buzzonetti L, Petrocelli G, Valente P, et al. Iontophoretic transepithelial cross-linking to halt keratoconus in pediatric cases: 15 month follow-up. Cornea. 2015;34:512–5.
33. Koppen C, Wouters K, Mathysen D, Rozema J, Tassignon MJ. Refractive and topographic results of benzalkonium chloride-assisted transepithelial cross-linking. J Cataract Refract Surg. 2012;38:1000–5.
34. Buzzonetti L, Petrocelli G. Transepithelial corneal cross linking in children. Early results. J Refract Surg. 2012;28:763–7.
35. Colin J. European clinical evaluation: use of Intacs for the treatment of keratoconus. J Cataract Refract Surg. 2006;32:747–55.
36. Zare MA, Hashemi H, Salari MR. Intracorneal ring segment implantation for the management of keratoconus: safety and efficacy. J Cataract Refract Surg. 2007;33:1886–91.
37. Vega-Estrada A, Alio JL, Brenner LF, Javaloy J, Plaza Puche AB, Barraquer RI, Teus MA, Murta J, Henriques J, Uceda-Montanes A. Outcome analysis of intracorneal ring segments for the treatment of keratoconus based on visual, refractive, and aberrometric impairment. Am J Ophthalmol. 2013;155: 575–84.

38. Kankariya VP, Kymionis GD, Diakonis VF, Yoo SH. Management of pediatric keratoconus—evolving role of corneal collagen cross-linking: an update. Indian J Ophthalmol. 2013;61:435–40.
39. Colby K. Changing times for pediatric keratoplasty. J APPOS. 2008;12:223–4.
40. Hovlykke M, Hjortdal J, Ehlers N, Nielsen K. Clinical results of 40 years of pediatric keratoplasty in a single university eye clinic. Acta Ophthalmol. 2013. doi:10.1111/aos.12198x.
41. Huang C, O'Hara M, Mannis MJ. Primary pediatric keratoplasty: indications and outcomes. Cornea. 2009;28:1003–8.
42. Aasuri MK, Garg P, Gokhle N, Gupta S. Penetrating keratoplasty in children. Cornea. 2000;19:140–4.
43. Vanathi M, Panda A, Vengayil S, Chaudhuri Z, Dada T. Pediatric keratoplasty. Surv Ophthalmol. 2009;54: 245–71.
44. Harding SA, Nishal KK, Upponi-Patil A, Fowler DJ. Indications and outcomes of deep anterior lamellar keratoplasty in children. Ophthalmology. 2010;117:2191–5.
45. Ashar JN, Pahuja S, Ramappa M, Vaddavalli PK, Chaurasia S, Garg P. Deep anterior lamellar keratoplasty in children. Am J Ophthalmol. 2013;155: 570–4.
46. Buzzonetti L, Laborante A, Petrocelli G. Standardized big-bubble technique in deep anterior lamellar keratoplasty assisted by femtosecond laser. J Cataract Refract Surg. 2010;36:1631.6.
47. Buzzonetti L, Petrocelli G, Valente P. Big-bubble deep anterior lamellar keratoplasty assisted by femtosecond laser in children. Cornea. 2012;31:1083–6.
48. Agarwal A, Brubaker JW, Mamalis N, Kumar DA, Jacob S, Chinnamuthu S, Nair V, Prakash G, Meduri A, Agarwal A. Femtosecond-assisted lamellar keratoplasty in atypical Avellino corneal dystrophy of Indian origin. Eye Contact Lens. 2009;35(5):272–4. doi:10.1097/ICL.0b013e3181b3859c.
49. Buzzonetti L, Petrocelli G, Laborante A. Anterior lamellar keratoplasty assisted by IntraLase femtosecond laser in pediatric patient. Two years follow up. J Pediatr Ophthalmol Strabismus. 2010. doi:10.3928/01913913-20100507-01.
50. Reinhart WJ, Musch DC, Jacobs DS, Lee WB, Kaufman SC, Shtein RM. Deep anterior lamellar keratoplasty as an alternative to penetrating keratoplasty. Ophthalmology. 2011;118:209–18.

Part II

Diagnostic Tools in Keratoconus

6 Instrumentation for Diagnosis of Keratoconus

Francesco Versaci and Gabriele Vestri

The current methods to detect, diagnose, and monitor the evolution of keratoconus morphologically are computerized videokeratoscopy, corneal tomography, and optical scanning tomography, both in the Scheimpflug configuration as well as based on optical coherence. For reference, a more detailed list would also include tools based on rasterstereography, Moiré interferometry, or laser interferometry [1, 2] but many of these instruments have remained at the prototype stage, and others have been used only in laboratory for research purposes.

The advent of computerized corneal topography has made it possible to gather considerable information about the shape and refractive behavior of the cornea affected by keratoconus. By means of some of these examination techniques it is also possible to measure both the shape of the front surface as well as the back surface thereby giving more accurate information about the location and shape of the cone, the extension of ectasia, and the refractive power localized in the ectatic area.

In-depth knowledge of the profile of the corneal surface is not only essential in the diagnosis or treatment of keratoconus but it is important in many other aspects of clinical practice. In fact, since the cornea alone is responsible for about 80 % of the refractive power of the eye [3], its form has extreme importance in the study of visual function: this surface, formed by the front face of the cornea and coated by the tear film, presents, in fact, the highest refractive index jump with respect to all other elements of the dioptric ocular system and small changes of its shape produce considerable effects on the optical quality of the entire ocular system. Therefore, a careful study of the corneal morphology, in addition to providing valuable information in the early diagnosis of all corneal diseases that change the shape of the surface (and first keratoconus), lends itself to many other clinical applications such as preoperative planning and postoperative assessment throughout the range of refractive surgery and keratoplasty, the application of rigid contact lenses, or the calculation of intraocular lenses in accordance with the formulas or other methods of calculation.

6.1 Videokeratoscopes

The study of the Purkinje–Sanson image dates from the mid-1800s and was the first method of investigation of catoptric images for diagnostic purposes. A Placido disk (consisting simply of a series of concentric black and white circles with a positive lens in the center) was used to observe

F. Versaci, M.S.E. (✉) • G. Vestri, M.S.E.
CSO srl, Via degli Stagnacci 12/E, Badia a Settimo, Firenze, Italy
e-mail: F.Versaci@csoitalia.it; G.Vestri@csoitalia.it

J.L. Alió (ed.), *Keratoconus*, Essentials in Ophthalmology, DOI 10.1007/978-3-319-43881-8_6

the appearance of images reflected from the corneal surface and evaluate approximately and qualitatively, on the basis of the deformation of the reflections of the circles, aberrations borne by the cornea as shown in Fig. 6.1.

The objective measurement of the radius of curvature of the anterior surface of the cornea, also through mire projected on the cornea and reflected by it, dates back to 1854 [4]. Assuming known dimensions of an object (mires) and its distance from the specular surface (cornea), measuring the size of the images formed by the mirror and applying the catadioptric laws, the shape of the specular surface that has reflected upon is obtained: this principle is based on the elementary keratometry measurement.

It is already clear from this brief history that reflection-based devices or videokeratoscopes do not directly measure the elevation data of the cornea, but rather analyze the physical phenomenon that occurs on the anterior corneal surface: specular reflection.

6.2 The Sagittal Curvature

Conceptually, we can consider modern videokeratoscopes as a derivative of ophthalmometers, so much so that the first method developed in this regard is based on the same principles of the ophthalmometer [5]. Indeed, we can consider a topographic measure as many keratometries with ever larger fixed mires, centered on the same axis. The corneal curvature so measured is called the *sagittal* (or *axial*) curvature and can be defined as the radius of an arc of a circle, centered on the optical axis of videokeratoscope (or the keratometer) when this is well aligned to the corneal vertex, which has the same tangent as the cornea to the point concerned, as shown in Fig. 6.2 on the left. In the branches of topography this measure was carried out essentially for comparison: once the device has been calibrated by acquiring spheres (calibration spheres) with known curvature, the curvature of a sample is estimated by comparing the position of the mires reflected by its surface and the ones obtained from the calibration spheres [6].

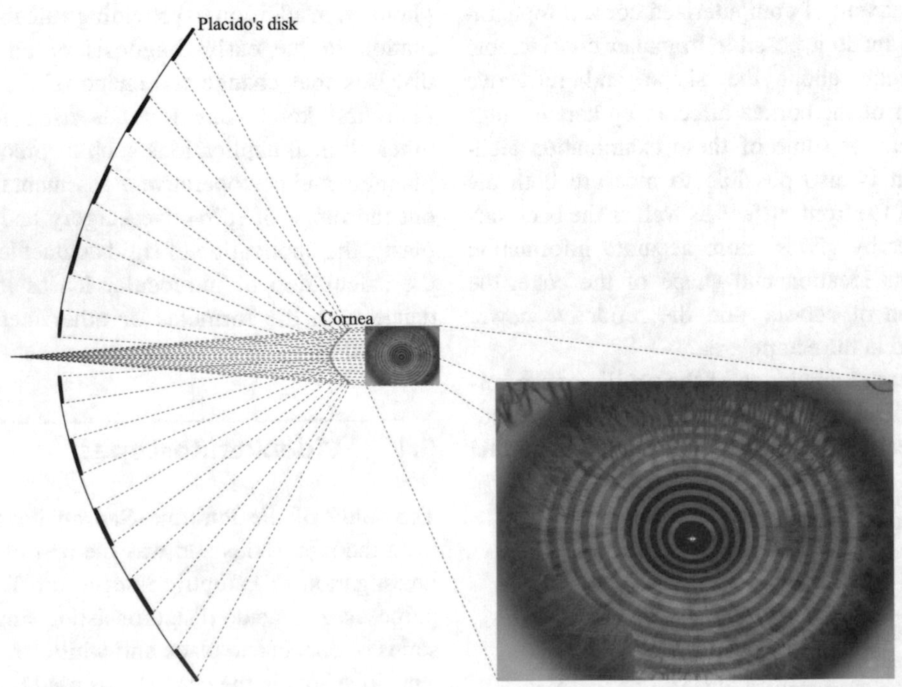

Fig. 6.1 Process of formation of the first Purkinje image from a Placido disk

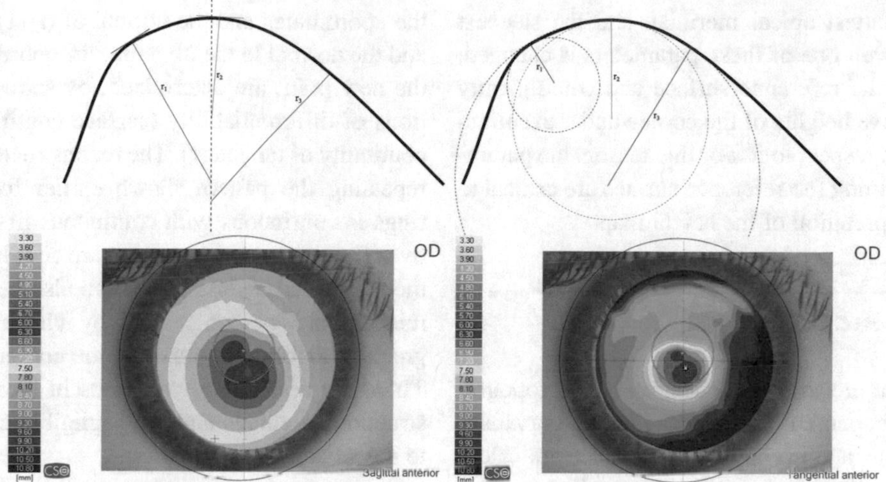

Fig. 6.2 *Left map* of sagittal curvature, *right map* of tangential curvature

The curvature as defined earlier suffers from a low sensitivity for determining shape variations localized in the peripheral cornea. A map of sagittal curvature expressed in diopters, while not being the direct expression of the real refractive power, can represent quite well the optical characteristics of the corneal surface, but it is not able to accurately describe the morphological aspects of the cornea. For this reason, it is felt necessary to support the sagittal curvature with magnitudes which best show the details of the shape of the corneal surface.

6.3 The Tangential Curvature

The *tangential curvature* (sometimes called *instantaneous* or *local*) is the geometric unit that describes the steepening of the cornea, for a given point and in a given direction: it is therefore defined as the radius of the osculating circle for each point belonging to the meridian in question, as shown in Fig. 6.2 on the right. Unlike the sagittal curvature, the center of tangential curvature is not constrained to lie on a reference axis: this condition does not occur unless the cornea is not exactly spherical, and the tangential and the sagittal curvatures are different at every point and coincide only at the vertex. The tangential curvature of a surface is independent of the position of the reference axis along the meridian considered: its sagittal curvature is instead a function of this axis.

6.4 The Height Maps

Topographic maps that represent elevation data are probably more understandable, since they are similar to those used in geographic cartography to describe the elevations of the Earth's surface or the depth of the seabed. The corneal elevation maps are expressed in microns [μm] the position of each point of the cornea, in terms of the elevations along the z axis, with respect to a reference surface. As in geographic maps, where the reference surface is the mean sea level (the *geoid*), the elevation of the corneal surface needs to be expressed in respect to some reference surface: usually spherical, aspherical, or asphero-toric. The reference surfaces, with respect to which the height is measured, are almost always the best-fit surfaces (best approximating surfaces in the sense of the least square error) and have some parameters that characterize them: the spheres are defined by their radius of curvature, the aspherical surfaces by the apical radius of curvature and eccentricity, the asphero-toric surfaces by the apical radius of curvature, eccentricity, and by toricity, that is, the difference of curvature of the flattest apical meridian and the steepest one. If even one of these parameters is changed, it alters the reference surface and consequently the relative heights of the cornea under examination with respect to it. For this reason, the parameters defining the reference surface are critical to the interpretation of the height map.

6.5 Arc Step

In recent generation reflection-based topographers, tangential curvature, sagittal curvature, elevations, and normals to the surface are calculated simultaneously by a process called *arc step* [7–10]. For videokeratoscopies, the definition of this algorithm marked a real turning point, expanding the range of measurements possible, from only the sagittal curvature to all the morphological or refractive measurements arising from the shape of the cornea.

The arc-step algorithm is summarized as follows: for each point corresponding to the edge of a ring of each meridian, a ray-tracing procedure is carried out, which, from the known positions of the rings on the Placido disk and the detected positions of the keratoscopy rings, allows to derive normals of the surface to be measured. Such information depends on the correct positioning of the surface to be measured and the exact knowledge of the location of the rings of the Placido disk: the first condition is obtained by different methods (maximum sharpness algorithms on a focusing video stream, triangulations, or interruptions of light beams), while the second is known from construction data and is refined by means of instrument calibration. Once the normals to the corneal surface are known (and therefore its derivatives) an iterative algorithm is started. At step 0, the condition of zero derivative in correspondence of the corneal vertex is imposed and, setting the validity of the law of reflection for the first ring, an arc that meets the slope conditions is identified. The algorithm of arc step, as the name suggests, is iterative, and therefore cannot proceed without the knowledge of data obtained in the previous step (step $i-1$) to derive data for the current step (step i). Knowing the coordinates and the normal of $(i-1)$th point, and the normal to the ith point, the coordinates of the new point are determined, by setting conditions of differentiability (surface continuity and continuity of tangency). The reconstructed curve, repeating the pattern shown earlier for all the rings is continuous with continuous first derivative. The connecting functions are circular arcs in the traditional algorithm but can also be polynomial splines or conic arcs (by virtue of their greater flexibility in pursuing the corneal slope). There are essentially two limits in these reconstructions methods and are negligible compared to the advantages they offer:

- Assuming a continuous curve with a continuous derivative is not able to describe steps or cusps (interruption or discontinuity of the derivative). However, it can be reasonably admitted that stroma rarely has discontinuities that cannot be smoothed by the epithelium.
- Separating in fact the reconstruction for each hemi-meridian it is assumed that the normal belongs to the plane on which lays the hemi-meridian itself. This approximation is called *skew ray error* and was thoroughly discussed in the literature [11].

6.6 Optical Scanning Devices

The optical scanning instruments directly measure the sagittal height of the front surface and the back of the cornea (i.e., the corneal elevation with respect to a reference plane). Usually, the transverse field of view goes from limbus to limbus and the vertical is such as to include the entire anterior chamber limited by the iris and the visible part of the lens. The big advantage of this class of instruments is therefore, in addition to the high transverse coverage, the ability to view and measure the whole anterior chamber and all its surfaces (front cornea, posterior cornea, iris, and lens).

The optical scanning devices base their operation on the projection of beams or light slits which, due to scattering effects, diffuse in every direction part of the energy of the incident light.

Therefore, thanks to the scattering, the tissue crossed behaves like a real extended emitter: part of the back-diffused light radiation is captured by a suitable optics able to form the image on the CCD.

6.7 Corneal Thickness

The measurement of the two front and rear corneal surfaces allows agile deduction of pachymetry information: it is the measurement in microns of the distance between the front surface and posterior surface in the direction normal to the anterior corneal surface. It is very useful information from the clinical point of view: it can allow, for example, to assess the evolution of keratoconus or to decide whether a patient may undergo refractive surgery and what can be the maximum amount of the bearable correction of the cornea. In contact lens practice, differential pachymetry can also highlight possible edematous conditions due to the wearing of contact lenses.

6.8 Scheimpflug Camera

The simplest and most intuitive way to obtain the image of a corneal section is to project a luminous slit along a meridional plane of the cornea and to shoot the backscattered light through suitable optics, having its axis of at 90° with respect to this plane and its focus on the plane of the slit (Fig. 6.3 left). This configuration, however, in practice does not work because of obstacles to the path of the shot such as the nose or eyelids. These obstacles force the choice of a nonorthogonal axis of shot to lighting plane and consequently to have a good part of the image out of focus. The Scheimpflug method (see Fig. 6.4) is useful in this case (or Carpentier, or should we say by Scheimpflug's [12] own admission) that shows how to tilt the CCD in order to focus a plane inclined to the axis of the optical system shoot, as shown in Fig. 6.3 on the right. Once scanned the first image, the light blade and the Scheimpflug system can be rotated in order to acquire images of a succession of equidistant angular sections that allow to completely map the anterior segment of the eye. The anterior corneal surface is determined by identifying its edge on the image in section and correcting the distortion effect due to the optical configuration. The internal structures (posterior corneal surface, iris, angles) are determined by identifying the corresponding edges on images in section, correcting the effect of distortion due to the optics in Scheimpflug configuration and correcting the distorting effect given by the fact that they are seen through the overlying corneal surfaces.

- As previously mentioned this technology presents the substantial advantages of a wide coverage of the area measured and the possibility to extend the topographic analysis to the back surface. In considering real corneas meet however important limitations: sectioning the cornea in radial directions and not considering the azimuthal component, the optical scanning systems are also implicitly affected by skew ray error.
- The time required to scan is relatively long (approximately 1 s in the modern conception devices), and then there is the possibility of introducing errors due to the microsaccadic eye movements of the eye examined. Some systems use software corrections for realignment of the acquired sections to overcome this problem.
- The presence of nonperfectly transparent areas of the corneal tissue (such as a scar or opacity) produces a phenomenon known as hyper-backscattering of a certain area of the cornea. This results in the recognition of a false edge and an error in the measurement of the surface.
- These instruments directly measure the elevations, from which it is then possible to deduce mathematical derivation for the curvatures and the refractive data of the cornea: the resolution that can be achieved with this method, however, is significantly lower than that which can be achieved with reflection devices. For this reason, in the majority of cases manufacturers provided a hybrid Scheimpflug + Placido system, allowing a direct measurement of the curvatures of the anterior corneal surface.

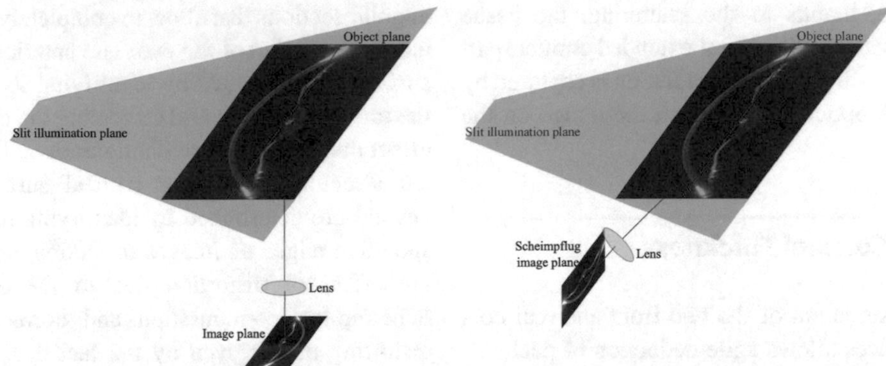

Fig. 6.3 *On the left*, an image system of a section of the cornea with the shooting plane parallel to the plane of illumination. *On the right*, an image system of a section of the cornea in Scheimpflug configuration

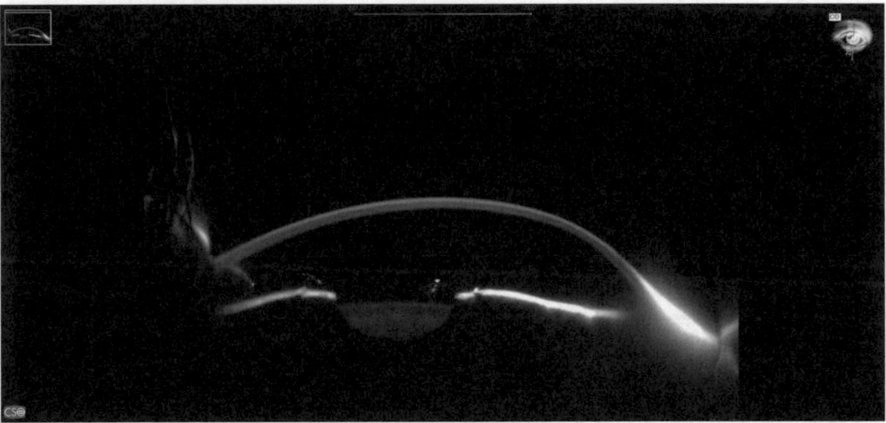

Fig. 6.4 Image of the corneal section of a cornea affected by pellucid obtained by Scheimpflug technology

6.9 AS-OCT (Anterior Segment Optical Coherence Tomography) [13]

Until now, optical tomography coherence has been applied with great success in ophthalmology for the study of the retina and for the measurement of the ocular distances, firstly of the axial length. Only recently industries have turned their attention to this for topography and tomography of the anterior segment of the eye. The reasons for this delay are to be found mainly in the complexity of this technology that is reflected at least for now in high prices of products, in their robustness, in the difficulty of obtaining images that contain the anterior segment in its entirety, and in the difficulty of obtaining accurate measurements comparable to those typical of the simplest techniques in spite of the promising quality of the images.

Optical tomography coherence is a technology based on the measurement of the interference of two beams of broadband radiation (typically infrared) from a reference arm and a sample arm [14–17].

In its simplest embodiment, the radiation emitted from a broadband source, usually an infrared super luminescent diode, is sent in part to a reference arm and in part to a sample arm. A mirror is placed at the end of the reference arm that reflects the beam back toward a fourth arm (detection arm) on which is placed a photodetector. Instead, the radiation sent to the arm of the sample is backscattered by the ocular tissues and also toward the detection arm, where it interferes with the return beam from the reference arm. If the reference mirror is moved, thereby altering the length of the reference arm, the interference due to the ocular structures encountered by the incident beam of the sample arm can be sampled at various depths. In practice, the photodiode reveals a peak signal at each backscattering element encountered by the beam incident on the sample at a position corresponding to that of the movable mirror of the reference arm.

This type of embodiment is that of the Time Domain OCT (TD-OCT) and is shown in Fig. 6.5a. It was the first to be applied in the field of ophthalmology for the measurement of distances, in particular the axial length of the eye and interdistances between the various ocular structures (thickness of the cornea, the anterior chamber height, thickness of the crystalline lens, etc.). Having this technique the need to move the reference mirror for obtaining a response from the structures at various depths, it presents the speed limit when it is necessary to make a scan of several contiguous axes (A-scan) to create an image of an ocular section (B-scan): eye movements during a slow scan lead to an unwanted and uncorrectable distortion of the scanned image.

A more complex implementation is that which goes under the name of Fourier Domain OCT (FD-OCT) [18], which eliminates the need of scanning the reference mirror to have a measurement at various depths. This allows for the possibility of acquiring slice images relatively quickly, thereby reducing artifacts due to eye movements. The Fourier Domain OCT, in addition to decreasing the time of acquisition, also presents advantages in terms of signal-to-noise ratio compared to the Time Domain. The basic idea is to measure the spectral interference between the radiation returning from the reference arm and the sample arm in a certain range of wavelengths emitted by the source. This means that each wavelength obtains an interference value of the return radiation by the two arms (sample and reference arms) in a single A-scan. The set of these values at various wavelengths is processed with more or less complicated algorithms, but basically containing a Fourier transformation, to obtain the profile of the reflectivity of the sample acquired along an axis.

The Fourier Domain OCT devices are in turn classifiable into the following two classes depending on how they get the interference at various wavelengths: Spectral Domain OCT (SD-OCT in Fig. 6.5b) and Swept Source OCT (SS-OCT in Fig. 6.5c).

The first class of instruments uses a source that emits a certain range of wavelengths all at the same time. The detection arm contains a spectrometer or a device suitable to decompose the returned signal from the sample and reference arms in their components at various wavelengths. In only one stroke the sensor of the spectrometer collects the spectrum necessary, after a sequence of processing, to determine the profile of reflectivity along an axis of the sample. An example of what is achieved with this technology is shown in Fig. 6.6.

The second class of devices uses instead a light source that is a tunable laser, i.e., laser whose wavelength can be changed very quickly [19]. This laser is driven so as to emit in sequence the various wavelengths and is synchronized with a photodiode, which replaces the spectrometer on the detection arm. A processor, which knows the wavelength emitted by the source associates the value measured by the photodiode, and reconstructs in a certain time interval the interference spectrum between the beams coming back from the reference arm and the sample arm.

6.10 Brief Introduction to Automated Systems for Keratoconus Screening

6.10.1 Objective Parameters for Quantifying the Ectasia

The first step toward the creation of systems for the recognition of keratoconus has been dictated by the need to objectify and quantify the morphological distortions caused by the onset of ectasia. Quantitative indicators may in fact exceed the

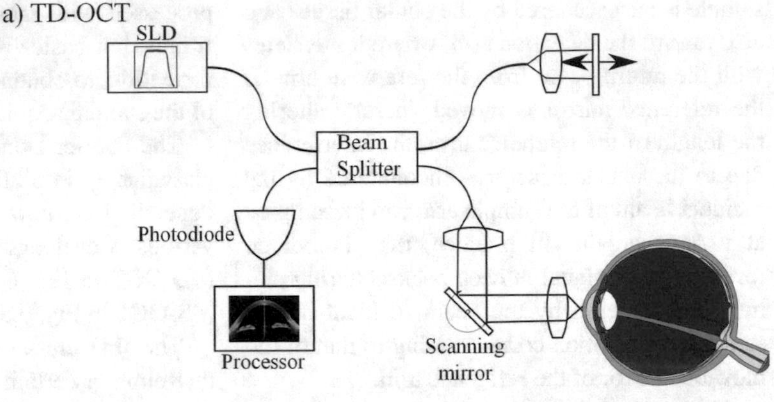

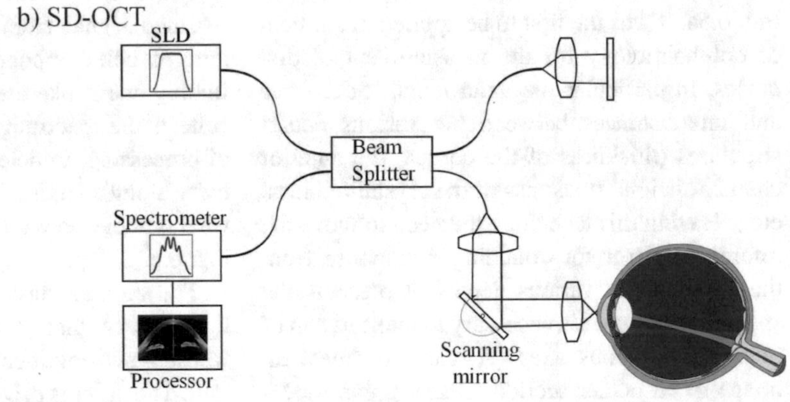

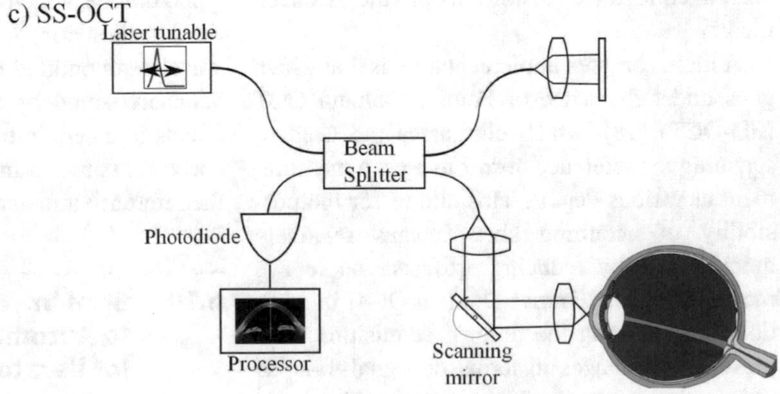

Fig. 6.5 (**a**) Time domain OCT, (**b**) spectral domain OCT, (**c**) swept source OCT

limits of a purely subjective and qualitative interpretation of the topographical framework of a cornea. The calculation of indices also makes possible the temporal interpretation of a case through the comparison of these parameters in the follow-up of the patient: it is in fact possible to monitor over time even very slight variations, so as to keep under observation in a detailed manner the evolution of the pathology.

Since the dawn of modern corneal topography, different authors have proposed different quantitative methods to represent the videokeratoscopic characteristics of keratoconus. The changes induced by the onset of a cone can be

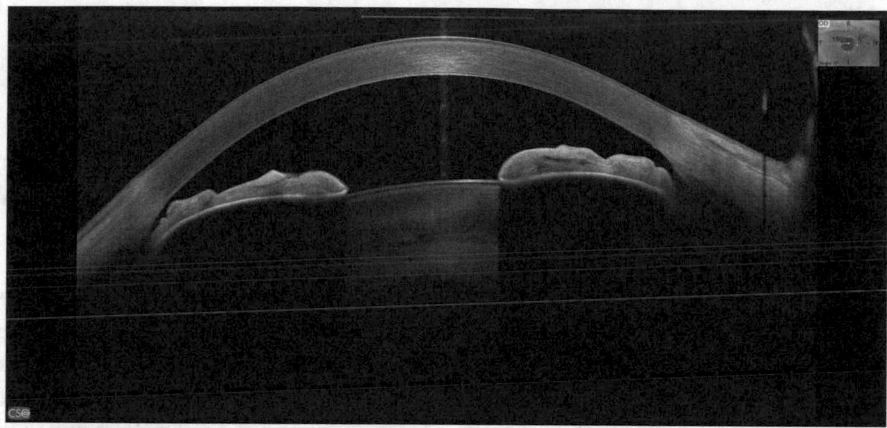

Fig. 6.6 Image of the corneal section of a healthy cornea obtained by technology ASOCT in configuration spectral domain

observed considering wide range of parameters derived from multiple morphological and refractive aspects.

Since the analysis of the anterior surface of the cornea is prior to that of the entire anterior segment, and given that the first topographers provided only sagittal data, the first screening systems for keratoconus and the first indices are based on the analysis of sagittal curvatures of the cornea front: quantitative descriptors derived mainly from sagittal data, such as the KISA% index proposed by Rabinowitz et al. [20–22], the Cone Location and Magnitude Index (CLMI) proposed by Mahmoud et al. [23], and the Keratoconus Prediction Index (KPI) and Keratoconus Index proposed by Maeda et al. [24, 25], have been and are being widely used for keratoconus detection.

Given the desirable characteristics of the tangential curvature in the representation of the shape of keratoconus some authors have abandoned the sagittal representation in favor of the more sensitive tangential representation. Calossi [26] developed some indices derived from the tangential curvature to determine the likelihood of compatibility with a topographic pattern of keratoconus, considering the symmetry and the change of curvature in the ectatic area.

Other indices based on decomposition into Zernike polynomials of the anterior surface of the cornea have been proposed by Schwiegerling and Greivenkamp [27] (Z3 index) and Langenbucher et al. [28], essentially the maps of elevation of a group of healthy patients and a group of patients with the cornea affected by keratoconus have been decomposed into a set of Zernike polynomials and the coefficients resulting from the fitting were compared. The statistical comparison showed that the coefficients that mainly discriminate healthy eyes from keratoconus are those of the third order, $c_3^{\pm 1}$ and $c_3^{\pm 3}$.

Posterior corneal curvature and pachymetry data provided by Scheimpflug imaging have been investigated by Ambrósio et al. [29], who showed that corneal-thickness spatial profile, corneal-volume distribution, percentage increase in thickness, and percentage increase in volume were different in keratoconus and normal eyes. Measurements obtained from the posterior corneal curvature using a Scheimpflug camera have been evaluated in several other papers [30, 31].

6.11 Modern Hybrid Systems Based Assisted Learning

The recognition of keratoconus by its morphological features is a daunting and challenging task and, given that there is no gold standard for the certainty of keratoconus and that there is no agreement on what the signs of topographic lows are, the interpretation of topographical frameworks is often subjective. In addition, if on the one hand modifications induced by the onset of a cone are such and so many that they can be observed considering a number of parameters resulting from multiple aspects both morphological and refractive, on the other, keratoconus shows itself in forms so different and heterogeneous that only one class of indices is not often enough to ensure its correct diagnosis and description. The combination of such parameters and the weight to be assigned to each of them is often so complicated that many authors, in order to take into account all the heterogeneous variables related to the presence of a corneal ectasia, thought of making use of assisted learning techniques and actually abstracting the problem of classification [24, 25, 28, 32, 33].

Assisted learning itself is a multidisciplinary field: it bases its roots on the results of studies in fields such as artificial intelligence, probability and statistics, computational complexity theory, information theory, and neurobiology. The main objective of a system based on assisted learning is actually to learn to automatically recognize complex patterns and make intelligent decisions based on data provided in a first stage (training) producing useful behavior (or in our case a correct classification) for new cases. Nowadays, we are not yet capable of reproducing automatic learning systems similar to that of humans. However, effective algorithms were invented for certain types of learning tasks.

In the field of classification patterns of corneal topography and recognition of frameworks of keratoconus, three types of systems have been mainly used: decision trees, artificial neural networks, and support vector machines [34, 35]. The first method is a method of learning in which the element that learns is representable by a set of rules if-else. An artificial neural network is instead an adaptive system that changes its structure based on external or internal information that flows through the network during the learning phase. In practical terms neural networks are nonlinear structures of statistical data organized as modeling tools. They can be used to simulate complex relationships between inputs and outputs that other analytic functions fail to represent. The SVM (Support Vector Machine) finally are a set of supervised learning methods used for classification. Given a set of training examples, each marked as belonging to two possible categories, a training SVM algorithm builds a model that can predict which category must be from a new sample input.

What is usually done is to collect a large series and classify them according to clinical experience in at least two classes (the sick and the healthy). Cutting across this division we shall proceed to divide the set into two groups the first of which will be used to train the expert system and the second to assess the performance of the classifier: the choice of cases to be used in the training set and the control set must be random, but the number and the ratio of cases to be used is a key parameter for the success of the training. The choice of parameters which will serve as input to the system is an essential step and requires experience and sensitivity.

The only drawback to this approach is that of a priori classification frameworks: as there is no fixed rule for the certainty of keratoconus and being the interpretation of the clinical frameworks still too arbitrary such arbitrariness is reflected in what the expert system learns, in a much stronger way when the diagnosis of keratoconus is precocious. In fact, the more prematurely topographers are able to read signs of ectasia the less agreement there will be on the interpretation of signs and classification.

Compliance with Ethical Requirements *Conflict of Interest*: Francesco Versaci and Gabriele Vestri are employees of CSO srl.

Informed Consent: No human studies were carried out by the authors for this article.

Animal Studies: No animal studies were carried out by the authors for this article.

References

1. Jongsma FHM, De Brabander J, Hendrikse F. Review and classification of corneal topographers. Lasers Med Sci. 1999;14(1):2–19.
2. Mejía-Barbosa Y, Malacara-Hernández D. A review of methods for measuring corneal topography. Optom Vis Sci. 2001;78(4):240–53.
3. Atchison DA, Smith G. Optics of the human eye. Oxford: Butterworth-Heinemann; 2000. p. 34–5.
4. von Helmholtz H. Graefe's Archiv für Ophthalmologie. 1854;2:3.

5. Wilson SE, Wang J-Y, Klyce SD. Quantification and mathematical analysis of photokeratoscopic images. In: Shanzlin DJ, Robin JB, editors. Corneal topography. New York: Springer; 1992. p. 1–9.
6. Klyce SD. Computer-assisted corneal topography. High-resolution graphic presentation and analysis of keratoscopy. Invest Ophthalmol Vis Sci. 1984;25(12): 1426–35.
7. Doss JD, et al. Method for calculation of corneal profile and power distribution. Arch Ophthalmol. 1981;99(7):1261–5.
8. van Saarloos PP, Constable IJ. Improved method for calculation of corneal topography for any photokeratoscope geometry. Optom Vis Sci. 1991;68(12):960–65.
9. Campbell C. Reconstruction of the corneal shape with the mastervue Corneal Topography System. Optom Vis Sci. 1997;74(11):899–905.
10. Mattioli R, Tripoli NK. Corneal geometry reconstruction with the Keratron videokeratographer. Optom Vis Sci. 1997;74(11):881–94.
11. Klein SA. Axial curvature and the skew ray error in corneal topography. Optom Vis Sci. 1997;74(11):931–44.
12. Merklinger HM. Focusing the view camera. Bedford: Seaboard Printing Limited; 1996. p. 5.
13. Izatt JA, et al. Micrometer-scale resolution imaging of the anterior eye in vivo with optical coherence tomography. Arch Ophthalmol. 1994;112(12):1584–9.
14. Fercher AF, et al. In-vivo dual-beam optical coherence tomography. In: Europto Biomedical Optics' 93. International Society for Optics and Photonics. 1994.
15. Fercher AF, et al. Measurement of intraocular distances by backscattering spectral interferometry. Opt Commun. 1995;117(1):43–8.
16. Huang D, et al. Optical coherence tomography. Science. 1991;254(5035):1178–81.
17. Swanson EA, et al. In vivo retinal imaging by optical coherence tomography. Opt Lett. 1993;18(21):1864–6.
18. Drexler W, et al. Ultrahigh-resolution ophthalmic optical coherence tomography. Nat Med. 2001;7(4):502–7.
19. Chinn SR, Swanson EA, Fujimoto JG. Optical coherence tomography using a frequency-tunable optical source. Opt Lett. 1997;22(5):340–2.
20. Rabinowitz YS. Videokeratographic indices to aid in screening for keratoconus. J Refract Surg. 1995;11(5):371.
21. Rabinowitz YS, Mcdonnell PJ. Computer-assisted corneal topography in keratoconus. Refract Cor Surg. 1988;5(6):400–8.
22. Rabinowitz YS, Rasheed K. KISA% index: a quantitative videokeratography algorithm embodying minimal topographic criteria for diagnosing keratoconus. J Cataract Refract Surg. 1999;25(10):1327–35.
23. Mahmoud AM, et al. CLMI the cone location and magnitude index. Cornea. 2008;27(4):480.
24. Maeda N, et al. Automated keratoconus screening with corneal topography analysis. Invest Ophthalmol Vis Sci. 1994;35(6):2749–57.
25. Maeda N, Klyce SD, Smolek MK. Neural network classification of corneal topography. Preliminary demonstration. Invest Ophthalmol Vis Sci. 1995;36(7):1327–35.
26. Calossi A. Screening by computerized videokeratography [in Italian]. In: Il Cheratocono. Canelli: SOI Publishing Group, Fabiano Group Ltd; 2004. p.114–7.
27. Schwiegerling J, Greivenkamp JE. Keratoconus detection based on videokeratoscopic height data. Optom Vis Sci. 1996;73(12):721–8.
28. Langenbucher A, et al. [Keratoconus screening with wave-front parameters based on topography height data]. Klin Monbl Augenheilkd. 1999;214(4):217–23.
29. Ambrósio R, et al. Corneal-thickness spatial profile and corneal-volume distribution: tomographic indices to detect keratoconus. J Cataract Refract Surg. 2006;32(11):1851–9.
30. Piñero DP, et al. Corneal volume, pachymetry, and correlation of anterior and posterior corneal shape in subclinical and different stages of clinical keratoconus. J Cataract Refract Surg. 2010;36(5):814–25.
31. Uçakhan ÖÖ, et al. Evaluation of Scheimpflug imaging parameters in subclinical keratoconus, keratoconus, and normal eyes. J Cataract Refract Surg. 2011;37(6).1116–24.
32. Chastang PJ, et al. Automated keratoconus detection using the EyeSys videokeratoscope. J Cataract Refract Surg. 2000;26(5):675–83.
33. Arbelaez MC, et al. Use of a support vector machine for keratoconus and subclinical keratoconus detection by topographic and tomographic data. Ophthalmology. 2012;119(11):2231–38.
34. Cortes C, Vapnik V. Support-vector networks. Mach Learn. 1995;20(3):273–97.
35. Cristianini N, Shawe-Taylor J. An introduction to support vector machines and other kernel-based learning methods. Cambridge: Cambridge University Press; 2000.

7 Analyzing Tomographic Corneal Elevation for Detecting Ectasia

Michael W. Belin and Renato Ambrósio Jr.

7.1 Introduction

The last decade has seen a dramatic change in the diagnosis and early identification of keratoconus and other ectatic disorders. As in other areas in ophthalmology, imaging techniques have played a large part in this change. This new information offered by anterior segment tomography not only allows for earlier identification of disease, but has altered our perception of what constitutes keratoconus. Tomographic imaging (Scheimpflug, ocular coherence tomography (OCT), scanning slit) offers significant advantages over traditional Placido-based curvature analysis (topography). Elevation-based imaging has advantages in that it allows for the measurement of both the anterior and posterior corneal surfaces. The accurate measurement of both the anterior and posterior corneal surfaces and the anterior lens allows for the creation of a three-dimensional reconstruction of the anterior segment which affords vastly more diagnostic information than was previously available [1–5]. Posterior measurements are often the first indicators of future ectatic disease, in spite of completely normal anterior curvature. Examination of the posterior corneal surface can often reveal pathology that would otherwise be missed if one was relying on anterior analysis alone [2, 4–7] (Fig. 7.1).

Although there is little disagreement in diagnosing clinically evident keratoconus, agreement on what constitutes 'form fruste' or subclinical keratoconus remains elusive. The ability of elevation-based topography to analyze both anterior and posterior corneal surfaces adds significantly to our ability to identify eyes believed to be 'at risk.' As more knowledge is gained, it is appreciated that a full understanding of the workings of the human eye requires knowledge obtained from more than just one surface. While other tomographic devices are available (OCT, scanning slit), the balance of this chapter will deal with Scheimpflug imaging (OCULUS GmbH Pentacam, Wetzlar, Germany) as this is the device most familiar to and used by the authors. For the most part, the general concepts presented here are applicable to other anterior segment tomographic instruments.

M.W. Belin, M.D. (✉)
Department of Ophthalmology and Vision Science, Southern Arizona VA Healthcare System, University of Arizona, Tucson, AZ, USA
e-mail: mwbelin@aol.com

R. Ambrósio Jr., M.D., Ph.D.
Department for Ophthalmology, Instituto de Olhos Renato Ambrósio, Rua Conde de Bonfim 211/712, Rio de Janeiro, RJ 20520-050, Brazil

Federal University, Sao Paulo, Brazil
e-mail: dr.renatoambrosio@gmail.com

J.L. Alió (ed.), *Keratoconus*, Essentials in Ophthalmology, DOI 10.1007/978-3-319-43881-8_7

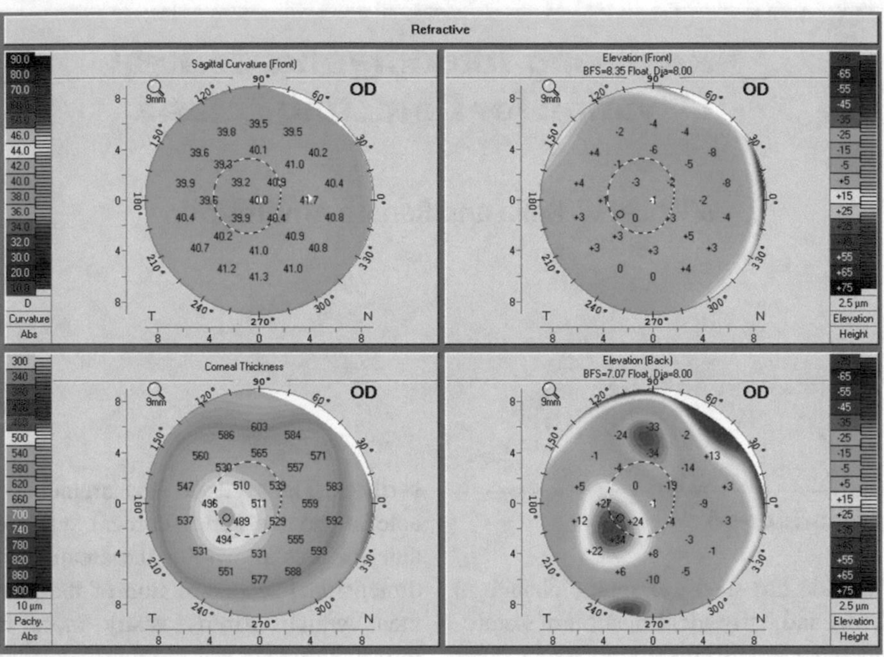

Fig. 7.1 Subclinical Keratoconus. Four map composite display (anterior sagittal curvature (*upper left*), anterior elevation (*upper right*), corneal thickness (*lower left*), posterior elevation (*lower right*)). While the anterior surface is normal, the posterior surface shows a prominent ectatic region and the corneal thickness map shows a corresponding displacement of the thinnest point (OCULUS Pentacam)

7.2 Background

True tomographic imaging requires the generation of an *X*, *Y*, and *Z* coordinate system and the measurement of true shape. The first commercially available elevation-based system was the PAR Corneal Topography System (PAR CTS) (PAR Technology, New Hartford, NY). The PAR CTS used a stereo-triangulation technique (rasterphotogrammetry) to make direct measurements on the anterior corneal surface. The PAR CTS used a grid pattern composed of horizontal and vertical lines projected onto the anterior surface at an angle (Fig. 7.2). In order to visualize the grid, the PAR system required a small amount of fluorescein in the tear film. From the known geometry of the grid and the change when projected onto the corneal surface the system was able to compute the *X*, *Y*, and *Z* coordinate in space. Because the system required a stained tear film to visualize the grid it was limited to measuring only the anterior corneal surface [8]. While, the PAR is no longer commercially available, it was the first system to utilize elevation data in a clinically useful form and had documented accuracy superior to the available Placido-based systems at that time [9].

The first elevation system with the capability to measure both anterior and posterior corneal surfaces utilized a scanning-slit technique of optical cross sectioning (Orbscan (formerly Orbtek) Bausch & Lomb, Rochester, NY). The ability to measure both corneal surfaces in space allowed for the generation of a corneal thickness map as corneal thickness is simply the spatial difference between the corresponding anterior and posterior corneal positions. A full corneal thickness map offers significant advantages over single point pachymetry (discussed in the following chapter). Numerous articles have demonstrated the limitations of the Orbscan, particularly in locating the posterior corneal surface after refractive surgery and subsequently underestimating the corneal thickness [10–13]. Currently, there are a number of different devices and differ-

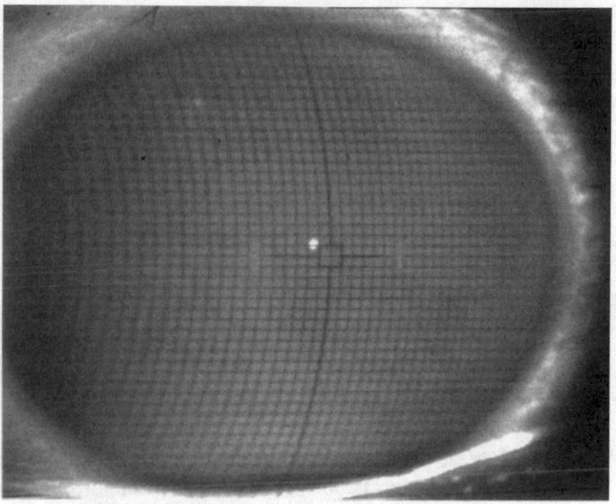

Fig. 7.2 Projected grid pattern onto the anterior corneal surface. The distortion of the grid pattern was analyzed to produce a front elevation map (PAR CTS, PAR Technology, New Hartford, NY)

ent technologies that produced tomographic data. Although some differences exist between systems, they all display elevation data in a similar fashion that was first introduced with the PAR CTS in 1990 [8].

7.3 How Elevation Is Displayed

While we refer to standard anterior and posterior corneal tomographic maps as elevation maps, that is somewhat of a misnomer. Rarely does the clinician view elevation data in its raw form and most systems do not offer the actual raw elevation data. The reason is that the raw elevation data from normal eyes and markedly ectatic corneas look remarkably similar (Fig. 7.3). In order to make the maps clinically useful and to allow for a rapid visual inspection, the raw data is compared to some reference surface. The purpose of the reference surface is to magnify or amplify the surface differences that would otherwise not be appreciated to the naked eye. The so-called elevation maps depict how the corneal surface differs from a defined reference shape. While the appearance of the map will vary greatly depending on the reference surface used, all maps are generated using the raw elevation data. The reference surface will affect the appearance, but not the accuracy of the actual data [14].

The choice of the reference surface will often depend on the clinical situation, the population being evaluated, and the specific pathology you are screening for. For most applications the best fit sphere (BFS) is the most qualitatively intuitive (easiest to read and understand) surface and the most commonly used. A BFS allows for the visualization of astigmatism as the flat meridian rises above the BFS, while the steep meridian drops below the BFS. The normal astigmatic pattern generated against a BFS is easily recognizable (Fig. 7.4). As opposed to a BFS, a best fit toric ellipsoid (BFTE) will better fit or mask an astigmatic cornea. When screening for ectatic disease one is trying to identify an abnormal conical protrusion. A focalized protrusion will appear as an elevated area against the BFS (Fig. 7.5). Since the cornea is normally aspherical, steeper in the center and flatter toward the periphery, normal corneas will display a central positive elevation. The goal of screening is to allow for a rapid visual inspection to separate normal from abnormal. This task is made more difficult by the fact that the normal cornea is aspherical and displays, to a smaller degree, a positive elevation ("positive island of elevation"), similar to what is seen with ectatic disease. The BFS and the resultant elevation map will vary depending on how much of the cornea is utilized to construct the reference surface. If the entire cornea is used to construct the BFS then the normal asphericity of the cornea will be clearly demonstrated. As the area (optical zone) utilized to compute the BFS is decreased the BFS steepens as less of the flatter periphery is incorporated into the

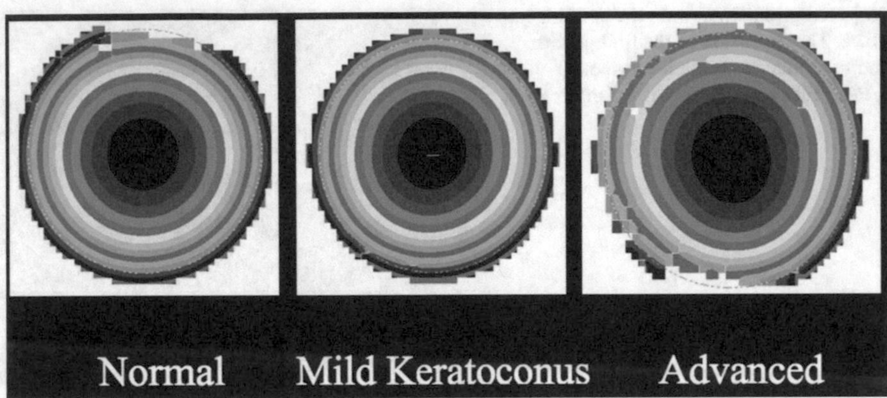

Fig. 7.3 Raw elevation maps of a normal eye (*left*), mild to moderate keratoconus (*center*), and advanced keratoconus (*right*). The maps appear remarkably similar and lack enough surface differences to allow a visual distinction between normal and ectatic corneas (PAR CTS)

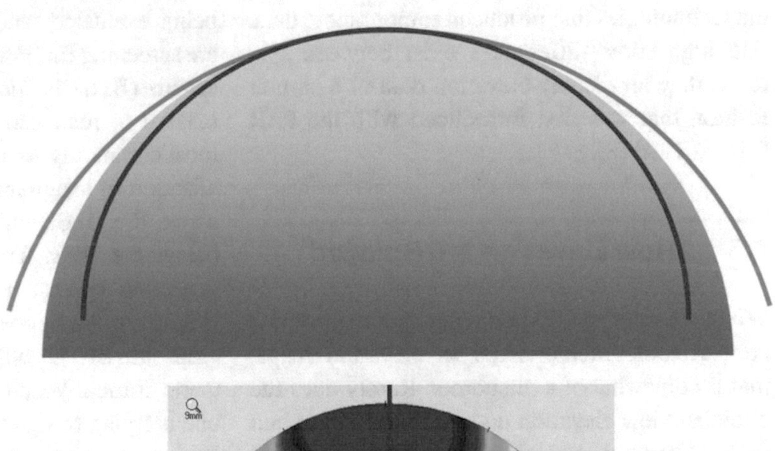

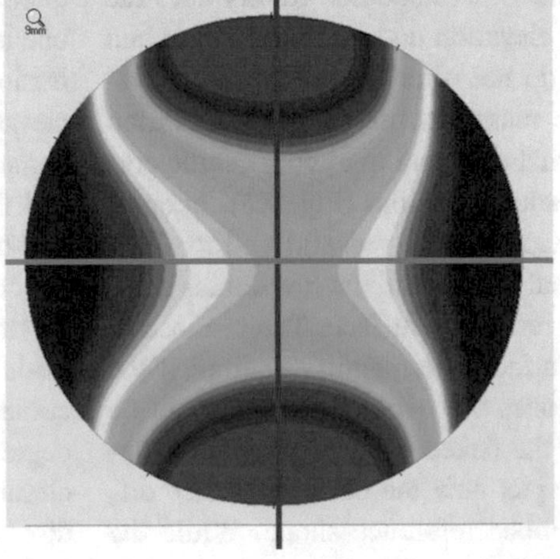

Fig. 7.4 Schematic representation (*above*) of the flat meridian rising above the best fit sphere (BFS) and the steep meridian falling below. This produces the typical astigmatic pattern when the reference surface is a BFS (*below*) (OCULUS Pentacam)

BFS. If only the central 3.0 mm of the cornea were to be utilized, the resultant BFS would be substantially steeper. It has been shown that taking the BFS from the central 8.0 mm optical zone steepens the BFS enough to effectively mask the normal asphericity (Fig. 7.6). Masking the normal asphericity makes screening for ectatic disease easier and allows for a rapid visual inspection looking for positive Island of elevation against the 8.0 mm derived BFS.

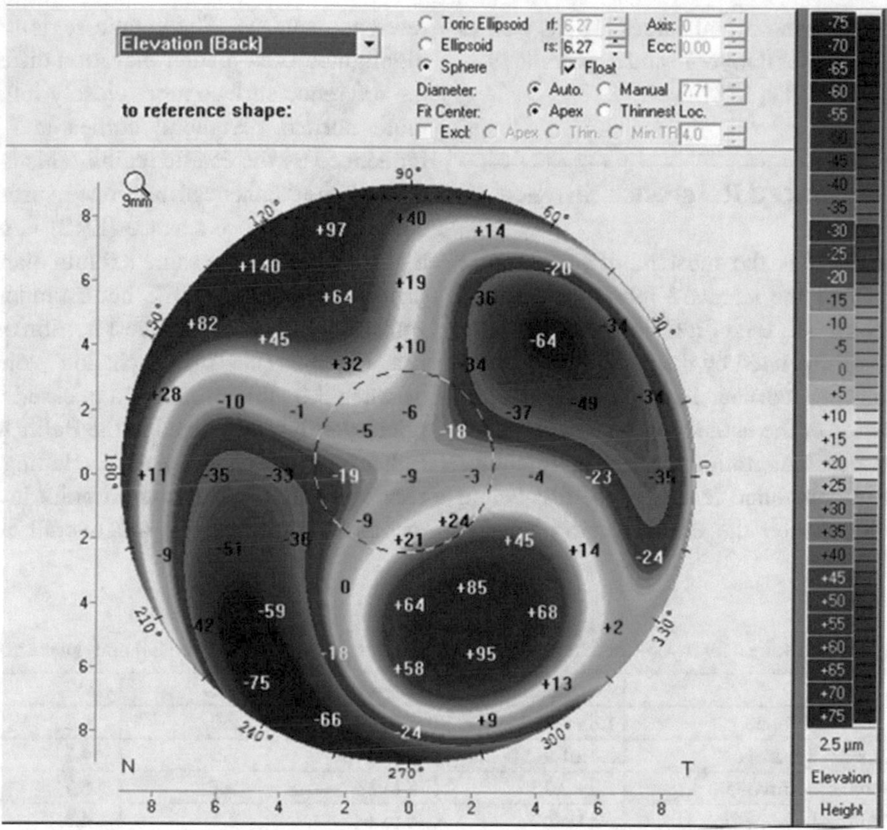

Fig. 7.5 Posterior elevation map against a BFS showing a prominent posterior ectasia. The positive "island of elevation" is supposed over an astigmatic pattern. This is typical for a keratoconic cornea (OCULUS Pentacam)

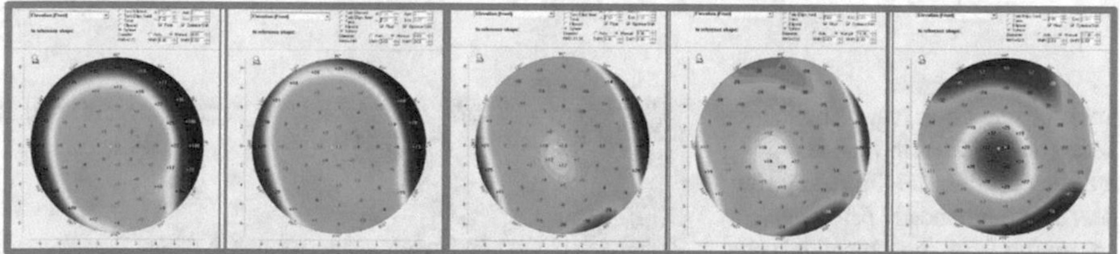

Fig. 7.6 A series of front elevation maps where the BFS is computed from increasing optical zones (4, 6, 8, 10, and 12 mm). As the area used to compute the BFS is increased the reference surface becomes flatter and the normal corneal asphericity is revealed (OCULUS Pentacam)

While a BFS derived from the central 8.0 mm zone allows for a rapid visual inspection, it should be understood that while the reference surface does not affect "accuracy," it does affect quantitative data and published normal values are all reference surface specific [15, 16]. Normal elevation values will not only vary based on which reference surface is utilized, but will vary based on where or what part of the cornea the values are measured from. Elevation normal values have been reported at the apex, maximal value within the central 4.0 mm zone, and at the thinnest point [15–17]. The thinnest point has some advantages as in the keratoconic cornea, the thinnest point usually corresponds to the center of the cone and this is where we normally quote our recommended normal values. Additionally, there is some geographic and/or ethnic variation in normal values [16] as well as differences between myopic and hyperopic individuals (Table 7.1) [15].

7.4 Enhanced Reference Surface

While the BFS is the most intuitive reference surface any of the standard reference surfaces (e.g., BFS, BFTE. Best Fit Ellipse (BFE)) suffer from being influenced by the pathologic portion of an abnormal cornea. In ectatic disease, the incorporation of the ectatic region into the reference surface computation causes the reference surface to steepen and results in the less height difference between the ectatic region and the reference surface. The ectatic region could be highlighted (i.e., greater elevation difference) if the reference surface more closely reflected the more normal peripheral cornea and was not influenced by the ectatic region. This is the concept of the "enhanced reference surface." The enhanced reference surface (ERS) is generated by incorporating the same 8.0 mm diameter utilized in the standard BFS but excludes a small zone surrounding the thinnest portion of the cornea (Fig. 7.7). This exclusion zone varies between 3.0 and 4.0 mm and is based on a proprietary program utilized in the Belin/Ambrosio Enhanced Ectasia Display. Excluding a small zone surrounding the thinnest point in the keratoconic cornea flattens the overall reference.

Table 7.1 Normal values for myopic and hyperopic eyes based on a best fit sphere from 8.0 mm optical zone

Location	Avg elevation	Range	+1 SD	+2 SD	+3 SD
Anterior apex—myope	1.6±1.3	−5 to +4	2.9	4.2	5.5
Anterior apex—hyperope	0.4±1.9	−3 to +13	2.3	4.2	6.2
Anterior thinnest—myope	1.7±2.0	−5 to +6	3.7	5.7	7.7
Anterior thinnest—hyperope	−0.1±2.2	−6 to +4	2.1	4.3	6.5
Posterior apex—myope	0.8±3.0	−6 to +6	3.8	6.8	9.8
Posterior apex—hyperope	5.7±3.6	−1 to +14	9.3	12.9	16.3
Posterior thinnest—myope	3.6±4.7	−6 to +18	8.3	13.0	17.7
Posterior thinnest—hyperope	10.6±5.7	−2 to +30	16.3	22.1	27.8

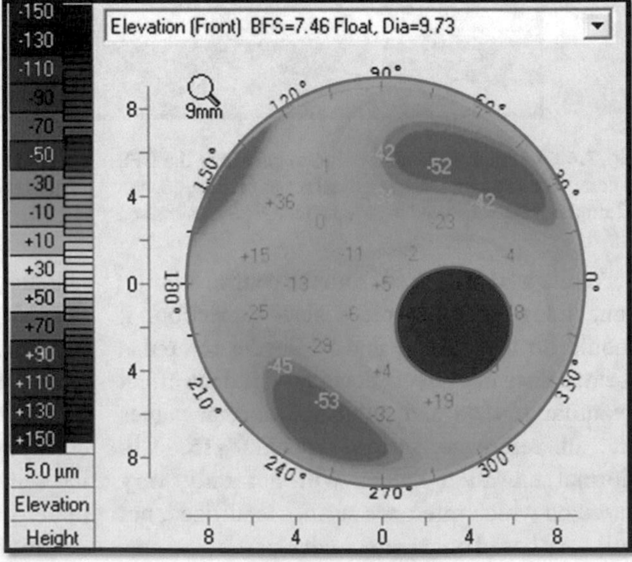

Fig. 7.7 Anterior elevation map. The exclusion zone (highlighted in *red*) is a 3.0 mm zone surrounding the thinnest point on the cornea. The "enhanced" reference surface is computed from the central 8.0 mm optical zone minus the area within the exclusion zone (OCULUS Pentacam)

The degree of flattening of the ERS compared to the standard BFS will vary greatly based on the presence or absence of a significant cone. Normal eyes undergo very little change from BFS to ERS resulting in little if any elevation change, but in ectatic eyes eliminating the zone surrounding the ectatic region (thinnest portion of the cornea) flattens the reference surface and allows the ectatic region to be more prominent (greater height off the reference surface) and so easier to differentiate by visual inspection (Fig. 7.8). The change in elevation going from a standard BFS to the ERS has also been shown to have discriminatory ability, as eyes with ectatic change have a statistically greater change in elevation (p, 0.001) compared to normal eyes (Table 7.2).

Screening for ectatic disease by tomography derived elevation data can be accomplished in a multitude of ways. The simplest is by comparison to established normal values (Table 7.1). As noted earlier, normal values are reference surface specific and screening by normal values is typically more time consuming than visual inspection. If one standardizes both the reference surfaces, the elevation scale and the colors scales then the user can become acclimated to the normal and abnormal appearance and in as such should be able to make a more rapid visual inspection (Fig. 7.9). For elevation data on the OCULUS Pentacam, the authors recommend a BFS from the 8.0 mm optical zone, an elevation scale of ±75 μm, and the "Intuitive" color bars.

An ectasia screening display (Belin/Ambrosio Enhanced Ectasia Display (BAD)) is currently offered on the OCULUS Pentacam. The BAD display is a comprehensive screening program that combines both elevation and pachymetric parameters into a regression analysis and then compares the data to a large normative database. In addition to showing the anterior and posterior elevation maps with the standard BFS and ERS, the BAD also reports the front

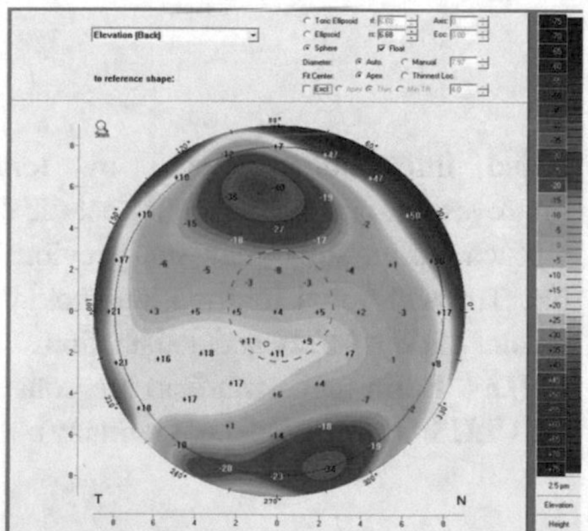

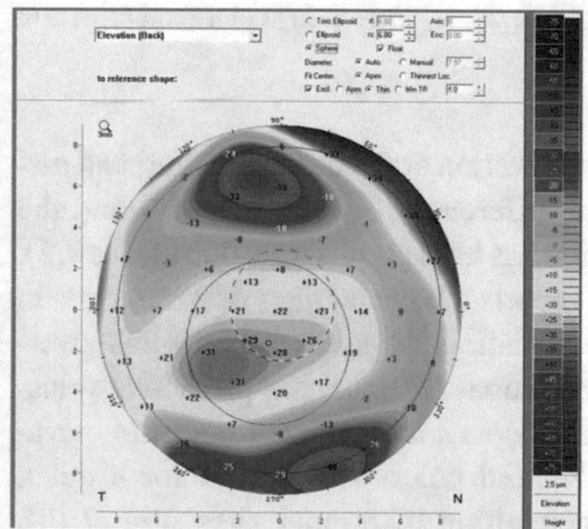

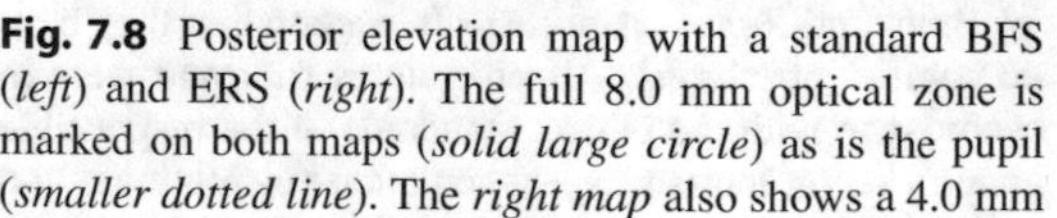

Fig. 7.8 Posterior elevation map with a standard BFS (*left*) and ERS (*right*). The full 8.0 mm optical zone is marked on both maps (*solid large circle*) as is the pupil (*smaller dotted line*). The *right map* also shows a 4.0 mm circle which represents the exclusion zone. The ERS is flatter than the standard BFS which results in greater elevation for the ectatic region and one that is much easier to visualize (OCULUS Pentacam)

Table 7.2 Change in elevation using enhanced reference surface compared to standard best fit sphere

	Anterior apex change	Anterior max change	Posterior apex change	Posterior max chance
Normal eyes	1.63 ± 1.4 μm	1.86 ± 1.9 μm	2.27 ± 1.1 μm	2.86 ± 1.9 μm
Keratoconic eyes	20.4 ± 23.1 μm	20.9 ± 21.9 μm	39.9 ± 38.1 μm	45.7 ± 35.9 μm

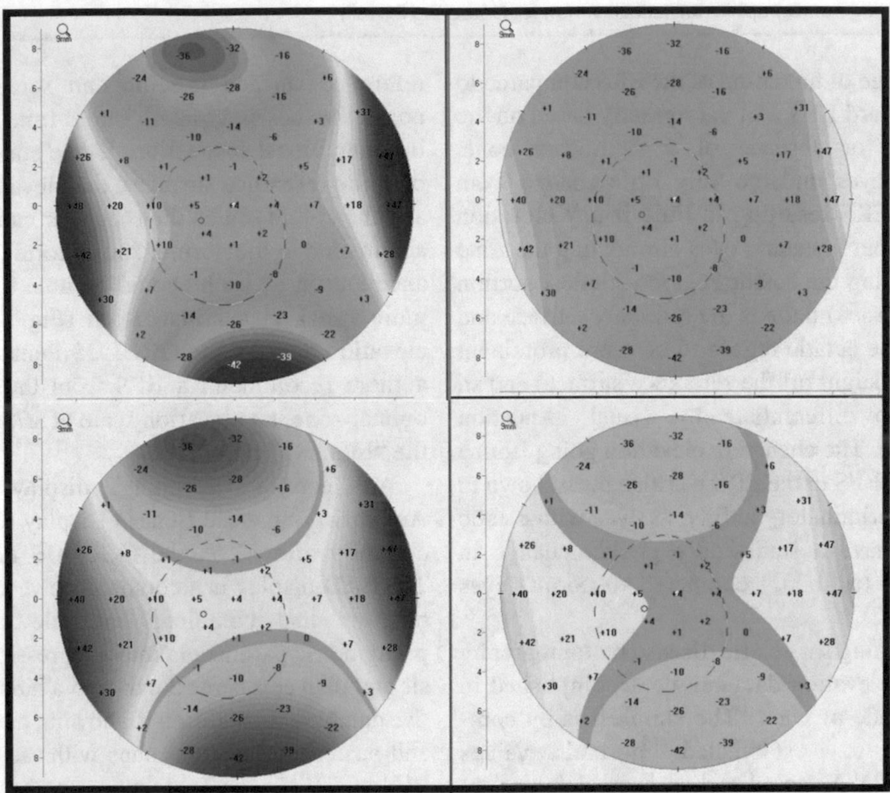

Fig. 7.9 Anterior elevation maps of the same cornea using different scales and different color bars (±75 μm, intuitive color (*upper left*), ±300 μm, intuitive color (*upper right*), ±75 μm, "American" color (comparable to Orbscan default) (*lower left*), ±300 μm, "American" color (*lower right*)). While all the elevation values are identical, the appearance of the maps varies greatly

and back elevation at the thinnest point, and displays the difference between the BFS and the ERS which has high predictive value (Table 7.2). While it reports a large number of parameters in standard deviation form, it is only the final overall analysis (final "D") that has predictive value. The BAD display standardizes both the elevation scales and colors and allows for a quick visual recognition of normal eyes (Fig. 7.10), subclinical keratoconus (Fig. 7.11), and advanced ectatic disease (Fig. 7.12).

Modern comprehensive preoperative refractive screening mandates evaluation of both the anterior and posterior corneal surfaces. The added information offered by tomography improves our ability to identify ectatic disease at a much earlier stage than was previously possible. The additional information should result in greater patient safety and satisfaction.

(Drs. Belin and Ambrosio are consultants to OCULUS GmbH, Wetzlar, Germany).

Compliance with Ethical Requirements Michael W. Belin and Renato Ambrósio Jr. declare that they have no conflict of interest. All procedures followed were in accordance with the ethical standards of the responsible committee on human experimentation (institutional and national) and with the Helsinki Declaration of 1975, as revised in 2000. Informed consent was obtained from all

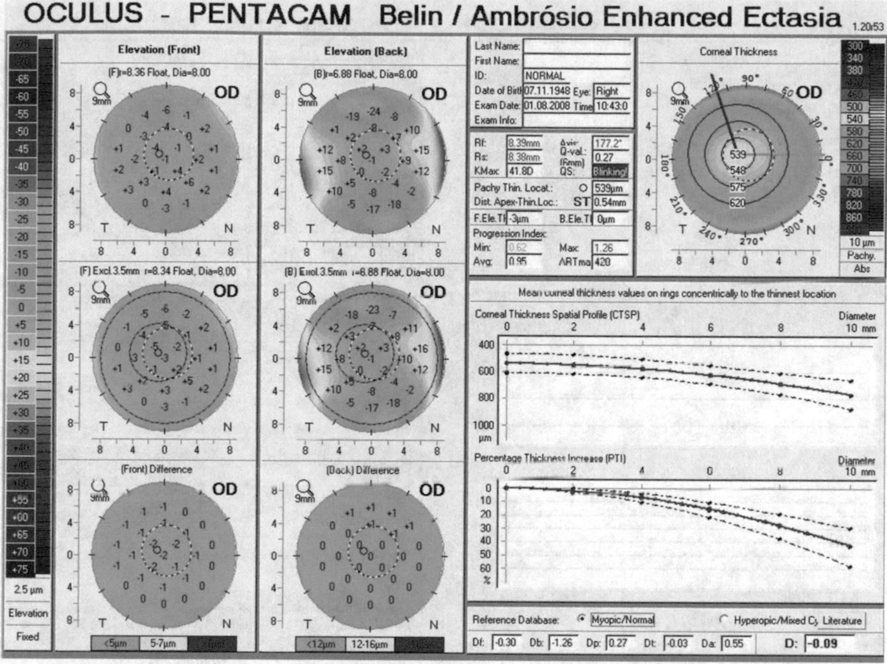

Fig. 7.10 BAD display of a normal cornea. The anterior and posterior elevation maps show a normal pattern and there is no significant difference between the elevation maps with the standard BFS and the ERS (OCULUS Pentacam)

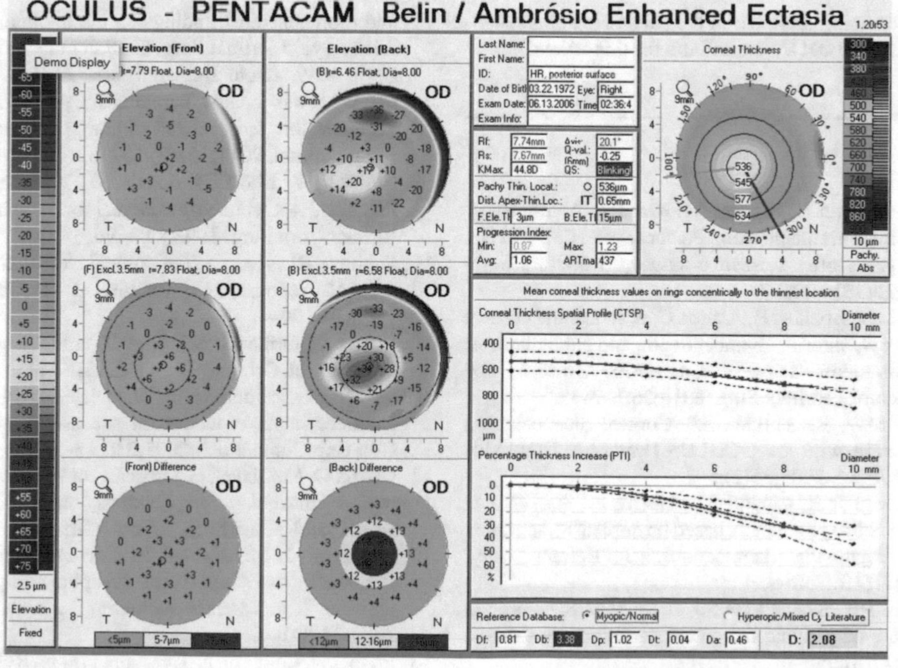

Fig. 7.11 BAD display depicting subclinical keratoconus. While the anterior surface appears normal the posterior surface shows a positive island of elevation on the standard BFS which is more prominent against the ERS. The *back difference map* shows a significant change going from the BFS to the ERS (OCULUS Pentacam)

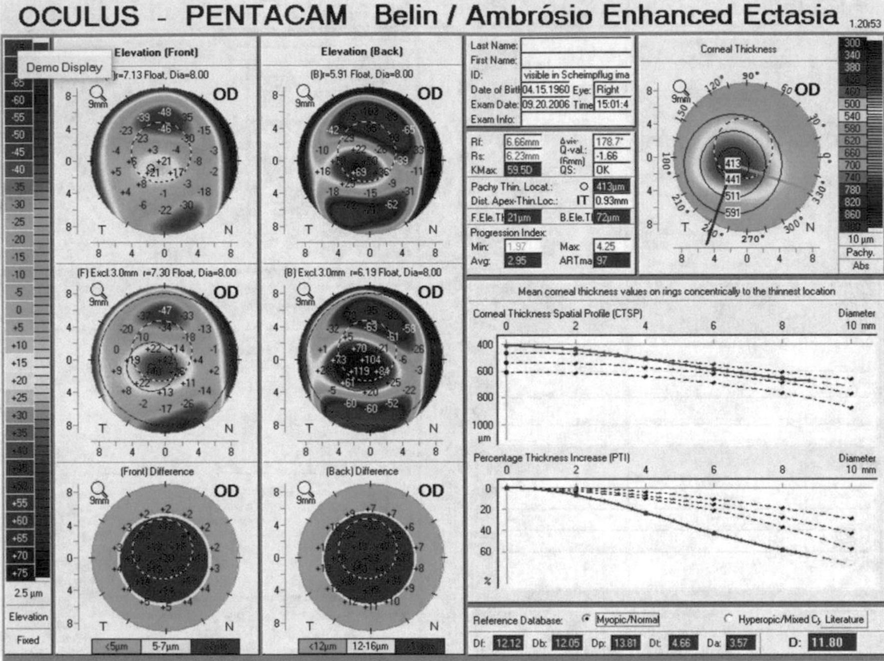

Fig. 7.12 BAD display of advanced keratoconus. Here changes can be seen on both the anterior and posterior corneal surfaces, in addition to elevation abnormalities at the thinnest point (OCULUS Pentacam)

patients for being included in the study. No animal studies were carried out by the authors for this article.

References

1. Kim SW, Sun HJ, Chang JH, Kim EK. Anterior segment measurements using Pentacam and Orbscan II 1 to 5 years after refractive surgery. J Refract Surg. 2009;25(12):1091–7.
2. Yazici AT, Bozkurt E, Alagoz C, et al. Central corneal thickness, anterior chamber depth, and pupil diameter measurements using Visante OCT, Orbscan, and Pentacam. J Refract Surg. 2010;26:127–33.
3. Belin MW, Khachikian SS. Corneal diagnosis and evaluation with the OCULUS Pentacam. Highlights Ophthalmol. 2007;35(2):5–7.
4. Ambrosio Jr R, Caiado AL, Guerra FP, et al. Novel pachymetric parameters based on corneal tomography for diagnosing keratoconus. J Refract Surg. 2011;27(10):753–8.
5. Walker RN, Khackikian SS, Belin MW. Scheimpflug imaging of pellucid margainal degeneration. Cornea. 2008;27(8):963–6.
6. Ambrosio Jr R, Dawson DG, Salomao M, et al. Corneal ectasia after LASIK despite low risk: evidence of enhanced sensitivity based on tomographic and biomechanical findings on the unoperated stable fellow eye. J Refract Surg. 2010;26(11):906–11.
7. Belin MW, Asota IM, Ambrosio Jr R, Khachikian SS. What's in a name: keratoconus, pellucid marginal degeneration and related thinning disorders. Am J Ophthalmol. 2011;152(2):157–62.
8. Belin MW, Litoff D, Strods SJ, Winn SS, Smith RS. The PAR technology corneal topography system. Refract Corn Surg. 1992;8:88–96.
9. Schultze RL. Accuracy of corneal elevation with four corneal topography systems. J Refract Surg. 1998;14:100–4.
10. Cairns G, Ormonde SE, Gray T, et al. Assessing the accuracy of Orbscan II post-LASIK: apparent keratectasia is paradoxically associated with anterior chamber depth reduction in successful procedures. Clin Exp Ophthalmol. 2005;33:147–52.
11. Cairns G, McGhee CH. Orbscan computerized topography: attributes, applications, and limitations. J Cataract Refract Surg. 2005;31:205–20.
12. Hashemi H, Mehravaran S. Corneal changes after laser refractive surgery for myopia: comparison of Orbscan II and Pentacam findings. J Cataract Surg. 2007;33:841–7.
13. Prisant O, Calderon N, Chastang P, et al. Reliability of pachymetric measurements using Orbscan after excimer refractive surgery. Ophthalmology. 2003;110:511–5.

14. Belin MW, Khachikian SS. An Introduction to understanding elevation-based topography: how elevation data are displayed—a review. Clin Exp Ophthalmol. 2009;37:14–29.
15. Kim JT, Cortese M, Belin MW, Khachikian SS, Ambrosio Jr R. Tomographic normal values for corneal elevation and pachymetry in a hyperopic population. J Clin Exp Ophthalmol. 2011;2:130–5.
16. Feng MT, Belin MW, Ambrosio R, et al. International values for corneal elevation in normal subjects by rotating Scheimpflug camera. J Cataract Refract Surg. 2011;37(10):1817–21.
17. Hashemi H, Mehravaran S. Day to day clinically relevant corneal elevation, thickness and curvature parameters using the Orbscan II scanning slit topographer and Pentacam Scheimpflug imaging device. Mid East Afr J Ophthalmol. 2010;17(1): 44–55.
18. Khachikian SS, Belin MW. Posterior elevation in keratoconus. Ophthalmology. 2009;116:816.
19. de Sanctus U, Loiacono C, Richiardi L, et al. Sensitivity and specificity of posterior corneal elevation measured by Pentacam in discriminating keratoconus/subclinical keratoconus. Ophthalmology. 2008;115:1534–9.

8 Analyzing Tomographic Thickness for Detecting Corneal Ectatic Diseases

Renato Ambrósio Jr., Fernando Faria Correia, and Michael W. Belin

8.1 Introduction

Corneal thickness is an important indicator of corneal health status, which is relevant in different clinical situations, such as evaluating and treating corneal ectatic diseases (ECD), keratorefractive surgeries, and corneal endothelium dehydrating function [1–7]. The need for accurate evaluation of corneal thickness was determined by the advent of keratorefractive surgery, leading to the development of new technologies [8].

The measurement of corneal thickness began with the development of the optical pachymeter by David Maurice, Ph.D., (1922–2002) in the early 1950s [9]. Ultrasound measurements were demonstrated to have higher repeatability than optical pachymetry, but still provided data from a single point [10]. Mandell and Polse proposed the study of the horizontal corneal thickness profile using a modified optical pachymeter and demonstrated the variation in thickness over the horizontal meridian as a powerful diagnostic feature of keratoconus [11]. However, it was only with the development of corneal tomography (CTm) that the evaluation of the thickness profile was possible from pachymetric mapping the whole cornea [12–14]. *Tomography* (from the Greek words *tomos* meaning slice and *graphia* meaning describing) is a better term for the evaluation of the three-dimensional reconstruction of the whole cornea that enables characterization of the front and back corneal surfaces along with thickness mapping. Different

R. Ambrósio Jr., M.D., Ph.D. (✉)
Department of Ophthalmology, Instituto de Olhos Renato Ambrósio, Rio de Janeiro, RJ, Brazil

VisareRio, Rio de Janeiro, Brazil

Universidade Federal de São Paulo, São Paulo, Brazil

Rio de Janeiro Corneal Tomography and Biomechanics Study Group, Rio de Janeiro, Brazil
e-mail: dr.renatoambrosio@gmail.com

F. Faria Correia, M.D.
Rio de Janeiro Corneal Tomography and Biomechanics Study Group, Rio de Janeiro, Brazil

Cornea and Refractive Surgery Department, Hospital de Braga, Braga, Portugal

Cornea and Refractive Surgery Department, Instituto CUF, Porto, Portugal

Life and Health Sciences Research Institute (ICVS), School of Health Sciences, University of Minho, Braga, Portugal

ICVS/3B's-PT Government Associate Laboratory, Braga/Guimarães, Portugal
e-mail: f.faria.correia@gmail.com

M.W. Belin, M.D.
Department of Ophthalmology and Vision Science, University of Arizona, Southern Arizona VA Healthcare System, Tucson, AZ, USA
e-mail: mwbelin@aol.com

J.L. Alió (ed.), *Keratoconus*, Essentials in Ophthalmology, DOI 10.1007/978-3-319-43881-8_8

technologies, such as horizontal slit scanning, rotational Scheimpflug, very high frequency ultrasound, and optical coherence tomography (OCT), are available in different commercial tools [12, 14].

8.2 Tomographic Corneal Thickness Assessment

There is a large variation in corneal thickness in the normal population [1, 15, 16]. For example, in a study using ultrasound pachymetry involving 1374 normal eyes from candidates for LASIK or PRK, mean central corneal thickness (US-CCT) was 556 μm with a standard deviation of 34 μm, ranging from 454 to 669 μm [1]. Ultrasonic central corneal thickness (US-CCT) measurements usually refer to the measurements at the corneal geometric center or at the apex, which is not the corneal thinnest point [17, 18]. In 12 % of normal patients, the difference from the thinnest point and the geometric central point is over 10 μm. Interestingly, there is also a significant correlation between the distance from these points (central and thinnest) and their difference. Also, the distance between the thinnest point and the geometric central point is significantly higher in keratoconus (1.51 ± 0.54 mm) when compared to normal corneas (0.79 ± 0.23 mm) ($p < 0.05$) [17]. Thereby, the need for a reliable pachymetric map for determining the localization and value of the cornea's thinnest point is well supported for proper calculations of the "Mathematics of LASIK" and other conditions.

The importance and advantages of CTm for the evaluation of corneal thickness are not limited to the evaluation of the "true" thinnest point (location and value). This tool enables the characterization of the corneal thickness profile. Considering the absolute central (or thinnest) value varies significantly among a normal population, the relationship of central and peripheral corneal thickness is an important indicator if the cornea has developed thinning, such as in keratoconus and pellucid marginal corneal degeneration, or thickening process, such as in cases with Fuchs' endothelial dystrophy [7, 17, 19].

8.3 The Corneal Thickness Spatial Profile (CSTP) and the Percentage Thickness Increase (PTI) Graphs

The CTSP graph displays the sequence of pachymetric values, starting on the TP, followed by the averages of thickness values of the points within imaginary circles centered on the TP. The original analysis was performed considering 22 circles with increased diameters at 0.4 mm steps (Fig. 8.1) [17]. In this study involving 46 eyes with mild to moderate keratoconus and 364 normal eyes, significant differences were found for all positions of the CTSP from normal eyes and keratoconus ($p < 0.01$), in which keratoconus had much lower (thinner) values. It was estimated that keratoconic corneas were, in average, 27.3 μm thinner than normals [17].

The percentage of thickness increase (PTI) from the TP is calculated using a simple formula: (CT@x − TP)/TP, where x represents the diameter of the imaginary circle centered on the TP with increased diameters as provided by the CTSP. In the original study, significant differences were also found for all positions of the PTI from normal eyes and keratoconus ($p < 0.0001$), in which keratoconus had much higher increase [17]. The CTSP and PTI graphs display the examined eye data in red and three broken lines, which represent the upper and lower double standard deviation (95 %—confidence interval) and the average values from a normal population (Fig. 8.2).

Considering the presented concepts on corneal thickness distribution, the CTSP and PTI graphs provide clinical information to distinguish between a normal thin cornea and ectasia (Fig. 8.3). In addition, the thickness profile also allows the detection of early corneal edema. In this situation, the pachymetric progression from the center toward the periphery is attenuated (Fig. 8.4). However, some very compact corneas (not necessarily thick) may also have a rectification of the CTSP and PTI lines [7, 20]. In such cases, it is also very important to evaluate the Scheimpflug images, searching for signs of edema (higher reflectivity) or the "Camel sing"—a second hump

Fig. 8.1 Pachymetric spatial profile analyses the averages of thickness values of the points within imaginary circles centered on the TP. The original analysis was performed considering 22 circles with increased diameters (0.4 mm-steps)

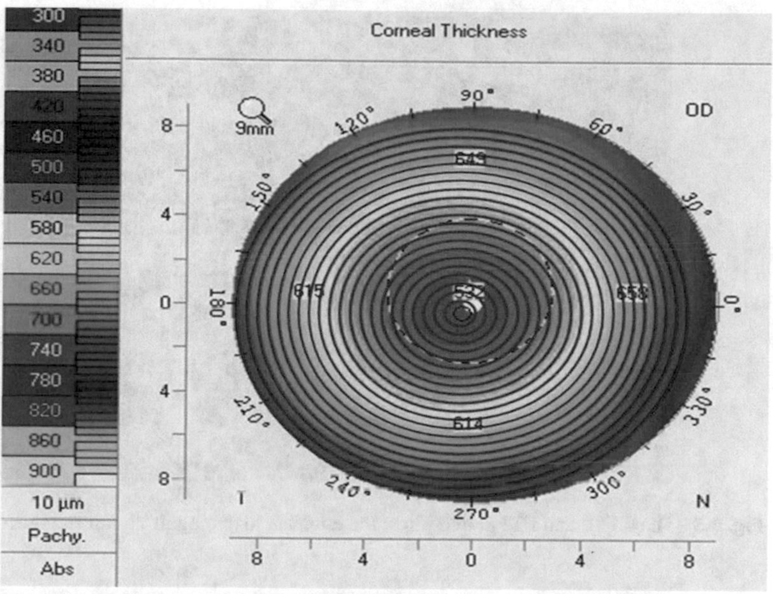

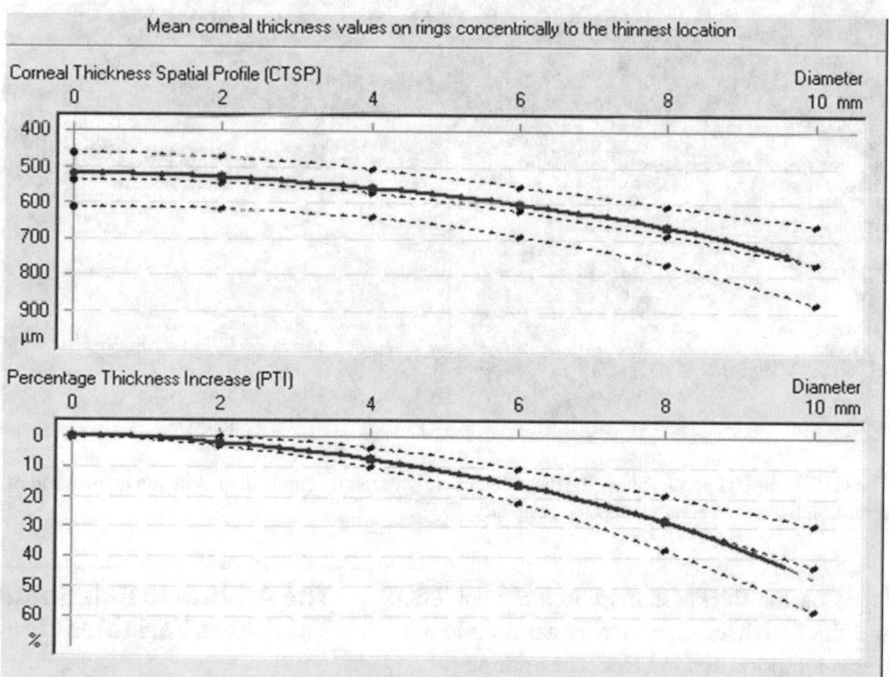

Fig. 8.2 The CTSP and PTI graphs display the examined eye data in *red* and *three broken lines*, which represent the upper and lower double standard deviation (95%—confidence interval) and the average values from a normal population

on the densitometry "green" graph, at the level of the Descemet's membrane. This finding on the Scheimpflug image correlates with the presence of corneal guttata (Figs. 8.5 and 8.6) [7].

The arithmetic average of the pachymetric values on each meridian enables the detection of the ones with maximal (fastest) progression and minimal (slowest) progression. The hemi-meridians

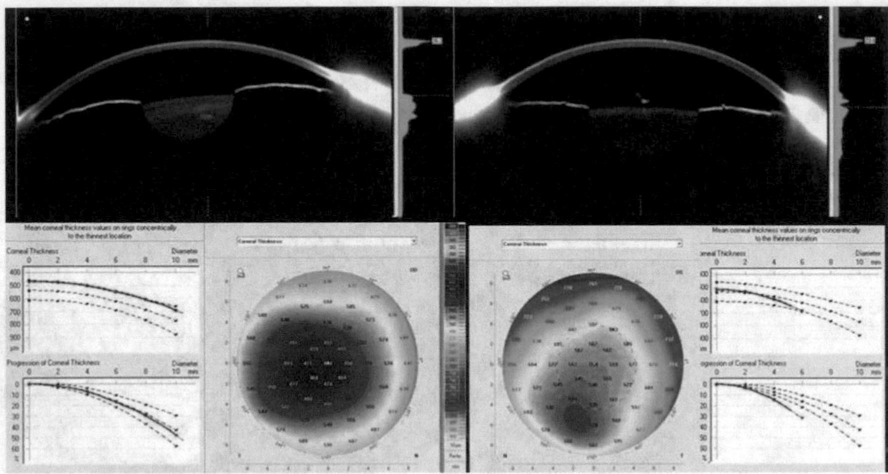

Fig. 8.3 The CTSP and PTI graphs allow the clinician to distinguish a normal thin cornea from ectasia

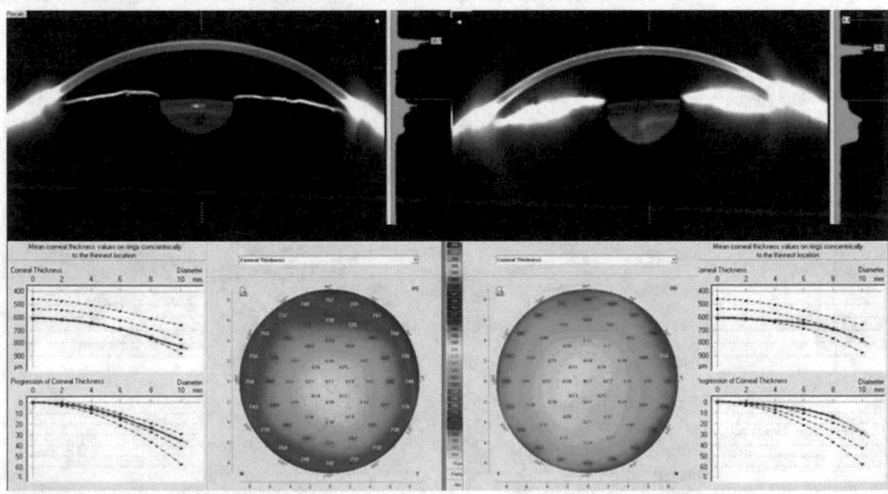

Fig. 8.4 The CTSP and PTI graphs allow the detection of early corneal edema, displaying an attenuation of the pachymetric progression from the center toward the periphery

are displayed on the thickness map. In a normal cornea, the thickest hemi-meridian is nasal and the thinnest is temporal and inferior. The arithmetic average of thickness on the 1, 2, 3, 4, and 5 mm diameter rings is represented as the average pachymetric progression index (PPI Ave). The maximum pachymetric progression index (PPI Max) considers the meridian with maximal pachymetric increase. Previous reports described that these metrics had a statistical significant difference among normal when compared to keratoconus, also demonstrating its usefulness in the diagnosis of ectasia [17].

8.4 The Ambrósio Relational Thickness Variables

Our study group described the concept of relational thickness, which considers the single-point metrics central corneal thickness (CCT) and TP with the PPI [13, 14, 18]. The combinations of pachymetric metrics TP and PPI were used in a simple ratio formula to provide a single metric that better describes corneal thickness. The ART ("Ambrósio Relational Thickness") can be calculated for the minimal (ART-Min), average (ART Ave), and maximal (ART Max) progression

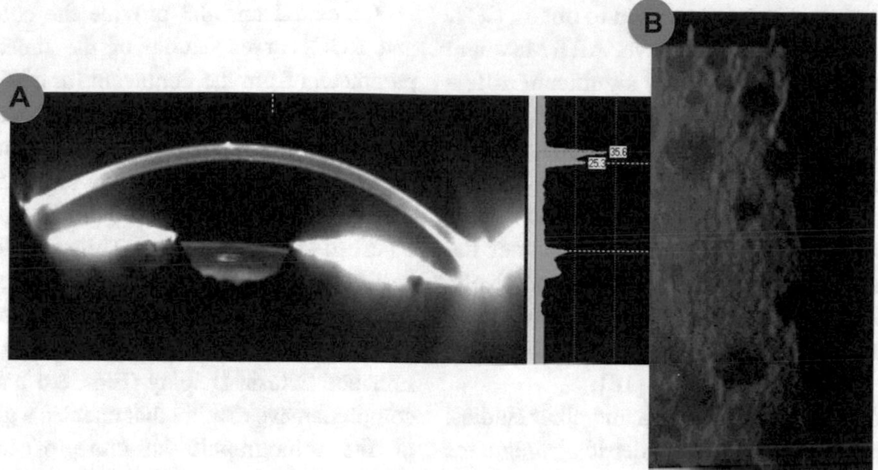

Fig. 8.5 (**a**) Scheimpflug image showing "Camel Sign," which consists of a second hump on the densitometry "*green*" graph, at the level of the Descemet's Membrane. (**b**) The presence of the "Camel Sign" on the Scheimpflug image correlates with the presence of corneal guttata

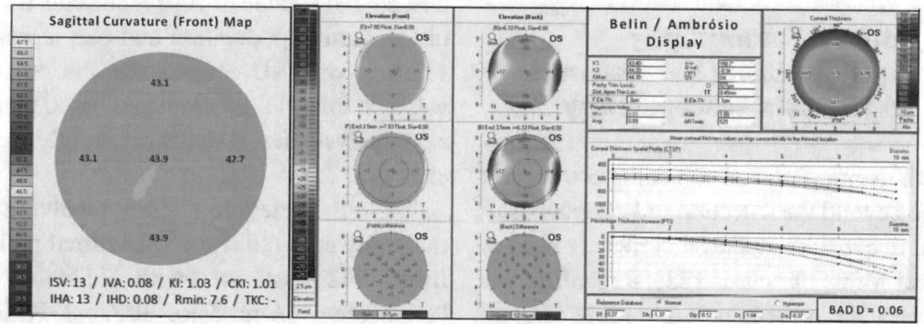

Fig. 8.6 Composite of a normal cornea, including front curvature map (axial or sagittal; Smolek-Klyce 1.5 absolute scale) and Belin Ambrósio Enhanced Ectasia Display. BAD D<1.45 and ART Max>412 are the most relevant findings. *ART* Ambrósio's relational thickness

indices. These parameters are obtained by dividing the thinnest pachymetric value by the respective pachymetric progression index [18].

8.5 Single-Point Pachymetry vs. Tomography-Derived Pachymetric Variables for Diagnosing Keratoconus

We published a study that enrolled 46 eyes diagnosed as mild to moderate keratoconus and 364 normal patients, which were evaluated by the Pentacam Comprehensive Eye Scanner (OCULUS, Wetzlar, Germany) [17]. Annular pachymetric distribution (CTSP and PTI) has been used successfully and validated statistically for the diagnosis of keratoconus, with higher accuracy than single-point CCT and TP. Significant differences were found for all positions of the CTSP from normal eyes and keratoconus ($p<0.01$), in which keratoconus had much lower (thinner) values. It was estimated that keratoconic corneas were, in average, 27.3 μm thinner than normal corneas. There were also significant differences for all positions of the PTI from normal eyes and keratoconus ($p<0.0001$), in which keratoconus had much higher increase. It was noticeable that normal corneas have a more homogeneous increase than in keratoconus [17].

Another study enrolled 113 individual eyes randomly selected from 113 normal patients and 44 eyes of 44 patients with keratoconus [18].

The Pentacam Scanner was used to obtain CCT, TP, PPI Min, PPI Max, PPI Ave, ART Max, and ATR Ave values. Statistically significant differences were noted between normal and keratoconic eyes for all parameters ($p<0.001$), except for horizontal position of TP ($p=0.79$). As shown in Table 8.1, the best parameters were ART Ave and ART Max with areas under the ROC curves of 0.987 and 0.983, respectively. Pachymetric progression indices and ART parameters had a greater area under the curve than TP and CCT ($p<0.001$) [18].

Based on the presented data and other studies, tomographic-derived pachymetric parameters provided a higher accuracy to differentiate normal and keratoconic corneas than single-point pachymetric measurements [17, 18, 21].

8.6 Corneal Tomography for Diagnosing Keratoconus and Ectasia Susceptibility

It is worth mentioning that screening ectasia risk should go beyond the detection of keratoconus; it is critical to consider studies that include mild or subclinical forms of ectasia [22]. Regarding this issue, one of the most important groups is composed by the eyes with relatively normal topography from patients with keratoconus detected in the fellow eye, referred as Forme Fruste Keratoconus (FFKC) [13, 23, 24].

Tables 8.2 and 8.3 provide the cutoff values and ROC curves details of the most effective parameters from the Pentacam for distinguishing normal from ectatic corneas [14]. We included parameters derived from the anterior curvature of the cornea (K Max as the point of maximum curvature), back elevation at the thinnest point using a best fit sphere (PostElev Thinnest BFS), and a best fit toric ellipsoid (PostElev Thinnest BFTE); ART Ave and Max; and Belin Ambrósio Final Deviation Value (BAD D). The Belin-Ambrósio Enhance Ectasia Display (Figs. 8.6 and 8.7) is a comprehensive display that enables a global view of the tomographic structure of the cornea through combination of the enhanced elevation approach, described by Belin, pachymetric, and curvature data [13]. The BAD considers the deviations of normality values for different parameters, so that a value of zero represents the average of the normal population and one represents the value is one SD toward the disease (ectasia) value. A final 'D' is calculated based on a regression analysis that weights differently the parameters [13, 25].

Table 8.2 refers to a study involving one eye randomly selected from 331 normal patients and from 242 patients with bilateral clinical keratoconus (Ambrósio, Ramos, Faria-Correa and Luz, unpublished data). Table 8.3 refers to a study that included 47 corneas with FFKC and the same normal control as in the study of Table 8.2 (Ambrósio, Ramos, Faria-Correa and

Table 8.1 Data summary from receiver operating characteristic curves of pachymetric parameters in normal and keratoconic eyes

Parameter	Cutoff	AUC	Sensitivity	Specificity	SE[a]	95 % CI[b]	*p* value[c]
ART Ave	424	0.987	95.5	96.5	0.00639	0.954–0.998	0.0001
ART Max	339	0.983	100	95.6	0.00961	0.945–0.997	0.0001
PPI Ave	1.06	0.980	97.7	98.5	0.00831	0.944–0.995	0.0001
PPI Max	1.44	0.977	100	93.8	0.0114	0.939–0.994	0.0001
TP	504	0.955	95.5	84.1	0.0165	0.910–0.982	0.0001
PPI Min	0.79	0.939	93.2	85.8	0.0304	0.890–0.971	0.0001
CCT	529	0.909	95.5	73.0	0.0251	0.853–0.949	0.0001

AUC area under the receiver operating characteristic curve, *SE* standard error, *CI* confidence interval, *ART* Ambrósio relational thickness, *Ave* average, *Max* maximum, *PPI* pachymetric progression indices, *CCT* central corneal thickness, *TP* thinnest point

[a]DeLong et al. [31]

[b]Binomial exact

[c]Area = 0.5

Table 8.2 Receiver operating characteristic results of Pentacam parameters (331 normal corneas randomly selected from 331 normal patients vs. 242 keratoconic corneas randomly selected from 242 patients with clinical bilateral keratoconus)

	Cutoff	AUC	SE[a]	95 % CI of AUC[b]	Sensitivity	95 % CI of sensitivity	Specificity	95 % CI of specificity
BAD D	>2.11	1	0.0000743	0.993–1000	99.59	97.7–100.0	100	98.9–100.0
PostElev thinnest BFS	>12	0991	0.00396	0.979–0.997	96.28	93.1–98.3	98.79	96.9–99.7
PostElev thinnest BFTE	>8	0.994	0.00218	0.984–0.999	95.04	91.5–97.4	99.09	97.4–99.8
ART Avg	≤474	0.999	0.000663	0.991–1.000	99.59	97.8–100.0	98.19	96.1–99.3
ART Max	≤386	0.999	0.000674	0.991–1.000	99.17	97.0–99.9	97.28	94.9–98.7
K Max	>47.8	0.978	0.00633	0.963–1.000	90.50	86.1–93.9	97.89	95.7–99.1

ART Ave Ambrósio's Relational Thickness to Average pachymetric progression increase, *ART Max* Ambrósio's Relational Thickness to maximal pachymetric progression increase, *BAD D* Belin/Ambrósio Enhanced Ectasia Deviation Value, *BFS* Best Fit Sphere, *BFTE* Best Fit Toric Ellipsoid, *K Max* maximal keratometric value, *SE* Standard error with DeLong, was calculated with binomial method

[a]Method for calculating the standard error (DeLong 1988), listed in the MedCalc software

[b]*95 % CI* confidence interval; *AUC* area under the receiver operating characteristic curve

Table 8.3 Receiver operating characteristic results of Pentacam parameters (331 normal corneas randomly selected from 331 normal patients vs. 47 cases with forme fruste keratoconus—eye with relatively normal topography from patient with keratoconus detected in the fellow eye)

	Cutoff	AUC	SE[a]	95 % CI of AUC[b]	Sensitivity	95 % CI of sensitivity	Specificity	95 % CI of specificity
BAD D	>1.22	0.975	0.0121	0.954–0.989	93.62	82.5–98.7	94.56	91.5–96.7
PostElev thinnest BFS	>5	0.825	0.0348	0.783–0.862	74.47	59.7–86.1	74.92	69.9–79.5
PostElev thinnest BFTE	>1	0.849	0.0324	0.809–0.883	80.85	66.7–90.9	72.51	67.4–77.2
ART Avg	≤521	0.956	0.0203	0.930–0.974	91.49	79.6–97.6	93.05	89.8–95.5
ART Max	≤416	0.959	0.0153	0.934–0.977	85.11	71.7–93.8	93.05	89.8–95.5
K Max	>45	0.635	0.0431	0.584–0.683	53.19	38.1–67.9	64.05	58.6–69.2

ART Ave Ambrósio's Relational Thickness to Average pachymetric progression increase, *ART Max* Ambrósio's Relational Thickness to maximal pachymetric progression increase, *BAD D* Belin/Ambrósio Enhanced Ectasia Deviation Value, *BFS* Best Fit Sphere, *BFTE* Best Fit Toric Ellipsoid, *K Max* maximal keratometric value, *SE* Standard error with DeLong, was calculated with binomial method

[a]Method for calculating the standard error (DeLong 1988), listed in the MedCalc software

[b]Method of calculating the 95 % CI of AUC (binomial exact)

Luz, unpublished data). It is of critical importance to adjust the cutoff values for identifying such mild cases of ectasia or susceptibility. For example, the BAD-D has a threshold of 2.11 for detecting keratoconus (99.59 % sensitivity and 100 % specificity, Table 8.2), but the best cutoff value for detecting FFKC is 1.22, with 93.62 % sensitivity and 94.56 % specificity. Although the adjustment of the cutoff value should be able to optimize the area under the ROC, minimal tolerable loss of specificity should be attempted. For example, some parameters that are very efficient for detecting keratoconus, such as K Max, may be found not useful for FFKC identification [14].

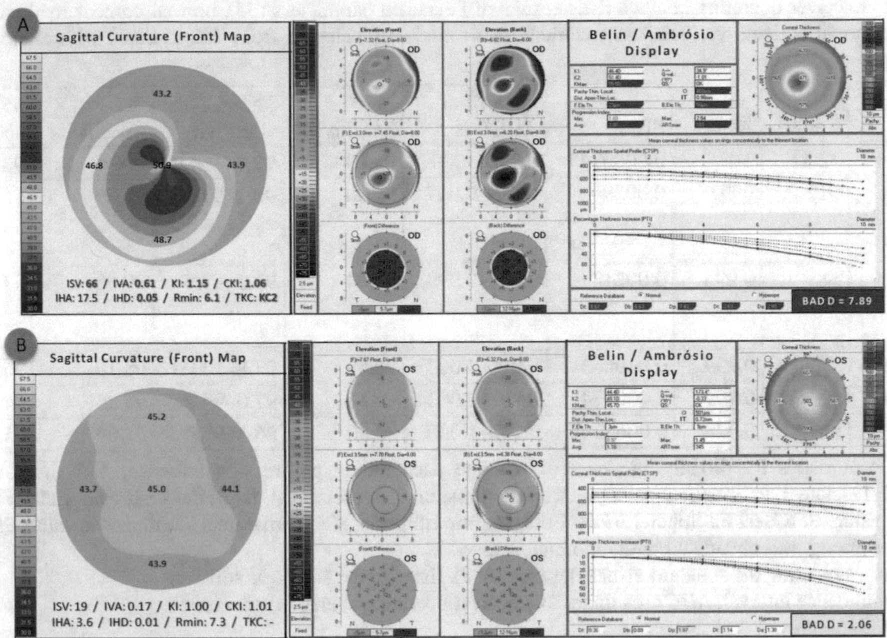

Fig. 8.7 Composite of both eyes from the same patient with very asymmetric keratoconus. (**a**) Typical keratoconic cornea on front curvature, with BAD D>2.5 and ART Max<360; (**b**) FFKC cornea with relatively normal front surface curvature map, but with BAD D>1.45 and ART Max<412. *ART* Ambrósio's relational thickness, *BAD* Belin-Ambrósio Enhance Ectasia Display, *FFKC* forme fruste keratoconus

8.7 New Concepts in Pachymetric Assessment

With the introduction of novel imaging technologies, such as the very-high frequency ultrasound and the anterior segment OCT, the corneal analysis progressed to a higher level [12]. With the segmental tomography, the analysis of individual corneal layers is possible, allowing precise epithelial and stromal mapping. Using a very-high frequency ultrasound prototype, Reinstein and coworkers demonstrated the usefulness of the epithelial mapping in the diagnosis of keratoconus. In this situation the pattern was different in keratoconic eyes compared to normal ones, showing a doughnut pattern derived from the epithelial thickening around the cone and the apical thinning [26–28]. Huang and coworkers used a Fourier-domain OCT for epithelial thickness mapping. Their studies showed that this technology mapped corneal epithelial thickness with good repeatability in both normal and keratoconic eyes. Apical epithelial thinning was also a feature in keratoconic corneas. The variables based on the pattern of the epithelial thickness profile provided good diagnostic accuracy to detect keratoconus [29, 30].

In summary, screening ectasia risk should go beyond the detection of keratoconus, since it is critical to identify mild or subclinical forms of ectasia. The standard screening criteria in keratorefractive surgery, based on corneal topography and CCT, has important limitations. Compared to single-point measurements, the indices generated from corneal thickness measurements over the entire cornea are useful for diagnosing ectatic corneas. Combination of these parameters with others derived from corneal tomography may enhance the accuracy for detecting mild forms of ectasia. Integration with biomechanical assessments may improve the understanding of the corneal architecture and shape.

Compliance with Ethical Requirements Renato Ambrosio, F. Faria Correia, and Michael W. Belin declare that they have no conflict of interest. All procedures followed were in accordance with the ethical standards of the responsible committee on human experimentation (institutional and national) and with the Helsinki

Declaration of 1975, as revised in 2000. Informed consent was obtained from all patients for being included in the study. No animal studies were carried out by the authors for this article.

Financial Disclosures: Ambrósio and Belin are consultants for OCULIS (Wetzlar, Germany); Ambrósio is consultant for Zeiss (Jena, Germany) and Alcon (Fort Worth, TX, USA)

References

1. Ambrosio Jr R, Klyce SD, Wilson SE. Corneal topographic and pachymetric screening of keratorefractive patients. J Refract Surg. 2003;19:24–9.
2. Jonsson M, Behndig A. Pachymetric evaluation prior to laser in situ keratomileusis. J Cataract Refract Surg. 2005;31:701–6.
3. Gromacki SJ, Barr JT. Central and peripheral corneal thickness in keratoconus and normal patient groups. Optom Vis Sci. 1994;71:437–41.
4. DeLong ER, DeLong DM, Clarke-Pearson DL (1988): Comparing the areas under two or more correlated receiver operating characteristic curves: a nonparametric approach. Biometrics 44:837-845..
4. Pflugfelder SC, Liu Z, Feuer W, Verm A. Corneal thickness indices discriminate between keratoconus and contact lens-induced corneal thinning. Ophthalmology. 2002;109:2336–41.
5. Ucakhan OO, Ozkan M, Kanpolat A. Corneal thickness measurements in normal and keratoconic eyes: Pentacam comprehensive eye scanner versus noncontact specular microscopy and ultrasound pachymetry. J Cataract Refract Surg. 2006;32:970–7.
6. Seitzman GD, Gottsch JD, Stark WJ. Cataract surgery in patients with Fuchs' corneal dystrophy: expanding recommendations for cataract surgery without simultaneous keratoplasty. Ophthalmology. 2005;112:441–6.
7. Ramos I, Belin M, Valbon B, et al. Keratoconus associated with Corneal Guttata. Int J Kerat Ect Corneal Dis. 2012;1:173–8.
8. Belin MW, Khachikian SS. New devices and clinical implications for measuring corneal thickness. Clin Exp Ophthalmol. 2006;34:729–31.
9. Maurice DM, Giardini AA. A simple optical apparatus for measuring the corneal thickness, and the average thickness of the human cornea. Br J Ophthalmol. 1951;35:169–77.
10. Salz JJ, Azen SP, Berstein J, Caroline P, Villasenor RA, Schanzlin DJ. Evaluation and comparison of sources of variability in the measurement of corneal thickness with ultrasonic and optical pachymeters. Ophthalmic Surg. 1983;14:750–4.
11. Mandell RB, Polse KA. Keratoconus: spatial variation of corneal thickness as a diagnostic test. Arch Ophthalmol. 1969;82:182–8.
12. Ambrosio Jr R, Belin MW. Imaging of the cornea: topography vs tomography. J Refract Surg. 2010;26:847–9.
13. Ambrosio Jr R, Nogueira LP, Caldas DL, et al. Evaluation of corneal shape and biomechanics before LASIK. Int Ophthalmol Clin. 2011;51:11–38.
14. Ambrosio Jr R, Valbon BF, Faria-Correia F, Ramos I, Luz A. Scheimpflug imaging for laser refractive surgery. Curr Opin Ophthalmol. 2013;24:310–20.
15. Shah S, Chatterjee A, Mathai M, et al. Relationship between corneal thickness and measured intraocular pressure in a general ophthalmology clinic. Ophthalmology. 1999;106:2154–60.
16. Konstas AG, Irkec MT, Teus MA, et al. Mean intraocular pressure and progression based on corneal thickness in patients with ocular hypertension. Eye (Lond). 2009;23:73–8.
17. Ambrosio Jr R, Alonso RS, Luz A, Coca Velarde LG. Corneal-thickness spatial profile and corneal-volume distribution: tomographic indices to detect keratoconus. J Cataract Refract Surg. 2006;32:1851–9.
18. Ambrosio Jr R, Caiado AL, Guerra FP, et al. Novel pachymetric parameters based on corneal tomography for diagnosing keratoconus. J Refract Surg. 2011;27:753–8.
19. Belin MW, Ambrosio R. Scheimpflug imaging for keratoconus and ectatic disease. Indian J Ophthalmol. 2013;61:401–6.
20. Kwon RO, Price MO, Price Jr FW, Ambrosio Jr R, Belin MW. Pentacam characterization of corneas with Fuchs dystrophy treated with Descemet membrane endothelial keratoplasty. J Refract Surg. 2010;26:972–9.
21. Faria-Correia F, Ramos IC, Lopes B, et al. Topometric and tomographic indices for the diagnosis of keratoconus. Int J Kerat Ect Cor Dis. 2012;1:92–9.
22. Ambrosio Jr R, Randleman JB. Screening for ectasia risk: what are we screening for and how should we screen for it? J Refract Surg. 2013;29:230–2.
23. Amsler M. The "forme fruste" of keratoconus. Wien Klin Wochenschr. 1961;73:842–3.
24. Klyce SD. Chasing the suspect: keratoconus. Br J Ophthalmol. 2009;93:845–7.
25. Ambrosio Jr R, Dawson DG, Salomao M, Guerra FP, Caiado AL, Belin MW. Corneal ectasia after LASIK despite low preoperative risk: tomographic and biomechanical findings in the unoperated, stable, fellow eye. J Refract Surg. 2010;26:906–11.
26. Reinstein DZ, Archer TJ, Gobbe M. Stability of LASIK in topographically suspect keratoconus confirmed non-keratoconic by Artemis VHF digital ultrasound epithelial thickness mapping: 1-year follow-up. J Refract Surg. 2009;25:569–77.
27. Reinstein DZ, Archer TJ, Gobbe M. Corneal epithelial thickness profile in the diagnosis of keratoconus. J Refract Surg. 2009;25:604–10.
28. Reinstein DZ, Gobbe M, Archer TJ, Silverman RH, Coleman DJ. Epithelial, stromal, and total corneal thickness in keratoconus: three-dimensional display with artemis very-high frequency digital ultrasound. J Refract Surg. 2010;26:259–71.
29. Li Y, Meisler DM, Tang M, et al. Keratoconus diagnosis with optical coherence tomography pachymetry mapping. Ophthalmology. 2008;115:2159–66.
30. Li Y, Tan O, Brass R, Weiss JL, Huang D. Corneal epithelial thickness mapping by Fourier-domain optical coherence tomography in normal and keratoconic eyes. Ophthalmology. 2012;119:2425–33.

9 Diagnostic Approach of Corneal Topography Maps

Francisco Cavas-Martínez, Ernesto De la Cruz Sánchez, José Nieto Martínez, Francisco J. Fernández Cañavate, and Daniel García Fernández-Pacheco

9.1 Introduction

The geometrical characterization of the morphology of the ocular globe, and specifically of the cornea, has become a fundamental analysis in the clinical practice in ophthalmology due to any change in its morphology can affect the patients' visual acuity [1]. Moreover, the knowledge of its morphology is critical when deciding the adequate corrective treatment [2].

During the last years, several imaging techniques have been developed for the detection and diagnosis of different pathologies that can be present in the biological structures [3]. Corneal topography is currently one of the most important tools in the ophthalmology field for the imaging diagnosis of corneal diseases related to the alteration of corneal morphology, and more concretely with the diagnosis of keratoconus.

F. Cavas-Martínez, Ph.D. (✉) • J. Nieto Martínez, Ph.D.
F.J. Fernández Cañavate, Ph.D.
D.G. Fernández-Pacheco, Ph.D.
Department of Graphical Expression,
Technical University of Cartagena, C/Doctor
Fleming s/n, Cartagena, Murcia 30202, Spain
e-mail: francisco.cavas@upct.es; jose.nieto@upct.es; francisco.canavate@upct.es; daniel.garcia@upct.es

E. De la Cruz Sánchez, Ph.D.
Faculty of Sports Science, University of Murcia,
C/Santa Alicia s/n, Santiago de la Ribera,
Murcia 30720, Spain
e-mail: erneslacruz@um.es

This noninvasive technique provides a series of indices that permit a new diagnostic approach from corneal topographies, which are based on the univariate and multivariate quantitative detection systems. Furthermore, the use of these corneal topographies permits to define new diagnosis techniques based on geometric models, mathematical models, biomechanical models, and neural networks systems.

The present chapter describes the technologies on which the current corneal topographers are based, the maps and biometric indices that these devices provide for the diagnosis of keratoconus, and the new diagnosis techniques based on different systems: univariate quantitative diagnosis systems, multivariate quantitative diagnosis systems, systems based on variables obtained by the aid of graphical geometry, and systems based on neural networks.

9.2 Actual Trends for the Geometrical Characterization of Corneal Anatomy

The corneal topography is considered a noninvasive technology that, using image processing, maps the corneal surface for its reconstruction and is later compared with a reference surface (see Fig. 9.1). The obtained topography is used for clinical diagnosis of the corneal pathologies related to an alteration of its corneal morphology.

J.L. Alió (ed.), *Keratoconus*, Essentials in Ophthalmology, DOI 10.1007/978-3-319-43881-8_9

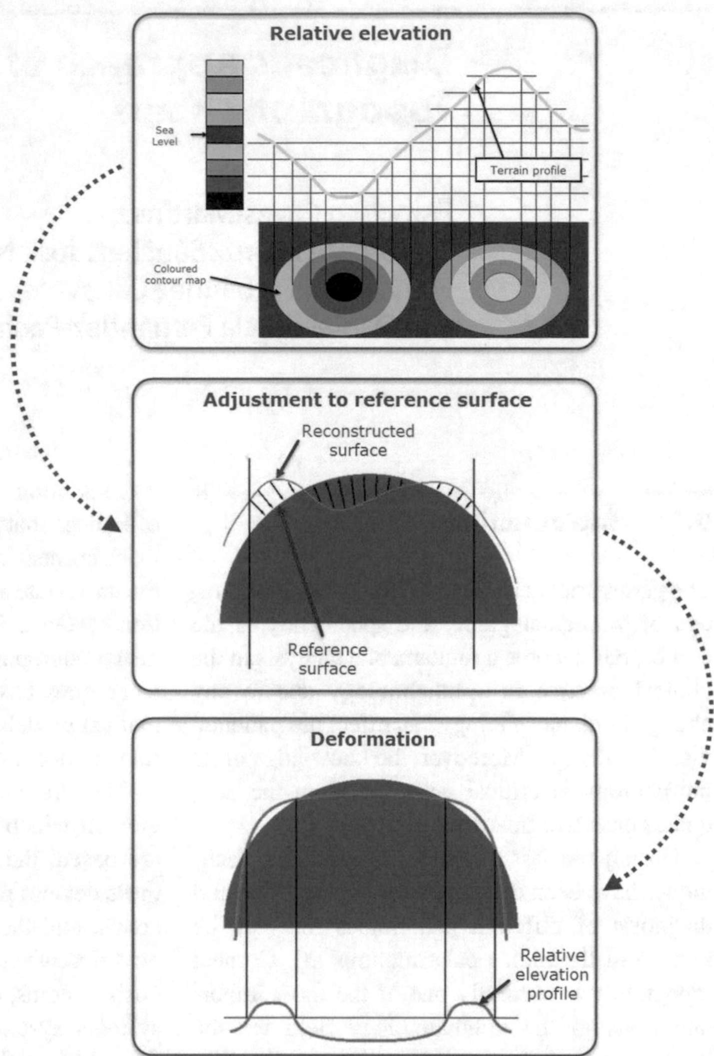

Fig. 9.1 Corneal topography

Cornea is responsible for more than 2/3 of the total refractive power of the human eye, so its morphology is of vital importance to determine the quality of the ocular optic system and therefore the vision quality. For this reason it must be understood that quantifying corneal topography is fundamental in clinical practice and helps to decide the corrective (invasive or not) treatment for the corneal disease.

Current corneal topographers are based on three technologies: (1) systems based on the light reflection on the cornea, (2) systems based on the projection of a slit light on the cornea, and (3) systems based on the asymmetric reflection of multicolor LEDs. All of these technologies provide different topographical maps of the anterior and posterior surfaces, as well as pachymetric maps and a series of indices for monitoring and clinic assessment of the corneal topographies.

9.2.1 Systems Based on the Light Reflection on the Cornea

Corneal topographers based on this technology, also called videokeratoscopes, are based on the application of the principles of convex mirrors' geometrical optics to an instrument in which the rings or Placido discs, with known size and spacing, are reflected on the anterior surface of the cornea. This image is initially captured by a digital camera and then processed by a computer [4]. From identifying the edges of the rings, each topographer uses an algorithm reconstruction of the corneal curvature, which accuracy depends on how the programming architecture is defined. The so-called arc step algorithms are the most used and are based on an iterative process that uses a sequence of arcs from point to point, covering the entire corneal region from the apex to the periphery. This process does not ignore data obtained in the previous step (step $i-1$) for obtaining current data (step i) [5]. Moreover, this reconstruction algorithm has an error lower than 0.25 μm in the central 3 mm and less than 1 μm for the rest of the corneal surface [6]. This precision is important since the minimum abnormal morphology due to keratoconus may impair the corneal homeostasis [7].

Height and slope data derived from the radial curvature of the corneal surface are presented by topographers as corneal keratometric data of the entire surface by a series of maps that follow a color scale developed by the University of Louisiana [8] (see Fig. 9.1).

- Cool colors correspond to flat curves and elevation values below the reference sphere (blue or violet colors).
- Mild colors correspond to medium curvature and elevation values equal to the reference sphere (green or yellow colors).
- Warm colors correspond to high curvature and elevation values above the reference sphere.

In addition, depending on the size of the Placido disc rings there are two commercial options [4]:

- Corneal topographers based on large diameter Placido disc rings. These devices are less susceptible to error associated with the misalignment between examiner and patient because they work at a large distance from the eye. However, because of this distance, it is possible to lose representative points because of the patient's facial morphology, produced by the shadow of the patient's nose and eyelashes.
- Corneal topographers based on small diameter Placido disc rings. These devices are most susceptible to alignment errors between the examiner and patient because they work in short distances, very close to the human eye. However, it mitigates the loss of information produced by patient's facial morphology, reducing the shadow that the nose and eyelashes could cause.

However, both systems have an important limitation that results from the use of internal algorithms that do not allow an accurate characterization of the corneal morphology in case of high levels of irregularity. In some cases, it is possible to obtain mistakes up to 4 diopters in corneas that present a very curved morphology, as it occurs in keratoconus disease [9].

9.2.2 Systems Based on the Projection of a Slit Light on the Cornea

Corneal topographers that use this technology are based on the integration of a dual technology. The first process involves projecting a Placido disc, obtaining the mirror image by reflection and representing the curvature and refractive power, which is obtained by an arc-step algorithm. The second phase is the projection of a slit light onto the cornea: due to the transparent structure of the cornea, and using Rayleigh scattering, it is possible to photograph it. These images will provide accurate data of corneal elevations for the entire anterior segment (see Fig. 9.2) [10].

Furthermore, this technology has two variants, depending on the spatial arrangement of the photographic system:

- System based on the principle of standard or normal photography. Its main feature is that the plane of the camera lens is located in parallel with the image. It means that only a small region is focused (the imaginary extensions of the film planes, the lens, and the focal plane

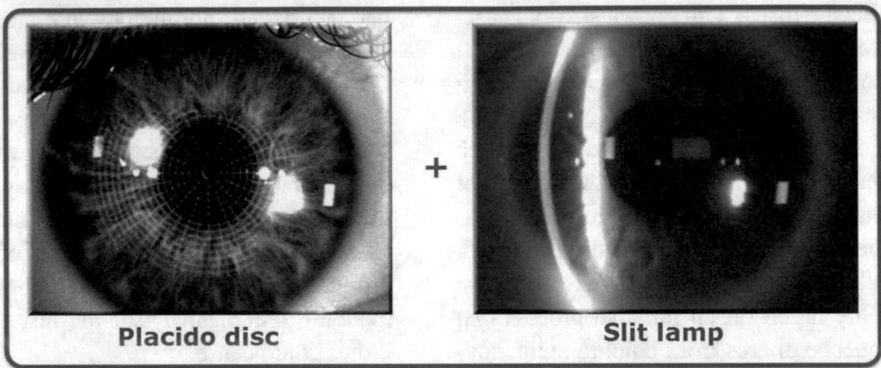

Fig. 9.2 Systems based on the projection of a slit light on the cornea

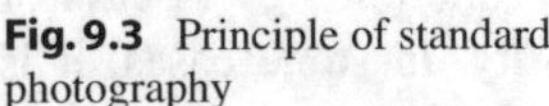
Fig. 9.3 Principle of standard photography

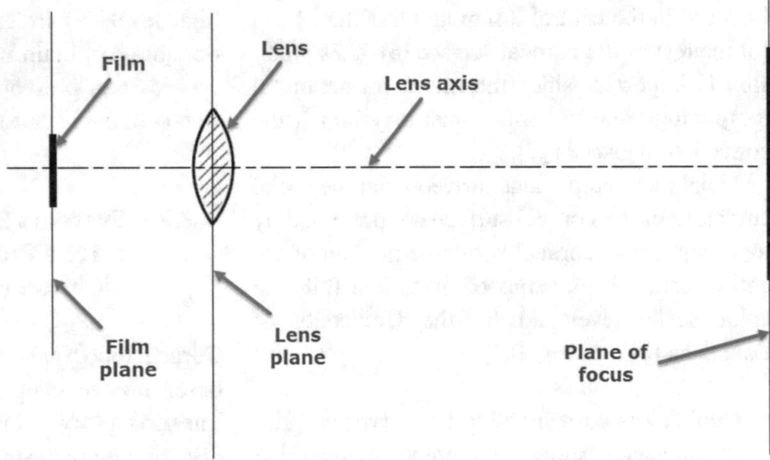

are parallel) (Fig. 9.3) [11, 12]. The most common system is the Orbscan (Bausch & Lomb Incorporated, USA), which was the first commercial device that assessed the posterior corneal surface in a noninvasive and quick way. This system provides different maps of the anterior and posterior corneal surfaces, and also pachymetric data; however, several authors from scientific literature present a strong controversy due to the reliability of the measurements performed by this device on the posterior surface, and also the limited repeatability [8, 13, 14].

- Systems based on the principle of Scheimpflug photography. Its main feature is that the plane of the camera lens is placed sideways to the image (the imaginary extensions of the planes of the film, the lens, and the focal plane are not parallel (Fig. 9.4) [12], and therefore the focused region is increased and the image sharpness is improved) [15–17]. The main commercial systems based on this principle are Pentacam (Oculus, USA), Galilei (Ziemer, Switzerland), and Sirius (CSO, Italy), which offer repeatable measurements of the corneal curvature and other anatomical measurements of the anterior segment. However, several authors question the degree of concordance between the measurements provided by these devices [18–20].

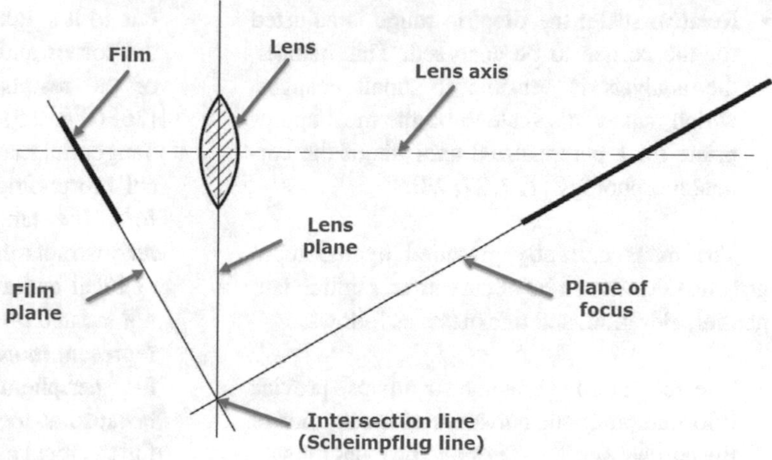

Fig. 9.4 Principle of Scheimpflug photography

9.2.3 Systems Based on the Asymmetric Reflection of Multicolor LEDs

These systems are based on the same optical principle than convex mirrors previously described in Sect. 9.2.1, but in this case the emitters are multicolor light-emitting diodes (LEDs).

More specifically, this system uses a panel formed with an asymmetric distribution of more than 700 LEDs in colors red, yellow, and green, which reflection on the cornea provides a more accurate reconstruction of the corneal surface if compared with the lack of detail obtained when projecting a monochromatic light [21–23].

The main novelty of this system is the use of a unique reconstruction algorithm for the reflection of each LED projection; this one being independent of the algorithm used for the other LED projections. This new approach has one main difference with respect to the systems previously described where the rest of them were based on the projection of a monochromatic light and use the same reconstruction algorithm for all the points of the corneal surface. Moreover, the new device permits redefining at the local level, every three points identified in the corneal surface, its curvature or elevation.

The unique commercial equipment based on this principle and currently available is the Cassini color LED Corneal Analyzer (i-Optics, The Netherlands) [21–23].

9.3 Corneal Topography

Corneal topography is considered a noninvasive exploratory technique that permits to analyze both qualitatively and quantitatively the morphology of the cornea, differentiating standard patterns from those potentially devastating for vision disorders caused by pathological ectatic conditions [1, 7, 15, 24, 25].

Corneal topographers present different maps to represent the measurements that characterize the corneal surface, but previously to the description of these maps, it is fundamental to take into account the dimension or scale to be adopted during the assessment of the topographical test to obtain the maximum information from the clinical point of view. In this regard, two scales can be distinguished [26]:

- Absolute scale: the entire dioptric range that the topographer can measure is assigned to a color scale, so sensitivity decreases with small alterations.

- Relative scale: the dioptric range is adjusted for the cornea to be analyzed. This manner, the analysis is sensible to small changes, which makes this scale to be the most appropriate for a personalized analysis of the corneal morphology [1, 7, 27, 28].

The maps currently provided by the topographic devices can be of curvature, sagittal, tangential, elevation, and thickness, as follows:

- The curvature keratometric maps provide information about curvature at each point of the corneal surface. They can be axial (or sagittal) and tangential (or instant). Although both types report information about focal curvature, there exist significant differences between them [1, 29]:
  - Sagittal maps fix the curvature centers on the optical axis and considers the corneal surface to have a spherical geometry, achieving a marked overall smoothing of the corneal periphery. This results in a larger and more peripheral curving area than the actual area of the cone; however, this consideration is erroneous and only true in the paraxial approach since the cornea has a spherical surface. Therefore, it distorts the true picture of the cornea and provides quantitatively inaccurate values [1, 26, 29, 30]. However, this map is useful for a qualitative assessment through colors due to it softens the geometric contours of the cornea and facilitates the interpretation of the results by less-experienced users [26] (Fig. 9.5).
  - Tangential maps do not assume the spherical morphology of the cornea and therefore, the tangential curvature algorithm reconstructs the corneal surface by means of local curvature radii whose centers are not located on the optical axis. These maps represent more accurately the curvature of the peripheral corneal region. This is because at local level the area which best fits the focal curve is considered, which has not been imperatively placed on the optical axis, as occurs in the axial maps (Fig. 9.6) [26]. This map shows a high sensitivity to data obtained, being suitable for monitoring the conical shape of the ectatic disease; however, it is less intuitive than the axial map and its interpretation may be more complex.
- Elevation maps do not represent data directly measured by the corneal topographer, but are obtained by comparing the reconstruction of the anterior or posterior corneal surface to the best fitted surface, typically a sphere, a toroid, a revolution ellipsoid or a non-revolution ellipsoid. The difference between both surfaces is provided by altimetry data that correspond to the elevation maps (Fig. 9.7) [4, 31, 32]. Furthermore, typical dimensions of the refer-

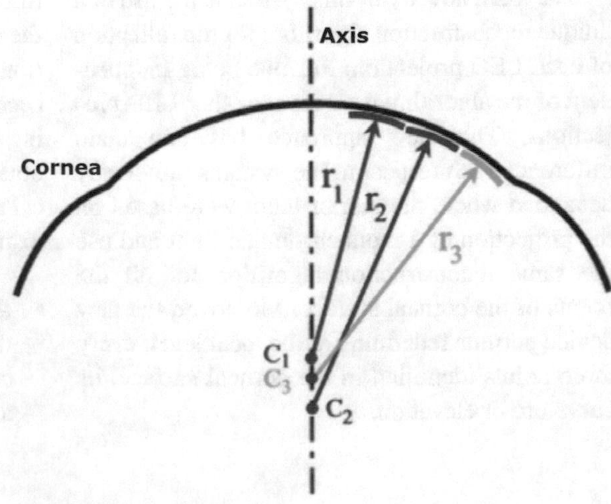

Fig. 9.5 Geometric reconstruction of the corneal sagittal map

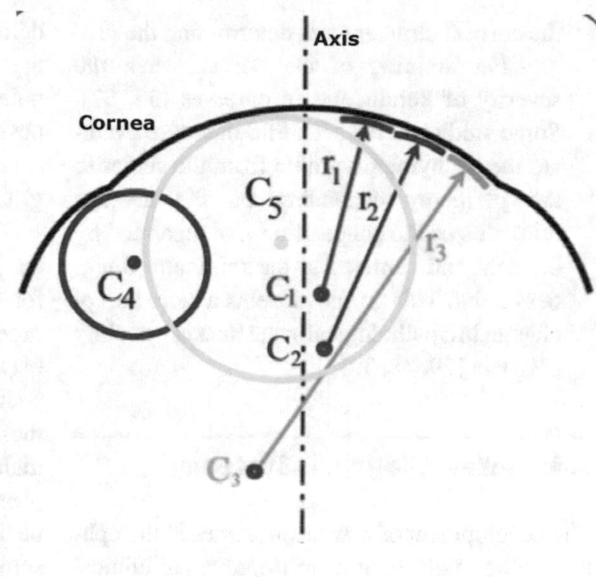

Fig. 9.6 Geometric reconstruction of the corneal tangential map

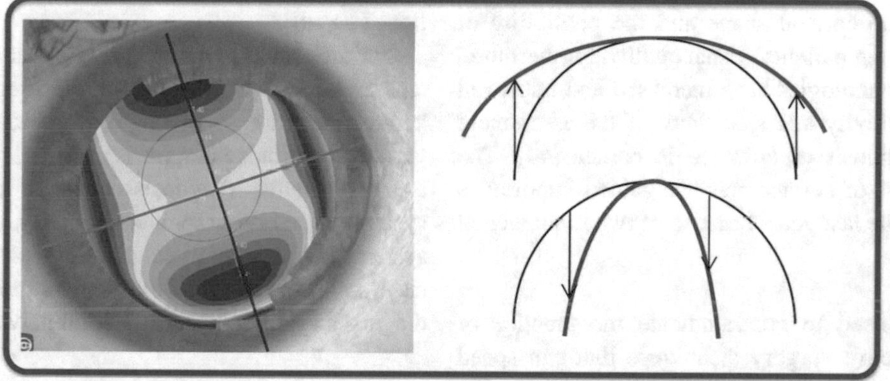

Fig. 9.7 Altimetry elevation map

ence surface are around 8 mm in diameter, thereby scenarios that may influence the data acquisition process, such as shadows generated by eyelashes, are avoided [33]. These maps present several advantages: data are presented quantitatively in μm, so they are highly accurate and have a high sensitivity to small changes that can occur in the corneal morphology as a result of keratoconus [1]; also, topographers allow the selection of the best suited surface to perform the elevation map, which results in a sensitivity increase of the clinical diagnosis. This map provides, for both corneal surfaces, the elevation of the corneal apex, the elevation of the minimum thickness point [34] and the elevation of the center of the central region [35]. As the posterior surface is not altered by the excimer laser photoablation or by the generation of the corneal flap, nor is adulterated by the hyperplastic effect of corneal epithelium, data from the posterior surface could be very useful for the clinical diagnosis of keratoconus [1, 8, 26, 34, 35].

- The thickness map does not show data directly measured by the corneal topographer, but must be precisely reconstructed using the anterior and posterior corneal surfaces. This map gives information of the minimum thickness point and its position on the center of the cornea. This point is essential for maintaining the corneal structure and determining the progressive thinning of the cornea when the severity of keratoconus progresses [36, 37]. Some studies in the scientific literature evaluate the pachymetric profile from the center to the periphery depending on the average thickness of the concentric rings separated by 0.1 mm and centered at the minimum thickness point. This profile presents a more abrupt change in a pathological stage than in a healthy scenario [29, 38, 39].

9.4 New Diagnosis Systems

The development of new technologies in the ophthalmology field permits to improve the clinical diagnosis capability providing an accurate analysis of the corneal shape and the possibility of quantifying patients' visual quality. Furthermore, these technologies have increased and improved the sensitivity and specificity of the assessment and diagnosis of keratoconic cornea [40]. The diagnosis of keratoconus has gained importance during the last years because of two fundamental reasons:

- The need to contraindicate the practice of refractive surgery techniques that can speed up the development of keratoconus [41, 42]. In this case, it is fundamental to carry to an extreme the sensitivity of the diagnosis process even at the cost of sacrificing specificity, which most negative consequence would be to contraindicate a suitable candidate for a refractive surgery.
- The possibility of using therapies that can stop or delay the severity grade of keratoconus, such as cross-linking [43] or implantation of intrastromal rings [44, 45]. In this case, it is fundamental to ensure specificity in order to avoid unnecessary treatments in healthy eyes.

The different analysis methods based on assessment indices of the corneal surface that are available in the clinical practice try to diagnosis the presence of the keratoconus disease by using a quantitative and qualitative detection of this deformation in the cornea. Although the methods that are going to be referenced do not achieve individually a diagnostic accuracy of 100 % (real positives + real negatives/number of cases), the sum of all of them does provide the ophthalmologist a diagnostic accuracy of 100 %.

These evaluation indices are obtained from the topographical maps previously described, and for this reason several clinical studies have proposed determined cutoff values to distinguish between normal corneas and corneas with keratoconus [40]. However, the main problem with these indices lies in the fact that each index has a high degree of specificity for the corneal topographer for which it has been developed, and cannot be directly extrapolated to other devices. Even in some cases, the results obtained from those devices do not coincide with the published equations [40, 46].

For the above-mentioned reasons, it is important to know the systems for the diagnosis of keratoconus disease, distinguishing between univariate quantitative diagnosis systems, multivariate quantitative diagnosis systems, diagnosis systems based on graphical geometry, diagnosis systems based on mathematical models, diagnosis systems based on biomechanical models, and diagnosis systems based on neural networks.

9.4.1 Univariate Quantitative Diagnosis Systems

These indices are based on a unique variable and are used to characterize the corneal irregularity from corneal topographies. Some of the most used indices are the following:

- *Asphericity coefficient* (*Q*). It is an index that describes how the corneal curvature changes from the central region to the peripheral region. Its value depends on the diameter of study, so it is necessary to indicate it when expressing a particular index [47]. The most common parameter used in literature is *Q*. In a natural or non-pathological stage, the section of the cornea is a prolate ellipse with an average *Q* value setting –20 ± 0.12 DS [48, 49].

This is physically interpreted as the cornea is more curved in the center than at the periphery. For keratoconic corneas, Savini et al. [19] reported Q values in the corneal region that comprise a 8 mm diameter of −0.84 for the anterior surface and −1.10 for the posterior surface [19]. Another study comprising the same diameter and the same corneal region reports Q values of the anterior surface between −0.65 and −1.18 and between −1.17 and −0.66 for the posterior surface [50], according to the severity of keratoconus using the Amsler–Krumeich classification [51]. The values of asphericity describing the geometry of the cornea showed that the central and paracentral regions are more curved than the peripheral region, and this difference is greater in keratoconus disease than in normal corneas. Moreover, these values are higher when the severity of keratoconus increases. However, due to asphericity is measured in the central region (4–5 mm), if protrusion is located in the peripheral region, topographer may provide normal or even positive values of asphericity. Therefore, this quantitative index is not very specific for the diagnosis of keratoconus, and must be considered in relation to the apex position in the cone.

- *Inferior–Superior Value (I–S).* This index is defined as the power difference between five points of the inferior hemisphere and five points of the superior hemisphere of the corneal region located at 3 mm from the corneal apex at spatial intervals of 30°. A positive value indicates higher inferior curvature, while a negative value indicates higher superior curvature. I–S values between 1.4 and 1.8 D are defined as cutoff points for suspected keratoconus and I–S values higher than 1.8 D as cutoff points for clinical keratoconus [52, 53].
- *Simulated keratometry (SIMK).* This index provides information on the diopter power of the flattest and most curved meridians in the so-called useful region of the topographer (ring diameters between 3 and 9 mm). Numerically, it is expressed as $K1$ and $K2$, and the difference between the two values provides a quantitative value of corneal astigmatism. A clinical study provided SIMK mean values of 43.53 ± 1.02 D for a group of normal corneas, and established a cutoff value for keratoconus group twice the value of the standard deviation of the control group [4, 54].
- *Central Keratometry (K Central).* This is the average value of corneal power for the rings with diameter of 2, 3, and 4 mm. Values below 47.2 D are considered normal, while values between 47.2 and 48.7 D are considered probable keratoconus. Values above 48.7 D are clinical keratoconus [4, 53].
- *Average corneal power (ACP).* This index indicates an average power value of various points in the central region [53].
- *Effective refractive power (EffRP).* Index averaging the power in the central area of 3 mm diameter. It considers Styles–Crawford effect [47].
- *Apex curvature (AK).* It corresponds to an index that provides a value of the instantaneous curvature in the corneal apex. Values below 48 D indicate normality, values between 48 and 50 D are suspect, and values above 50 D denote abnormally high curvature [40].
- *Surface asymmetry index (SAI).* It is an index that indicates an average value of the power differences between the points spatially located at 180° from 128 equidistant meridians. A radially symmetrical surface has a value of zero, and this value increases as the degree of asymmetry is greater [4, 40, 55].
- *Surface Regularity index (SRI).* It is a local descriptor of regularity in a central area of 4.5 mm diameter (it comprises the central ten rings of Placido Disc). It quantifies power gradient differences between successive pairs of rings in 256 equidistant semimeridians. It correlates well with the value of visual acuity ($p = 0.80$, $P < 0.001$), assuming the cornea as the only limiting factor for vision. A normal cornea presents SRI values below 0.56 (this value would be 0 in a perfectly regular cornea) [4, 40, 56].
- *Different sector index (DSI).* It is an index that quantifies the average power difference between sectors of 45° with the highest and lowest power [40, 53].

- *Opposite industry index (OSI).* This is another index indicating in terms of average power difference between opposing sectors of 45° [40, 53].
- *Irregular astigmatism index (IAI).* It is a measure of dioptric variables along each semimeridian, which is normalized by the mean power of the cornea and the number of measured points [40, 53].
- *Corneal Irregularity Measurement (CIM).* This is a numeric index representing the degree of irregularity in the morphology of the corneal surface. It quantifies the standard deviation between the corneal surface and the best-fit reference surface, which in this case is a toric surface. High values of this ratio indicate a greater possibility of the cornea to present a pathology related to a morphological abnormality. A healthy cornea has CIM values from 0.03 to 0.68 μm, while a value from 0.69 to 1 μm is considered as suspect or normal limit, and a value from 1.10 to 5.00 μm as pathological or unusual [4].
- *Analyzed area (AA).* It is the ratio of the data area interpolated by the area circumscribed by the outermost peripheral ring [40, 53] area.
- *Centre Surround index (CSI).* It is an index that quantifies the average power difference between the central zone of 3 mm diameter and a half-peripheral ring comprised between 3 and 6 mm diameters [40, 53].
- *Corneal uniformity index (CU).* It corresponds to an index that quantifies the distortion uniformity in the central area with 3 mm diameter. It is expressed as a percentage, that is, a value of 100 % indicates that the cornea has a perfect consistency [47].
- *Predicted Corneal Acuity (PC Acuity).* It quantifies the optical quality in Snellen units (with a range of 20/10 to 20/200) in the central zone of the cornea with 3 mm diameter [40, 47].
- *Skew of steepest radial axis (SRAX).* It measures the angle between the more curved superior semimeridian and more curved inferior semimeridian. The more curved semimeridian for each hemisphere is determined by averaging the powers of the rings from 5 mm to 16 mm diameter. The smallest angle between these semimeridians is subtracted from 180°, and the result, in degrees, is the SRAX index. A value greater than 20° is considered indicative of keratoconus, but due to the high dispersion of values in some astigmatic corneas, this value is only valuable if corneal astigmatism is greater than 1.5 D [40].
- *Topographic irregularity (TI).* It is the root mean square (RMS) value of the difference between the actual topography data and a geometric reference surface, which in this case is a spherical cylinder that best fits the corneal surface of the study [40].
- *Calossi–Foggi Apex curvature gradient (ACG).* This index quantifies the average difference per length unit of the corneal power in relation to the apical power. Values greater than 2 D/mm can indicate keratoconus, between 1.5 and 2 suspect, and less than 1.5 is considered a normal value [40].
- *Calossi–Foggi Inferior-Superior Index.* It is a vertical asymmetry index similar to I–S value, but this indicates the difference in terms of average power between the superior area and a inferior area. This last is determined according to a major probability of presence of the cone. A positive value means that inferior area is more curved, and vice versa. A value less than 1.5 is considered normal, a value between 1.5 and 2 considered suspect, and values greater than 2 are considered abnormal [40].
- *Orbscan surface irregularity.* It is a coefficient calculated from the standard deviations of the mean curvature and mean astigmatism in the zones comprised between the center rings of 3 mm and 5 mm diameters. Values greater than 1.5 in the area of 3 mm and/or 2 in the area of 5 mm are indicative of high irregularity. This value is not specific for keratoconus, but merely indicates irregularity [40].
- *Mean toric keratometry (MTK).* This index is obtained from the data of the elevation map of the cornea. It compares and analyzes the elevation values of the cornea calculated by means of the best adjustment to a toric reference surface. If the MTK value is high, the cornea acquires a geometrical behavior similar to a

toric surface, which is clinically interpreted as a major probability of suffering ectatic alterations. The MTK index follows a Gaussian probability distribution, with an average value of 44.5 D, and the range defined for the values from 41.25 D to 47.25 D contains 96 % of the population. [57]

9.4.2 Multivariate Quantitative Diagnosis Systems

The diagnosis of keratoconus has been facilitated by the application of different quantitative detection systems using multivariate combinations of the topographic indices described above. Each topographer incorporates a different strategy and it is essential for the user to understand the sensitivity and specificity of each software. These systems can be:

- *Rabinowitz and McDonell Index*. It is one of the first multivariate indices based on the combination of the numerical values supplied by the I–S index, the value of the center K, and the difference of the central *K* between both eyes of the patient. This multivariate system combines the information obtained from the central curvature values with the inferior-superior asymmetry values as diagnostic parameters of keratoconus that can occur in both central and peripheral regions. However, this indicator is unable to quantify the amount of irregular astigmatism associated with the keratoconus disease [40, 52].
- *PathFinder Corneal Analysis*. It is a system which uses three different indices (CIM, Q and MTK) for detecting the morphological alterations that corneal topographies present. In the case of a normal cornea, the three indicators give values within normal limits. In the case of molding due to contact lenses, there is also a corneal distortion known as pseudokeratoconus, where the CIM index is outside the normal range, but the other two indicators are within normal limits. In the case of a subclinical keratoconus, central curvature values and inferior–superior asymmetry cause both the CIM and the MTK to have abnormal values, while asphericity remains normal or borderline normal. In the case of keratoconus, the three indicators are outside the bounds of normality [4, 58].
- *Keratoconus prediction index (KPI)*. It is a calculated by a combination of eight topographic indices and uses a linear discriminant function. These indices are: Sim *K*1, Sim *K*2, UPS, DSI, OSI, CSI, IAI, and AA. A value greater than 0.23 is suggestive of keratoconus. In a validation group of a hundred eyes with different clinical conditions, this method showed a sensitivity of 68 % and a specificity of 99 %. The KPI multivariate method along with DSI, OSI, GSI and Sim K2 indices were implemented using an expert computational algorithm based on a binary decision tree [40].
- *Keratoconus Index (KCI)*. This is a method commonly known in the ophthalmology field as the Klyce–Maeda method. This method can differentiate a healthy cornea from a kerato conic cornea, and also distinguish between keratoconus developed in the central or the peripheral regions.
- *Keratoconus severity index (KSI)*. This index is also known in the ophthalmology field as the Smolek–Klyce method [76]. This multivariate system calculates the severity of keratoconus, which possibly distinguishes between a healthy cornea, a suspected keratoconic cornea, and a cornea with keratoconus. The algorithm used is based on a neural network with ten topographic indices as inputs. A KSI value <15 % is considered normal, values between 15 % and 30 % as suspected keratoconus, and above this value is considered subclinical keratoconus [4, 40, 54].
- *KISA%*. It is calculated from four indices: Central K, SIMK, I-S and SRAX. It is a very effective index in the identification of keratoconus, but may have a significant number of false negatives in the clinical diagnosis and in incipient keratoconus cases, which can suppose a major risk in its use as a screening tool in refractive surgery. A value between 60 and 100 is indicative of suspected keratoconus, while a value greater than 100 is diagnostic of keratoconus; for this last

value the KISA index has a high sensitivity and specificity [4, 40, 59].

- *Chastang method.* Combines SDSD and Asph indices, developing a primary decision tree. This method is not applicable for defining the grade or severity of keratoconus, so incipient or early cases are not identified [40, 60].
- *Belin/Ambrósio Enhanced Ectasia Display III (BAD III).* This method combines the following nine parameters: anterior elevation at the minimum thickness point, posterior elevation at the minimum thickness point, change in anterior elevation, change in posterior elevation, corneal thickness at minimum thickness point, location of thinnest point, pachymetric progression, Ambrósio relational thickness, and Kmax. The BAD III index provides individual information for every parameter and then performs a discriminant analysis combined with a regression of the nine indices, which permits the discrimination between healthy and keratoconic corneas [61].

9.4.3 Systems Based on Graphical Geometry

Generation of virtual models has experienced during the last years an important technological advance thanks to the development of new computational tools for the image acquisition and processing [62], making possible the generation of 3D shapes [16] and the formulation of behavioral models that faithfully reproduce the geometry of a solid structure [63]. One of this tools is Computer-Aided Geometric Design (CAGD), which permits to study geometric and computational aspects of any complex physical entity, such as surfaces and volumes, for generating virtual models [64].

One of the last studies in this field is the work carried out by Cavas et al. [51, 65], where a new method based on graphical geometry is described for the diagnosis of keratoconus. The proposed diagnosis procedure consists of the following stages (Fig. 9.8):

1. Geometric modeling of the cornea. In this phase the human cornea is scanned with the aid of a corneal topographer and the information provided is used to reconstruct a 3D geometrical virtual model of the cornea. The following subprocesses are performed:
   (a) Measurement of corneal topography and preparation of the point cloud. In this process the corneal topography of the eye is obtained using the Sirius device (CSO, Florence, Italy), which is an instrument that combines the rotation of two Scheimpflug cameras with the projection of a Placido disc on the cornea to obtain the corneal topography, obtaining measures with a good consistency. After measurements are made by the corneal topographer, spatial point clouds formatted in Cartesian coordi-

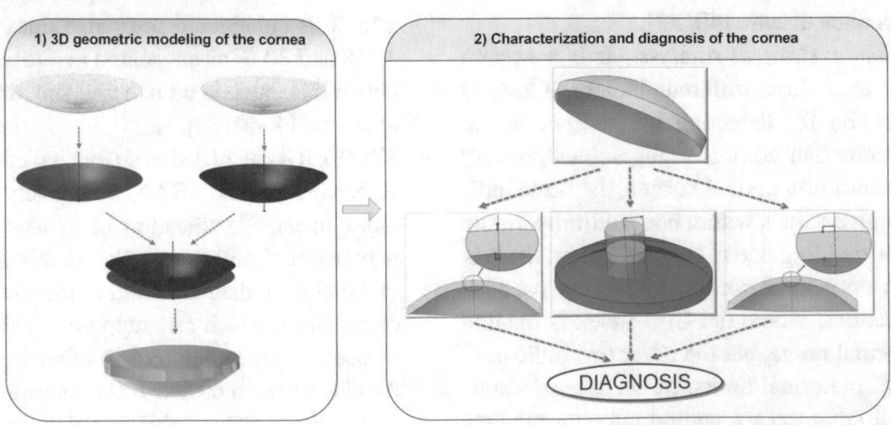

Fig. 9.8 Scheme of the method based on graphical geometry for the diagnosis of keratoconus

nates (*X*,*Y*,*Z*) and representative of the anterior and posterior corneal surfaces are generated using the altimetry data generated by the topographer and a specific algorithm developed in Matlab software.

(b) Geometric surface reconstruction. The point clouds previously obtained are then imported to the geometric surface reconstruction software Rhinoceros V5.0. This software uses a mathematical model to generate the surfaces for both corneal surfaces basing on nonuniform rational B-spline (NURBS) functions, which have been generated with the highest goodness of fit that the software can provide. The anterior and posterior corneal surfaces obtained from this process are then positioned by the aid of their geometrical center and the peripheral surface (bonding surface between both sides in the *Z*-axis direction) is calculated, forming a single surface.

(c) Generation of the solid model. The surfaces obtained are then exported to the geometric modeling software SolidWorks V2012 and the solid model representative of the corneal morphology is generated.

2. Geometric analysis of the cornea. In this phase determined geometric variables are extracted from the virtual model and analyzed to classify the studied cornea as healthy or keratoconic. Some of these variables are the following (these variables are described with more detail in the following chapter): total corneal volume, anterior/posterior corneal surface area, total corneal surface area, sagittal plane area in apex, anterior/posterior apex deviation, sagittal plane area at minimum thickness point, anterior/posterior minimum thickness point deviation, centre of mass coordinates (*X*,*Y*,*Z*), net deviation from the center of mass in *XY*, and volume of corneal cylinder with radius-x.

9.4.4 Diagnosis Systems Based on Biomechanical Models

The use of mathematical modeling in the field of ophthalmology is almost universal [66]. The latest technological advances encourage more accurate models that sometimes are ignored by the professionals of this area [67].

A fundamental tool in the clinical practice for the diagnosis of keratoconus is the corneal topography, which, independently of the technology on which it is based, rebuilds the corneal surface by means of modal methods and provide the corneal topography by comparing this surface with a reference one [4].

A broadly accepted standard in ophthalmology as modal method is the use of Zernike polynomials [68–71]. Furthermore, there exist other methods such as the ones based on Fourier Transform [72–74], least squares adjustment [71], non-linear reconstruction by rational functions [70], or reconstruction by means of contour problems [75, 76]. However, these methods are limited to the reconstruction of the corneal surface.

There exists other modal method based on radial basis functions [77, 78] that proposes a series of indices for clinical diagnosis of keratoconus based on mathematical geometry of a 2D space [79].

9.4.5 Diagnosis Systems Based on Neural Networks

Artificial neural networks (ANN) are mathematical algorithms which try to simulate the behavior of the biological neural networks of the human brain. A neural network is considered as a processor distributed in a parallel structure that has a natural trend to store experimental knowledge making it suitable for its use. It has two similarities with respect to the human brain: on one hand, knowledge is acquired by the net by means of a learning process; and on the other hand, that knowledge is stored in synoptic weights or connections between neurons. Current ANNs only try to reproduce, in a simplified manner, the basic mechanisms of the human brain, not attempting to reproduce the brain in its totality and focusing on possible mechanisms to resolve individual problems. Therefore, the aim of these nets is to provide them with the possibility of understanding the manner in which the human being resolves problems and use them to complement the capacities of the artificial intelligent systems. There exist different types of neural networks depending on several items: the organization of the neurons that conform the net, the self-training procedure, the association between input and output information, and display of the information [26].

These neural networks have been used with success in the ophthalmology field for the diagnosis of keratoconus by using the classification of topographical patterns [53, 80–84].

Compliance with Ethical Requirements *Conflict of Interest*: F. Cavas-Martínez, E. De la Cruz Sánchez, J. Nieto Martínez, F.J. Fernández Cañavate and D.G. Fernández-Pacheco declare that they have no conflict of interest.

Informed Consent: No human studies were carried out by the authors for this article.

No animal studies were carried out by the authors for this article.

References

1. Piñero DP, Nieto JC, Lopez-Miguel A. Characterization of corneal structure in keratoconus. J Cataract Refract Surg. 2012;38(12):2167–83. doi:10.1016/j.jcrs.2012.10.022.
2. Oie Y, Nishida K. Regenerative medicine for the cornea. Biomed Res Int. 2013;2013:428247. doi:10.1155/2013/428247.
3. Lohfeld S, Barron V, McHugh PE. Biomodels of bone: a review. Ann Biomed Eng. 2005;33(10):1295–311. doi:10.1007/s10439-005-5873-x.
4. Montalbán R. Caracterización y validación diagnóstica de la correlación de la geometría de las dos superficies de la córnea humana. Alicante: Universidad de Alicante; 2013.
5. Goldberg AV, Tarjan RE. Efficient maximum flow algorithms. Commun ACM. 2014;57(8):82–9. doi:10.1145/2628036.
6. Sicam VA, Snellenburg JJ, van der Heijde RG, van Stokkum IH. Pseudo forward ray-tracing: a new method for surface validation in cornea topography. Optom Vis Sci. 2007;84(9):915–23. doi:10.1097/OPX.0b013e3181559d70.
7. Maldonado MJ, Nieto JC, Piñero DP. Advances in technologies for laser-assisted in situ keratomileusis (LASIK) surgery. Exp Rev Med Dev. 2008;5(2):209–29. doi:10.1586/17434440.5.2.209.
8. Maldonado MJ, Nieto JC, Diez-Cuenca M, Piñero DP. Repeatability and reproducibility of posterior corneal curvature measurements by combined scanning-slit and placido-disc topography after LASIK. Ophthalmology. 2006;113(11):1918–26. doi:10.1016/j.ophtha.2006.05.053.
9. Rand RH, Howland HC, Applegate RA. Mathematical model of a Placido disk keratometer and its implications for recovery of corneal topography. Optom Vis Sci. 1997;74(11):926–30.
10. Karpecki PM. Bausch & Lomb Orbscan II/IIz anterior segment analysis system. In: Wang M, editor. Corneal topography in the wavefront era. Thorofare: Slack Inc.; 2006.
11. Fernandez-Garcia P, Cervino A, Quiles-Guinau L, Albarran-Diego C, Garcia-Lazaro S, Sanchis-Gimeno JA. Corneal thickness differences between sexes after oxybuprocaine eye drops. Optom Vis Sci. 2015;92(1):89–94. doi:10.1097/opx.0000000000000449.
12. Merklinger HM. Focusing the view camera: a scientific way to focus the view camera and estimate depth of field. Canada: Paperback; 1993.
13. Cheng AC, Rao SK, Lam DS. Accuracy of Orbscan II in the assessment of posterior curvature in patients with myopic LASIK. J Refract Surg. 2007;23(7):677–80.
14. Nawa Y, Masuda K, Ueda T, Hara Y, Uozato H. Evaluation of apparent ectasia of the posterior surface of the cornea after keratorefractive surgery. J Cataract Refract Surg. 2005;31(3):571–3. doi:10.1016/j.jcrs.2004.05.050.
15. Piñero DP. Technologies for anatomical and geometric characterization of the corneal structure and anterior segment: a review. Semin Ophthalmol. 2013;30(3):161–70. doi:10.3109/08820538.2013.835844.
16. Dubbelman M, Sicam VA, Van der Heijde GL. The shape of the anterior and posterior surface of the aging human cornea. Vis Res. 2006;46(6–7):993–1001. doi:10.1016/j.visres.2005.09.021.
17. Piñero DP, Saenz Gonzalez C, Alió JL. Intraobserver and interobserver repeatability of curvature and aberrometric measurements of the posterior corneal surface in normal eyes using Scheimpflug photography. J Cataract Refract Surg. 2009;35(1):113–20. doi:10.1016/j.jcrs.2008.10.010.
18. Nasser CK, Singer R, Barkana Y, Zadok D, Avni I, Goldich Y. Repeatability of the Sirius imaging system and agreement with the Pentacam HR. J Refract Surg. 2012;28(7):493–7. doi:10.3928/1081597x-20120619-01.
19. Savini G, Barboni P, Carbonelli M, Hoffer KJ. Repeatability of automatic measurements by a new Scheimpflug camera combined with Placido topography. J Cataract Refract Surg. 2011;37(10):1809–16. doi:10.1016/j.jcrs.2011.04.033.
20. Salouti R, Nowroozzadeh MH, Zamani M, Fard AH, Niknam S. Comparison of anterior and posterior elevation map measurements between 2 Scheimpflug imaging systems. J Cataract Refract Surg. 2009;35(5):856–62. doi:10.1016/j.jcrs.2009.01.008.
21. Kanellopoulos AJ, Asimellis G. Forme fruste keratoconus imaging and validation via novel multi-spot reflection topography. Case Rep Ophthalmol. 2013;4(3):199–209. doi:10.1159/000356123.
22. Kanellopoulos AJ, Asimellis G. Clinical correlation between Placido, Scheimpflug and LED color reflection topographies in imaging of a scarred cornea. Case Rep Ophthalmol. 2014;5(3):311–7. doi:10.1159/000365962.

23. Klijn S, Reus NJ, Sicam VA. Evaluation of keratometry with a novel color-LED corneal topographer. J Refract Surg. 2015;31(4):249–56. doi:10.3928/1081597x-20150212-01.
24. Ambrosio Jr R, Caiado AL, Guerra FP, Louzada R, Roy AS, Luz A, et al. Novel pachymetric parameters based on corneal tomography for diagnosing keratoconus. J Refract Surg. 2011;27(10):753–8. doi:10.3928/1081597x-20110721-01.
25. Ambrosio Jr R, Valbon BF, Faria-Correia F, Ramos I, Luz A. Scheimpflug imaging for laser refractive surgery. Curr Opin Ophthalmol. 2013;24(4):310–20. doi:10.1097/ICU.0b013e3283622a94.
26. Buey Salas MA, Peris MC. Biomecánica y arquitectura corneal. Barcelona: Elsevier; 2014.
27. Wilson SE, Klyce SD, Husseini ZM. Standardized color-coded maps for corneal topography. Ophthalmology. 1993;100(11):1723–7.
28. Smolek MK, Klyce SD, Hovis JK. The Universal Standard Scale: proposed improvements to the American National Standards Institute (ANSI) scale for corneal topography. Ophthalmology. 2002;109(2):361–9.
29. Ambrosio Jr R, Nogueira LP, Caldas DL, Fontes BM, Luz A, Cazal JO, et al. Evaluation of corneal shape and biomechanics before LASIK. Int Ophthalmol Clin. 2011;51(2):11–38. doi:10.1097/IIO.0b013e31820f1d2d.
30. Rabinowitz YS. Tangential vs sagittal videokeratographs in the "early" detection of keratoconus. Am J Ophthalmol. 1996;122(6):887–9.
31. Chan JS, Mandell RB, Burger DS, Fusaro RE. Accuracy of videokeratography for instantaneous radius in keratoconus. Optom Vis Sci. 1995;72(11):793–9.
32. Szczotka LB, Thomas J. Comparison of axial and instantaneous videokeratographic data in keratoconus and utility in contact lens curvature prediction. CLAO J. 1998;24(1):22–8.
33. Hamano T. Lacrimal duct occlusion for the treatment of dry eye. Semin Ophthalmol. 2005;20(2):71–4. doi:10.1080/08820530590931133.
34. Khachikian SS, Belin MW. Posterior elevation in keratoconus. Ophthalmology 2009;116(4):816.e1; author reply -7. doi:10.1016/j.ophtha.2009.01.009.
35. de Sanctis U, Loiacono C, Richiardi L, Turco D, Mutani B, Grignolo FM. Sensitivity and specificity of posterior corneal elevation measured by Pentacam in discriminating keratoconus/subclinical keratoconus. Ophthalmology. 2008;115(9):1534–9. doi:10.1016/j.ophtha.2008.02.020.
36. Emre S, Doganay S, Yologlu S. Evaluation of anterior segment parameters in keratoconic eyes measured with the Pentacam system. J Cataract Refract Surg. 2007;33(10):1708–12. doi:10.1016/j.jcrs.2007.06.020.
37. Alió JL, Piñero DP, Aleson A, Teus MA, Barraquer RI, Murta J, et al. Keratoconus-integrated characterization considering anterior corneal aberrations, internal astigmatism, and corneal biomechanics. J Cataract Refract Surg. 2011;37(3):552–68. doi:10.1016/j.jcrs.2010.10.046.
38. Ambrosio Jr R, Alonso RS, Luz A, Coca Velarde LG. Corneal-thickness spatial profile and corneal-volume distribution: tomographic indices to detect keratoconus. J Cataract Refract Surg. 2006;32(11):1851–9. doi:10.1016/j.jcrs.2006.06.025.
39. Saad A, Gatinel D. Topographic and tomographic properties of forme fruste keratoconus corneas. Invest Ophthalmol Vis Sci. 2010;51(11):5546–55. doi:10.1167/iovs.10-5369.
40. Albertazzi R. Queratocono: pautas para su diagnóstico y tratamiento. Buenos Aires: Ediciones Científicas Argentinas; 2010.
41. Seiler T, Quurke AW. Iatrogenic keratectasia after LASIK in a case of forme fruste keratoconus. J Cataract Refract Surg. 1998;24(7):1007–9.
42. Binder PS, Lindstrom RL, Stulting RD, Donnenfeld E, Wu H, McDonnell P, et al. Keratoconus and corneal ectasia after LASIK. J Refract Surg. 2005;21(6):749–52.
43. Wollensak G, Spoerl E, Seiler T. Riboflavin/ultraviolet-a-induced collagen crosslinking for the treatment of keratoconus. Am J Ophthalmol. 2003;135(5):620–7.
44. Colin J, Cochener B, Savary G, Malet F. Correcting keratoconus with intracorneal rings. J Cataract Refract Surg. 2000;26(8):1117–22.
45. Torquetti L, Ferrara G, Almeida F, Cunha L, Araujo LP, Machado A, et al. Intrastromal corneal ring segments implantation in patients with keratoconus: 10-year follow-up. J Refract Surg. 2014;30(1):22–6.
46. Mahmoud AM, Roberts C, Lembach R, Herderick EE, McMahon TT. Simulation of machine-specific topographic indices for use across platforms. Optom Vis Sci. 2006;83(9):682–93. doi:10.1097/01.opx.0000232944.91587.02.
47. Holladay JT. Corneal topography using the Holladay Diagnostic Summary. J Cataract Refract Surg. 1997;23(2):209–21.
48. Calossi A. The optical quality of the cornea. In: Caimi F, Brancato R, editors. The aberrometers: theory, clinical and surgical applications. Canelli: Fabiano Editore; 2003.
49. Carney LG, Mainstone JC, Henderson BA. Corneal topography and myopia. A cross-sectional study. Invest Ophthalmol Vis Sci. 1997;38(2):311–20.
50. Piñero DP, Alió JL, Aleson A, Escaf Vergara M, Miranda M. Corneal volume, pachymetry, and correlation of anterior and posterior corneal shape in subclinical and different stages of clinical keratoconus. J Cataract Refract Surg. 2010;36(5):814–25. doi:10.1016/j.jcrs.2009.11.012.
51. Cavas-Martínez F, Fernández-Pacheco DG, De La Cruz-Sánchez E, Nieto Martínez J, Fernández Cañavate FJ, Vega-Estrada A, et al. Geometrical custom modeling of human cornea in vivo and its use for the diagnosis of corneal ectasia. PLoS One 2014;9(10):e110249. doi:10.1371/journal.pone.0110249.
52. Rabinowitz YS, McDonnell PJ. Computer-assisted corneal topography in keratoconus. Refract Corneal Surg. 1989;5(6):400–8.
53. Maeda N, Klyce SD, Smolek MK, Thompson HW. Automated keratoconus screening with corneal

topography analysis. Invest Ophthalmol Vis Sci. 1994;35(6):2749–57.
54. Smolek MK, Klyce SD. Current keratoconus detection methods compared with a neural network approach. Invest Ophthalmol Vis Sci. 1997;38(11):2290–9.
55. Dingeldein SA, Klyce SD, Wilson SE. Quantitative descriptors of corneal shape derived from computer-assisted analysis of photokeratographs. Refract Corneal Surg. 1989;5(6):372–8.
56. Wilson SE, Lin DT, Klyce SD. Corneal topography of keratoconus. Cornea. 1991;10(1):2–8.
57. Toprak I, Yaylali V, Yildirim C. A combination of topographic and pachymetric parameters in keratoconus diagnosis. Cont Lens Anterior Eye. 2015; 38(5):357–62. doi:10.1016/j.clae.2015.04.001.
58. Abad JC, Rubinfeld RS, Del Valle M, Belin MW, Kurstin JM. Vertical D: a novel topographic pattern in some keratoconus suspects. Ophthalmology. 2007;114(5): 1020–6. doi:10.1016/j.ophtha.2006.10.022.
59. Rabinowitz YS, Rasheed K. KISA% index: a quantitative videokeratography algorithm embodying minimal topographic criteria for diagnosing keratoconus. J Cataract Refract Surg. 1999;25(10):1327–35.
60. Chastang PJ, Borderie VM, Carvajal-Gonzalez S, Rostene W, Laroche L. Automated keratoconus detection using the EyeSys videokeratoscope. J Cataract Refract Surg. 2000;26(5):675–83.
61. Belin MW, Ambrosio R. Scheimpflug imaging for keratoconus and ectatic disease. Indian J Ophthalmol. 2013;61(8):401–6. doi:10.4103/0301-4738.116059.
62. Eklund A, Dufort P, Forsberg D, LaConte SM. Medical image processing on the GPU—past, present and future. Med Image Anal. 2013;17(8):1073–94. doi:10.1016/j.media.2013.05.008.
63. Sun W, Darling A, Starly B, Nam J. Computer-aided tissue engineering: overview, scope and challenges. Biotechnol Appl Biochem. 2004;39(1):29–47.
64. Farin G, Hoschek J, Kim MS. Handbook of computer aided geometric design. North Holland: Elsevier; 2002.
65. Cavas-Martínez F, Fernández-Pacheco DG, De La Cruz-Sánchez E, Nieto-Martínez J, Fernández-Cañavate F, Alió JL. Virtual biomodelling of a biologic structure: the human cornea. DYNA 2015;90(6):648–52. http://dx.doi.org/10.6036/7689.
66. Harris A, Guidoboni G, Arciero JC, Amireskandari A, Tobe LA, Siesky BA. Ocular hemodynamics and glaucoma: the role of mathematical modeling. Eur J Ophthalmol. 2013;23(2):139–46. doi:10.5301/ejo.5000255.
67. Velten K. Mathematical modeling and simulation: introduction for scientists and engineers. Weinheim: Wiley; 2008.
68. ANSI Z80.28-2004. Methods for reporting optical aberrations of eyes. New York: American National Standards Institute;2004.
69. Klyce SD, Karon MD, Smolek MK. Advantages and disadvantages of the Zernike expansion for representing wave aberration of the normal and aberrated eye. J Refract Surg. 2004;20(5):S537–41.
70. Schneider M, Iskander DR, Collins MJ. Modeling corneal surfaces with rational functions for high-speed videokeratoscopy data compression. IEEE Trans Biomed Eng. 2009;56(2):493–9. doi:10.1109/tbme.2008.2006019.
71. Espinosa J, Mas D, Perez J, Illueca C. Optical surface reconstruction technique through combination of zonal and modal fitting. J Biomed Opt. 2010;15(2):026022. doi:10.1117/1.3394260.
72. Dai GM. Comparison of wavefront reconstructions with Zernike polynomials and Fourier transforms. J Refract Surg. 2006;22(9):943–8.
73. Wang L, Chernyak D, Yeh D, Koch DD. Fitting behaviors of Fourier transform and Zernike polynomials. J Cataract Refract Surg. 2007;33(6):999–1004. doi:10.1016/j.jcrs.2007.03.017.
74. Yoon G, Pantanelli S, MacRae S. Comparison of Zernike and Fourier wavefront reconstruction algorithms in representing corneal aberration of normal and abnormal eyes. J Refract Surg. 2008;24(6):582–90.
75. Okrasiński W, Płociniczak Ł. A nonlinear mathematical model of the corneal shape. Nonlinear Anal Real World Appl. 2012;13(3):1498–505. doi:10.1016/j.nonrwa.2011.11.014.
76. Płociniczak L, Okrasiński W, Nieto JJ, Domínguez O. On a nonlinear boundary value problem modeling corneal shape. J Math Anal Appl. 2014;414(1):461–71. doi:10.1016/j.jmaa.2014.01.010.
77. Martinez-Finkelshtein A, Delgado AM, Castro GM, Zarzo A, Alió JL. Comparative analysis of some modal reconstruction methods of the shape of the cornea from corneal elevation data. Invest Ophthalmol Vis Sci. 2009;50(12):5639–45. doi:10.1167/iovs.08-3351.
78. Martinez-Finkelshtein A, Lopez DR, Castro GM, Alió JL. Adaptive cornea modeling from keratometric data. Invest Ophthalmol Vis Sci. 2011;52(8):4963–70. doi:10.1167/iovs.10-6774.
79. Ramos-Lopez D, Martinez-Finkelshtein A, Castro-Luna GM, Piñero D, Alió JL. Placido-based indices of corneal irregularity. Optom Vis Sci. 2011;88(10):1220–31. doi:10.1097/OPX.0b013e3182279ff8.
80. Accardo PA, Pensiero S. Neural network-based system for early keratoconus detection from corneal topography. J Biomed Inform. 2002;35(3):151–9.
81. Klyce SD, Karon MD, Smolek MK. Screening patients with the corneal navigator. J Refract Surg. 2005;21(5 Suppl):S617–22.
82. Souza MB, Medeiros FW, Souza DB, Garcia R, Alves MR. Evaluation of machine learning classifiers in keratoconus detection from Orbscan II examinations. Clinics (Sao Paulo). 2010;65(12):1223–8.
83. Arbelaez MC, Versaci F, Vestri G, Barboni P, Savini G. Use of a support vector machine for keratoconus and subclinical keratoconus detection by topographic and tomographic data. Ophthalmology. 2012;119(11):2231–8. doi:10.1016/j.ophtha.2012.06.005.
84. Valdes-Mas MA, Martin-Guerrero JD, Ruperez MJ, Pastor F, Dualde C, Monserrat C, et al. A new approach based on machine learning for predicting corneal curvature (K1) and astigmatism in patients with keratoconus after intracorneal ring implantation. Comput Methods Prog Biomed. 2014;116(1):39–47. doi:10.1016/j.cmpb.2014.04.003.

Geometrical Analysis of Corneal Topography

10

Francisco Cavas-Martínez, Ernesto De la Cruz Sánchez, José Nieto Martínez, Francisco J. Fernández Cañavate, and Daniel García Fernández-Pacheco

10.1 Introduction

Increased life expectancy has led to a growing demand of new technologies in the ophthalmologic clinic field, such as new medical imaging devices or increasing computer performance. All this makes the integration of engineering into clinical practice very appealing to, for instance, comprehend how organisms function [1], or to geometrically characterise tissues from a structural point of view [2].

The complexity of the cornea structure and its ocular globe shape, especially its singular architecture and metrics at both microscopically and macroscopically, are particularly challenging when developing a personalised geometric model of the cornea to represent any morphological variation that may occur when moving from a natural scenario to a pathological one [3].

Therefore, it is essential to know the geometry of the anterior and posterior corneal surfaces to diagnose any pathology related to morphological cornea alterations [4], and to thus decide posterior corrective treatment by either invasive or non-invasive techniques [5].

This chapter first describes the geometry of the cornea, then presents the topography concept and includes a brief description of the stages required to generate corneal topography. It ends by proposing a new geometrical analysis of the cornea, obtained from a personalised virtual solid model of the cornea.

10.2 Geometrical Analysis of the Cornea

Demand of the geometrical characterisation of the cornea in clinical practice has increasingly grown given the importance of its study for understanding that certain changes in the cornea can affect not only patients' visual acuity [6], evolution, diagnosis and treatment of determined corneal pathologies [7–9], but also planning ophthalmologic surgery [10, 11].

For this reason, the cornea must be studied in two different scenarios:

- Natural scenario, that is, absence of anomalous alterations (see Fig. 10.1). Here the tissues that form part of the corneal architecture are subjected to dynamic balance between intracorneal

F. Cavas-Martínez, Ph.D. (✉) • J. Nieto Martínez, Ph.D.
F.J. Fernández Cañavate, Ph.D.
D.G. Fernández-Pacheco
Department of Graphical Expression, Technical University of Cartagena, C/Doctor Fleming s/n, Cartagena, 30202 Murcia, Spain
e-mail: francisco.cavas@upct.es; jose.nieto@upct.es; francisco.canavate@upct.es; daniel.garcia@upct.es

E. De la Cruz Sánchez, Ph.D.
Faculty of Sports Science, University of Murcia, C/Santa Alicia s/n, Santiago de la Ribera, 30720, Murcia, Spain
e-mail: erneslacruz@um.es

J.L. Alió (ed.), *Keratoconus*, Essentials in Ophthalmology, DOI 10.1007/978-3-319-43881-8_10

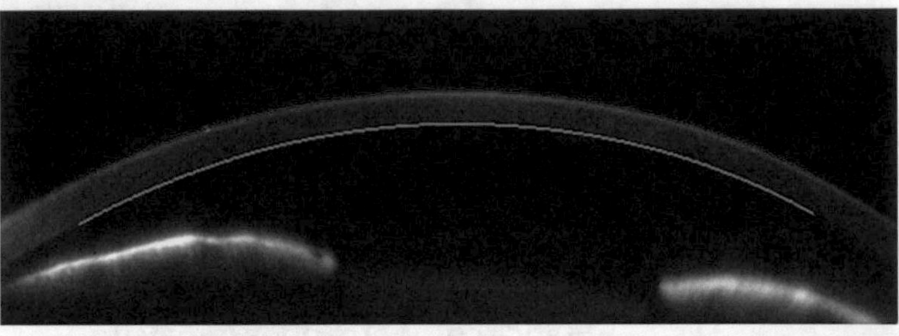

Fig. 10.1 Cornea in a natural scenario

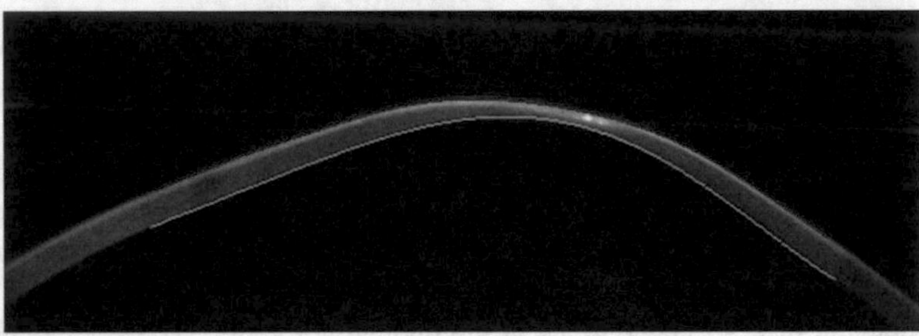

Fig. 10.2 Cornea in a pathological scenario

eye factors (apex, corneal thickness, etc.) and extracorneal eye factors (intraocular pressure, atmospheric pressure of the corneal anterior surface, etc.), when a balanced stress–strain behaviour is maintained (minimum energy status) and a singular geometrical style is achieved with a stable corneal surface curvature and optimum optical power [12].

- Pathological scenario, that is, presence of anomalous alterations (see Fig. 10.2), in which the tissues that form part of the corneal architecture display structural weakness due to a pathological process, as in ectatic pathological diseases like keratoconus [13]. This weakened structure is manifested clinically by an alteration to the cornea's surface morphology. This implies redistributing the corneal pachymetry, changes in the surface geometry and loss of optical power [14].

10.2.1 Geometry of the Cornea: Natural Scenario

In the natural scenario (see Fig. 10.1), the cornea presents corneal surface regularity, which makes it act as a lens and confers the cornea the ability to act as the most important refractive element of the eye scheme. Thus, the anterior corneal surface is responsible for two-thirds of the human eye's total optical power at the highest point of the cornea, known as the corneal apex (see Fig. 10.3).

A healthy cornea presents the following morphological characteristics:

- On the anterior surface, its surface presents an average curvature of between 7.75 and 7.89 mm [14–16], with an average curvature of 7.79 mm in the centre [17].
- On the posterior surface, its surface presents an average curvature of between 6.34 and 6.48 mm [14–16], and an average curvature of 6.53 mm in the centre [17, 18].

Between both surfaces, pachymetry or corneal thickness is defined with an average value in its geometrical centre of about 0.54 mm [14, 18, 19].

Several works in the scientific literature have demonstrated that the average curvature and corneal thickness values remain stable in the natural scenario [18].

Besides the aforementioned parameters, cornea characterisation implies knowing the morphology

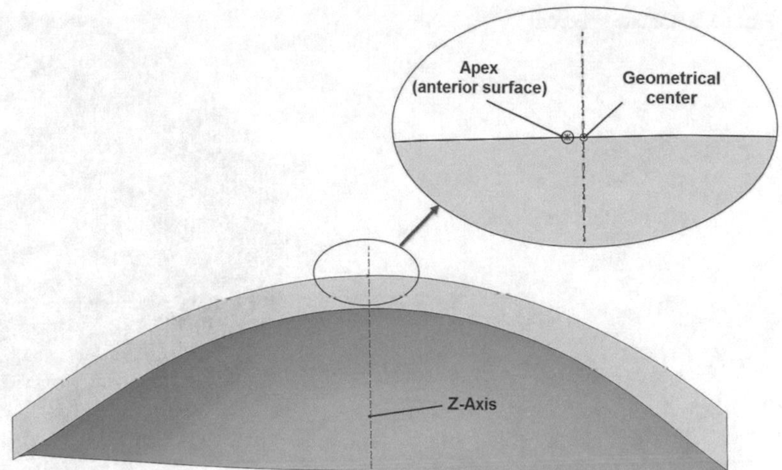

Fig. 10.3 Corneal apex

of the anterior and posterior cornea surfaces. From a geometrical point of view, surfaces are similar to a spheroid, which is a geometrical shape whose generatrix is obtained when an ellipse revolves around one of its main axes. This shape has two axes: the symmetry axis, located on the Cartesian coordinate axis, denoted with a letter 'c'; the axis perpendicular to the symmetry axis, denoted with a letter 'a'. Letters 'c' and 'a' are defined on the spheroid by international convention (see Fig. 10.4).

The spheroid can simulate three different configurations according to the relation between its main axes '*c*' and '*a*':

- Oblate spheroid: if $a>c$, the symmetry axis is the smallest (see Fig. 10.5).
- Prolate spheroid: if $a<c$, the symmetry axis is the largest (see Fig. 10.6).
- Sphere: if $a=c$; the symmetry axis is equal (see Fig. 10.7). This is a special case because the surface generated by the generatrix is a sphere; consequently, this curve is not an ellipse, but a circumference.

All this can be extrapolated to the ophthalmology field, where the cornea displays similar geometrical behaviour to an elliptic profile [6]:

$$X^2 - Y^2 + (1+Q)\, Z^2 - 2ZR = 0 \quad (10.1)$$

This equation presents three spatial coordinates (*X*, *Y*, *Z*), on the basis of which the cornea can be

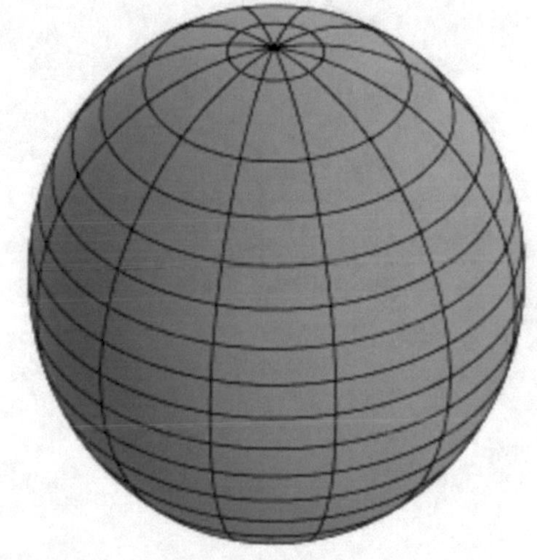

Fig. 10.4 Spheroid

interpreted as a three-dimensional refractive element by the following three parameters (see Fig. 10.8):

- Corneal asphericity (*Q*): a parameter that characterises the nature of the conical curve, represented by the mathematical expression.
- The known revolution axis (*Z*).
- Conoid radius (*R*): the radius of the highest point of the anterior corneal surface (corneal apex).

Corneal asphericity is defined as the degree of curvature, or slope, of the cornea from the central

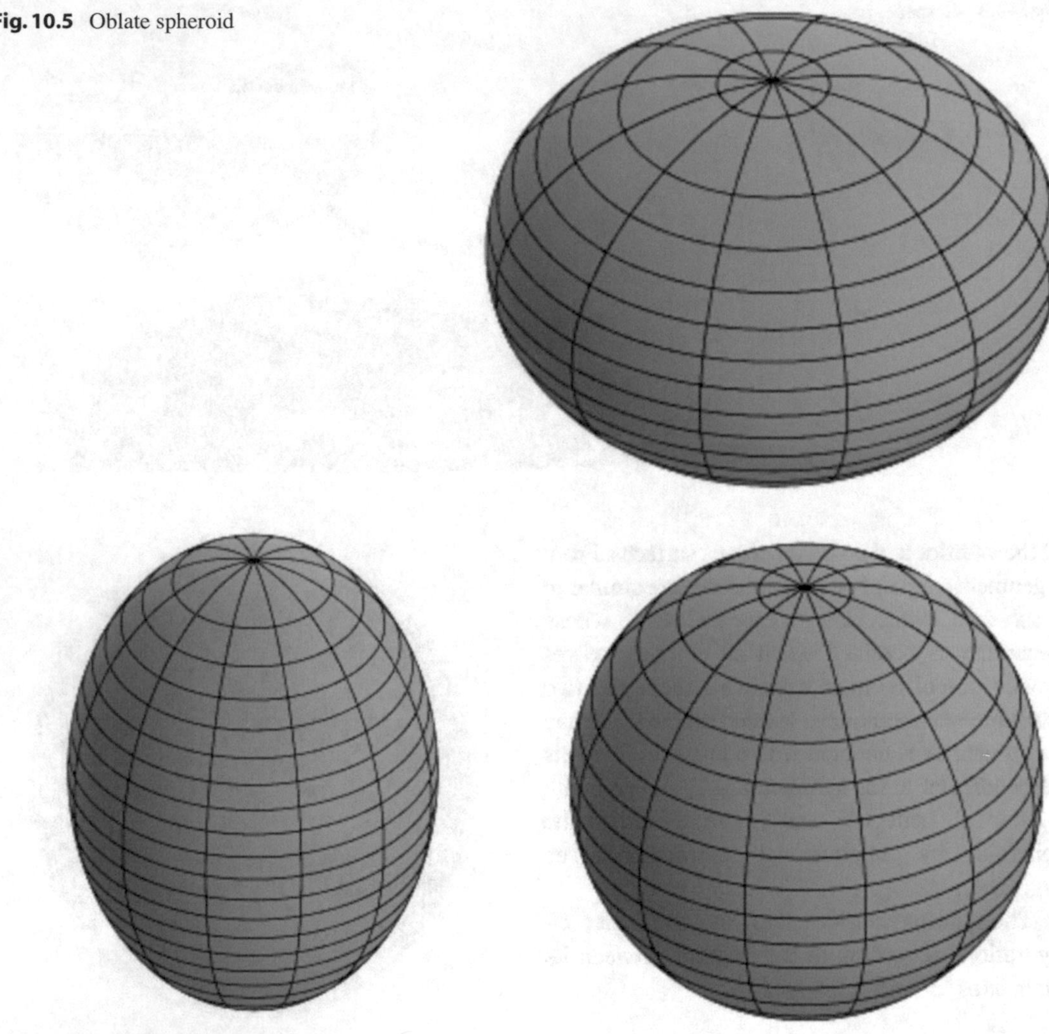

Fig. 10.5 Oblate spheroid

Fig. 10.6 Prolate spheroid

Fig. 10.7 Sphere

region to the peripheral region. This slope can present a plainer tendency (a geometrical scenario for a healthy cornea) or a more curved state (a geometrical scenario for a pathological cornea) (see Fig. 10.9).

The corneal asphericity coefficient (Q) can be mathematically calculated using the relation between the central (b) and peripheral (a) hemiaxes of the corneal elliptic profile (see Fig. 10.9).

In light of the earlier, the elliptic profile of the corneal surface can be classified as:

- Spherical ($Q=0$). A singular case in which the horizontal or peripheral (a), and central or vertical (b) hemi-axes of the ellipse are equal, that is, the corneal surface has the same curvature in the central region as in the peripheral zone.
- Prolate ellipse ($0>Q>-1$). In this case the elliptic profile of the corneal surface flattens as it moves away from the highest point of the corneal surface (the apex). This behaviour occurs in a natural scenario which, from a refractive point of view, implies the cornea having a low spherical aberration.
- Oblate ellipse ($Q>0$). In this other case, the elliptic profile of the corneal surface becomes more curved as it moves away from

the corneal apex. This behaviour occurs in a pathological scenario which, from a refractive point of view, implies the cornea having a spherical aberration, which is proportional to the Q factor.

- Parabola or hyperbola ($Q \leq -1$). This is an exceptional case in healthy eyes and is exclusive in central ectatic cornea pathologies. From the refractive surface viewpoint, the cornea has a negative spherical aberration index, which is also proportional to Q factor.

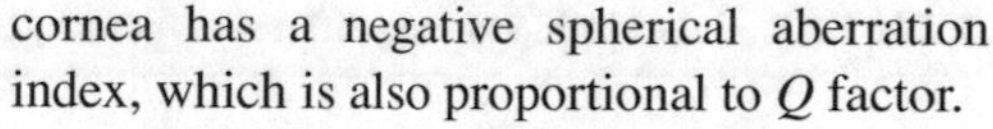

Apart from the aforementioned asphericity, the degree of cornea curvature can also be expressed according to other factors, for instance:

- Eccentricity factor (e):

$$e = -\sqrt{Q} \tag{10.2}$$

- Shape factor (p)

$$p = 1 - e^2 \text{ or } p = Q + 1 \tag{10.3}$$

They are all interrelated (see Table **10.1**).

In addition, the corneal elliptical cross-section profile is defined according to the central curvature radius (Rc) (see Fig. 10.10), thus:

$$p = \left(\frac{b}{a}\right)^2 = \text{Rc} / a \tag{10.4}$$

$$Q = p - 1 \tag{10.5}$$

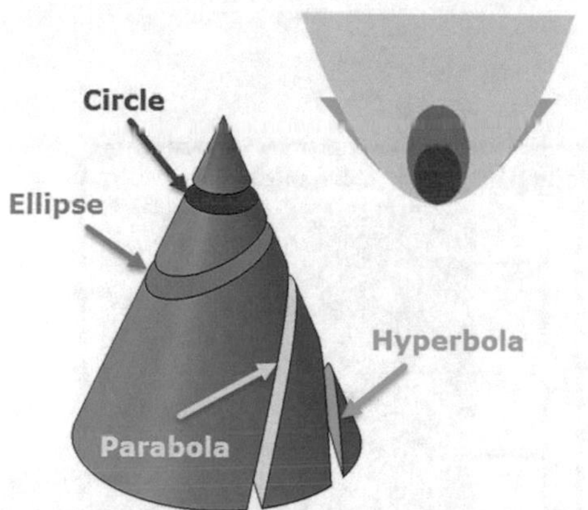

Fig. 10.8 Sections for different types of conical curves

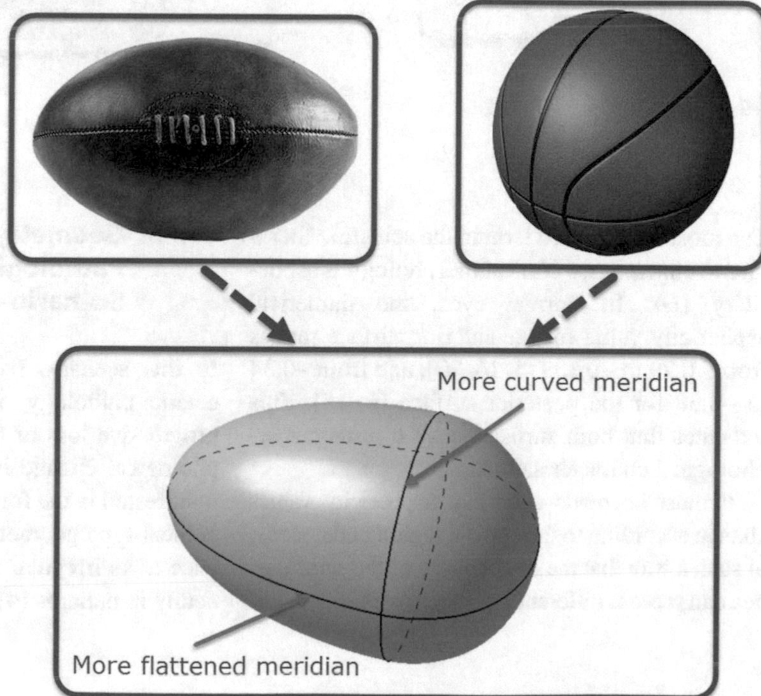

Fig. 10.9 Asphericity. Concept

Table 10.1 Relationship among different types of geometric curves of the cornea in function of several parameters

Cornea profile	Eccentricity e^2	Form factor $p=1-e^2$ $p=Q+1$	Asphericity $Q=-e^2$
Sphere	$e^2=1$	$p=1$	$Q=0$
Oblate ellipse	$e^2<1$	$p>1$	$Q>0$
Prolate ellipse	$0<e^2<1$	$0<p<1$	$1<Q<0$
Parabola	$e^2=1$	$p=0$	$Q=-1$
Hyperbola	$e^2>1$	$p<0$	$Q<-1$

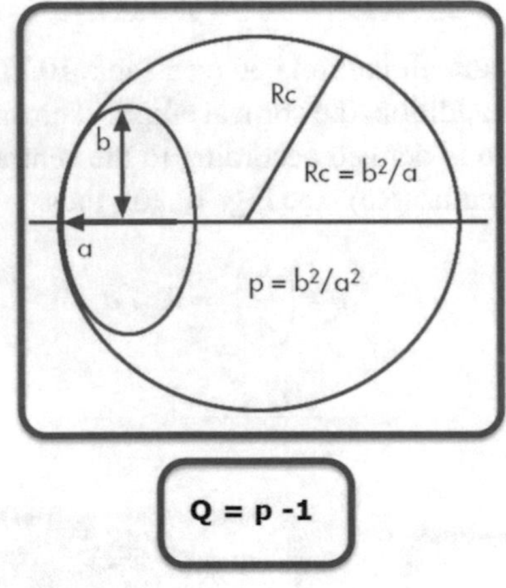

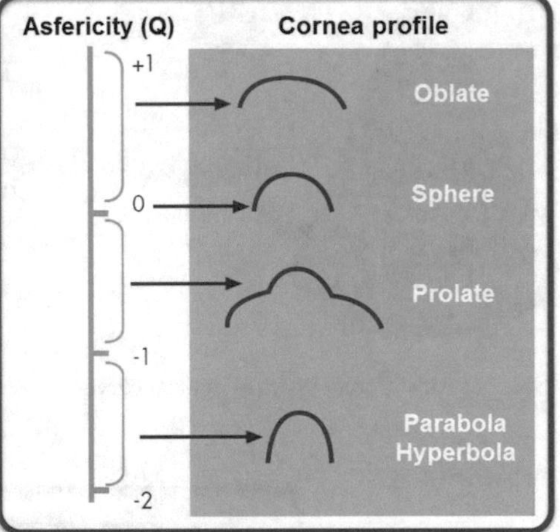

Fig. 10.10 Corneal asphericity

The most widely used term in the scientific literature to characterise corneal morphology is asphericity (Q). In normal eyes, the numerical asphericity value for the anterior surface ranges from −0.29 to −0.13 [15, 16, 20], and from −0.34 to −0.38 for the posterior surface [6, 15]. This indicates that both surfaces have a prolate morphological characterisation.

It must be made clear that asphericity values change according to the corneal region under study, in such a way that the morphology of the same cornea can present different asphericity values.

10.2.2 Geometry of the Cornea: Pathological Scenario—Keratoconus

In this scenario (see Fig. 10.2), the bilateral ectatic pathology, named keratoconus, causes progressive loss of corneal thickness. This morphological change in the corneal architecture is manifested in the form of protrusion. It presents a conical-type geometry which causes the appearance of an irregular astigmatism or loss of visual acuity in patients [4].

This protrusion creates thinning, which affects the tissues that form part of the corneal architecture. This situation occurs progressively as the degree of disease severity advances, leading to morphological changes that follow a characteristic pattern which is related to a structural weakening of the tissues that make up the cornea (see Fig. 10.11). From the geometric perspective, keratoconus may give way to several keratoconus subtypes according to cone size and shape [21], these being [4]:

- Nipple. The corneal topography analysis presents a cone-like morphology with a diameter of roughly 5 mm that affects at least 50 % of the corneal area. Its morphology becomes rounded and curved, but the rest of the corneal surface takes its natural form. The apex is located in the central or paracentral area, but can sometimes shift inferonasally.
- Oval. The corneal topography analysis presents a larger sized cone than the nipple kind; it affects one quadrant or two, and is generally located in the inferotemporal area. Its morphology is ellipsoid-type.
- Globe. This morphology practically covers the whole corneal area because it presents an extension of more than 6 mm in diameter. This morphology is characterised by generalised thinning.
- Astigmatism. This characterisation presents a conical protrusion characterised by vertical bow tie-type astigmatism whose asymmetry is inferosuperior, and frequently more curved in the upper area, thus affects less than 50 % of the corneal area.

This cone-based classification serves in particular to describe cone extension and to classify keratoconus according to its shape. However, it offers no information about corneal pathology severity.

The scientific literature offers many publications that employ corneal topography techniques to represent the typical topographical patterns of the disease [4, 13, 22–25] (see Fig. 10.12).

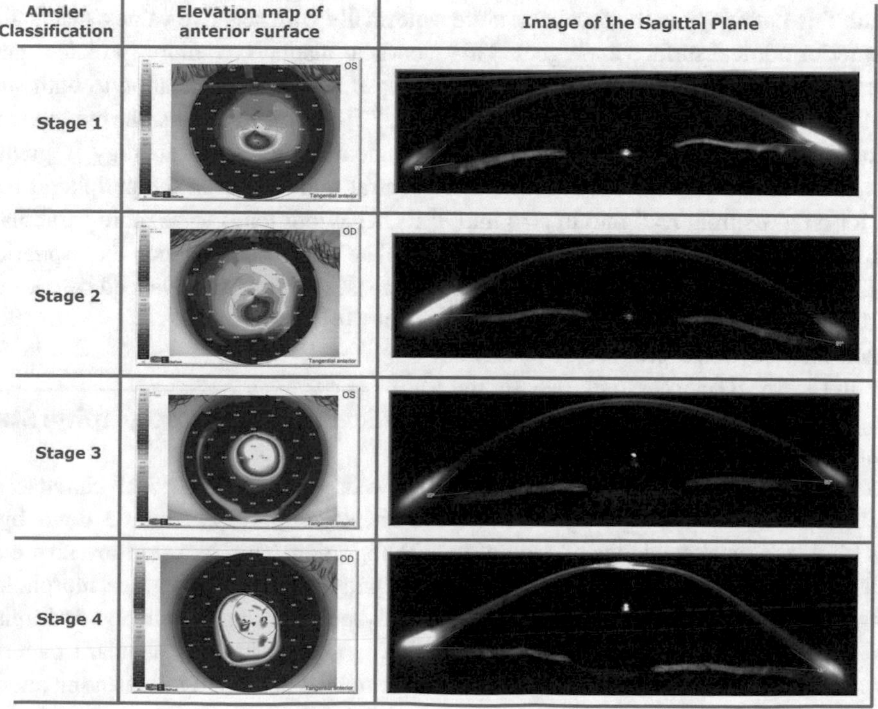

Fig. 10.11 Severity grade of keratoconus according Amsler-Krumeich classification [4]

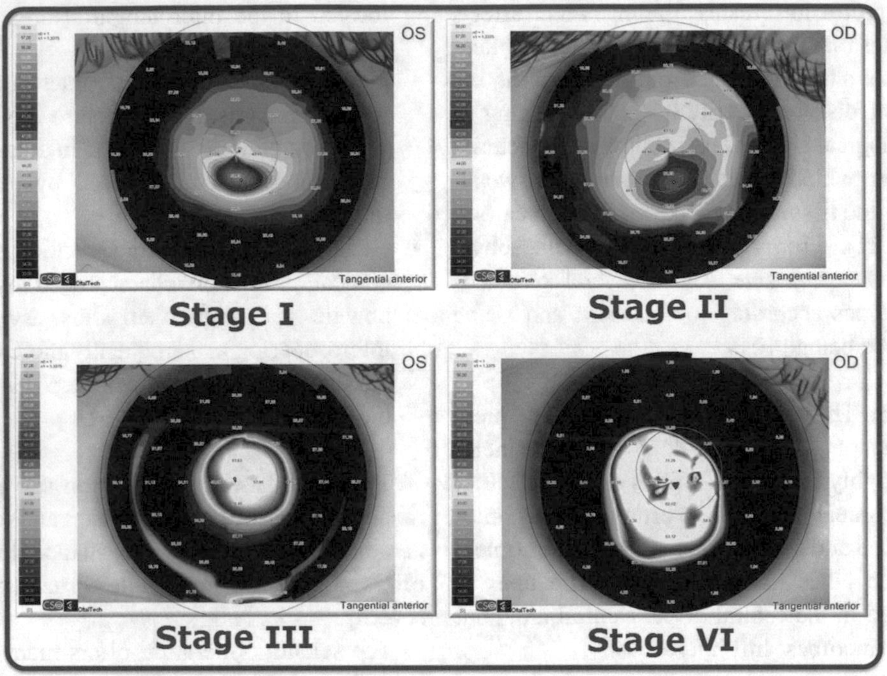

Fig. 10.12 Keratoconus characteristic topographical patterns

One of the main morphological characteristics that the corneal architecture presents and is related with this pathology is the focal curvature that the anterior corneal surface undergoes. This protrusion is more frequently manifested, in fact in 72 % of cases, in the paracentral region, and in the central region in around 25 % of cases. Therefore, 97 % of cases with keratoconus are localised for a radius from $r=0$ mm to $r=4$ mm, which include the central and paracentral corneal regions [24]. Presence of a protrusion in the peripheral region is considered unusual [26, 27].

The increased curvature produced by keratoconus in the corneal morphology due to the weakening of the tissues that form part of the corneal architecture not only affects the anterior corneal surface, but also the posterior corneal surface, even in incipient or early stage keratoconus cases [4, 27]. Thus, knowledge of geometric behaviour of posterior corneal surface is most interesting in the ophthalmology field to early diagnose keratoconus [28–30] (see Fig. 10.2).

Another differentiating element of the keratoconic cornea exists: a parameter that characterises the nature of the conical curve or asphericity. In this scenario, variation in asphericity occurs on the anterior/posterior corneal surfaces, and normally with negative values; that is, the healthy cornea displays a more prolated geometrical ellipse behaviour in relation to both surfaces [6, 31, 32]. Based on all this, the curvature of a pathological cornea's morphology is greater in the central region than in the peripheral region, and its behaviour tends to be more parabola like than prolate ellipse like. Hence the asphericity value increases with more advanced degrees of keratoconus [4].

10.3 Corneal Topography: Stages

Nowadays, the geometrical characterisation of corneal morphology can be done by Corneal Topography. This is a non-invasive exploratory technique that allows cornea morphology to be analysed both quantitatively and qualitatively and is able to identify standard patterns and to rule out the potentially devastating alterations for eyesight that derive from ectatic pathological disorders [9, 33–36].

Topography is performed with equipment known as corneal topographers (see Fig. 10.13). These instruments are widely used by the ophthalmological medical community and allow anatomical and geometrical corneal characterisation based on its surface reconstruction [35].

Today's corneal topographers are based on two technologies: (1) systems based on light reflected on the cornea; (2) systems based on slit light projected on the cornea. In turn, they both present a standard photographic system or are based on Scheimpflug's photography principle.

Corneal topographers are based on the above-described technologies (see Fig. 10.13) and provide different topographic maps of the anterior and posterior corneal surfaces, pachymetry maps, and summary indices to follow-up and clinically evaluate corneal topographies.

They also contemplate two clearly different stages to present the data obtained from corneal topography to doctors, who can use them as a basis to clinically diagnose corneal ectasis:

- The first stage corresponds to the internal data collection and processing procedure.
- The second stage corresponds to geometric corneal surface reconstruction and to corneal topography generation.

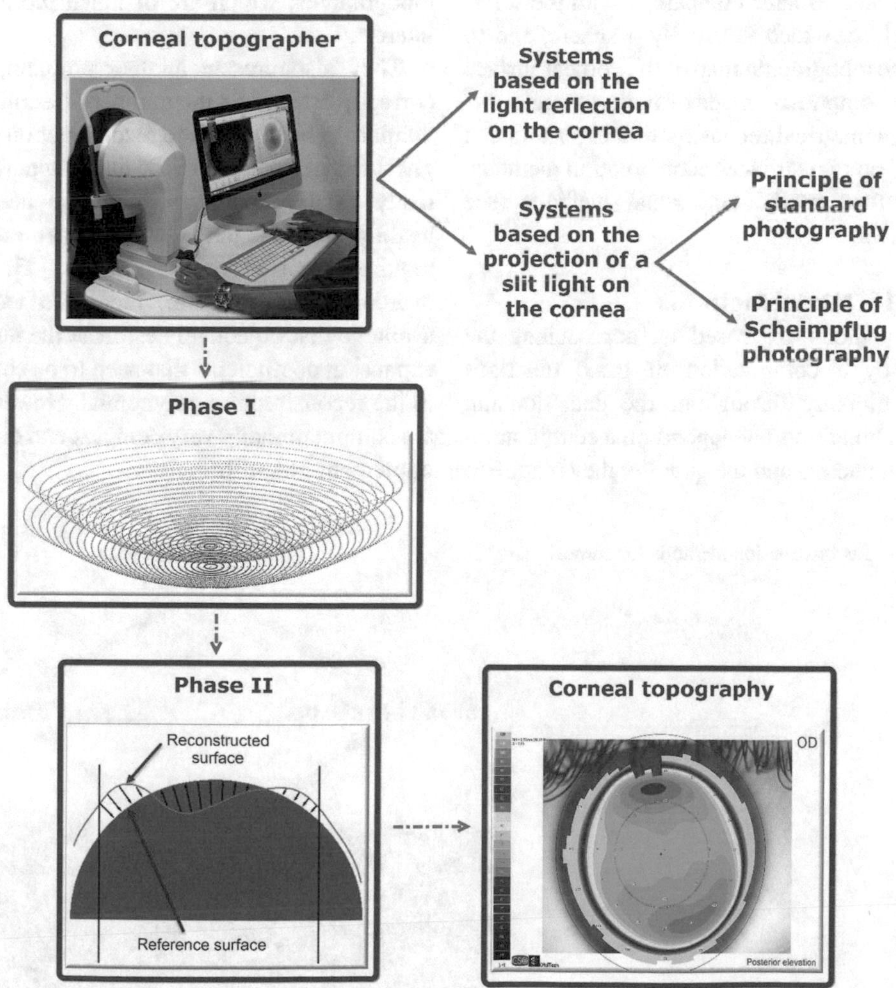

Fig. 10.13 Phases of a corneal topographer

10.3.1 Stage I: Internal Data Collection and Processing

In this stage topographers obtain altimetry data, as a matrix of elevations, on a discrete and finite set of points that is representative of the corneal surface, known as raw data.

10.3.2 Stage II: Geometric Corneal Surface Reconstruction—Corneal Topography Generation

In this second stage, by using the data that form the matrix of elevations, the corneal surface is reconstructed to later compare it with the reference surface, which is usually a sphere, and to obtain the topographic map of the corneal surface from the comparison made of both surfaces.

The geometrical reconstruction algorithm can be based on two surface reconstruction methods: the so-called modal and zonal methods (see Fig. 10.14).

10.3.2.1 Modal Methods

Modal methods are based on approaching the surface by a combination of basic functions defined globally throughout the data domain. This combination may depend on a certain number of parameters and the quantity they require to retrieve relevant information about the surface in an attempt to avoid overfitting their measurement error [37].

In the ophthalmology field, most of the modal methods used for surface reconstruction from standard heights employ Zernike's polynomials-based developments [38–40], where expansion coefficients are interpreted in terms of the basic aberrations or degradation in the image in optic systems [41, 42].

However, this procedure entails a series of problems that have been well discussed in the scientific literature [37, 43–45]. In particular, there is growing concern about this method being inaccurate in abnormal situations as it does not obtain a reliable reconstruction in complex topographies, which are of much more clinical interest.

They also present another problem, that of correctly estimating the number of Zernike polynomials to be used in the reconstruction process: given the general nature of their support, a relatively small number of them are needed for healthy corneas, but a much larger number is required for pathological corneas [43, 46]. To overcome this problem, there are techniques available that objectively estimate the number of expansion coefficients that need to be considered in the reconstruction polynomial. However, they are computationally very complex and difficult to implement [47, 48].

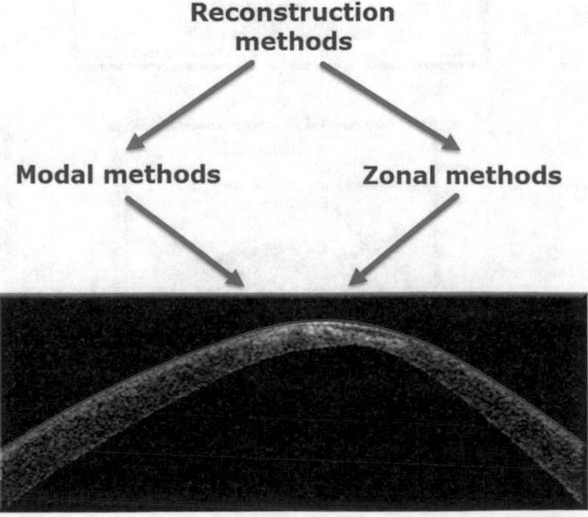

Fig. 10.14 Reconstruction methods for corneal surface

Regarding the earlier problems, some alternative techniques have been proposed in the literature:

- Reconstruction by discrete or continuous Fourier transform [49–51].
- Reconstruction using least squares model fitting [40].
- Non-linear reconstruction by rational functions [39].
- Reconstruction based on radial basis functions [37, 52, 53].
- Reconstruction using contour problems to model the corneal surface [54, 55].

However, they all entail the same problems as Zernike, and even with other ones, such as high computational complexity when dealing with residual errors, or obtaining controversial results.

10.3.2.2 Zonal Methods

In zonal methods the data domain is divided into more elemental subdomains, and the surface is approached in each subdomain, defined independently of the others [37, 40].

This reconstruction method is characterised as it presents a flexible and accurate fitting when considering data inside a zone delimited for the calculation of a surface point. This means that representation is local, and therefore local irregularities do not affect the global surface representation, unlike the global functions adopted in modal reconstruction as high-order quadratic or polynomial surfaces, which lack local information. Hence local surface irregularities or defects cannot be suitably represented by these approaches [3, 56].

The mostly widely used tool is Splines [57], especially B-Splines [3, 45, 58], which are numerically stable and flexible functions that offer good fit accuracy [59, 60].

B-Spline functions have been widely used in engineering to solve geometrical and computational problems which appear when we wish to use entities that are highly complex in geometric terms [59, 60].

In the ophthalmology field, these B-Spline functions have been successfully employed in the following applications:

- Topographical corneal surface characterisation [3, 56, 61–63].
- Eye ball characterisation [64].
- Designing optic lenses to treat keratoconus [65].
- Designing an ocular surface prosthesis for a so-called keratoglobus corneal pathology [66].

In short, depending on the descriptions of the models and the previously mentioned purposes, and given the singular nature of corneal surface morphology, creating a model that offers the advantages of zonal reconstruction models by B-Spline functions based on Computer-Aided Geometrical Design (CAGD) is interesting for real corneal morphology characterisation. This model could, in turn, also be used to diagnose certain pathologies that relate to corneal morphology modifications, such as keratoconus.

10.4 Geometrical Model of the Cornea

Generating a geometric corneal model using CAGD tools requires representative points of corneal morphology for the reconstruction of the whole corneal surface and the subsequent generation of a solid representative model of the human cornea.

Some corneal topographers can export these points, specifically from the aforementioned first data collection stage. Such data correspond to a matrix of elevations that is representative of the corneal surface, known in the scientific literature as raw data, which can be obtained by an internal vision algorithm of the corneal topographer [2, 3, 37, 67–69].

Some authors have conducted works using these raw data, e.g. geometrical cornea characterisation done by evaluating corneal symmetry with shape and position parameters [68]; developing a personalised biomechanical model by obtaining the patient's geometry [2, 67, 69]. Both these works were performed using Cartesian coordinates (*x*, *y*, *z*), provided by a Pentacam topographer. However, in both cases, raw data were interpolated given the above-cited extrinsic examiner–team–patient trinomial problems, which affected the measurement process. In order to obtain the representative spatial points of the whole corneal area, such data interpolation would imply them being biased. This would imply that throughout the process of reconstructing the whole corneal surface, minor morphological alterations caused by an incipient degree of the corneal pathology, such as keratoconus, not to be reliably reproduced.

To date, only raw spatial data obtained from the EyeTop 2005 corneal topographer (CSO, Italy) without them being interpolated have been considered in anterior cornea surface reconstructions [37], and also in the reconstruction of the anterior and posterior corneal surfaces [3] conducted with the data supplied by the Sirius corneal topographer (CSO, Italy).

Therefore with these data and CAGD tools, the corneal surface is reconstructed and the solid model of a human cornea is generated.

10.4.1 Computer-Aided Geometrical Design

In recent years, major technological progress has been made thanks to both the generation of virtual models and new computation tools to acquire and process images [1]. These have enabled 3D shapes to be produced [70], and performance models to be formulated that more reliably reproduce the geometry of a solid structure [71].

One of these tools is CAGD, which emerged when attempting to meet the technological requirements of companies in the automobile and aeronautics sectors. CAGD allows us to study geometrical and computational aspects of any complex physical entity, e.g. surfaces and volumes, to produce virtual models [72], which differ from physical models as they do not imply a destructive process, and reduce both production and time costs [73, 74].

In the bioengineering field, the development of virtual models by CAGD allows the characterisation of biological structures by establishing new experimental procedures in the field of medicine [71] for different purposes:

- Clinical diagnosis and subsequent treatment of a pathology using either invasive or non-invasive techniques [75–77].
- Analysis of behaviour in a pathological scenario by numerical methods [78–80].
- Educational purposes by generating virtual 3D models [81] or by obtaining a physical model with 3D printers [82].

In the optics field, some models have been found which propose using CAGD to generate only the corneal surface and to perform its posterior optical analysis with the spatial points obtained by corneal topographers to be used later by the aforementioned conical or biconical functions [83–85], or using the images taken of the incisions made ex vivo to chicken eyes [86, 87]. In both cases, however, the produced cornea model was incomplete because, in order to generate the cloud of the points that constitute the corneal surface, which will be subsequently reconstructed by CAGD, data were interpolated, and only the corneal surface of optic interest was reconstructed. The use of CAGD tools allowed us to define and adopt a new methodology [3], which guarantees that the data employed for geometric reconstruction did not undergo any type of preprocessing or interpolation, which that could avoid quite accurately detecting minor distortions formed on both corneal surfaces due to keratoconus.

10.5 Geometric Reconstruction of the Cornea

The geometric reconstruction process of the cornea defined by the authors proposes carrying out the following stages in sequence (Fig. 10.15): (1) Obtaining the representative point clouds of the

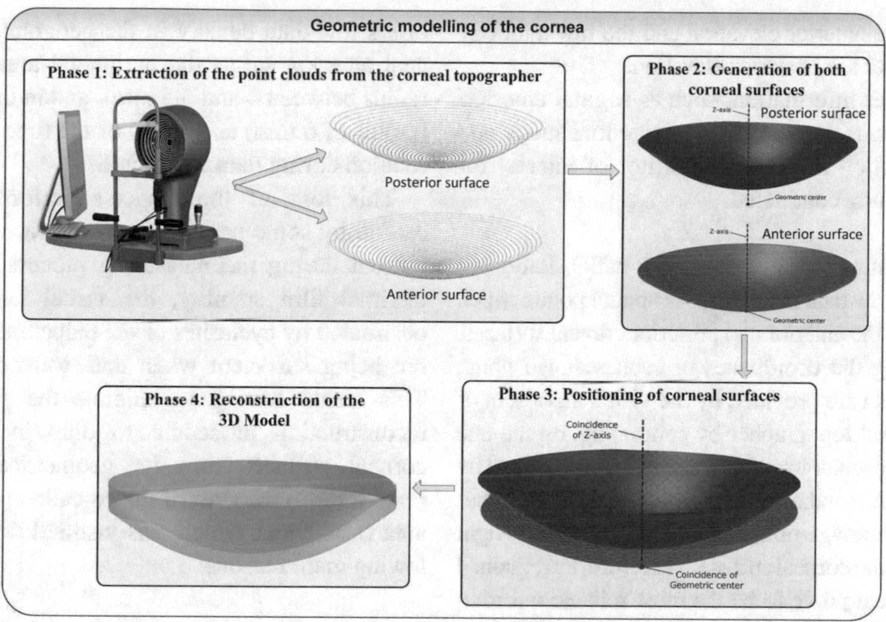

Fig. 10.15 Scheme for 3D geometric reconstruction of the cornea

corneal surfaces, (2) geometrically reconstructing the corneal surfaces and (3) generating a representative solid model of the cornea.

10.5.1 Obtaining the Point Clouds

The reconstruction process is based on generating a surface using the geometry that the point cloud presents in a system of three-dimensional coordinates in space, which normally takes a Cartesian coordinates format. This geometric reconstruction technique is not new to the biomedical engineering domain as it has already been successfully used to reconstruct other parts of the human body [88, 89].

For this process to reconstruct the point clouds of the geometry of the anterior and posterior corneal surfaces, a Sirius corneal topographer (CSO, Italy) was resorted to, which provides a CSV file that contains the following information for each patient:

- The radii of Placido's disc rings (in mm). This measurement includes 31 radii values taken in 0.2-mm intervals which cover the whole corneal area, that is, from $r=0$ mm to $r=6$ mm.
- Raw altimetry data of the anterior elevation (in µm). This is a matrix of elevations formed by the 31 rows that correspond to 31 radii of Placido's disc rings, and by the 256 columns that correspond to the 256 points that the topographer measures per ring. In all, the matrix provides 7936 altimetry values that are representative of the anterior corneal surface.
- Raw altimetry data of the posterior elevation (in µm). This is a matrix of elevations formed by the 31 rows that correspond to 31 radii of Placido's disc rings, and by the 256 columns that correspond to the 256 points that the topographer measures per ring. In all, the matrix provides 7936 altimetry values that are representative of the posterior corneal surface.
- Corneal thickness data (in µm). This is a matrix formed by the 31 rows that correspond to 31 radii of Placido's disc rings, and by the 256 columns that correspond to the 256 points that can be measured by each ring. In all, the matrix provides 7936 corneal thickness values, obtained by the difference between the raw altimetry data

for the anterior elevation and the raw altimetry data for the posterior elevation.

- Further information, such as sagittal anterior/posterior corneal maps, tangential maps and refraction maps, which is not of interest for the study conducted.

A Sirius corneal topographer (CSO, Italy) can provide raw data in the form of spatial points which make up the anterior and posterior corneal surfaces, indicating the coordinates of each scanned point. These data are provided by the vision algorithm of the corneal topographer by combining, on the one hand, a specular image of Placido's disc obtained by a reflection on the corneal surface and, on the other hand, the image obtained by projecting a slit light on the same corneal surface. Therefore, the obtained spatial data prove to be the most reliable information that can be used for geometric modelling since they have not been manipulated or processed by any of the equipment's internal software algorithms [37]. For this reason the described reconstruction procedure employs only raw data.

However, the topographic data in the CSV file take a polar format, where each row represents a circle or a ring on the map, and each column represents a semi-meridian, providing 256 points for each cornea radius (from $r=0$ to 6 mm in 0.2-mm intervals). Thus, each ith row samples a map on a radius circle, i*0.2 mm, and each jth column samples a map on a semi-meridian in the j*360/256° direction. So each Z value in the $[i, j]$ matrix represents point P (i*0.2, j*360/256°) in the polar coordinates.

For the purpose of converting the data supplied by the CSV file with a polar format into a point cloud with a Cartesian format (X, Y, Z), which is representative of both the anterior and posterior corneal surfaces, an algorithm was implemented in Matlab.

During the conversion process it was verified that not all the points provided by the CSV file correctly represented the anterior and posterior corneal surfaces since some points were detected whose elevation value appeared with an out-of-range value ($Z=-1000$), which indicated that the point had not been properly scanned.

This demonstrates something previously known: a Sirius corneal topographer (CSO, Italy) offers low data density in the geographical corneal area known as the peripheral area (with a radius between 4 and 5.5 mm), and in the limbus (radius of 6 mm) as a result of the time spent on rotation during data collection.

This loss of the device's performance is caused by some patient's extrinsic factors being present during the measuring process, such as lacrimal film stability, the visual field being obstructed by eyelashes or the palpebral aperture not being sufficient when data were collected. This meant having to redefine the geometric reconstruction procedure to only include the corneal surface from its geometrical centre ($r=0$ mm) to the start of the so-called peripheral area ($r=4$ mm), which was justified for the following main reasons:

- Geometrical principle. A Sirius corneal topographer allows all the points making up the corneal geometry in the region defined for the reconstruction to be obtained ($r=0$ to 4 mm). It specifically permitted 10,752 spatial points to be obtained, which corresponded to both the anterior and posterior corneal surfaces (5376 points each surface) per patient, which included both healthy and diseased corneas.
- Clinical principle. The defined corneal surface ($r=0$ to 4 mm) was considered to present more information about the corneal morphology for both healthy and diseased eyes. This area included both the so-called central zone ($r=0$ to 2 mm), which corresponded to the most spherical zone with the best visual repercussion and concentrated 25 % of keratoconus cases, and the so-called paracentral zone ($r=2$ to 4 mm), which corresponded to the zone where the cornea starts to flatten and concentrated 72 % of keratoconus cases [24]. All in all, the morphology of the area to undergo geometric reconstruction ($r=0$ to 4 mm) was irregular on both the anterior and posterior surfaces, and comprised 97 % of keratoconus cases.

Having obtained the representative point clouds of both corneal surfaces, from $r=0$ mm to

$r = 4$ mm, the next stage was to import this point clouds to a software that allows the reliable and accurate reconstruction of both surfaces.

10.5.2 Geometric Reconstruction of Corneal Surfaces

The point clouds representative of cornea geometry are later imported by the surface reconstruction software Rhinoceros®, v5.0 (Fig. 10.16). This software uses a mathematical model to generate surfaces based on non-uniform rational B-splines (NURBS) [60], where the surface generated from these spatial points is characterised by progressing in two parametric directions, *u* and *v*. These types of surfaces are invariant with similar transformations—or perspective transformations—and offer flexibility to design a wide range of surfaces with very little computational cost if compared with other methods.

Among the functions that the earlier software offers, the so-called "Patch" surface reconstruction function is that which offers the best fit to the point cloud. This is a reconstruction function that fits a surface by curves, meshes, point objects, and previously provided point clouds [90]. This function aims to minimise the nominal distance between the spatial point cloud and the solution surface. For this purpose, configuring this function by fixing the spacing between the sampling points to 256 (the number of points per data ring) is recommended, done by defining 255 surface segments for both directions *U* and *V* (the maximum number of segments that the software allows), and by fixing solution surface rigidity to 10^{-3} mm, a parameter that provides information about the degree that the best fitting plane can be distorted to guarantee it containing the input points.

After applying the "Patch" function to the point clouds of both corneal surfaces, two similar surfaces to those shown in Fig. 10.17 are obtained.

To verify the deviation between the finally reconstructed surface and the point cloud to generate it, the Rhinoceros® software has a function known as "Point Cloud Deviation", which calculates the average value of the error of the distance for the solution surface in relation to the point cloud to generate it.

This is seen in Fig. 10.18a, where the upper view of the point cloud of the anterior surface of a healthy cornea is represented. An average distance error is obtained, this being $7.23 \times 10^{-6} \pm 1.536 \times 10^{-5}$ mm (mean ± standard deviation).

Figure 10.18b shows the deviation error for the anterior corneal surface in an advanced keratoconus case. Here the average distance error is

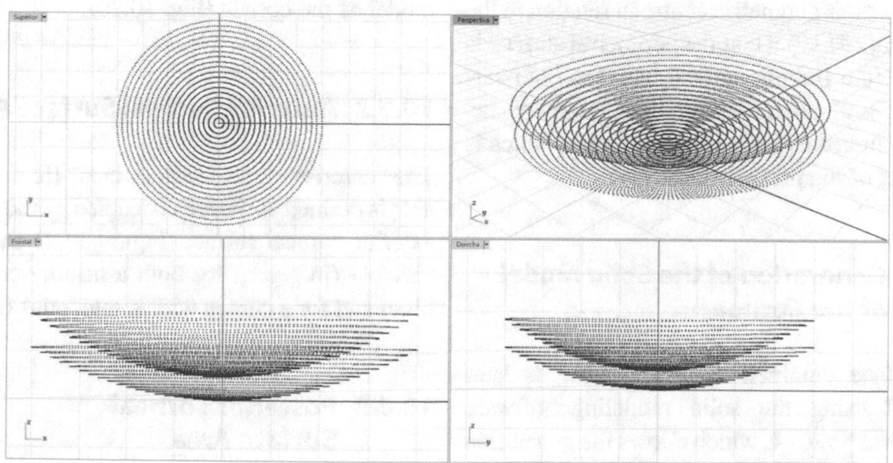

Fig. 10.16 Importing the point clouds for both corneal surfaces

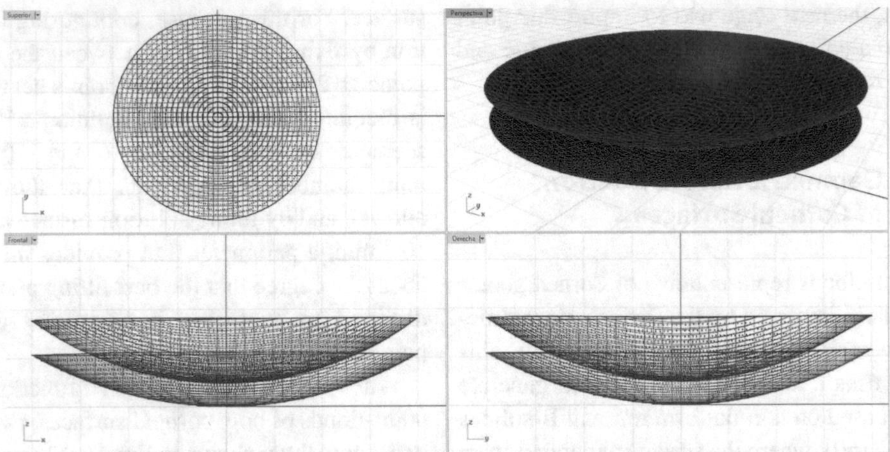

Fig. 10.17 Final surfaces generated by "Patch" function

$3.54 \times 10^{-4} \pm 6.36 \times 10^{-4}$ mm (mean ± standard deviation).

In both figures the same threshold values were configured to consider which points were valid and which were not by fixing 10^{-3} mm for invalid points (in red) and 10^{-4} mm for valid points (in blue). These figures also show how the points are distributed in perfectly circular rings with radii from $r=0$ mm to $r=4$ mm in 0.2-mm intervals. As mentioned previously, this is due to the conversion of the data provided by the corneal topographer from a polar format into a Cartesian format $[X, Y, Z]$.

The anterior and posterior corneal surfaces are generated by this procedure, and they are connected by their geometric centre in relation to the Z axis (Fig. 10.19). Next the perimetral surface is obtained (the linking surface between both surfaces in the Z axis direction), and the three surfaces are linked to form a single surface, which is the object of the present study.

10.5.3 Generation of the Solid Model of the Cornea

The surface obtained by Rhinoceros® is later imported using the solid modeling software SolidWorks® v2014, which allows the generation of the solid model that is representative of the real and customised geometry of the cornea (Fig. 10.20).

10.6 Characterisation of the Cornea

After obtaining the 3D solid model of the cornea, it can be used to calculate certain geometrical variables, which will characterise the analysed cornea. Following are some geometrical variables which can be obtained from the model.

10.6.1 Total Corneal Volume

The "total corneal volume" (in mm^3) variable is defined as the volume among the anterior, posterior and perimetral surfaces of the generated solid model of the cornea (Fig. 10.20).

10.6.2 Anterior Corneal Surface Area

The "anterior corneal surface area" (in mm^2) variable is defined as the area occupied by the anterior/exterior corneal surface. Figure 10.21 shows this variable (in green) for both a healthy cornea (in blue) and for a cornea with keratoconus (in red).

10.6.3 Posterior Corneal Surface Area

The "posterior corneal surface area" (in mm^2) variable is defined as the area occupied by the

Fig. 10.18 Point-surface deviation analysis for the reconstruction of anterior surface in: (**a**) a healthy cornea, (**b**) a cornea with advanced-state keratoconus

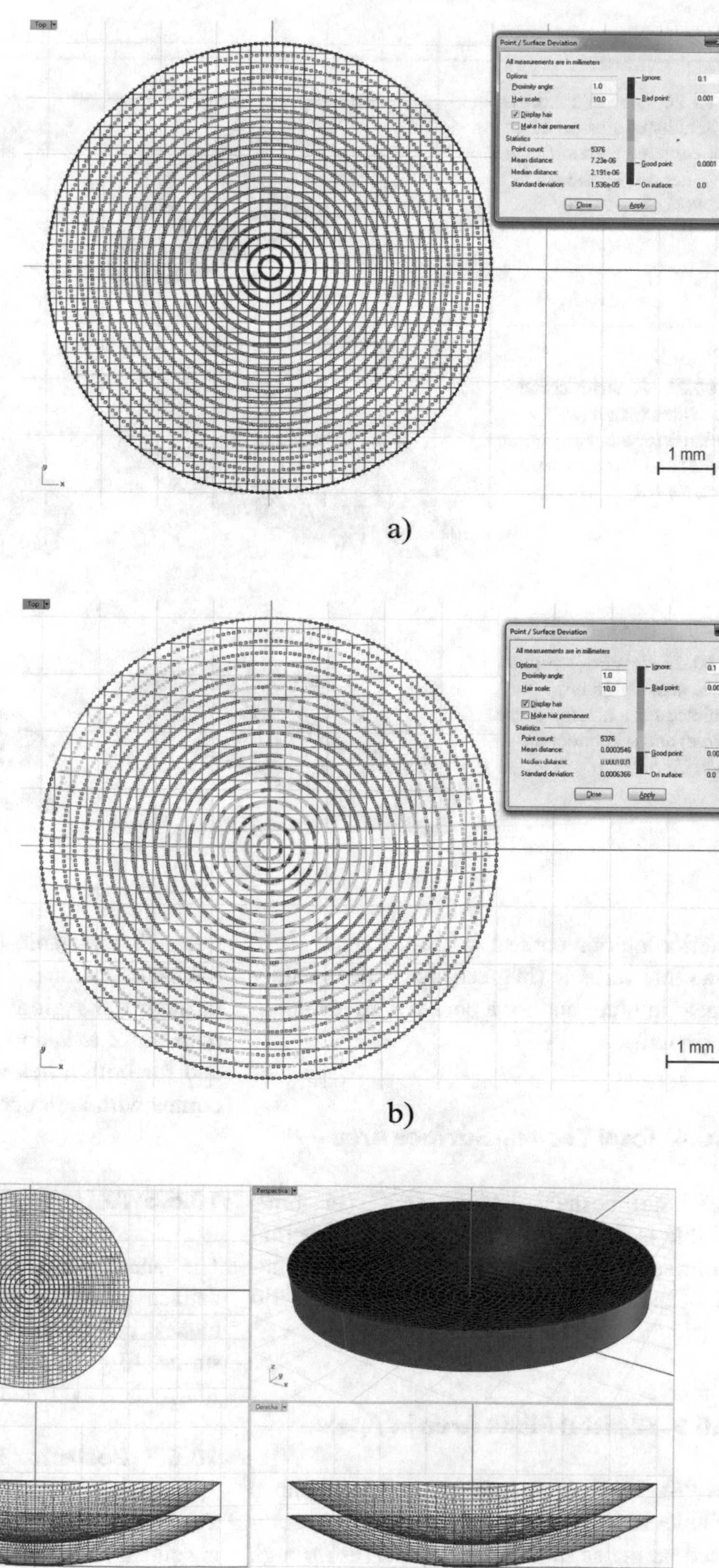

Fig. 10.19 Creation of peripheral surface and welding in a unique surface

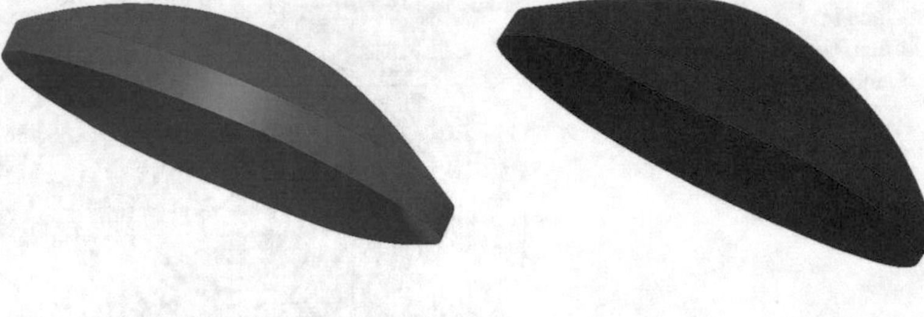

Fig. 10.20 3D solid models of a healthy cornea (*in blue*) and a keratoconic cornea (*in red*) generated by the aid of Solidworks® software

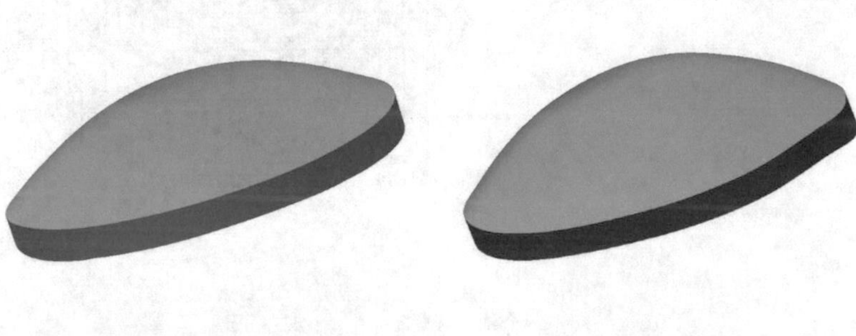

Fig. 10.21 Anterior corneal surface area (*in green*) calculated for a healthy cornea (*in blue*) and a keratoconic cornea (*in red*)

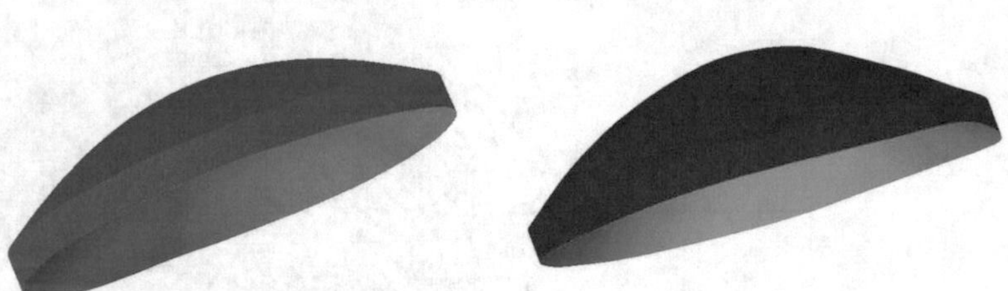

Fig. 10.22 Posterior corneal surface area *(in green)* calculated for a healthy cornea (*in blue*) and a keratoconic cornea (*in red*)

posterior/interior corneal surface. Figure 10.22 shows this variable (in green) for both a healthy cornea (in blue) and for a cornea with keratoconus (in red).

10.6.4 Total Corneal Surface Area

The "total corneal surface area" (in mm^2) variable is defined as the sum of the area that comprises the anterior, posterior and perimetral corneal surfaces of the generated solid model.

10.6.5 Sagittal Plane Area in Apex

The "Sagittal plane area in apex" (in mm^2) variable is defined as the cornea area comprised on the sagittal plane that passes through the Z axis and the highest point (apex) of the anterior corneal surface. Figure 10.23 illustrates this variable (in green) after making a three-dimensional incision in the cornea through the sagittal plane that passes through both the Z axis and the anterior surface apex, and for both a healthy cornea (in blue) and a cornea with keratoconus (in red).

10.6.6 Anterior Apex Deviation

The "anterior apex deviation" (in mm) variable is defined as the distance from the Z axis to the highest point (the apex) of the anterior corneal surface (Fig. 10.24).

10.6.7 Posterior Apex Deviation

The "posterior apex deviation" (in mm) variable is defined as the distance from the Z axis to the highest point (apex) of the posterior corneal surface (Fig. 10.25).

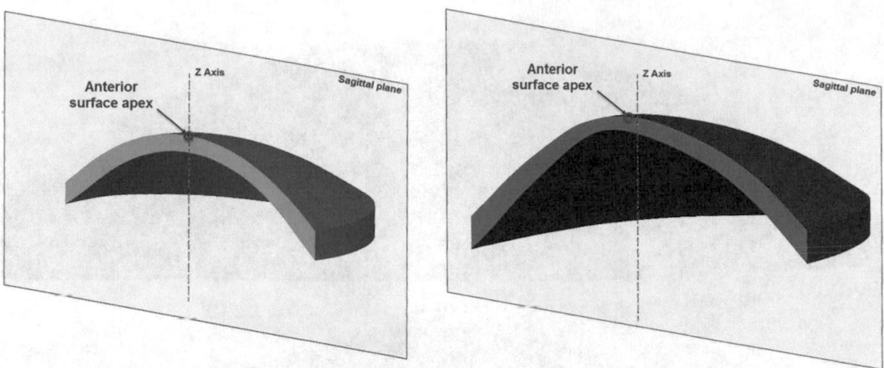

Fig. 10.23 Area of the sagittal plane that passes through the apex of the anterior surface (*in green*) calculated for a healthy cornea (*in blue*) and a keratoconic cornea (*in red*)

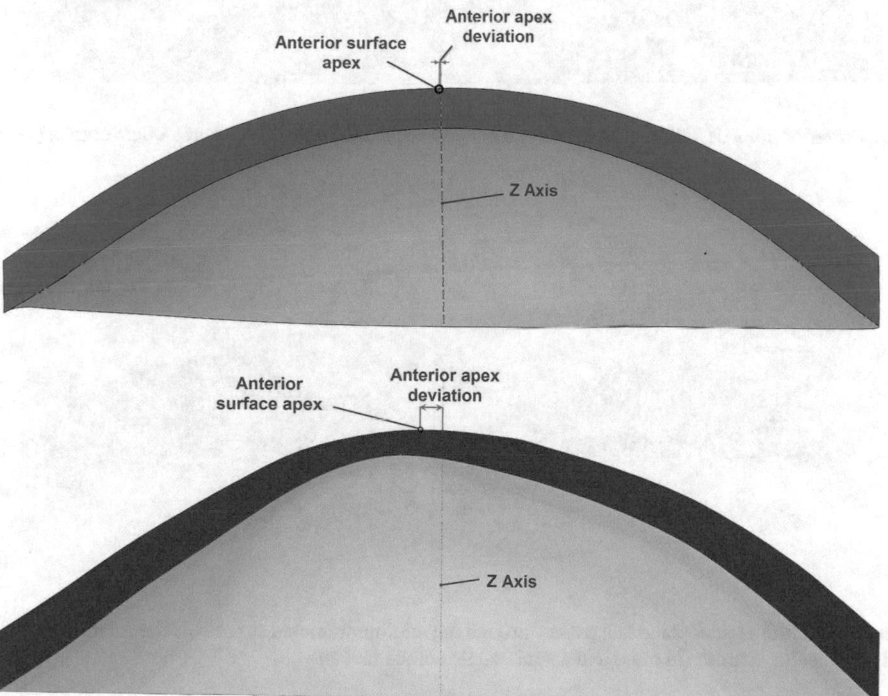

Fig. 10.24 Anterior apex deviation calculated for a healthy cornea (*in blue*) and a keratoconic cornea (*in red*)

10.6.8 Sagittal Plane Area at the Minimum Thickness Point

The "sagittal plane area at the minimum thickness point" (in mm^2) variable is defined as the corneal area that comprises the sagittal plane that passes through the *Z* axis and the minimum thickness point (maximum curvature) of the anterior corneal surface. Figure 10.26 depicts this variable (in green) after making a three-dimensional incision in the cornea through the sagittal plane, which passes through both the *Z* axis and the minimum thickness point of the anterior surface, for both a healthy cornea (in blue) and a cornea with keratoconus (in red).

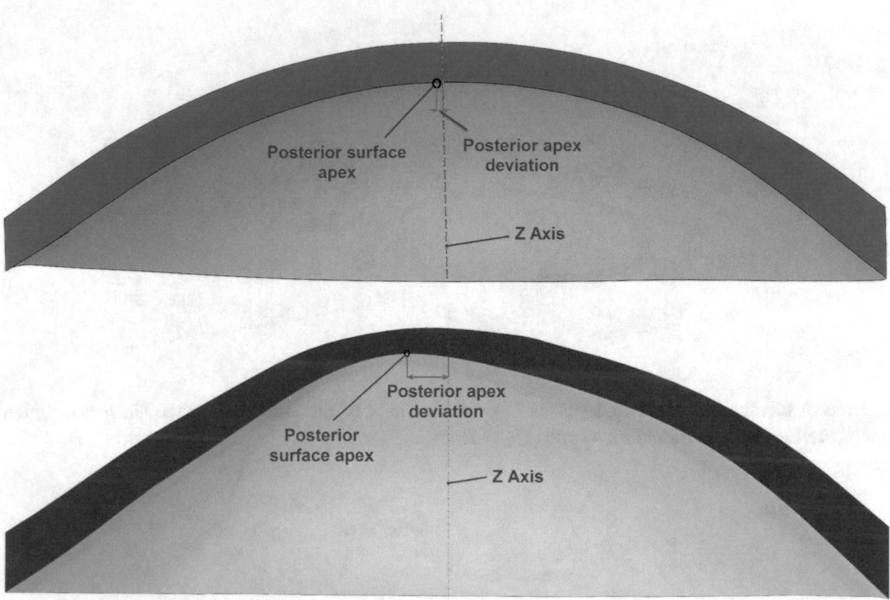

Fig. 10.25 Posterior apex deviation calculated for a healthy cornea (*in blue*) and a keratoconic cornea (*in red*)

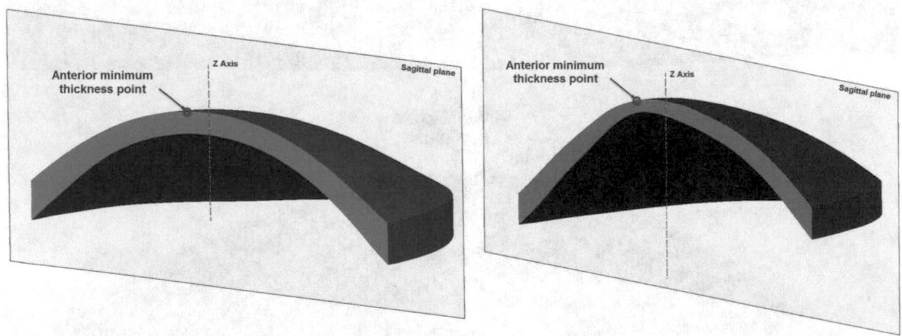

Fig. 10.26 Area of the sagittal plane that passes through the minimum thickness point of the anterior surface (*in green*) calculated for a healthy cornea (*in blue*) and a keratoconic cornea (*in red*)

10.6.9 Anterior Minimum Thickness Point Deviation

The "anterior minimum thickness point deviation" (in mm) variable is defined as the distance from the *Z* axis to the minimum thickness point (maximum curvature) of the anterior corneal surface (Fig. 10.27).

10.6.10 Posterior Minimum Thickness Point Deviation

The "posterior minimum thickness point deviation" (in mm) variable is defined as the distance from the *Z* axis to the minimum thickness point (maximum curvature) of the posterior corneal surface (Fig. 10.28).

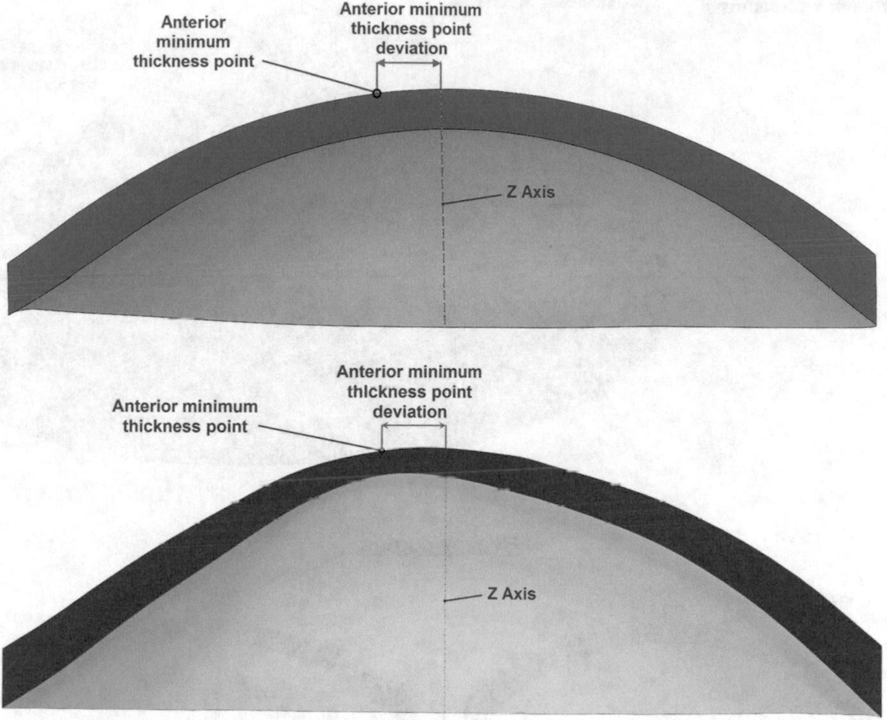

Fig. 10.27 Anterior minimum thickness point deviation calculated for a healthy cornea (*in blue*) and a keratoconic cornea (*in red*)

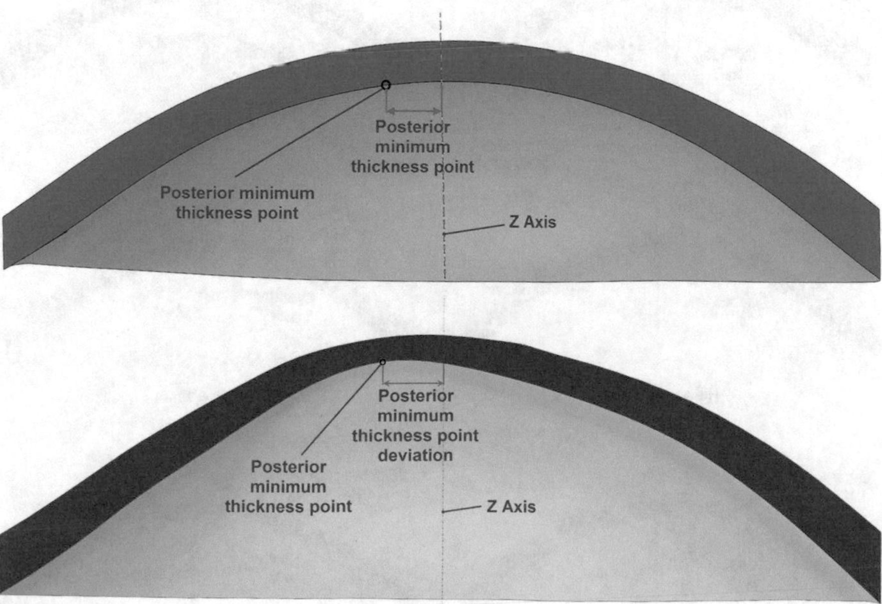

Fig. 10.28 Posterior minimum thickness point deviation calculated for a healthy cornea (*in blue*) and a keratoconic cornea (*in red*)

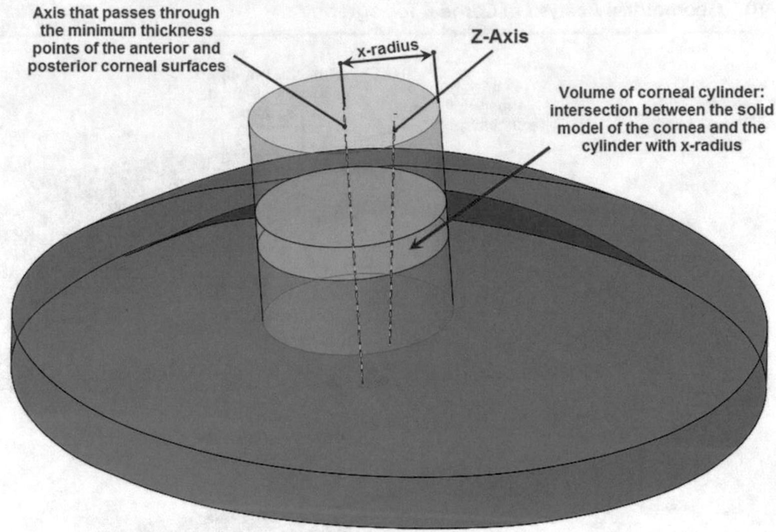

Fig. 10.29 Procedure for calculating the volume of the corneal cylinder with radius-x

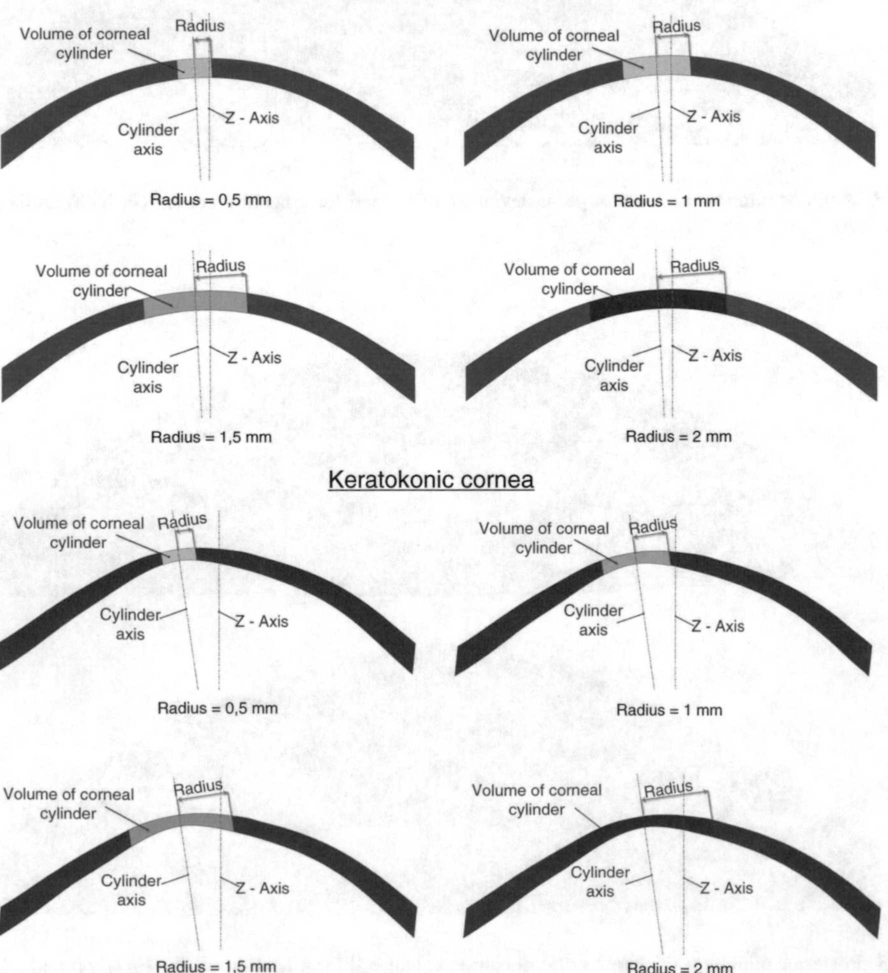

Fig. 10.30 Different volumes of corneal cylinders with radii 0.5, 1.0, 1.5 and 2.0 mm calculated for a healthy cornea (*in blue*) and a keratoconic cornea (*in red*)

10.6.11 Centre of Mass

The "Centre of mass" (in mm) variable is defined as the centre of mass' position, expressed in Cartesian coordinates *X, Y, Z*.

10.6.12 Net Deviation from the Centre of Mass in *XY*

The "net deviation from the centre of mass in *XY*" (in mm) variable is defined as the projective *XY* modulus of the centre of mass.

10.6.13 Volume of Corneal Cylinder *R–x*

The "volume of corneal cylinder *R–x*" (in mm^3) variable is defined as the volume of the 3D intersection between the generated solid model of the cornea and one cylinder of radius $r=x$ mm, whose axis passes through the minimum thickness points (maximum curvature) of the anterior and posterior corneal surfaces (Fig. 10.29). The following radii were used for this study: 0.5, 1.0, 1.5 and 2.0 mm. Figure 10.30 depicts the calculation of these radii for both a healthy cornea (in blue) and a cornea with keratoconus (in red).

Compliance with Ethical Requirements *Conflict of Interest*: F. Cavas-Martínez, E. De la Cruz Sánchez, J. Nieto Martínez, F.J. Fernández Cañavate and D.G. Fernández-Pacheco declare that they have no conflict of interest.

Informed Consent: All procedures followed were in accordance with the ethical standards of the responsible committee on human experimentation (institutional and national) and with the Helsinki Declaration of 1975, as revised in 2000. Informed consent was obtained from all patients for being included in the study.

No animal studies were carried out by the authors for this chapter.

References

1. Eklund A, Dufort P, Forsberg D, LaConte SM. Medical image processing on the GPU—past, present and future. Med Image Anal. 2013;17(8):1073–94. doi:10.1016/j.media.2013.05.008.
2. Ariza-Gracia MA, Zurita JF, Pinero DP, Rodriguez-Matas JF, Calvo B. Coupled biomechanical response of the cornea assessed by non-contact tonometry. A simulation study. PLoS One 2015;10(3):e0121486. doi:10.1371/journal.pone.0121486.
3. Cavas-Martínez F, Fernández-Pacheco DG, De La Cruz-Sánchez E, Nieto Martínez J, Fernández Cañavate FJ, Vega-Estrada A, et al. Geometrical custom modeling of human cornea in vivo and its use for the diagnosis of corneal ectasia. PLoS One 2014;9(10). doi:10.1371/journal.pone.0110249.
4. Montalbán R. Caracterización y validación diagnóstica de la correlación de la geometría de las dos superficies de la córnea humana. Alicante: Universidad de Alicante; 2013.
5. Oie Y, Nishida K. Regenerative medicine for the cornea. Biomed Res Int. 2013;2013:428247. doi:10.1155/2013/428247.
6. Pinero DP, Alio JL, Barraquer RI, Michael R, Jimenez R. Corneal biomechanics, refraction, and corneal aberrometry in keratoconus: an integrated study. Invest Ophthalmol Vis Sci. 2010;51(4):1948–55. doi:10.1167/iovs.09-4177.
7. Levy D, Hutchings H, Rouland JF, Guell J, Burillon C, Arne JL, et al. Videokeratographic anomalies in familial keratoconus. Ophthalmology. 2004;111(5):867–74. doi:10.1016/j.ophtha.2003.12.024.
8. Vryghem JC, Devogelaere T, Stodulka P. Efficacy, safety, and flap dimensions of a new femtosecond laser for laser in situ keratomileusis. J Cataract Refract Surg. 2010;36(3):442–8. doi:10.1016/j.jcrs.2009.09.030.
9. Ambrosio Jr R, Caiado AL, Guerra FP, Louzada R, Roy AS, Luz A, et al. Novel pachymetric parameters based on corneal tomography for diagnosing keratoconus. J Refract Surg. 2011;27(10):753–8. doi:10.3928/1081597x-20110721-01.
10. Alessio G, Boscia F, La Tegola MG, Sborgia C. Topography-driven excimer laser for the retreatment of decentralized myopic photorefractive keratectomy. Ophthalmology. 2001;108(9):1695–703.
11. Ribeiro FJ, Castanheira-Dinis A, Dias JM. Personalized pseudophakic model for refractive assessment. PLoS One. 2012;7(10), e46780. doi:10.1371/journal.pone.0046780.
12. Buey Salas MA, Peris MC. Biomecánica y Arquitectura Corneal. Amsterdam: Elsevier; 2014.
13. Rabinowitz YS. Keratoconus. Surv Ophthalmol. 1998;42(4):297–319.
14. Pinero DP, Alio JL, Aleson A, Escaf Vergara M, Miranda M. Corneal volume, pachymetry, and correlation of anterior and posterior corneal shape in subclinical and different stages of clinical keratoconus. J Cataract Refract Surg. 2010;36(5):814–25. doi:10.1016/j.jcrs.2009.11.012.
15. Dubbelman M, Weeber HA, van der Heijde RG, Volker-Dieben HJ. Radius and asphericity of the posterior corneal surface determined by corrected Scheimpflug photography. Acta Ophthalmol Scand. 2002;80(4):379–83.
16. Ho JD, Tsai CY, Tsai RJ, Kuo LL, Tsai IL, Liou SW. Validity of the keratometric index: evaluation by the

Pentacam rotating Scheimpflug camera. J Cataract Refract Surg. 2008;34(1):137–45. doi:10.1016/j.jcrs.2007.09.033.
17. Dubbelman M, Sicam VA, Van der Heijde GL. The shape of the anterior and posterior surface of the aging human cornea. Vis Res. 2006;46(6–7):993–1001. doi:10.1016/j.visres.2005.09.021.
18. Atchison DA, Markwell EL, Kasthurirangan S, Pope JM, Smith G, Swann PG. Age-related changes in optical and biometric characteristics of emmetropic eyes. J Vis. 2008;8(4):29.1. doi:10.1167/8.4.29.
19. Calossi A. Corneal asphericity and spherical aberration. J Refract Surg. 2007;23(5):505–14.
20. Yebra-Pimentel E, Gonzalez-Jeijome JM, Cervino A, Giraldez MJ, Gonzalez-Perez J, Parafita MA. Corneal asphericity in a young adult population. Clinical implications. Arch Soc Esp Oftalmol. 2004;79(8): 385–92.
21. Perry HD, Buxton JN, Fine BS. Round and oval cones in keratoconus. Ophthalmology. 1980;87(9):905–9.
22. Kennedy RH, Bourne WM, Dyer JA. A 48-year clinical and epidemiologic study of keratoconus. Am J Ophthalmol. 1986;101(3):267–73.
23. Rabinowitz YS, McDonnell PJ. Computer-assisted corneal topography in keratoconus. Refract Cor Surg. 1989;5(6):400–8.
24. Wilson SE, Lin DT, Klyce SD. Corneal topography of keratoconus. Cornea. 1991;10(1):2–8.
25. Auffarth GU, Wang L, Volcker HE. Keratoconus evaluation using the Orbscan Topography System. J Cataract Refract Surg. 2000;26(2):222–8.
26. Prisant O, Legeais JM, Renard G. Superior keratoconus. Cornea. 1997;16(6):693–4.
27. Schlegel Z, Hoang-Xuan T, Gatinel D. Comparison of and correlation between anterior and posterior corneal elevation maps in normal eyes and keratoconus-suspect eyes. J Cataract Refract Surg. 2008;34(5):789–95. doi:10.1016/j.jcrs.2007.12.036.
28. Smolek MK, Klyce SD. Current keratoconus detection methods compared with a neural network approach. Invest Ophthalmol Vis Sci. 1997;38(11):2290–9.
29. Tomidokoro A, Oshika T, Amano S, Higaki S, Maeda N, Miyata K. Changes in anterior and posterior corneal curvatures in keratoconus. Ophthalmology. 2000;107(7):1328–32.
30. Wolffsohn JS, Safeen S, Shah S, Laiquzzaman M. Changes of corneal biomechanics with keratoconus. Cornea. 2012;31(8):849–54. doi:10.1097/ICO.0b013e318243e42d.
31. Savini G, Carbonelli M, Barboni P, Hoffer KJ. Repeatability of automatic measurements performed by a dual Scheimpflug analyzer in unoperated and post-refractive surgery eyes. J Cataract Refract Surg. 2011;37(2):302–9. doi:10.1016/j.jcrs.2010.07.039.
32. Savini G, Barboni P, Carbonelli M, Hoffer KJ. Repeatability of automatic measurements by a new Scheimpflug camera combined with Placido topography. J Cataract Refract Surg. 2011;37(10):1809–16. doi:10.1016/j.jcrs.2011.04.033.
33. Maldonado MJ, Nieto JC, Pinero DP. Advances in technologies for laser-assisted in situ keratomileusis (LASIK) surgery. Exp Rev Med Dev. 2008;5(2):209–29. doi:10.1586/17434440.5.2.209.
34. Pinero DP, Nieto JC, Lopez-Miguel A. Characterization of corneal structure in keratoconus. J Cataract Refract Surg. 2012;38(12):2167–83. doi:10.1016/j.jcrs.2012.10.022.
35. Pinero DP. Technologies for anatomical and geometric characterization of the corneal structure and anterior segment: a review. Semin Ophthalmol. 2013;30(3):161–70. doi:10.3109/08820538.2013.835844.
36. Ambrosio Jr R, Valbon BF, Faria-Correia F, Ramos I, Luz A. Scheimpflug imaging for laser refractive surgery. Curr Opin Ophthalmol. 2013;24(4):310–20. doi:10.1097/ICU.0b013e3283622a94.
37. Ramos-Lopez D, Martinez-Finkelshtein A, Castro-Luna GM, Piñero D, Alio JL. Placido-based indices of corneal irregularity. Optom Vis. 2011;88(10):1220–31. doi:10.1097/OPX.0b013e3182279ff8.
38. Klyce SD, Karon MD, Smolek MK. Advantages and disadvantages of the Zernike expansion for representing wave aberration of the normal and aberrated eye. J Refract Surg. 2004;20(5):S537–41.
39. Schneider M, Iskander DR, Collins MJ. Modeling corneal surfaces with rational functions for high-speed videokeratoscopy data compression. IEEE Trans Biomed Eng. 2009;56(2):493–9. doi:10.1109/tbme.2008.2006019.
40. Espinosa J, Mas D, Perez J, Illueca C. Optical surface reconstruction technique through combination of zonal and modal fitting. J Biomed Opt. 2010;15(2):026022. doi:10.1117/1.3394260.
41. Tyson RK. Conversion of Zernike aberration coefficients to Seidel and higher-order power-series aberration coefficients. Opt Lett. 1982;7(6):262–4.
42. Conforti G. Zernike aberration coefficients from Seidel and higher-order power-series coefficients. Opt Lett. 1983;8(7):407–8.
43. Smolek MK, Klyce SD. Goodness-of-prediction of Zernike polynomial fitting to corneal surfaces. J Cataract Refract Surg. 2005;31(12):2350–5. doi:10.1016/j.jcrs.2005.05.025.
44. Carvalho LA. Accuracy of Zernike polynomials in characterizing optical aberrations and the corneal surface of the eye. Invest Ophthalmol Vis Sci. 2005;46(6):1915–26. doi:10.1167/iovs.04-1222.
45. Ares M, Royo S. Comparison of cubic B-spline and Zernike-fitting techniques in complex wavefront reconstruction. Appl Opt. 2006;45(27):6954–64.
46. Schwiegerling J, Greivenkamp JE. Keratoconus detection based on videokeratoscopic height data. Optom Vis Sci. 1996;73(12):721–8.
47. Iskander DR, Alkhaldi W, Zoubir AM, editors. On the computer intensive methods in model selection. In: ICASSP, IEEE International conference on acoustics, speech and signal processing—proceedings; 2008.
48. Alkhaldi W, Iskander DR, Zoubir AM, Collins MJ. Enhancing the standard operating range of a Placido

disk videokeratoscope for corneal surface estimation. IEEE Trans Biomed Eng. 2009;56(3):800–9. doi:10.1109/tbme.2008.2005997.
49. Dai GM. Comparison of wavefront reconstructions with Zernike polynomials and Fourier transforms. J Refract Surg. 2006;22(9):943–8.
50. Wang L, Chernyak D, Yeh D, Koch DD. Fitting behaviors of Fourier transform and Zernike polynomials. J Cataract Refract Surg. 2007;33(6):999–1004. doi:10.1016/j.jcrs.2007.03.017.
51. Yoon G, Pantanelli S, MacRae S. Comparison of Zernike and Fourier wavefront reconstruction algorithms in representing corneal aberration of normal and abnormal eyes. J Refract Surg. 2008;24(6):582–90.
52. Martinez-Finkelshtein A, Delgado AM, Castro GM, Zarzo A, Alio JL. Comparative analysis of some modal reconstruction methods of the shape of the cornea from corneal elevation data. Invest Ophthalmol Vis Sci. 2009;50(12):5639–45. doi:10.1167/iovs.08-3351.
53. Martinez-Finkelshtein A, Lopez DR, Castro GM, Alio JL. Adaptive cornea modeling from keratometric data. Invest Ophthalmol Vis Sci. 2011;52(8):4963–70. doi:10.1167/iovs.10-6774.
54. Okrasiński W, Płociniczak Ł. A nonlinear mathematical model of the corneal shape. Nonlinear Anal Real World Appl. 2012;13(3):1498–505. doi:10.1016/j.nonrwa.2011.11.014.
55. Płociniczak L, Okrasiński W, Nieto JJ, Domínguez O. On a nonlinear boundary value problem modeling corneal shape. J Math Anal Appl. 2014;414(1):461–71. doi:10.1016/j.jmaa.2014.01.010.
56. Zhu Z, Janunts E, Eppig T, Sauer T, Langenbucher A. Iteratively re-weighted bi-cubic spline representation of corneal topography and its comparison to the standard methods. Z Med Phys. 2010;20(4):287–98. doi:10.1016/j.zemedi.2010.07.002.
57. Wahba G. Spline models for observational data. Philadelphia: SIAM; 1990.
58. Liu X, Gao Y. B-spline based wavefront reconstruction for lateral shearing interferometric measurement of engineering surfaces. Key Engineering Materials2003. p. 169–74.
59. Piegl L. On NURBS: a survey. IEEE Comput Graph Appl. 1991;11(1):55–71. doi:10.1109/38.67702.
60. Piegl L, Tiller W. The NURBS book. Washington: U.S. Government Printing Office; 1997.
61. Turuwhenua J, Henderson J. A novel low-order method for recovery of the corneal shape. Optom Vis Sci. 2004;81(11):863–71. doi:10.1097/01.OPX.0000145023.74460.EE.
62. Turuwhenua J. An improved low order method for corneal reconstruction. Optom Vis Sci. 2008;85(3):E211–8. doi:10.1097/OPX.0b013e318164ee9b.
63. Zhu Z, Janunts E, Eppig T, Sauer T, Langenbucher A. Tomography-based customized IOL calculation model. Curr Eye Res. 2011;36(6):579–89. doi:10.3109/02713683.2011.566978.
64. Xing Q, Wei Q. Human eyeball model reconstruction and quantitative analysis. Conference proceedings: In: Annual international conference of the IEEE engineering in medicine and biology society, 26–30 Aug. 2014. p. 2460–3. doi:10.1109/embc.2014.6944120
65. Rosenthal P, Cotter JM. Clinical performance of a spline-based apical vaulting keratoconus corneal contact lens design. CLAO J. 1995;21(1):42–6.
66. Mahadevan R, Fathima A, Rajan R, Arumugam AO. An ocular surface prosthesis for keratoglobus and Terrien's marginal degeneration. Optom Vis Sci. 2014;91(4 Suppl 1):S34–9. doi:10.1097/opx.0000000000000200.
67. Roy AS, Dupps Jr WJ. Patient-specific computational modeling of keratoconus progression and differential responses to collagen cross-linking. Invest Ophthalmol Vis Sci. 2011;52(12):9174–87. doi:10.1167/iovs.11-7395.
68. Bao F, Chen H, Yu Y, Yu J, Zhou S, Wang J, et al. Evaluation of the shape symmetry of bilateral normal corneas in a Chinese population. PLoS One. 2013;8(8), e73412. doi:10.1371/journal.pone.0073412.
69. Simonini I, Pandolfi A. Customized finite element modelling of the human cornea. PLoS One. 2015;10(6), e0130426. doi:10.1371/journal.pone.0130426.
70. Sun W, Darling A, Starly B, Nam J. Computer-aided tissue engineering: overview, scope and challenges. Biotechnol Appl Biochem. 2004;39(1):29–47.
71. Lohfeld S, Barron V, McHugh PE. Biomodels of bone: a review. Ann Biomed Eng. 2005;33(10):1295–311. doi:10.1007/s10439-005-5873-x.
72. Farin G, Hoschek J, Kim MS. Handbook of computer aided geometric design. North Holland: Elsevier; 2002.
73. Pottmann H, Leopoldseder S, Hofer M, Steiner T, Wang W. Industrial geometry: recent advances and applications in CAD. Comput Aided Des Appl. 2005;37(7):751–66. doi:10.1016/j.cad.2004.08.013.
74. Cui J, Tang M, Liu H. Dynamic shape representation for product modeling in conceptual design. Jisuanji Fuzhu Sheji Yu Tuxingxue Xuebao/J Comput Aided Des Comput Graph. 2014;26(10):1879–85.
75. Lee T, Choi JB, Schafer BW, Segars WP, Eckstein F, Kuhn V, et al. Assessing the susceptibility to local buckling at the femoral neck cortex to age-related bone loss. Ann Biomed Eng. 2009;37(9):1910–20. doi:10.1007/s10439-009-9751-9.
76. Almeida HA, Bártolo PJ, editors. Computational technologies in tissue engineering. WIT transactions on biomedicine and health. Southampton: WIT Press; 2013.
77. Wu Z, Fu J, Wang Z, Li X, Li J, Pei Y, et al. Three-dimensional virtual bone bank system for selecting massive bone allograft in orthopaedic oncology. Int Orthopaed. 2015;39(6):1151–8. doi:10.1007/s00264-015-2719-5.
78. Brand M, Avrahami I, Einav S, Ryvkin M. Numerical models of net-structure stents inserted into arteries. Comput Biol Med. 2014;52:102–10. doi:10.1016/j.compbiomed.2014.06.015.
79. Chiang CI, Shyh-Yuan L, Ming-Chang W, Sun CW, Jiang CP. Finite element modelling of implant designs

and cortical bone thickness on stress distribution in maxillary type IV bone. Comput Methods Biomech Biomed Eng. 2014;17(5):516–26. doi:10.1080/10255842.2012.697556.

80. Schmidt T, Pandya D, Balzani D. Influence of isotropic and anisotropic material models on the mechanical response in arterial walls as a result of supra-physiological loadings. Mech Res Commun. 2015;64:29–37. doi:10.1016/j.mechrescom.2014.12.008.
81. Rocha M, Pereira JP, De Castro AV, editors. 3D modeling mechanisms for educational resources in medical and health area. In: Proceedings of the 6th Iberian conference on information systems and technologies, CISTI 2011; 2011.
82. Schubert C, van Langeveld MC, Donoso LA. Innovations in 3D printing: a 3D overview from optics to organs. Br J Ophthalmol. 2014;98(2):159–61. doi:10.1136/bjophthalmol-2013-304446.
83. Donnelly III W. The Advanced Human Eye Model (AHEM): a personal binocular eye modeling system inclusive of refraction, diffraction, and scatter. J Refrac Surg. 2008;24(9):976–83.
84. Talu S, Stach S, Sueiras V, Ziebarth NM. Fractal analysis of AFM images of the surface of Bowman's membrane of the human cornea. Ann Biomed Eng. 2015;43(4):906–16. doi:10.1007/s10439-014-1140-3.
85. Giovanzana S. A virtual environment for modeling and analysis of human eye. Padua: Universidad de Padua; 2011.
86. Genest R. Effect of intraocular pressure on chick eye geometry, finite element modeling, and myopia. Ontario: Universidad de Waterloo; 2010.
87. Wong A, Genest R, Chandrashekar N, Choh V, Irving EL. Automatic system for 3D reconstruction of the chick eye based on digital photographs. Comput Methods Biomech Biomed Eng. 2012;15(2):141–9. doi:10.1080/10255842.2010.518566.
88. Ding S, Ye Y, Tu J, Subic A. Region-based geometric modelling of human airways and arterial vessels. Comput Med Imaging Graph. 2010;34(2):114–21. doi:10.1016/j.compmedimag.2009.07.005.
89. Duan CY, Lü HB, Hu JZ. In vivo study on three-dimensional structure of lumbar facet joints based on computer-assisted medical image processing method. Yiyong Shengwu Lixue/J Med Biomech. 2012;27(2):159–65.
90. Cheng RKC. Inside Rhinoceros 5. Stamford: Cengage Learning; 2014.

Early Keratoconus Detection Enhanced by Modern Diagnostic Technology

11

Francisco Cavas-Martínez, Pablo Sanz Díez, Alfredo Vega Estrada, Ernesto De la Cruz Sánchez, Daniel García Fernández-Pacheco, Ana Belén Plaza Puche, José Nieto Martínez, Francisco J. Fernández Cañavate, and Jorge L. Alió

11.1 Introduction

Early detection of corneal ectasia is a main concern for clinical ophthalmologists, in order to prevent the iatrogenic effects of several surgical procedures such as laser-assisted in situ keratomileusis (LASIK), lamellar cut, or excimer laser ablation. One retrospective study in 1364 patients has found a total of 69 eyes with a corneal topography suggesting forme fruste keratoconus (FFKC) after LASIK procedure [1]. Although it is a rare complication, the probability of an ectatic disease due to the surgically induced alteration of the corneal biomechanical structures is always present, and not only for those patients who have a previous ectatic cornea: in the same study, the rate of iatrogenic post-LASIK ectasia was 0.05 % (1/1992 eyes), and the total rate of post-LASIK ectasia for the entire study was 0.25 % (1/398). The rate of eyes with unrecognized preoperative FFKC that developed post-LASIK ectasia was 5.8 % (1/17) [1]. So even the use of the most conservative screening recommendations would not have precluded some patients from LASIK, as the one case of post-LASIK ectasia previously described, with no identifiable preoperative risk factors. Maybe in some cases it is not possible to elucidate how surgical procedures will lead to a biomechanical failure in response to forces from intraocular pressure (IOP), forces from the three antagonistic pairs of muscles that control eye movements (lateral and medial rectus muscles, the superior and inferior rectus muscles, and the superior and inferior oblique muscles), as well as other forces. But with a higher rate of surgical-related corneal ectasia development in those patients with previous ectatic signs, as observed before, there is a great interest in the development of new

F. Cavas-Martínez, Ph.D. (✉)
D.G. Fernández-Pacheco, P.h. D.
J. Nieto Martínez, Ph.D. • F.J. Fernández Cañavate, Ph.D.
Department of Graphical Expression, Technical University of Cartagena, Murcia, Spain
e-mail: francisco.cavas@upct.es; daniel.garcia@upct.es; jose.nieto@upct.es; francisco.canavate@upct.es

A. Vega Estrada, Ph.D. • A.B. Plaza Puche, Ph.D.
Keratoconus Unit, Vissum Alicante, Alicante, Spain
e-mail: alfredovega@vissum.com; abplaza@vissum.com

E. De la Cruz Sánchez, Ph.D.
Faculty of Sports Science, University of Murcia
Santiago de la Ribera, Murcia, Spain
e-mail: erneslacruz@um.es

J.L. Alió, M.D., Ph.D., F.E.B.O. • P. Sanz Díez, O.D., M.Sc.
Keratoconus Unit, Department of Refractive Surgery, Vissum Alicante, Alicante, Spain

Division of Ophthalmology, Miguel Hernández University, Alicante, Spain
e-mail: jlalio@vissum.com; pablosanz9143@gmail.com

J.L. Alió (ed.), *Keratoconus*, Essentials in Ophthalmology, DOI 10.1007/978-3-319-43881-8_11

approaches for the improvement of sensitivity and specificity of the clinical diagnostic tools for subclinical stages of the ectatic disease detection. This chapter is aimed to explain how it is possible to establish new criteria for the subclinical keratoconus detection using a custom, geometrical approach, for an in vivo corneal analysis.

11.2 Materials and Methods

11.2.1 Sampling Procedures

We developed an observational case series study, evaluating a total of 120 eyes from 120 subjects with normal best spectacle corrected visual acuity, using one eye per patient, following a numerical sequence (dichotomous sequence 0 and 1) created by computer software in order to avoid interference potential correlations that could exist between the eyes of the same person. Participants with any ocular or corneal pathology, or those whose eyes had undergone any previous procedure, were excluded.

Sample was divided into two groups: healthy and subclinical keratoconus corneas. The first group (eyes with healthy cornea) did not present any ocular pathology and consisted of 89 healthy eyes of 89 patients with ages ranging from 7 to 66 years (mean age of 37.49 ± 15.11 years). The second group was formed by eyes with ocular pathology and consisted of 31 eyes of 31 patients diagnosed with subclinical keratoconus, with ages ranging from 16 to 55 years (mean age of 34.72 ± 11.12 years). The classification protocol for healthy or subclinical keratoconus cases was performed based on reported state-of-the-art clinical and topography evaluation [2]: healthy eyes had spectacle correction visual acuity ≥1 on the decimal scale (Snellen 20/20), no clinical signs of keratoconus, no scissoring on retinoscopy, no asymmetric bowtie (AB), inferior steepening (IS), skewed axes (SRAX), or asymmetric bowtie with skewed axes (AB/SRAX) pattern on topography. Subclinical keratoconus had spectacle correction visual acuity ≥1 on the decimal scale (Snellen 20/20); no slit-lamp findings; no scissoring on retinoscopy; and presence of AB, IS, SRAX, or AB/SRAX pattern on topography only.

All clinical data and corneal examinations were performed in Vissum Corporation (Alicante, Spain). Prior to the examination, informed consent was obtained from each patient, and the study was conducted in accordance with the ethical standards stated in the Declaration of Helsinki and approved by the local clinical research ethics committee.

11.2.2 Eye Exam

The preoperative examination of all selected eyes included the following tests: uncorrected distance visual acuity (UDVA), corrected distance visual acuity (CDVA), manifest refraction, Goldmann tonometry, biometry (IOLMaster, Carl Zeiss Meditec AG), and corneal topographic analysis with Sirius System® (CSO, Florence, Italy). All measurements were performed by the same experienced optometrist certified in Good Clinical Practice (GCP). Regarding the corneal topographic analysis, three consecutive measurements were performed and the average values were calculated for posterior analysis. A high performance corneal topographer with a combination between rotating Scheimpflug camera and Placido disk was used during the study to obtain the corneal topography, achieving accurate measurement of elevations, curvature, power, and thickness for the whole cornea. This topographer has a good level of consistency for taking measurements of sagittal and tangential curvature of both faces of the corneal refractive power, points of the anterior and posterior corneal surface, corneal pachymetry, and estimations of other biometric structures. This consistency has been previously proved to be accurate [3]. During the study, the Phoenix® (Phoenix, CSO, Florence, Italy) software was used for data registration.

This topographer works in two clearly differentiated stages. The first stage performs a mapping of spatial data of the surface morphology of the anterior and posterior corneal surfaces.

The second stage uses an internal algorithm, whose performance is unknown. This proceeds to the reconstruction of the corneal surface by an elevation map, a topographic map, and a map of curvature (tangential or sagittal) from both sides of the corneal surface, and later makes a qualitative analysis of these maps using different index rates. For the study performed in this paper, only raw data extracted from the first stage of the topographer was used, which warranties that no manipulation of the data by any software algorithm was executed.

11.2.3 Corneal Modeling and Geometrical Characterization Proposals

The procedure proposed consists of two main stages: the reconstruction of a 3D geometrical model of the cornea through computational geometry techniques and using raw data from a Sirius (CSO) corneal topographer, and the determination and calculation of several geometric variables from this model.

Geometrical modeling and analysis. The geometric reconstruction of the cornea was performed by executing the following steps, described with more detail in chapter 10 [4]: extraction of the point clouds from the corneal topographer, geometric surface reconstruction, and solid modeling. The resulting solid model of the cornea is then used to perform an analysis of determined geometric variables. The variables studied in this study are as follows: total corneal volume [mm^3], anterior corneal surface area [mm^2], posterior corneal surface area [mm^2], total corneal surface area [mm^2], sagittal plane area in apex [mm^2], anterior and posterior apex deviation [mm], sagittal plane area at minimum thickness point (maximum curvature) [mm^2], anterior and posterior minimum thickness point deviation (maximum curvature) [mm], centre of mass coordinates *X, Y, Z* of the solid model [mm], net deviation from the centre of mass in *XY* [mm], and volume of corneal cylinder $R–x$ [mm^3]. A more detailed description of these variables can be found in Table 11.1.

11.2.4 Data Analysis

According to data engagement scores (K-S test), a Student's *t*-test or U-Mann–Whitney Wilcoxon test was employed, as appropriate. ROC curves were established in order to determine what parameters could be used to classify diseased corneas, calculating optimal cutoffs, sensitivity, and specificity. All analyses were performed using Graphpad Prism 6 and SPSS 17.0 software.

11.3 Results

Table **11.2** summarizes the main outcomes of the variables analyzed in this study. The majority of modeled variables have statistically significant differences when comparing healthy with diseased corneas, as presented in Table 11.2.

11.3.1 Importance of Volumetric Variables

Patients in the early keratoconus group showed a statistically significant decrease in total corneal volume when compared with healthy eyes ($p<0.05$). This behavior is also found in the area of highest corneal irregularity. The volume of corneal cylinder with radius x is where there are statistically higher values for healthy eyes, with a similar trend for all radii adopted in the study, ($x=0.5$, 1.0, 1.5, and 2.0 mm) ($p<0.05$).

11.3.2 Surface and Area-Related Variables

Regarding the corneal surfaces, the areas for both anterior and posterior corneal surfaces are statistically lower in subjects with healthy corneas ($p<0.05$). On the other hand, the total corneal surface area is higher in healthy corneas ($p<0.05$), as well as the area of the sagittal plane that passes through the apex of the anterior surface ($p<0.05$) and the area of the sagittal plane through the minimum thickness point of the anterior surface ($p<0.05$).

Table 11.1 Geometric variables analyzed in the study

Geometric variable	Description	Figure in which is represented
Total corneal volume [mm^3]	Volume limited by front, back, and peripheral surfaces of the solid model generated	1
Anterior corneal surface area [mm^2]	Area of the front/exterior surface	1
Posterior corneal surface area [mm^2]	Area of the rear/interior surface	1
Total corneal surface area [mm^2]	Sum of anterior, posterior, and perimetral corneal surface areas of the solid model generated	1
Sagittal plane area in apex [mm^2]	Area of the cornea within the sagittal plane passing through the *Z* axis and the highest point (apex) of the anterior corneal surface	2
Anterior and posterior apex deviation [mm]	Average distance from the *Z* axis to the highest point (apex) of the anterior/posterior corneal surfaces	2
Sagittal plane area at minimum thickness point [mm^2]	Area of the cornea within the sagittal plane passing through the *Z* axis and the minimum thickness point (maximum curvature) of the anterior corneal surface	3
Anterior and posterior minimum thickness point deviation [mm]	Average distance in the *XY* plane from the *Z* axis to the minimum thickness points (maximum curvature) of the anterior/posterior corneal surfaces	3
Centre of mass *X, Y, Z* [mm]	Centre of mass coordinates *X, Y, Z* of the solid	–
Net deviation from centre of mass in *XY* [mm]	Projective *XY* Modulus of the centre of mass	–
Volume of corneal cylinder *R–x* [mm^3]	Volume of the intersection in 3D between the solid model of the cornea generated and a cylinder with *x* radius whose axis passes through the minimum thickness points (maximum curvature) of the anterior and posterior corneal surfaces. Radii adopted for this study were 0.5, 1, 1.5, and 2 mm	4

11.3.3 Deviations of Several Geometrical Parameters

As expected, a minor deviation from the apex of the anterior and posterior surfaces, and also a minor deviation at minimum thickness points of both surfaces in the group of normal corneas were observed ($p<0.05$). Regarding net deviation from the centre of mass in *x*, *y*, no significant differences between the groups of this study were observed ($p<0.05$). The only parameter with no statistically significant differences between groups was the centre of mass (*x*, *y*, *z*) ($p>0.05$). Therefore, it would not be a good predictor of differences between healthy corneas and corneas with subclinical keratoconus.

11.3.4 Sensitivity and Specificity for This Method

The predictive value of the modeled variables has been established through a ROC analysis (Fig. 11.1). A total of six variables have been identified with an area under the curve above 0. 63: Posterior apex deviation (area: 0.883, $p<0.000$, std. error: 0.041, 95 % CI: 0.800–0.964), the cutoff value obtained was 0.0655 mm, with a sensitivity and specificity associated of 90.32 % and 34.83 %, respectively; anterior apex deviation (area: 0.758, $p<0.000$, std. error: 0.059, 95 % CI: 0.641–0.875), the cutoff value obtained was 0.0010 mm, with a sensitivity and specificity associated of 64.52 % and 100.00 %, respectively; posterior minimum thickness point

Table 11.2 Descriptive values (mean, standard deviation, 95 % CI, minimum, maximum, and 25th, 50th, and 75th percentiles) and differences between normal and subclinical keratoconus corneal variables modeled

Measurement	Normal group, $n=89$							Subclinical keratoconus group, $n=31$							p (statistical test)
	M	SD	(95 % CI)	Min–Max	P_{25}	P_{50}	P_{75}	M	SD	(95 % CI)	Min–Max	P_{25}	P_{50}	P_{75}	
Total corneal volume [mm³]	25.79	1.60	(24.45–26.13)	21.36–29.47	24.62	25.93	26.82	24.01	1.71	(23.38–24.63)	19.82–28.10	22.96	23.82	24.60	0.000 (*t*-test)
Anterior corneal surface area [mm²]	43.08	0.15	(43.05–43.11)	42.73–43.39	42.98	43.07	43.20	43.19	0.17	(43.12–43.25)	42.81–43.50	43.05	43.21	43.33	0.002 (*t*-test)
Posterior corneal surface area [mm²]	44.23	0.28	(44.17–44.29)	43.49–44.87	44.04	44.24	44.41	44.38	0.29	(44.28–44.49)	43.83–44.80	44.13	44.40	44.63	0.011 (*t*-test)
Total corneal surface area [mm²]	103.93	1.27	(103.67–104.19)	100.73–106.16	103.10	103.91	105.09	103.24	1.18	(102.81–103.67)	101.28–105.57	102.35	103.30	104.02	0.010 (*t*-test)
Sagittal plane are a in apex [mm²]	4.33	0.27	(4.27–4.38)	3.58–5.00	4.13	4.35	4.50	4.01	0.30	(3.90–4.12)	3.27–4.77	3.85	3.98	4.10	0.000 (*t*-test)
Sagittal plane area at minimum thickness point [mm²]	4.27	0.53	(4.16–4.39)	0.00–5.00	4.11	4.35	4.48	4.00	0.30	(3.89–4.11)	3.27–4.76	3.84	3.98	4.10	0.000 (Mann–Whitney)
Anterior apex deviation [mm]	0.00	0.00	(0.00–0.00)	0.00–0.00	0.00	0.00	0.00	0.01	0.03	(−0.0009–0.0198)	0.00–0.16	0.00	0.01	0.01	0.000 (Mann–Whitney)
Posterior apex deviation [mm]	0.08	0.02	(0.07–0.08)	0.03–0.14	0.06	0.07	0.09	0.16	0.08	(0.13–0.19)	0.06–0.39	0.11	0.14	0.21	0.000 (Mann–Whitney)
Anterior minimum thickness point deviation [mm]	0.88	0.27	(0.82–0.93)	0.46–2.18	0.70	0.82	0.99	1.15	0.33	(1.02–1.27)	0.59–1.81	0.85	1.14	1.42	0.000 (Mann–Whitney)
Posterior minimum thickness point deviation [mm]	0.81	0.25	(0.76–0.86)	0.44–1.95	0.65	0.77	0.90	1.07	0.31	(0.96–1.19)	0.54–1.72	0.79	1.08	1.33	0.000 (Mann–Whitney)
Net deviation from centre of mass *XY* [mm]	0.06	0.02	(0.05–0.06)	0.01–0.10	0.04	0.06	0.07	0.07	0.02	(0.06–0.07)	0.03–0.11	0.05	0.06	0.08	0.042 (*t*-test)
Centre of mass *X* [mm]	0.04	0.02	(0.04–0.05)	0.01–0.09	0.03	0.04	0.05	0.05	0.02	(0.04–0.05)	0.00–0.07	0.04	0.05	0.06	0.281 (*t*-test)

(continued)

Table 11.2 (continued)

Measurement	Normal group, $n=89$							Subclinical keratoconus group, $n=31$							p (statistical test)
	M	SD	(95 % CI)	Min–Max	P_{25}	P_{50}	P_{75}	M	SD	(95 % CI)	Min–Max	P_{25}	P_{50}	P_{75}	
Centre of mass *Y* [mm]	0.03	0.02	(0.03–0.04)	0.00–0.09	0.03	0.03	0.05	0.04	0.02	(0.03–0.05)	0.00–0.09	0.02	0.04	0.06	0.135 (*t*-test)
Centre of mass *Z* [mm]	0.77	0.03	(0.77–0.78)	0.71–0.81	0.75	0.77	0.79	0.76	0.02	(0.75–0.77)	0.71–0.80	0.74	0.76	0.78	0.078 (*t*-test)
Volume of corneal cylinder (mm^3) with Radius 0.5 (mm)	0.46	0.30	(0.39–0.52)	0.36–3.25	0.40	0.43	0.44	0.38	0.03	(0.37–0.39)	0.30–0.47	0.36	0.38	0.40	0.000 (Mann–Whitney)
Volume of corneal cylinder (mm^3) with radius 1 (mm)	1.71	0.11	(1.69–1.74)	1.44–2.01	1.63	1.72	1.78	1.55	0.13	(1.50–1.59)	1.22–1.88	1.46	1.54	1.62	0.000 (*t*-test)
Volume of corneal cylinder (mm^3) with Radius 1.5 (mm)	3.95	0.43	(3.86–4.04)	3.27–7.26	3.74	3.92	4.08	3.56	0.28	(3.46–3.67)	2.84–4.29	3.38	3.55	3.71	0.000 (Mann–Whitney)
Volume of corneal cylinder (mm^3) with Radius 2 (mm)	7.10	0.44	(7.01–7.19)	5.92–8.29	6.79	7.10	7.37	6.53	0.48	(6.35–6.70)	5.23–7.78	6.26	6.52	6.74	0.000 (*t*-test)

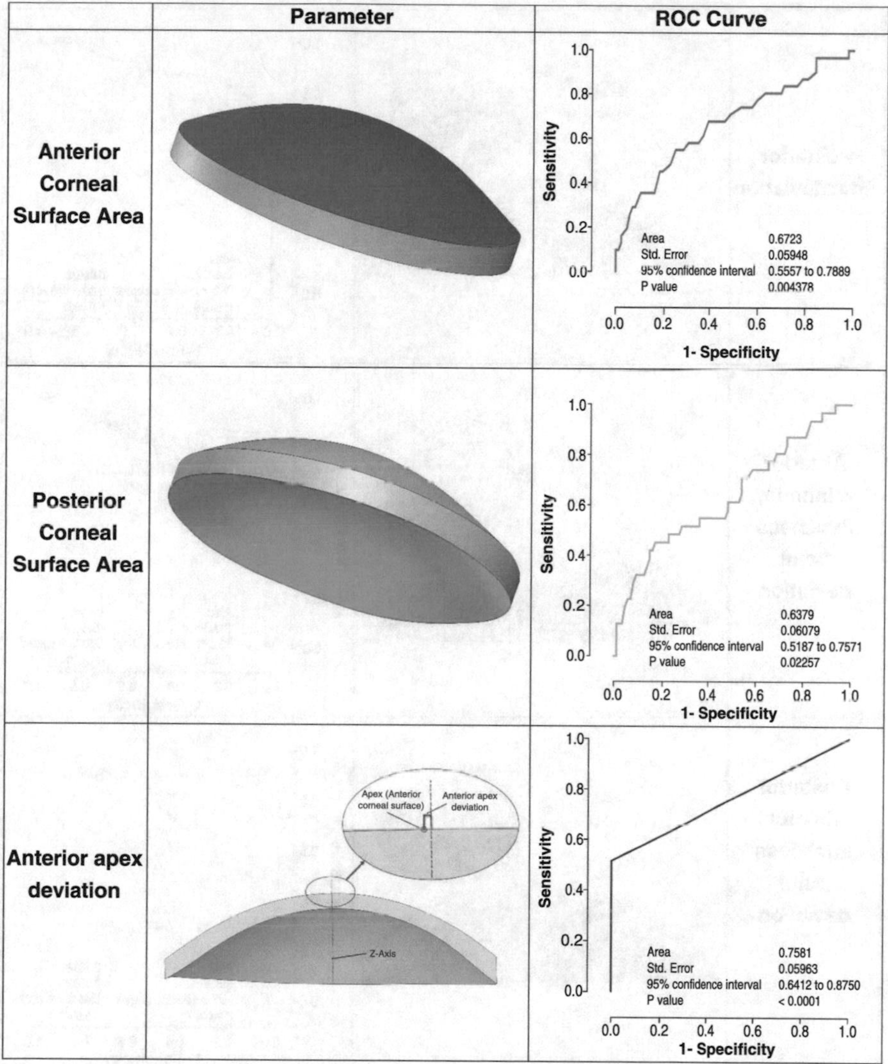

Fig. 11.1 ROC curve modeling the sensitivity versus 1-specificity for variables diagnosing the existence of subclinical keratoconus disease (plotted only selected variables with area under the curve over 0.63)

deviation (area: 0.758, $p<0.000$, std. error: 0.053, 95 % CI: 0.654–0.862), the cutoff value obtained was 0.6215 mm, with a sensitivity and specificity associated of 90.32 % and 20.22 %, respectively; anterior minimum thickness point deviation (area: 0.744, $p<0.000$, std. error: 0.054, 95 % CI: 0.638–0.851), the cutoff value obtained was 0.6795 mm, with a sensitivity and specificity associated of 90.32 % and 21.35 %, respectively; anterior corneal surface area (area: 0.672, $p<0.004$, std. error: 0.059, 95 % CI: 0.557–0.790), the cutoff value obtained was 42.9460 mm^2, with a sensitivity and specificity associated of 90.32 % and 15.73 %, respectively. Finally, the posterior corneal surface area (area: 0.638, $p<0.022$, std. error: 0.061, 95 % CI: 0.519–0.757), the cutoff value obtained was 44.9985 mm^2, with a sensitivity and specificity associated of 90.32 % and 19.10 %, respectively. Looking at these six variables, it can be concluded that the parameter that provides a higher rate of discrimination between normal corneal and corneas with subclinical keratoconus is the posterior apex deviation.

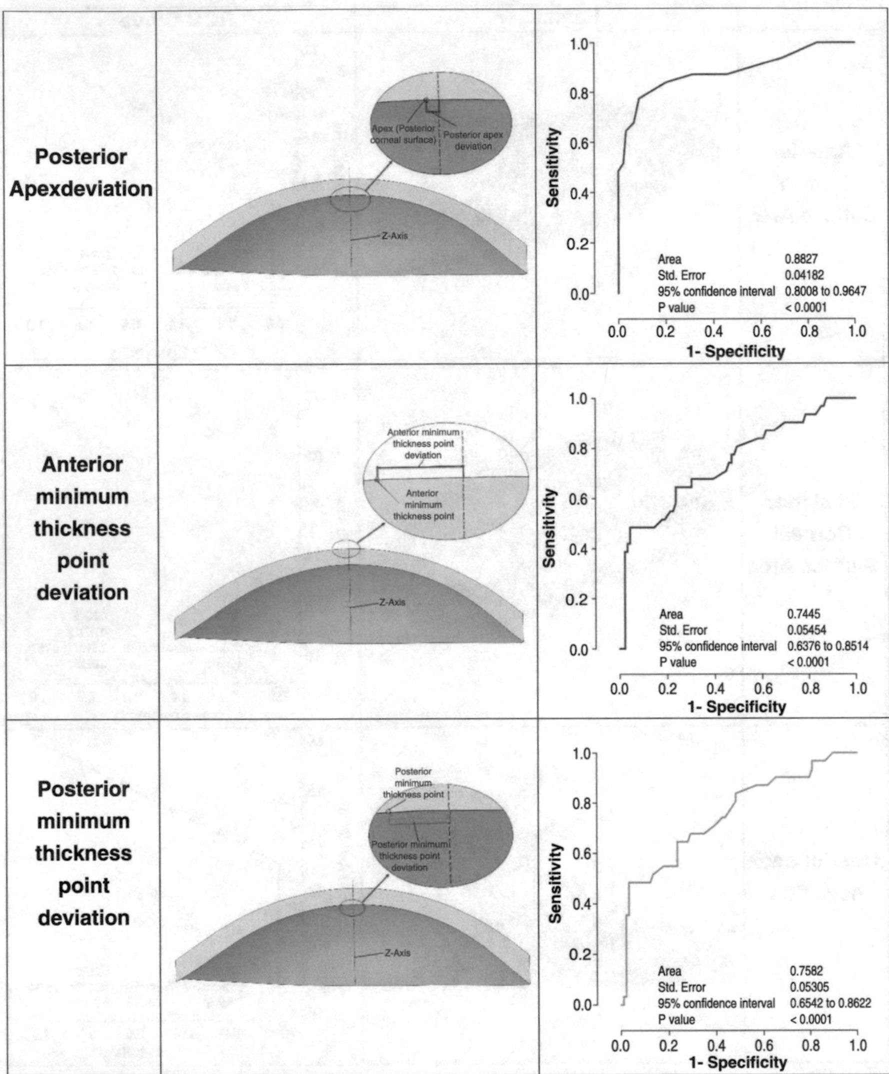

Fig. 11.1 (continued)

11.4 Discussion

Most of the indices employed by classic Placido disc topographers and tomographers devices use complicated formulas based on corneal curvature and thickness profiles for the detection of keratoconus. However, these devices have a number of limitations for analyzing completely the corneal topography, and their sensitivity and accuracy of the measurements are quite low in some cases, and therefore relevant information could be lost. Data are obtained directly from mathematical calculations that sometimes carry implicit assumptions to simplify the computation, and therefore, measurement error may increase. Due to this, it results of great interest to have detection indices for subclinical keratoconus that are based on the primary source of information, for example in the digitized data of the Placido rings, and that permit to improve the capacity of discrimination of this disease. Moreover, the independent analysis of the posterior and anterior corneal surfaces is not performed in an integrated way and requires the analysis of either surfaces separately, including also its aberrometric analysis, which provides a lot of different data that many times is redundant and sometimes difficult to interpret. This new method has shown new findings for the distinction between normal eyes and eyes with subclinical keratoconus, employing volumetric, pachymetric, surface area parameters, and deviations in the *XY* plane. Such parameters integrate both corneal surfaces and make aberrometric analysis of either of them unnecessary, creating a new, more simple, and global understanding of the limits of normality and early corneal pathology in the keratoconic eye.

Regarding volumetric parameters, the pathological group showed a statistically significant decrease of total corneal volume compared to healthy eyes. The same behavior was found in the volume of the corneal cylinders analyzed, detecting lower volumes for pathologic eyes. This trend was similar in all the radii studied (from 0.5 to 2 mm). Such changes may be due to the process of deterioration in keratoconus [5], which is triggered by the alteration of corneal collagen fibers, thus causing stromal thinning and breaks in Bowman membrane, initially in the subclinical degree. This way, the presence of orthogonality and homogeneity of the collagen fibers in healthy corneas is altered to an irregular distribution [6] and the bridges of collagen are affected in the pathological group. The analysis of this volumetric reduction has been identified in several studies as a parameter for the differentiation between normal and keratoconic eyes [7–11], where significant differences in the volume of the cornea were observed. In the case of this study, this difference is significantly compared to eyes with subclinical keratoconus where the degree of corneal protrusion is lower than in moderate cases, thus supporting the accuracy of the method proposed.

With regard to the area of the corneal surfaces, eyes with subclinical keratoconus show significant differences for both surfaces when compared with healthy corneas, being these areas higher in the pathological group. This result was expected because of the protrusion and existence of an irregular corneal area [5, 12, 13], due to an increment in the radius of curvature that causes an increase in the surface area. However, this behavior was not found when the total corneal surface area was obtained. Significant differences of the area of the total corneal surface were found between both groups, being higher in the group of healthy corneas. As previously mentioned in the section of solid modeling, anterior, posterior, and peripheral surfaces were considered for the calculation of the total corneal surface area. In the healthy corneas the peripheral corneal area is the possible cause of this fact, achieving a higher total corneal surface area. These values are consistent with those published by different studies on subclinical keratoconus, which report that the geometry and surface area of both corneal surfaces are affected because of the decreased number of stromal lamellae and lower interconnection lamellar surface at the level of the irregular corneal area [14, 15]. However, the presence of a higher total surface area in the healthy group is not as important as a higher total corneal volume accompanied by a high-density network of collagen fibers, making the cornea more resistant to the forces and therefore delaying the progression of keratoconus. This trend can also be appreciated with respect to the area of the sagittal plane that passes through the apex point of the anterior corneal surface, as well as to the area of the sagittal plane that passes through the minimum thickness point of the anterior surface. Statistically significant differences of these area parameters were found between groups, obtaining higher values for both parameters in the group of healthy corneas. The higher corneal volume in the healthy group previously mentioned may be the possible cause of these outcomes.

In addition, when analyzing the deviation of the apex points of both surfaces (average distance from the Z axis to the apex of the anterior/posterior corneal surfaces), significant differences between groups were observed, obtaining the largest deviation in the group of eyes with subclinical keratoconus [5, 16]. Concretely, in the case of deviation of the apex of the anterior surface, no observations were made in healthy corneas (0.00 ± 0.00 mm) and a minimal deviation with subclinical keratoconic corneas was detected (0.01 ± 0.03 mm). This might be related to the stage of lethargy in which the pathology can still be found in the anterior corneal surface. On the contrary, a deviation of the apex on the posterior surface of the cornea does exist in healthy corneas (0.08 ± 0.02 mm), possibly due to the existence of the toricity manifested in subjective refraction [17]. However, this deviation is significantly higher in eyes with subclinical keratoconus (0.16 ± 0.08 mm). This variation of the curvature could be detected by corneal tomography or topography [18]. On the other hand, the results showed by the deviation of the minimum thickness (maximum curvature) points of both surfaces (average distance from the Z axis to the minimum thickness points of the anterior/posterior corneal surfaces) were statistically different between groups, being higher in eyes with subclinical keratoconus (1.15 ± 0.33 mm for anterior surface and 1.07 ± 0.31 mm for posterior surface) with respect to healthy eyes (0. 88 ± 0.27 mm for anterior surface and 0.81 ± 0.25 mm for posterior surface). This fact is influenced by the presence of an irregular corneal surface creating a protrusion in the keratoconic case, thus increasing corneal curvature and therefore incrementing the distance of deviation [19]. Some researchers have evaluated certain ratios of corneal irregularity, concluding that they were significantly higher in keratoconic corneas than in normal corneas [20]. Saad et al. showed the comparison of a group of normal eyes with subclinical keratoconic eyes, demonstrating that only the combination of all indices of irregularity, extracted from the minimum thickness area of the cornea, allows a 92 % of accuracy in differentiation of these groups [11].

In this sense, we attempt to understand the performance provided by this technique for discrimination of both groups by each of these variables. The best results in the determination of the disease were obtained by the posterior apex deviation variable (area: 0.883, $p < 0.000$, std. error: 0.041, 95 % CI: 0.800–0.964). This variable, having a higher area under the ROC curve, provided a more discriminatory capacity. This may be due to the existence of structural instability in subclinical keratoconic corneas. For instance, the decrease of corneal volume in these cases was observed. The posterior corneal surface is more susceptible to variations due to the forces that are exerted on the tissue and for this reason the posterior apex deviation is one of the variables that most reliably represents the early changes in patients with early forms of the disease. Several studies conclude the great importance and interest regarding the posterior corneal surface. At the beginning of the disease, structural changes occur at the rear face of the cornea and an efficient analysis of this surface would be very useful to perform a positive and early identification of the subclinical keratoconus. These findings suggest that important clinical analysis of posterior corneal surface clearly contributes to early manifestation of subclinical keratoconus.

Compliance with Ethical Requirements *Conflict of Interest*: F. Cavas, P. Sanz, A. Vega, E. De la Cruz, D.G. Fernández-Pacheco, A.B. Plaza, J. Nieto, F.J. Fernández and J.L. Alió declare that they have no conflict of interest.

Informed Consent: All procedures followed were in accordance with the ethical standards of the responsible committee on human experimentation (institutional and national) and with the Helsinki Declaration of 1975, as revised in 2000. Informed consent was obtained from all patients for being included in the study.

No animal studies were carried out by the authors for this chapter.

References

1. Moshirfar M, Smedley JG, Muthappan V, Jarsted A, Ostler EM. Rate of ectasia and incidence of irregular topography in patients with unidentified preoperative risk factors undergoing femtosecond laser-assisted LASIK. Clin Ophthalmol. 2014;8:35–42. doi:10.2147/opth.s53370.
2. Lasko TA, Bhagwat JG, Zou KH, Ohno-Machado L. The use of receiver operating characteristic curves in biomedical informatics. J Biomed Inform. 2005; 38(5):404–15. doi:10.1016/j.jbi.2005.02.008.
3. Montalban R, Pinero DP, Javaloy J, Alio JL. Intrasubject repeatability of corneal morphology measurements obtained with a new Scheimpflug photography-based system. J Cataract Refract Surg. 2012;38(6):971–7. doi:10.1016/j.jcrs.2011.12.029.
4. Cavas-Martinez F, Fernandez-Pacheco DG, De la Cruz-Sanchez E, Nieto Martinez J, Fernandez Canavate FJ, Vega-Estrada A, et al. Geometrical custom modeling of human cornea in vivo and its use for the diagnosis of corneal ectasia. PLoS One. 2014;9(10), e110249. doi:10.1371/journal.pone.0110249.
5. Rabinowitz YS. Keratoconus. Surv Ophthalmol. 1998; 42(4):297–319. doi:10.1016/s0039-6257(97)00119-7.

6. Cervino A, Gonzalez-Meijome JM, Ferrer-Blasco T, Garcia-Resua C, Montes-Mico R, Parafita M. Determination of corneal volume from anterior topography and topographic pachymetry: application to healthy and keratoconic eyes. Ophthalmic Physiol Opt. 2009;29(6):652–60. doi:10.1111/j.1475-1313.2009.00642.x.
7. Ambrosio Jr R, Alonso RS, Luz A, Coca Velarde LG. Corneal-thickness spatial profile and corneal-volume distribution: tomographic indices to detect keratoconus. J Cataract Refract Surg. 2006;32(11):1851–9. doi:10.1016/j.jcrs.2006.06.025.
8. Cavas-Martinez F, Fernandez-Pacheco DG, De La Cruz-Sanchez E, Nieto-Martínez J, Fernandez-Cañavate F, Alió JL. Virtual biomodelling of a biologic structure: the human cornea. DYNA-Ingeniería e Industria. 2015;90(6):648–52. doi:10.6036/7689.
9. Pinero DP, Alio JL, Aleson A, Escaf Vergara M, Miranda M. Corneal volume, pachymetry, and correlation of anterior and posterior corneal shape in subclinical and different stages of clinical keratoconus. J Cataract Refract Surg. 2010;36(5):814–25. doi:10.1016/j.jcrs.2009.11.012.
10. Mannion LS, Tromans C, O'Donnell C. Reduction in corneal volume with severity of keratoconus. Curr Eye Res. 2011;36(6):522–7. doi:10.3109/02713683.2011.553306.
11. Saad A, Lteif Y, Azan E, Gatinel D. Biomechanical properties of keratoconus suspect eyes. Invest Ophthalmol Vis Sci. 2010;51(6):2912–6. doi:10.1167/iovs.09-4304.
12. Amsler M. Le kératocône fruste au Javal. Ophthalmologica. 1938;96(2):77–83. doi:10.1159/000299577.
13. Amsler M. Kératocône classique et kératocône fruste; arguments unitaires. Ophthalmologica. 1946;111(2–3):96–101. doi:10.1159/000300309.
14. de Sanctis U, Loiacono C, Richiardi L, Turco D, Mutani B, Grignolo FM. Sensitivity and specificity of posterior corneal elevation measured by Pentacam in discriminating keratoconus/subclinical keratoconus. Ophthalmology. 2008;115(9):1534–9. doi:10.1016/j.ophtha.2008.02.020.
15. Schlegel Z, Hoang-Xuan T, Gatinel D. Comparison of and correlation between anterior and posterior corneal elevation maps in normal eyes and keratoconus-suspect eyes. J Cataract Refract Surg. 2008;34(5):789–95. doi:10.1016/j.jcrs.2007.12.036.
16. Wilson SE, Lin DT, Klyce SD. Corneal topography of keratoconus. Cornea. 1991;10(1):2–8.
17. Montalban R, Pinero DP, Javaloy J, Alio JL. Correlation of the corneal toricity between anterior and posterior corneal surfaces in the normal human eye. Cornea. 2013;32(6):791–8. doi:10.1097/ICO.0b013e31827bf898.
18. de Rojas Silva V. Clasificación del queratocono. In: Albertazzi R, editor. Queratocono: pautas para su diagnostico y tratamiento. Buenos Aires, Argentina: Ediciones Científicas Argentinas; 2010. p. 33–97.
19. Daxer A, Fratzl P. Collagen fibril orientation in the human corneal stroma and its implication in keratoconus. Invest Ophthalmol Vis Sci. 1997;38(1):121–9.
20. Li X, Yang H, Rabinowitz YS. Keratoconus: classification scheme based on videokeratography and clinical signs. J Cataract Refract Surg. 2009;35(9):1597–603. doi:10.1016/j.jcrs.2009.03.050.

Role of Corneal Biomechanics in the Diagnosis and Management of Keratoconus

12

FangJun Bao, Brendan Geraghty, QinMei Wang, and Ahmed Elsheikh

12.1 Introduction

Keratoconus (KC), the most prevalent form of idiopathic corneal ectasia, is a progressive degenerative eye disease characterised by localised thinning and conical protrusion of the cornea. The cone typically develops in the inferior-temporal and central zones [1] although superior localisations can also occur [2]. Consequently, visual acuity is reduced due to irregular astigmatism and high myopia resulting from the corneal topographical changes. KC affects both genders and all ethnicities [3–6]; however, higher incidence has been reported in Asians when compared to Caucasians [7, 8]. Onset usually occurs during puberty and progresses until the fourth decade of life [3]. With 50 % of unilateral cases progressing to bilateral KC within 16 years [9], experts now agree that true unilateral KC does not exist [10].

Although the aetiology and pathology of the disease is still not fully understood, various biochemical, cellular and microstructural differences have been reported in the literature. For instance, biochemical changes include increased activity of proteolytic enzymes and a decrease in their inhibitors [11, 12]. A progressive reduction in collagen producing keratocytes has also been observed [13] and it has been suggested that variations in collagen type XIII [14], XV and XVIII [15] may alter the healing properties of keratoconic corneas. Stromal ultrastructural abnormalities comprise altered spatial distribution of proteoglycans [16], changes in collagen organisation and uneven distribution of collagen mass [17] as well as decreased fibril diameter and interfibrillar spacing, undulation of collagen lamellae [18], reduced lamellar interweaving and loss of lamellae inserting into Bowman's layer [19]. Moreover, the observed thinning of the stroma in KC has been associated with the uneven distribution of collagen mass with inter- and possibly intra-lamellar displacement and slippage resulting in changes in corneal curvature [20, 21].

F. Bao, Ph.D., M.D. (✉) • Q. Wang, M.D.
Eye Hospital, WenZhou Medical University, Wenzhou 325027, China

The Institution of Ocular Biomechanics, Wenzhou Medical University, Wenzhou, Zhejiang 325027, China
e-mail: bfjmd@126.com

B. Geraghty, Ph.D.
School of Engineering, University of Liverpool, Liverpool L69 3GH, UK

A. Elsheikh, Ph.D.
School of Engineering, University of Liverpool, Liverpool L69 3GH, UK

NIHR Biomedical Research Centre for Ophthalmology, Moorfields Eye Hospital NHS Foundation Trust and UCL Institute of Ophthalmology, Liverpool, UK
e-mail: B.Geraghty@liverpool.ac.uk; ahmed.elsheikh@liverpool.ac.uk

J.L. Alió (ed.), *Keratoconus*, Essentials in Ophthalmology, DOI 10.1007/978-3-319-43881-8_12

12.2 Clinical Tools for the Study of Corneal Biomechanics in Keratoconus: Diagnostic Techniques

With the disruption of the collagen network, the intraocular pressure causes a weakened cornea to bulge from its normal shape and become progressively conical. Consequently, corneal topography has become the most widely used tool to detect KC. Abnormal corneal tomography parameters such as atypical pachymetry profile, irregular anterior curvature and increased posterior surface elevation have all been used to detect KC at different stages of the disease. While topography analysis is well suited to characterising KC when clear geometrical changes have occurred in the cornea, its robustness reduces when attempting to assess mild, pathologic cases, especially in subclinical or early KC [22]. The reduced efficacy of these techniques stems from the fact that changes in corneal geometric features are secondary signs of KC whereas the earliest initiating changes of the disease occur within the microstructure and hence the biomechanical properties of tissue. Since KC is thought to be associated with a "weaker" cornea, a technique capable of determining in vivo biomechanical behaviour of this ocular component may be an important tool which could be used in the detection of subclinical KC [23].

12.2.1 Corneal Biomechanical Properties

The cornea exhibits complex biomechanical behaviour characteristics, namely hyperelasticity (a nonlinear stress increase with a linear strain increase), viscoelasticity (hysteresis, creep and stress relaxation) and anisotropy (directionally dependent response to applied loads). Non-enzymatic glycosylation, or "cross-linking", of collagen molecules also results in age-dependent stiffening of the tissue. Furthermore, medical history and diseases such as KC as well as treatment methods can also affect the biomechanical characteristics of the tissue. As a result, accurately determining the biomechanical behaviour of the cornea requires significant effort and its difficulty is exasperated when in vivo characterisation is considered. Nevertheless, there has been significant scientific interest in assessing corneal biomechanical properties due to potential clinical applications in recent years, particularly in the diagnosis and management of KC.

Since biomechanical stability is dependent on the regulation and organisation of structural components within the cornea, the biochemical, cellular and microstructural changes observed in keratoconic corneas would be expected to have negative consequences on structural integrity of the tissue and alter its biomechanical properties [24]. Tensile properties of soft biological tissues are determined by the size and organisation of collagen fibrils. Therefore, the observed alterations in alignment, diameter and spatial order of fibrils in KC would undoubtedly have implications on the cornea's response to intraocular pressure (IOP) induced stress. The corneal epithelium undergoes the earliest pathological changes in KC and proteolytic enzymes released by degenerating basal epithelial cells cause instability of Bowman's layer and loss of stromal collagen fibrils. In cases of acute corneal hydrops in KC, abnormalities in Descemet's membrane and endothelium have been noted. All of these combined may be responsible for the biomechanical instability of the tissue in keratoconus.

Experimental studies of ex vivo KC corneas have reported abnormalities in biomechanical response to applied loads when compared to normal corneas [25, 26]. However, in vivo measurement of corneal biomechanics still remains a difficult task. There are currently only two commercially available instruments capable of quantifying in vivo biomechanical metrics that can be used to assist in the diagnosis of the KC. These instruments are summarised as follows.

12.2.2 Ocular Response Analyser

The Ocular Response Analyser (ORA) became commercially available in 2005 and was the first device capable of evaluating the biomechanical response of the cornea in vivo. The device quantifies the dynamics of corneal deformation and recovery during a variable air-puff pressure application over a 20 ms period. In addition to intraocular pressure and pachymetry readings, the device also provides two biomechanical metrics: corneal hysteresis (CH) and corneal resistance factor (CRF). CH is the difference between the two applanation pressures (P_1 and P_2) recorded while applying the air puff. CRF, on the other hand, is an indicator of the overall resistance of the cornea to the applied air-puff pressure and is significantly correlated with central corneal thickness (CCT). Both of these biomechanical metrics are influenced by the viscoelastic behaviour of the corneal tissue [27]. Clinically measured metrics provided by ORA have been widely used to assess the biomechanical response of the cornea in order to help identify potential cases of KC. Compared with normal patients, both CH and CRF are usually reduced in KC corneas indicating a mechanical weakening of the stroma [28]. However, a wide substantial overlap exists in the biomechanical metrics of normal and keratoconic corneas [29, 30] and so they have not been as effective in identifying KC as first anticipated. Furthermore, the exact correlation between these metrics and the established mechanical properties of tissue (such as tangent modulus) is still unknown [22]. Thus, the ORA must be complemented with other diagnostic imaging tools to obtain a reliable diagnosis of KC. With the introduction of a software update (version 2.0) in 2009, the ORA now computes 37 new parameters that describe the waveform of the ORA applanation signal. These parameters show promise in providing additional biomechanical information about KC corneas [31, 32]. However, the manufacturers have not yet provided a specific explanation of the meaning of each parameter and so they still require thorough clinical validation before they can be commonly used in clinical practise.

12.2.3 Corvis ST

The Corvis ST (CVS) is another representative non-contact device that was first introduced in 2010. The CVS employs a similar deformation technique to the ORA, but with a non-varying maximum air pressure and provides information about the biomechanical response of the cornea using dynamic Scheimpflug imaging analysis. The CVS captures approximately 140 cross-sectional images of the cornea during the air-puff-induced dynamic deformation [33] using its high-speed camera system. This information is then used to characterise the morphological response of the cornea to the instrument's air-puff pressure using ten deformation parameters, some of which are strongly correlated with the tissue's mechanical stiffness. As shown in a previous study, the maximum deformation amplitude of keratoconic corneas is much greater than that of normal corneas [34]. Further analysis of the CVS data may yet be used to yield additional metrics about the biomechanical status of the cornea. However, the usefulness of CVS to evaluate KC severity and diagnose subclinical KC is yet to be determined. The inclusion of a high-speed Scheimpflug camera allows for precise monitoring of in vivo cornea cross-sectional deformation under the applied air pressure. This deformation data provides biomedical engineers with invaluable information that can be used to determine more precise biomechanical properties of the tissue. Work is now progressing to utilise this device to produce regional estimations of in vivo corneal stiffness, which may allow for better planning of the treatment and management of KC.

12.2.4 Other Devices

Several other technologies have also been developed to evaluate corneal biomechanical parameters in vivo such as optical coherence tomography [35], supersonic shear wave imaging (SSI) [36], confocal microscopy [37], applanation resonance tonometer (ART) [38], acoustic radiation force (ARF) [39] and scanning acoustic microscopy [40]. However, the validation of these technologies in human eyes will be essential before using the findings of studies to help improve the accuracy of KC diagnosis. Lack of reliable in vivo measurements or devices capable of characterising true corneal material properties has meant that KC biomechanics have only been investigated to a limited extent. It is now becoming apparent that the bulk biomechanical assessment of the cornea may not be sufficient to fully characterise this typically asymmetric disease. Spatial location of focal weakening in the cornea may be necessary to detect the disease at its earliest stages as well as fully characterise its progression.

12.3 Keratoconus Treatment Techniques: Implications of Corneal Biomechanics

KC is currently managed using a number of methods ranging from non-invasive options capable of providing short-term results to invasive techniques for more long-term outcomes. However, the method of treatment used is highly dependent on the severity of the ectasia. In early stages for instance, spectacles can sufficiently correct refractive errors although this method becomes unsuitable for correcting the irregular astigmatism associated with KC as the disease progresses [3]. In mild to moderate KC, contact lenses, especially rigid gas permeable (RGP) lenses, are the most common and successful method of treatment providing improved visual acuity whilst decreasing the need for surgical interventions [41]. In contrast to the aforementioned short-term solutions, which aim to improve visual acuity by improving the anterior curvature of the cornea, more long-term invasive clinical interventions are also available. Intrastromal corneal ring segment (ICRS) implants and corneal cross-linking (CXL) aim to improve the shape of the cornea or halt the progression of the cone. For advanced cases, which cannot be successfully managed with regular treatment, deep anterior lamellar keratoplasty (DALK) and penetrating keratoplasty (PK) were introduced to replace either the anterior layers of the stroma or the entire cornea with healthy donor tissue, respectively.

12.3.1 Contact Lenses

Contact lenses aim to improve the anterior curvature of the cornea and increase visual acuity. Nevertheless, all options interact mechanically with the cornea to varying degrees. While several lens options are available, the most commonly used materials include soft hydrogel and silicone hydrogel, and RGP polymethylmethacrylate (PMMA). Although soft lenses provide increased comfort for the wearer, rigid lenses are more prevalent since high levels of irregular astigmatism cannot be corrected with other lens types [42, 43].

Soft lenses interact mechanically with the cornea as surface tension forces arising from the tear film at the lens periphery and a negative pressure within the tear reservoir between the lens and cornea attract the lens towards the eye [44, 45]. Bespoke lens options, such as the KeraSoft® lens, are individually lathe cut to fit the specific irregularity of a patient's cornea resulting in a close fit between the lens and eye while improving the anterior curvature. The Young's modulus of current silicone hydrogel lenses is typically in the region of 0.3–1.0 MPa [46] which is similar to the tangent modulus of the cornea under normal IOP [47]. Consequently, the effect of the forces acting between the contact lens and eye influences the final lens topography and hence affect the patient's visual acuity. However, this mechanical interaction and subsequent change in lens topography is not yet considered when designing soft lenses.

As with soft lenses, RGP lenses are held in place by forces generated between the tear film, lens and eye but the degree of fit between the lens and eye varies. In mild KC an ideal fit can be achieved and the lens is usually intended to rest on the apex of the cone. However, as the cone progresses a compromised fit may need to be accepted as long as it does not cause damage to the cornea. In this instance, additional mechanical action occurs between the lens and cornea as the lens presses against the cone and temporarily changes its shape [48]. The Young's modulus of the PMMA material used in RGP lenses is also three orders of magnitude higher than that of soft lenses. Consequently, mechanical interaction with the cornea would be unlikely to cause any significant changes in lens shape. Originally it was hoped that the lens bearing pressure on the cornea could correct or stabilise the ectasia by flattening the cone [49]. However, it was later found that this can result in abrasion and scarring of the cornea [50].

12.3.2 Intrastromal Corneal Ring Segments

ICRS implants are designed to reshape abnormal corneal topographies based on an 'arc-shortening effect' when introduced into the stroma. This method was first developed to correct low myopia during its early stages [51] but has now become a treatment option for KC patients with significant irregular astigmatism and an intolerance to RGP lenses [52]. It has been shown that eyes with varying severities of KC respond differently to ICRS placement with the greatest effect shown in mild to moderate KC [53]. ICRS implants are inserted into the stroma by creating an incision using a femtosecond laser or a mechanical tunnelling technique in the peripheral region of the cornea with the aim of decreasing asymmetrical astigmatism and convexity of the cone [54, 55]. However, the incisions required to insert the implants would be expected to lead to a relaxation of the anterior stromal tissue resulting in an altered shape. Furthermore, the effect of wound healing may lead to a possible increase in membrane stiffness of the cornea whereas tissue separation caused by the introduction of the implant could result in changes in flexural stiffness. Although there have been no statistically significant differences observed in cornea hysteresis (CH) and corneal resistance factor (CRF) parameters obtained from the ORA [56], the introduction of rigid components to the stroma would be expected to affect the biomechanical behaviour of the tissue. This could be due to tissue scarring within the stroma resulting from the introduction of the ICRS implants or changes in the overall mechanical response of the tissue particularly in the peripheral region where the implant has been introduced.

12.3.3 Cornea Collagen Cross-Linking

CXL is achieved via saturation of the stroma with riboflavin followed by irradiation of the central region of the cornea using ultraviolet-A light at 365–370 nm [57]. While stromal saturation originally required the removal of the corneal epithelium, more recent advances in techniques allow for transepithelial application of riboflavin. Nevertheless, in all cases UVA is applied centrally with uniform distribution and in the same form for all patients despite their disease state. The procedure activates riboflavin generating reactive oxygen species that induce cross-links at the surface of collagen fibrils and within the proteoglycan-rich coating surrounding them [58] as well as limited linkages among collagen molecules and among proteoglycan core proteins [59]. The outcome of this procedure is an overall increase in mechanical stiffness [60] which usually halts the progression of the cone [61]. While various options are now available for the management of KC, CXL is fast becoming the most commonly used technique. This technique can be used to halt progression of the cone at all stages of the disease [10] provided that the minimum stromal thickness is at least 400 μm, thereby reducing further degradation of visual acuity and limiting the need for corneal transplants. With the development of CXL, some patients who might otherwise have required penetrating keratoplasty are now able to undergo a relatively well-tolerated procedure to potentially stabilise the progression of their disease. However, the uniform application of the CXL treatment to the diseased cornea will result in an over-stiffening of the regions unaffected by KC, something that is not yet considered in the patient treatment.

12.3.4 Keratoplasty

Advanced cases of keratoconus, such as keratometry values steeper than 55 D, corneal astigmatism >10 D, corrected visual acuity worse than 6/12 (20/40), the presence of corneal scarring or poor contact lens tolerance may require PK [62–64]. The procedure entails removing the entire thickness of the cornea, which is then replaced with donor tissue [3, 62]. DALK, in which anterior corneal layers are removed and replaced with healthy donor tissue while Descemet's membrane and the endothelium remain intact [65, 66], was employed in KC management in recent years.

Compared with PK, DALK has a lower risk of endothelial cell loss and graft rejection [65], avoids the risk associated with open sky surgery such as expulsive haemorrhage, endophthalmitis, iris and/or lens damage, and offers superior wound strength [67, 68]. For corneal pathologies not affecting the endothelium and Descemet's membrane, DALK is a reasonable alternative to PK [67]. However, normal stromal architecture cannot be fully recovered in full-thickness graft wounds [69–71]. Abnormalities in collagen fibril orientation and spatial organisation have been found around the entire graft margin following PK which may affect corneal biomechanical behaviour and graft stability in the long term [72].

12.4 Biomechanical Changes Induced by the Use of the Different Therapeutic Modalities

Although all current KC management techniques involve mechanical interaction with or mechanical changes to the cornea, the design and planning of these interventions do not consider the mechanical properties of the cornea either pre- or post-intervention. For instance, hypoxia-related corneal oedema can occur as a result of prolonged soft lens wear [73] even though the materials used have high oxygen permeability. From a biomechanical perspective, this oedema can lead to a decrease in corneal stiffness and hence an increase in corneal deformation [74]. In rigid lens wear, where the interaction between the lens and cornea can be even more pronounced, changes in corneal shape with possible biochemical, cellular and microstructural responses may have subsequent consequences for the overall biomechanical integrity of the cornea.

Surgical interventions can also result in biomechanical changes to the cornea. Recent studies using the ORA have found that CH and CRF values from DALK-treated corneas are similar to normal corneas whereas the corresponding values for PK-treated corneas are significantly lower [75, 76]. This reduction in the values of these metrics indicates a softer cornea. It has been suggested that this weakening is the result of lasting changes in collagen fibril orientation in and around the PK wounds caused by incomplete stromal wound remodelling. Conversely, the improved structural integrity of DALK-treated eyes may be the result of combined healing at the deep interface and graft margin as well as the intact Descemet's membrane.

The most significant iatrogenic changes in KC corneal biomechanics are those observed when a patient has been treated using CXL. Experimental cross-linking studies have reported human corneal stiffness increases in the region of 300 % using riboflavin/UVA treatment [60] but surprisingly no change in interlaminar cohesion [77]. However, in vivo assessments of corneal biomechanical stress–strain behaviour properties have not yet been determined as it is currently not possible to obtain this information. Consequently, this has meant that clinicians have to make assumptions about the post-procedure mechanics of the tissue, which can result in outcomes that are less than perfect. Furthermore, when riboflavin is combined with UVA irradiation, the cytotoxic effect is ten times greater than UVA irradiation alone [78]. It is therefore important to ensure that sufficient increases in tissue stiffness are achieved without damaging cellular components as complications from the procedure may result in the need for keratoplasty.

Since the deformation of the cornea in KC is not symmetric, optimum planning, treatment and management of the disorder would require patient-specific information. This would have to include information not only related to the cornea as a whole, but also the stiffness in the area affected by the disease. However, this lack of patient-specific information on the biomechanical properties of the diseased cornea has made it necessary to apply the CXL procedure uniformly over the central portion of the cornea, despite the fact that the keratoconic cone is usually eccentric. Applying a uniform distribution of UVA in the CXL treatment would also induce cross-linking in the unaffected regions of the cornea possibly leading to over-stiffening. The same is true for corneal implants where a concentric distribution is adopted potentially leading to a stiffness increase that is not compatible with the stiffness deterioration experienced in KC.

Over-stiffening of the cornea may have negative effects, which have not been considered before in the planning of the CXL treatment. In comparison to the sclera, the stiffness of the cornea is lower due to differences in microstructure such as smaller collagen fibril diameter and changes in fibril organisation in the peripheral cornea. As the eye is subjected to continuous changes in IOP due to typical diurnal variation [79], physical exertion or ocular pulse amplitude [80], these pressure changes are mainly absorbed by the cornea due to its large surface area and low mechanical stiffness. The majority of corneal deformation during these changes takes place in the peripheral region [81] where the fibril directions transition from an orthogonal to circumferential alignment [82]. Meanwhile, the central portion stretches while retaining its curvature to maintain its refractive power and sustain clear vision. However, since the increases in cornea stiffness due to CXL are significantly higher, the accommodating behaviour of this ocular component to changes in IOP would be greatly reduced and likely transferred to another region of lower stiffness such as the lamina cribrosa located in the optic nerve head. As a result, the risk of developing glaucoma in the long term may be increased since this region of the eye would be subjected to higher stresses and strains. Furthermore, experimental studies have reported stiffness increases in the cornea of 7–11 % per decade between the ages of 30 and 99 [47]. Similarly, increases in sclera stiffness due to ageing have also been reported [83, 84]. Therefore, the need to consider these changes may be more important now that CXL is also being used in young KC patients.

12.5 Conclusion

Progressive degeneration with localised thinning and conical protrusion of the cornea are the main clinical features of KC. Changes in corneal microstructure and uneven distribution of collagen mass also result in altered corneal biomechanical properties. The current inability to measure in vivo corneal biomechanical properties has been a major obstacle in the diagnosis of KC as well as the planning and assessment of clinical interventions. While diagnosis techniques rely on abnormal cornea tomography parameters, changes in corneal geometry are secondary signs of the disease. Consequently, the efficacy of using these parameters is reduced when attempting to assess mild and subclinical cases. Since the earliest changes to KC corneas occur within the microstructure, in vivo assessment of corneal biomechanics may be a more appropriate approach to detecting subclinical KC. The disease is managed using a number of methods depending on the severity of the ectasia. However, corneal biomechanics is not considered in the planning of these management techniques. Although several technologies have been developed to evaluate in vivo corneal biomechanical parameters, only two devices are commercially available to clinicians, namely the ORA and CVS. Unfortunately, substantial overlap exists between ORA metrics obtained from normal corneas and those affected by KC resulting in the need for further imaging tools to obtain reliable diagnoses. Furthermore, there is no exact correlation between ORA metrics and the mechanical properties of the tissue. The CVS, on the other hand, is capable of recording in vivo cross-sectional deformation of the cornea during the application of an air pulse using a high-speed Scheimpflug camera. Additional analysis of this data may be used to characterise biomechanical properties and identify the spatial location of focal weakening. Regional information about corneal biomechanical properties could then be used to guide CXL treatments and avoid over-stiffening of unaffected tissue. Work is now progressing to utilise this device in overcoming the obstacle of producing regional estimations of in vivo corneal biomechanical properties. Completion of this work will allow for better planning of the treatment and management of KC.

Compliance with Ethical Requirements FangJun Bao, Brendan Geraghty, QinMei Wang and Ahmed Elsheikh declare that they have no conflict of interest. No human or animal studies were carried out by the authors for this article.

References

1. Auffarth GU, Wang L, Völcker HE. Keratoconus evaluation using the Orbscan topography system. J Cataract Refract Surg. 2000;26(2):222–8.
2. Weed KH, McGhee CN, MacEwen CJ. Atypical unilateral superior keratoconus in young males. Cont Lens Anterior Eye. 2005;28(4):177–9.
3. Rabinowitz YS. Keratoconus. Surv Ophthalmol. 1998;42(4):297–319.
4. Wagner H, Barr JT, Zadnik K. Collaborative Longitudinal Evaluation of Keratoconus (CLEK) study: methods and findings to date. Cont Lens Anterior Eye. 2007;30(4):223–32.
5. Weed KH, MacEwen CJ, Giles T, et al. The Dundee University Scottish Keratoconus study: demographics, corneal signs, associated diseases, and eye rubbing. Eye (Lond). 2008;22(4):534–41.
6. Owens H, Gamble GD, Bjornholdt MC, et al. Topographic indications of emerging keratoconus in teenage New Zealanders. Cornea. 2007;26(3):312–8.
7. Pearson A, Soneji B, Sarvananthan N, Sandford-Smith J. Does ethnic origin influence the incidence or severity of keratoconus? Eye (Lond). 2000; 14(Pt4):625–8.
8. Georgiou T, Funnell CL, Cassels-Brown A, O'Conor R. Influence of ethnic origin on the incidence of keratoconus and associated atopic disease in Asians and white patients. Eye (Lond). 2004;18(4):379–83.
9. Li X, Rabinowitz Y, Rasheed K, Yang H. Longitudinal study of the normal eyes in unilateral keratoconus patients. Ophthalmology. 2004;111(3):440–6.
10. Gomes JA, Tan D, Rapuano CJ, et al. Global consensus on keratoconus and ectatic diseases. Cornea. 2015;34(4):359–69.
11. Cristina Kenney M, Brown DJ. The cascade hypothesis of keratoconus. Cont Lens Anterior Eye. 2003;26(3):139–46.
12. Kenney MC, Chwa M, Atilano SR, et al. Increased levels of catalase and cathepsin V/L2 but decreased TIMP-1 in keratoconus corneas: evidence that oxidative stress plays a role in this disorder. Invest Ophthalmol Vis Sci. 2005;46(3):823–32.
13. Ku JY, Niederer RL, Patel DV, et al. Laser scanning in vivo confocal analysis of keratocyte density in keratoconus. Ophthalmology. 2008;115(5):845–50.
14. Maatta M, Vaisanen T, Vaisanen MR, et al. Altered expression of type XIII collagen in keratoconus and scarred human cornea: increased expression in scarred cornea is associated with myofibroblast transformation. Cornea. 2006;25(4):448–53.
15. Maatta M, Heljasvaara R, Sormunen R, et al. Differential expression of collagen types XVIII/endostatin and XV in normal, keratoconus, and scarred human corneas. Cornea. 2006;25(3):341–9.
16. Fullwood NJ, Tuft SJ, Malik NS, et al. Synchrotron x-ray diffraction studies of keratoconus corneal stroma. Invest Ophthalmol Vis Sci. 1992;33(5): 1734–41.
17. Meek K, Tuft S, Huang Y, et al. Changes in collagen orientation and distribution in keratoconus corneas. Invest Ophthalmol Vis Sci. 2005;46(6):1948–56.
18. Akhtar S, Bron AJ, Salvi SM, et al. Ultrastructural analysis of collagen fibrils and proteoglycans in keratoconus. Acta Ophthalmol. 2008;86(7):764–72.
19. Morishige N, Wahlert AJ, Kenney MC, et al. Second-harmonic imaging microscopy of normal human and keratoconus cornea. Invest Ophthalmol Vis Sci. 2007;48(3):1087–94.
20. Meek KM, Blamires T, Elliott GF, et al. The organisation of collagen fibrils in the human corneal stroma: a synchrotron X-ray diffraction study. Curr Eye Res. 1987;6(7):841–6.
21. Sherwin T, Brookes NH. Morphological changes in keratoconus: pathology or pathogenesis. Clin Experiment Ophthalmol. 2004;32(2):211–7.
22. Pinero DP, Nieto JC, Lopez-Miguel A. Characterization of corneal structure in keratoconus. J Cataract Refract Surg. 2012;38(12):2167–83.
23. Pinero DP, Alio JL, Barraquer RI, et al. Corneal biomechanics, refraction, and corneal aberrometry in keratoconus: an integrated study. Invest Ophthalmol Vis Sci. 2010;51(4):1948–55.
24. Edmund C. Corneal elasticity and ocular rigidity in normal and keratoconic eyes. Acta Ophthalmol. 1988;66(2):134–40.
25. Andreassen TT, Simonsen AH, Oxlund H. Biomechanical properties of keratoconus and normal corneas. Exp Eye Res. 1980;31(4):435–41.
26. Nash IS, Greene PR, Foster CS. Comparison of mechanical properties of keratoconus and normal corneas. Exp Eye Res. 1982;35(5):413–24.
27. Roberts CJ. Concepts and misconceptions in corneal biomechanics. J Cataract Refract Surg. 2014;40(6):862–9.
28. Seiler T, Huhle S, Spoerl E, Kunath H. Manifest diabetes and keratoconus: a retrospective case-control study. Graefes Arch Clin Exp Ophthalmol. 2000;238(10):822–5.
29. Fontes BM, Ambrosio Jr R, Velarde GC, Nose W. Ocular response analyzer measurements in keratoconus with normal central corneal thickness compared with matched normal control eyes. J Refract Surg. 2011;27(3):209–15.
30. Johnson RD, Nguyen MT, Lee N, Hamilton DR. Corneal biomechanical properties in normal, forme fruste keratoconus, and manifest keratoconus after statistical correction for potentially confounding factors. Cornea. 2011;30(5):516–23.
31. Mikielewicz M, Kotliar K, Barraquer RI, Michael R. Air-pulse corneal applanation signal curve parameters for the characterisation of keratoconus. Br J Ophthalmol. 2011;95(6):793–8.
32. Wolffsohn JS, Safeen S, Shah S, Laiquzzaman M. Changes of corneal biomechanics with keratoconus. Cornea. 2012;31(8):849–54.
33. Valbon BF, Ambrosio Jr R, Fontes BM, et al. Ocular biomechanical metrics by CorVis ST in healthy

Brazilian patients. J Refract Surg. 2014;30(7): 468–73.
34. Ali NQ, Patel DV, McGhee CN. Biomechanical responses of healthy and keratoconic corneas measured using a non contact Scheimpflug tonometer. Invest Ophthalmol Vis Sci. 2014;55(6):3651–9.
35. Ford MR, Dupps Jr WJ, Rollins AM, et al. Method for optical coherence elastography of the cornea. J Biomed Opt. 2011;16(1):016005.
36. Touboul D, Gennisson JL, Nguyen TM, et al. Supersonic shear wave elastography for the in vivo evaluation of transepithelial corneal collagen cross-linking. Invest Ophthalmol Vis Sci. 2014;55(3):1976–84.
37. Scarcelli G, Besner S, Pineda R, et al. In vivo biomechanical mapping of normal and keratoconus corneas. JAMA Ophthalmol. 2015;133(4):480–2.
38. Beckman Rehnman J, Behndig A, Hallberg P, Linden C. Increased corneal hysteresis after corneal collagen crosslinking: a study based on applanation resonance technology. JAMA Ophthalmol. 2014;132(12):1426–32.
39. Urs R, Lloyd HO, Silverman RH. Acoustic radiation force for noninvasive evaluation of corneal biomechanical changes induced by cross-linking therapy. J Ultrasound Med. 2014;33(8):1417–26.
40. Beshtawi IM, Akhtar R, Hillarby MC, et al. Biomechanical changes of collagen cross-linking on human keratoconic corneas using scanning acoustic microscopy. Curr Eye Res. 2015;41(5):609–15.
41. Bilgin LK, Yilmaz S, Araz B, et al. 30 years of contact lens prescribing for keratoconic patients in Turkey. Cont Lens Anterior Eye. 2009;32(1):16–21.
42. Zadnik K, Barr JT, Edrington TB, et al. Baseline findings in the Collaborative Longitudinal Evaluation of Keratoconus (CLEK) study. Invest Ophthalmol Vis Sci. 1998;39(13):2537–46.
43. Lim N, Vogt U. Characteristics and functional outcomes of 130 patients with keratoconus attending a specialist contact lens clinic. Eye (Lond). 2002;16(1):54–9.
44. Hayashi T, Fatt I. Forces retaining a contact lens on the eye between blinks. Am J Optom Physiol Opt. 1980;57(8):485–507.
45. Jenkins JT, Shimbo M. The distribution of pressure behind a soft contact lens. J Biomech Eng. 1984;106(1):62–5.
46. Horst CR, Brodland B, Jones LW, Brodland GW. Measuring the modulus of silicone hydrogel contact lenses. Optom Vis Sci. 2012;89(10):1468–76.
47. Elsheikh A, Geraghty B, Rama P, et al. Characterization of age-related variation in corneal biomechanical properties. J R Soc Interface. 2010;7(51):1475–85.
48. McMonnies CW. Keratoconus fittings: apical clearance or apical support? Eye Contact Lens. 2004;30(3):147–55.
49. Hartstein J. Keratoconus that developed in patients wearing corneal contact lenses. Report of four cases. Arch Ophthalmol. 1968;80(3):345–6.
50. Korb DR, Finnemore VM, Herman JP. Apical changes and scarring in keratoconus as related to contact lens fitting techniques. J Am Optom Assoc. 1982; 53(3):199–205.
51. Schanzlin DJ, Asbell PA, Burris TE, Durrie DS. The intrastromal corneal ring segments. Phase II results for the correction of myopia. Ophthalmology. 1997;104(7):1067–78.
52. Rabinowitz YS. Intacs for keratoconus. Curr Opin Ophthalmol. 2007;18(4):279–83.
53. Alfonso JF, Lisa C, Fernandez-Vega L, et al. Intrastromal corneal ring segment implantation in 219 keratoconic eyes at different stages. Graefes Arch Clin Exp Ophthalmol. 2011;249(11):1705–12.
54. Akaishi L, Tzelikis PF, Raber IM. Ferrara intracorneal ring implantation and cataract surgery for the correction of pellucid marginal corneal degeneration. J Cataract Refract Surg. 2004;30(11):2427–30.
55. Zare MA, Hashemi H, Salari MR. Intracorneal ring segment implantation for the management of keratoconus: safety and efficacy. J Cataract Refract Surg. 2007;33(11):1886–91.
56. Dauwe C, Touboul D, Roberts CJ, et al. Biomechanical and morphological corneal response to placement of intrastromal corneal ring segments for keratoconus. J Cataract Refract Surg. 2009;35(10):1761–7.
57. Wollensak G, Spoerl E, Seiler T. Riboflavin/ultraviolet-a-induced collagen crosslinking for the treatment of keratoconus. Am J Ophthalmol. 2003;135(5):620–7.
58. Hayes S, Kamma-Lorger CS, Boote C, et al. The effect of riboflavin/UVA collagen cross-linking therapy on the structure and hydrodynamic behaviour of the ungulate and rabbit corneal stroma. PLoS One. 2013;8(1), e52860.
59. Zhang Y, Conrad AH, Conrad GW. Effects of ultraviolet-A and riboflavin on the interaction of collagen and proteoglycans during corneal cross-linking. J Biol Chem. 2011;286(15):13011–22.
60. Wollensak G. Crosslinking treatment of progressive keratoconus: new hope. Curr Opin Ophthalmol. 2006;17(4):356–60.
61. Caporossi A, Mazzotta C, Baiocchi S, Caporossi T. Long-term results of riboflavin ultraviolet a corneal collagen cross-linking for keratoconus in Italy: the Siena eye cross study. Am J Ophthalmol. 2010;149(4):585–93.
62. Sray WA, Cohen EJ, Rapuano CJ, Laibson PR. Factors associated with the need for penetrating keratoplasty in keratoconus. Cornea. 2002;21(8):784–6.
63. Tuft SJ, Moodaley LC, Gregory WM, et al. Prognostic factors for the progression of keratoconus. Ophthalmology. 1994;101(3):439–47.
64. Reeves SW, Stinnett S, Adelman RA, Afshari NA. Risk factors for progression to penetrating keratoplasty in patients with keratoconus. Am J Ophthalmol. 2005;140(4):607–11.
65. Watson SL, Ramsay A, Dart JK, et al. Comparison of deep lamellar keratoplasty and penetrating kerato-

plasty in patients with keratoconus. Ophthalmology. 2004;111(9):1676–82.
66. Funnell CL, Ball J, Noble BA. Comparative cohort study of the outcomes of deep lamellar keratoplasty and penetrating keratoplasty for keratoconus. Eye (Lond). 2006;20(5):527–32.
67. Sugita J, Kondo J. Deep lamellar keratoplasty with complete removal of pathological stroma for vision improvement. Br J Ophthalmol. 1997;81(3):184–8.
68. Shimazaki J. The evolution of lamellar keratoplasty. Curr Opin Ophthalmol. 2000;11(4):217–23.
69. Hayes S, Young R, Boote C, et al. A structural investigation of corneal graft failure in suspected recurrent keratoconus. Eye (Lond). 2010;24(4):728–34.
70. Farley MK, Pettit TH. Traumatic wound dehiscence after penetrating keratoplasty. Am J Ophthalmol. 1987;104(1):44–9.
71. Pettinelli DJ, Starr CE, Stark WJ. Late traumatic corneal wound dehiscence after penetrating keratoplasty. Arch Ophthalmol. 2005;123(6):853–6.
72. Boote C, Dooley EP, Gardner SJ, et al. Quantification of collagen ultrastructure after penetrating keratoplasty—implications for corneal biomechanics. PLoS One. 2013;8(7), e68166.
73. Holden BA, Mertz GW. Critical oxygen levels to avoid corneal edema for daily and extended wear contact lenses. Invest Ophthalmol Vis Sci. 1984; 25(10):1161–7.
74. Kling S, Marcos S. Effect of hydration state and storage media on corneal biomechanical response from in vitro inflation tests. J Refract Surg. 2013;29(7):490–7.
75. Hosny M, Hassaballa MA, Shalaby A. Changes in corneal biomechanics following different keratoplasty techniques. Clin Ophthalmol. 2011;5:767–70.
76. Abdelkader A. Influence of different keratoplasty techniques on the biomechanical properties of the cornea. Acta Ophthalmol. 2013;91(7):e567–72.
77. Wollensak G, Sporl E, Mazzotta C, et al. Interlamellar cohesion after corneal crosslinking using riboflavin and ultraviolet A light. Br J Ophthalmol. 2011; 95(6):876–80.
78. Wollensak G, Spoerl E, Reber F, Seiler T. Keratocyte cytotoxicity of riboflavin/UVA-treatment in vitro. Eye (Lond). 2004;18(7):718–22.
79. Liu JH, Medeiros FA, Slight JR, Weinreb RN. Diurnal and nocturnal effects of brimonidine monotherapy on intraocular pressure. Ophthalmology. 2010;117(11): 2075–9.
80. Dastiridou AI, Ginis HS, De Brouwere D, et al. Ocular rigidity, ocular pulse amplitude, and pulsatile ocular blood flow: the effect of intraocular pressure. Invest Ophthalmol Vis Sci. 2009;50(12):5718–22.
81. Boyce BL, Grazier JM, Jones RE, Nguyen TD. Full-field deformation of bovine cornea under constrained inflation conditions. Biomaterials. 2008;29(28): 3896–904.
82. Muller LJ, Pels E, Schurmans LR, Vrensen GF. A new three-dimensional model of the organization of proteoglycans and collagen fibrils in the human corneal stroma. Exp Eye Res. 2004;78(3):493–501.
83. Coudrillier B, Tian J, Alexander S, et al. Biomechanics of the human posterior sclera: age- and glaucoma-related changes measured using inflation testing. Invest Ophthalmol Vis Sci. 2012;53(4):1714–28.
84. Geraghty B, Jones SW, Rama P, et al. Age-related variations in the biomechanical properties of human sclera. J Mech Behav Biomed Mater. 2012;16: 181–91.

13 Diagnosing Keratoconus Using VHF Digital Ultrasound Epithelial Thickness Profiles

Dan Z. Reinstein, Timothy J. Archer, Marine Gobbe, Raksha Urs, and Ronald H. Silverman

13.1 Introduction

Keratoconus is a progressive corneal dystrophy which manifests as corneal thinning and formation of a cone-shaped protrusion. Because laser refractive surgery may lead to accelerated post-operative ectasia in patients with keratoconus [1, 2], the accurate detection of early keratoconus is a major safety concern. The prevalence of keratoconus in the Caucasian population is approximately 1/2000 [3]. The incidence of undiagnosed keratoconus presenting to refractive surgery clinics tends to be much higher than this, as keratoconics develop astigmatism that is more difficult to correct by contact lenses or glasses, leading them to consider refractive surgery [4]. The challenge for keratoconus screening is to have high sensitivity, but for this to be combined with high specificity to minimize the number of atypical normal patients who are denied surgery.

As has been described in other chapters, there have been significant efforts made to develop methods for screening of early keratoconus over the last 30 years. In 1984, Klyce [5] introduced color-coded maps derived from computerized front surface placido topography, which have made the diagnosis of keratoconus easier, as patterns including inferior steepening, asymmetric bow-tie and skew bow-tie typical of keratoconus can be seen early in the progression of the disease [6, 7]. Placido-based instruments producing maps of anterior surface topography and curvature became available by the early 1990s and their use in keratoconus screening demonstrated [7–16]. Characterization of corneal thickness and topography of both corneal surfaces using scanning-slit tomography was introduced commercially in the mid-1990s by the Orbscan scanning slit system (Bausch & Lomb, Rochester, NY) [17–19] and later by the Pentacam rotating Scheimpflug-based system (Oculus Optikgeräte, Wetzlar, Germany) [20, 21] and other tomogra-

D.Z. Reinstein, M.D., M.A.(Cantab), F.R.C.S.C., F.R.C. Ophth (✉)
London Vision Clinic, London, UK

Columbia University Medical Center, New York, NY, USA

Centre Hospitalier National d'Ophtalmologie, Paris, France

School of Biomedical Sciences, University of Ulster, Coleraine, UK
e-mail: dzr@londonvisionclinic.com

T.J. Archer, M.A.(Oxon), DipCompSci(Cantab)
M. Gobbe, M.S.T.(Optom), Ph.D.
London Vision Clinic, London, UK
e-mail: tim@londonvisionclinic.com; marine@londonvisionclinic.com

R.Urs, Ph.D.
Department of Ophthalmology, Columbia University Medical Center, New York, NY

R. H. Silverman, Ph.D.
Department of Ophthalmology, Columbia University Medical Center, New York, NY

F.L. Lizzi Center for Biomedical Engineering, Riverside Research, New York, NY

J.L. Alió (ed.), *Keratoconus*, Essentials in Ophthalmology, DOI 10.1007/978-3-319-43881-8_13

phy scanners. Wavefront assessment [22] and the Ocular Response Analyzer (Reichert, Depew, NY) [23] have been employed as a means for detecting early keratoconus.

Topographic and tomographic evaluation has evolved from qualitative observation [7] to quantitative measurements, and many parameters have been described to aid the differentiation of normal from keratoconus eyes [7–16]. Several statistical and machine-based or computerized learning models have been employed for keratoconus detection, and automated systems for screening based on front and back surface topography and whole corneal tomography and pachymetric profile have been developed [20, 24–31].

Although these approaches have improved the effectiveness of keratoconus screening, there still remain equivocal cases where a confident diagnosis cannot be made and undiagnosed keratoconus remains probably the leading cause of corneal ectasia after LASIK [32–44]. The addition of quantitative parameters that are independent of those now obtained by topographic and tomographic analysis could potentially improve screening.

The corneal epithelial and stromal thickness profiles may represent such an independent parameter and will be the focus of this chapter. As will be described later, the corneal epithelium has the ability to alter its thickness profile to re-establish a smooth, symmetrical optical outer corneal surface and either partially or totally mask the presence of an irregular stromal surface from front surface topography [45, 46]. Therefore, the epithelial thickness profile would be expected to follow a distinctive pattern in keratoconus to partially compensate for the cone.

To formally distinguish abnormal from normal epithelial thickness profiles, we set out to study a population of normal eyes to define the normal epithelial thickness profile. In parallel, we also set out to study the epithelial thickness profile in a population of keratoconic eyes to describe epithelial changes with keratoconus. Knowing the epithelial thickness profile in each population, we aimed to qualitatively assess the differences to be able to discriminate between the two populations. Any departure from a normal epithelial thickness profile might be used as a very sensitive indicator of stromal surface irregularity and therefore as a tool to detect early keratoconus.

13.2 VHF Digital Ultrasound Arc Scanning

All of the epithelial thickness data that is described in this chapter was obtained using the Artemis very high-frequency digital ultrasound arc scanner (ArcScan Inc., Golden, CO), which has been previously described in detail [47–49]. Briefly, Artemis VHF digital ultrasound is carried out using an ultrasonic standoff medium. The patient sits and positions the chin and forehead into a headrest while placing the eye in a soft rimmed eyecup. Warm sterile normal saline (33 °C) is filled into the darkened scanning chamber. The patient fixates on a narrowly focused aiming beam which is coaxial with the infrared camera, the corneal vertex and the centre of rotation of the scanning system. The technician adjusts the centre of rotation of the system until it is coaxial with the corneal vertex. In this manner, the position of each scan plane is maintained about a single point on the cornea and corneal mapping is therefore centred on the corneal vertex. The Artemis VHF digital ultrasound uses a broadband 50 MHz VHF ultrasound transducer (bandwidth approximately 10–60 MHz) which is swept by a reverse arc high-precision mechanism to acquire B-scans as arcs that follow the surface contour of anterior or posterior segment structures of interest. Performing a 3D scan set with the Artemis 1 takes approximately 2–3 min per each eye.

Using VHF digital ultrasound, interfaces between tissues are detected at the location of the maximum change in acoustic impedance (the product of the density and the speed of sound). It was first demonstrated in 1993 that acoustic interfaces being detected in the cornea were located spatially at the epithelial surface and at the interface between epithelial cells and the anterior surface of Bowman's layer [50]. This indicated that stromal thickness measurement with VHF digital ultrasound includes Bowman's layer. The posterior boundary of the stroma with VHF digital ultrasound is located at the interface between the endothelium and the aqueous as this is the location of the maximum change in acoustic impedance. This indicated that stromal thickness measurement with VHF digital ultrasound includes Descemet's and the endothelium.

13.2.1 Three-Dimensional Epithelial Pachymetric Topography

For three-dimensional scan sets, the scan sequence consisted of four meridional B-scans at 45° intervals. Each scan sweep takes about 0.25 s and consisted of 128 scan lines or pulse echo vectors. Ultrasound data are digitized and stored. The digitized ultrasound data are then transformed using patented Cornell University digital signal processing technology which includes auto-correlation of back surface curvatures to centre and align the meridional scans. A speed of sound constant of 1640 m/s was used. A linear polar radial interpolation function is used to interpolate between scan meridians to produce a Cartesian matrix over a 10 mm diameter in 0.1 mm steps.

13.3 Epithelial Thickness Profile in Normal Eyes

We set out to characterize the in vivo epithelial thickness profile in a population of normal eyes with no ocular pathology other than refractive error. We obtained the epithelial thickness profile across the central 10 mm diameter of the cornea for 110 normal eyes of 56 patients and averaged the data in the population. Epithelial thickness values for left eyes were reflected in the vertical axis and superimposed onto the right eye values so that nasal/temporal characteristics could be combined [49].

The average epithelial thickness map revealed that the epithelium was not a layer of homogeneous thickness as had previously been thought but followed a very distinct pattern (Fig. 13.1a); on average the epithelium was 5.7 μm thicker inferiorly than superiorly, and 1.2 μm thicker temporally than nasally. The pattern of thicker epithelium inferiorly than superiorly and thicker epithelium nasally than temporally was consistent across a majority of eyes in the population sampled. The average central epithelial thickness was 53.4 μm and the standard deviation was only 4.6 μm [49]. This indicated that there was little variation in central epithelial thickness in the population. The thinnest epithelial point within

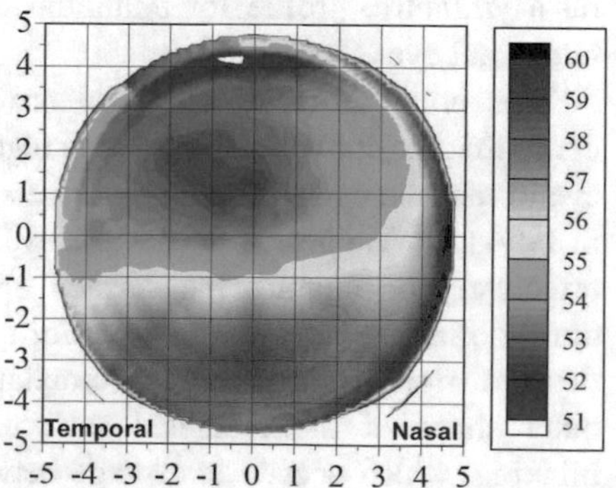

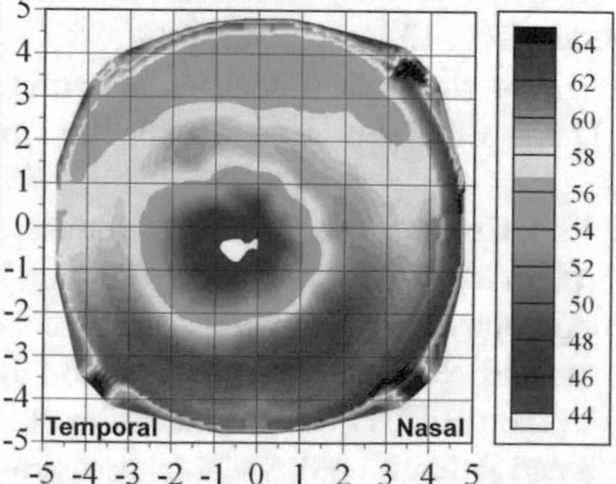

Fig. 13.1 Mean epithelial thickness profile for a population of 110 normal eyes and a population of 54 keratoconic eyes. The epithelial thickness profiles for all eyes in each population were averaged using mirrored left eye symmetry. The colour scale represents epithelial thickness in microns. A Cartesian 1-mm grid is superimposed with the origin at the corneal vertex. *Reprinted with permission from SLACK Incorporated: Reinstein, DZ., Archer, T., Gobbe M. (2009). "Corneal Epithelial Thickness Profile in the Diagnosis of Keratoconus." Journal or Refractive Surgery, 25, 604–610*

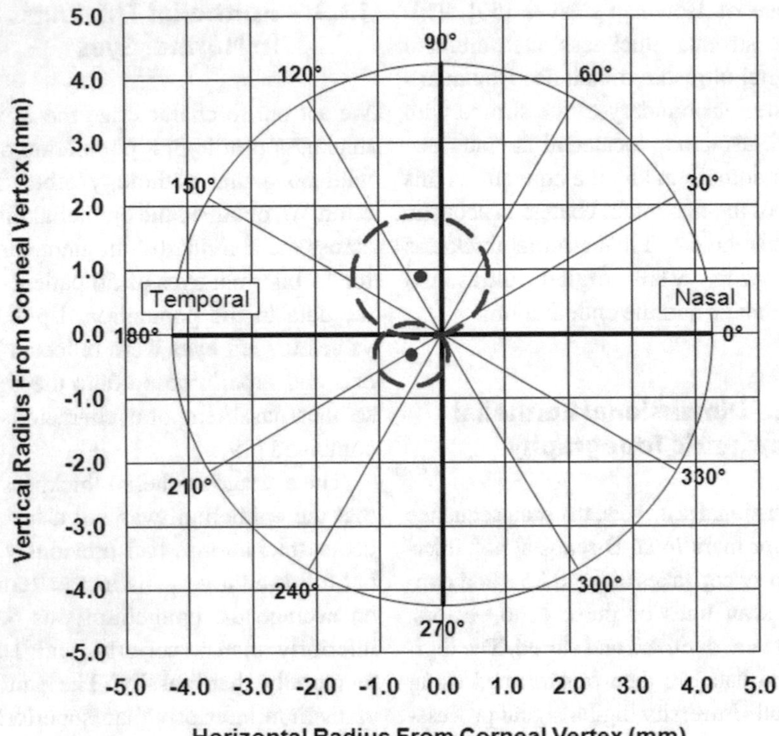

Fig. 13.2 Plot showing the mean location of the thinnest epithelium in a population of 110 normal eyes and 54 keratoconic eyes. The blue dot represents the mean location of the thinnest point for the normal population and the dotted blue line represents one standard deviation. The red dot represents the mean location of the thinnest point for the keratoconic population and the dotted red line represents one standard deviation. *Reprinted with permission from SLACK Incorporated: Reinstein, DZ., Gobbe, M., Archer, T., Silverman, R., Coleman, J. (2010). "Epithelial, Stromal and Total Corneal Thickness in Keratoconus." Journal or Refractive Surgery, 26, 259–271*

the central 5 mm of the cornea was displaced on average 0.33 mm (±1.08) temporally and 0.90 mm (±0.96) superiorly with reference to the corneal vertex (Fig. 13.1).

Figure 13.2a shows a B-scan of a normal cornea. The epithelium appears regular in thickness.

Figure 13.4, Column 1 shows the keratometry, Atlas 995 (Carl Zeiss Meditec, Jena, Germany) corneal topography map and PathFinder™ corneal analysis, Orbscan II (software version 3.00) anterior elevation BFS, Orbscan II posterior elevation BFS and Artemis epithelial thickness profile of a normal eye.

Epithelial thickness can now also be measured using some optical coherence tomography systems, notably the RTVue (Optovue, Fremont, CA) [51–53]. These studies have confirmed this superior–inferior and nasal-temporal asymmetric profile for epithelial thickness in normal eyes [53].

This non-uniformity seems to provide evidence that the epithelial thickness is regulated by eyelid mechanics and blinking, as we suggested in 1994 [50]. We postulated that the eyelid might effectively be chafing the surface epithelium during blinking and that the posterior surface of the semi-rigid tarsus provides a template for the outer shape of the epithelial surface. During blinking, which occurs on average between 300 and 1500 times per hour [54], the vertical traverse of the upper lid is much greater than that of the lower lid. Doane [55] studied the dynamics of eyelid anatomy during blinking and found that during a blink the descent of the upper eyelid reaches its maximum speed at about the time it crosses the visual axis. As a consequence, it is likely that the eyelid applies more force on the superior than inferior cornea. Similarly, the friction on the cornea during lid closure is likely to be greater temporally than nasally as the outer can thus is higher than the inner can thus (mean intercanthal angle = 3°), and the temporal portion of the lid is higher than the nasal lid (mean upper lid angle = 2.7°) [56]. Therefore, it seems that the nature of the eyelid completely explains the non-uniform epithelial thickness profile of a normal eye.

Further evidence for this theory is provided by the epithelial thickness changes observed in orthokeratology [57]. In orthokeratology, a shaped contact lens is placed on the cornea overnight that sits tightly on the cornea centrally but leaves a gap in the mid-periphery. Therefore, the natural template provided by the posterior surface of the semi-rigid tarsus of the eyelid is replaced by an artificial contact lens template designed to fit tightly to the centre of the cornea and loosely paracentrally. We found significant epithelial thickness changes with central thinning and mid-peripheral thickening showing that the epithelium had remodelled according to the template provided by the contact lens, i.e. the epithelium is chafed and squashed by the lens centrally while the epithelium is free to thicken paracentrally where the lens is not so tightly fitted.

13.4 Epithelial Thickness Profile in Keratoconic Eyes

It is well known that the epithelial thickness changes in keratoconus since extreme steepening leads to epithelial breakdown, as often seen clinically. Epithelial thinning over the cone has been demonstrated using histopathologic analysis of keratoconic corneas by Scroggs et al. [58] and later using custom software and a Humphrey-Zeiss OCT system (Humphrey Systems, Dublin, CA) by Haque et al. [59].

We have characterized the in vivo epithelial thickness profile in a population of keratoconic eyes. The subjects included for the study had previously been diagnosed with keratoconus, and the diagnosis was confirmed by clinical signs of keratoconus such as microscopic signs at the slit-lamp, corneal topographic changes, high refractive astigmatism, reduced best-corrected visual acuity and contrast sensitivity, and significant level of higher order aberrations, in particular vertical coma. We measured the epithelial thickness profile across the central 10 mm diameter of the cornea for 54 keratoconic eyes of 30 patients and averaged the data in the population [60]. Epithelial thickness values for left eyes were reflected in the vertical axis and superimposed onto the right eye values so that nasal/temporal characteristics could be combined.

The average epithelial thickness profile in keratoconus revealed that the epithelium was significantly more irregular in thickness compared to normals. The epithelium was thinnest at the apex of the cone and this thin epithelial zone was surrounded by an annulus of thickened epithelium (Fig. 13.1b). While all eyes exhibited the same epithelial doughnut pattern, characterized by a localized central zone of thinning surrounded by an annulus of thick epithelium, the thickness values of the thinnest point and the thickest point as well as the difference in thickness between the thinnest and thickest epithelium varied greatly between eyes. There was a statistically significant correlation between the thinnest epithelium and the steepest keratometry (D), indicating that as the cornea became steeper, the epithelial thickness minimum became thinner. In addition, there was a statistically significant correlation between the thickness of the thinnest epithelium and the difference in thickness between the thinnest and thickest epithelium. This indicated that as the epithelium thinned, there was an increase in the irregularity of the epithelial thickness profile, i.e. that there was an increase in the severity of the keratoconus. The location of the thinnest epithelium within the central 5 mm of the cornea was displaced on average 0.48 mm (±0.66 mm) tempo-

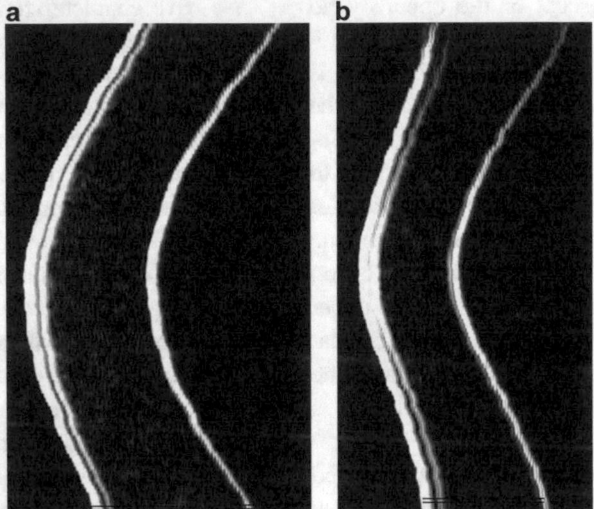

Fig. 13.3 (**a**) (*left*) Horizontal non-geometrically corrected B-scan of a normal cornea obtained using the Artemis very high-frequency digital ultrasound arc scanner. The epithelium appears uniform in thickness across the 10 mm diameter of the scan. (**b**) (*right*) Vertical non-geometrically corrected B-scan of a keratoconic cornea obtained using the Artemis very high-frequency digital ultrasound arc-scanner. The epithelium appears very thin centrally coincident with a visible cone on the back surface. The epithelium is clearly thicker either side of the cone. The central epithelium is much thinner and the peripheral epithelium is much thicker compared to that seen in the normal eye

rally and 0.32 mm (±0.67 mm) inferiorly with reference to the corneal vertex (Fig. 13.2). The mean epithelial thickness for all eyes was 45.7 ± 5.9 μm (range: 33.1–56.3 μm) at the corneal vertex, 38.2 ± 5.8 μm (range: 29.6–52.4 μm) at the thinnest point and 66.8 ± 7.2 μm (range: 54.1–94.4 μm) at the thickest point [60].

Figure 13.3b shows a B-scan for a keratoconic cornea which demonstrates the lack of homogeneity in epithelial thickness as well as central corneal thinning. There is epithelial thinning over the cone and relative epithelial thickening adjacent to the stromal surface cone.

Figure 13.4, Column 2 shows the keratometry, Atlas 995 corneal topography map and PathFinder™ corneal analysis, Orbscan II anterior elevation BFS, Orbscan II posterior elevation BFS and Artemis epithelial thickness profile of a keratoconic eye. As expected, the front surface topography shows infero-temporal steepening with steep average keratometry and high astigmatism; the anterior and posterior elevation BFS maps demonstrate that the apex of the cone is located infero-temporally; the epithelial thickness profile shows epithelial thinning at the apex of the cone surrounded by an annulus of thicker epithelium. The steepest cornea coincides with the apex of the anterior and posterior elevation BFS as well as with the location of the thinnest epithelium.

As for normal eyes, the epithelial thickness profile for keratoconus as described here has been confirmed by studies using OCT [53, 61–63]. The study by Laroche's group [63] elegantly described the different stages of advanced keratoconus demonstrating that as keratoconus moves into its latter stages, a very different epithelial thickness profile becomes apparent. In advanced keratoconus, there is stromal loss often in the location of the cone, for example due to hydrops. This means that rather than the cone being elevated relative to the rest of the stroma, this region is now a depression. Therefore, the epithelium changes from being thinnest over the cone to being thickest in this region, as it is compensating for a depression instead of an elevation (see next section). There can be significant stromal loss in such advanced keratoconus, so the epithelium can be as thick as 200 μm in some cases.

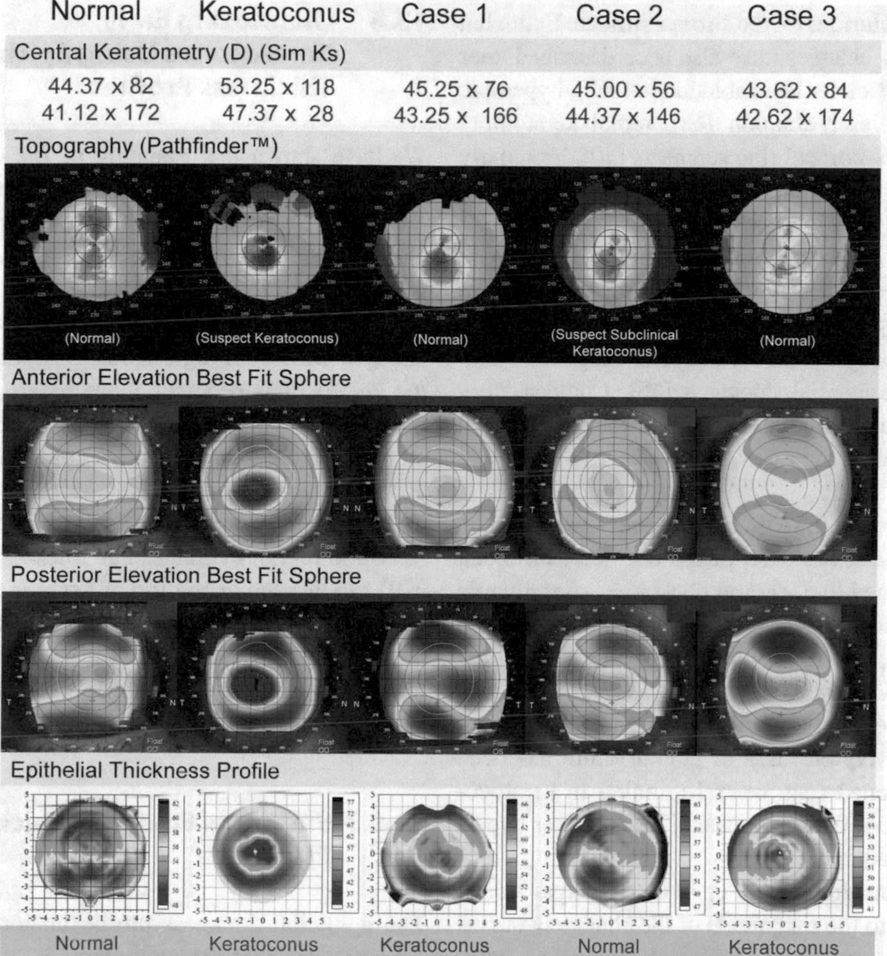

Fig. 13.4 Central keratometry, Atlas corneal topography and PathFinder™ corneal analysis, Orbscan anterior and posterior elevation BFS and Artemis epithelial thickness profile for one normal eye, one keratoconic eye, and three example eyes where the diagnosis of keratoconus might be misleading from topography. The final diagnosis based on the epithelial thickness profile is shown at the bottom of each example. *Reprinted with permission from SLACK Incorporated: Reinstein, DZ., Gobbe, M., Archer, T., Silverman, R., Coleman, J. (2010). "Epithelial, Stromal and Total Corneal Thickness in Keratoconus." Journal or Refractive Surgery, 26, 259–271*

Examples of this epithelial thickening were also reported by Rocha et al. [61] who concluded that focal central epithelial thinning was suggestive but not pathognomonic for keratoconus (i.e. the presence of an epithelial doughnut pattern did not prove beyond any doubt that an eye has keratoconus). However, as described by Laroche, these cases only appear in very advanced keratoconus, which means that they are of no interest with respect to keratoconus screening. Eyes with early keratoconus will never present with epithelial thickening in the location of the cone as by definition if there has been stromal loss, then the keratoconus must be more advanced and the cornea will be obviously abnormal.

13.5 Understanding the Predictable Behaviour of the Corneal Epithelium

Epithelial thickness changes in keratoconus provide another example of the very predictable mechanism of the corneal epithelium to compensate for irregularities on the stromal surface. Epithelial thickness changes have also been described after myopic excimer laser ablation [64–67], hyperopic excimer laser ablation [68], radial keratotomy [69], intra-corneal ring segments [70], irregularly irregular astigmatism after corneal refractive surgery [45, 71–75] and in ectasia [76].

In all of these cases, the epithelial thickness changes are clearly a compensatory response to the change to the stromal surface and can all be explained by the theory of eyelid template regulation of epithelial thickness [46]. Compensatory epithelial thickness changes can be summarized by the following rules:

1. The epithelium thickens in areas where tissue has been removed or the curvature has been flattened (e.g. central thickening after myopic ablation [64–66] or radial keratotomy [69] and peripheral thickening after hyperopic ablation [68]).
2. The epithelium thins over regions that are relatively elevated or the curvature has been steepened (e.g. central thinning in keratoconus [53, 60–63], ectasia [76] and after hyperopic ablation [68]).
3. The magnitude of epithelial changes correlates to the magnitude of the change in curvature (e.g. more epithelial thickening after higher myopic ablation [64, 65, 67], after higher hyperopic ablation [68] and in more advanced keratoconus [53, 60–63]).
4. The amount of epithelial remodelling is defined by the rate of change of curvature of an irregularity [46, 77]; there will be more epithelial remodelling for a more localized irregularity [45, 72, 73, 75]. The epithelium effectively acts as a low pass filter, smoothing local changes (high curvature gradient) almost completely, but only partially smoothing global changes (low curvature gradient). For example, there is almost twice as much epithelial thickening after a hyperopic ablation [68] compared with a myopic ablation [64, 65, 67], and there is almost total epithelial compensation for small, very localized stromal loss such as after a corneal ulcer [68].

13.6 Diagnosing Early Keratoconus Using Epithelial Thickness Profiles

We have shown that mapping of the epithelial thickness profile reveals a very distinct thickness profile in keratoconus compared to that of normal corneas, due to the compensatory mechanism of the epithelium for stromal irregularities. We have also shown that the epithelial thickness profile changes with the progression of the disease; as the keratoconus becomes more severe, the epithelium at the apex of the cone becomes thinner and the surrounding annulus of epithelium in the epithelial doughnut pattern becomes thicker. Therefore, the degree of epithelial abnormality in both directions (thinner and thicker than normal) can be used to confirm or exclude a diagnosis of keratoconus in eyes suggestive but not conclusive of a diagnosis of keratoconus on topography at a very early stage in the expression of the disease [78].

13.6.1 Pattern of Epithelial Thickness Profile

The epithelial thickness profile in normal eyes demonstrates that the epithelium is on average thicker inferiorly than superiorly and slightly thicker nasally than temporally. There is very little variation in epithelial thickness within both the inferior hemi-cornea and the superior hemi-cornea. In contrast, in keratoconic eyes, the average epithelial thickness map showed an epithelial doughnut pattern characterized by a localized central zone of thinning overlying the stromal cone, surrounded by an annulus of thick epithelium. In early keratoconus, we would expect to see the pattern of localized epithelial thinning surrounded by an annulus of thick epithelium coincident with a suspected cone on posterior elevation BFS. The coincidence of epithelial thinning together with an eccentric posterior elevation BFS apex may reveal whether or not to ascribe significance to an eccentric posterior elevation BFS apex occurring *concurrently with* a normal front surface topography. In other words, in the presence of normal front surface topography, thinning of the epithelium coincident with the location of the posterior elevation BFS apex would represent total masking or compensation for a sub-surface stromal cone and herald posterior elevation BFS changes which *do* represent keratoconus. Conversely, finding thicker epithelium over an area of topographic steepening or an eccentric posterior elevation BFS apex would imply that the steepening is *not* due to a keratoconic sub-surface stromal cone, but more likely due to localized epithelial thickening. Localized compensatory changes in epithelial thickness profiles can be detected by Artemis VHF digital ultrasound once they exceed 1–2 μm. In a way, examination of epithelial thickness profile irregularities provides a very sensitive method of examining stromal surface topography—by proxy. Therefore, this technique provides increased sensitivity and specificity to a diagnosis of keratoconus well in advance of any detectable corneal front surface topographic change.

Case Examples

Figure 13.4 shows three selected examples where epithelial thickness profiles helped to interpret and diagnose anterior and posterior elevation BFS abnormalities. In each case, the epithelial thickness profile appears to be able to differentiate cases where the diagnosis of keratoconus is uncertain, from normal [78].

Case 1 (OS) represents a 25-year-old male, with a manifest refraction of −1.00 −0.50 × 150 and a best spectacle-corrected visual acuity of 20/16. Atlas corneal topography demonstrated inferior steepening which would traditionally indicate keratoconus. The keratometry was 45.25/43.25 D × 76, and PathFinder™ corneal analysis classified the topography as normal. Orbscan II posterior elevation BFS showed that the posterior elevation BFS apex was decentred infero-temporally. Corneal pachymetry minimum by handheld ultrasound was 479 μm. Contrast sensitivity was slightly below the normal range measured using the CSV-1000 (Vector Vision Inc., Greenville, Ohio). There was −0.30 μm (OSA notation) of vertical coma on WASCA aberrometry. Corneal hysteresis was 7.5 mmHg and corneal resistance factor was 7.1 mmHg, which are low, but these could be affected by the low corneal thickness. The combination of inferior steepening, an eccentric posterior elevation BFS apex and thin cornea raised the suspicion of keratoconus although there was no suggestion of keratoconus by refraction, keratometry or PathFinder™ corneal analysis. Artemis epithelial thickness profile showed a pattern typical of keratoconus with an epithelial doughnut shape characterized by a localized zone of epithelial thinning displaced infero-temporally over the eccentric posterior elevation BFS apex, surrounded by an annulus of thick epithelium. The coincidence of an area of epithelial thinning with the apex of the posterior elevation BFS, as well as the increased irregularity of the epithelium confirmed the diagnosis of early keratoconus.

Case 2 (OD) represents a 31-year-old female, with a manifest refraction of −2.25 −0.50 × 88 and a best spectacle-corrected visual acuity of 20/16. Atlas corneal topography demonstrated a very similar pattern to case 1 of inferior steepening, therefore suggesting that the eye could also be keratoconic. The keratometry was 44.12/44.75 D × 148, and PathFinder™ corneal analysis classified the topography as suspect subclinical keratoconus. Orbscan II posterior elevation BFS showed that the apex was slightly decentred nasally. Corneal pachymetry minimum by handheld ultrasound was 538 μm. Contrast sensitivity was in the normal range. There was 0.32 μm (OSA notation) of vertical coma on WASCA aberrometry. Corneal hysteresis was 10.1 mmHg and corneal resistance factor was 9.8 mmHg, which are well within normal range. The combination of inferior steepening, against-the-rule astigmatism and high degree of vertical coma raised the suspicion of keratoconus, which was also noted by PathFinder™ corneal analysis. Artemis epithelial thickness profile showed a typical normal pattern with thicker epithelium inferiorly and thinner epithelium superiorly. Thicker epithelium inferiorly over the suspected cone (inferior steepening on topography) was inconsistent with an underlying stromal surface cone, and therefore the diagnosis of keratoconus was excluded. This patient would have been rejected for surgery given a documented PathFinder™ corneal analysis warning of suspect subclinical keratoconus, but given the epithelial thickness profile, this patient was deemed a suitable candidate for LASIK.

The anterior corneal topography in case 3 (OD) bears no features related to keratoconus. The patient is a 35-year-old female with a manifest refraction of −25 −0.50×4 and a best spectacle-corrected visual acuity of 20/16. The refraction had been stable for at least 10 years and the contrast sensitivity was within normal limits. The keratometry was 43.62/42.62 D×74 and PathFinder™ analysis classified the topography as normal. Orbscan II posterior elevation BFS showed that the apex was slightly decentred infero-temporally, but the anterior elevation BFS apex was well centred. Corneal pachymetry minimum by handheld ultrasound was 484 μm. Pentacam (Oculus, Wetzlar, Germany) keratoconus screening indices were normal. WASCA ocular higher order aberrations were low (RMS=0.19 μm) as well as the level of vertical coma (coma=0.066 μm). Corneal hysteresis was 8.9 mmHg and corneal resistance factor was 8.8 mmHg, both within normal limits. In this case, only the slightly eccentric posterior elevation BFS apex and the low–normal corneal thickness were suspicious for keratoconus, while all other screening methods gave no indication of keratoconus. However, the epithelial thickness profile showed an epithelial doughnut pattern characterized by localized epithelial thinning surrounded by an annulus of thick epithelium, coincident with the eccentric posterior elevation BFS apex. Epithelial thinning with surrounding annular thickening over the eccentric posterior elevation BFS apex indicated the presence of probable sub-surface keratoconus. In this case, it seems that the epithelium had fully compensated for the stromal surface irregularity so that the anterior surface topography of the cornea appeared perfectly regular. Given the regularity of the front surface topography and the normality of nearly all other screening parameters, it is feasible that this patient could have been deemed suitable for corneal refractive surgery and subsequently developed ectasia. As we were able to also consider the epithelial thickness profile, this patient was rejected for corneal refractive surgery. This kind of case may explain some reported cases of ectasia "without a cause" [79].

13.7 Automated Algorithm for Classification by Epithelium

Based on this qualitative diagnostic method, we then set out to derive an automated classifier to detect keratoconus using epithelial thickness data, together with Ron Silverman and his group at Columbia University [80]. We used stepwise linear discriminant analysis (LDA) and neural network (NN) analysis to develop multivariate models based on combinations of 161 features comparing a population of 130 normal and 74 keratoconic eyes. This process resulted in a six-variable model that provided an area under the receiver operating curve of 100 %, indicative of complete separation of keratoconic from normal corneas. Test-set performance averaged over ten trials, gave a specificity of 99.5 ± 1.5 % and sensitivity of 98.9 ± 1.9 %. Maps of the average epithelium and LDA function values were also found to be well correlated with keratoconus severity grade (see Figs. 13.5 and 13.6). Other groups have also been working on automated classification algorithms based on epithelial thickness data obtained by OCT [53, 81].

Following this study, we then applied the algorithm to a population of 10 patients with unilateral keratoconus (clinically and algorithmically topographically normal in the fellow eyes), on the basis that the fellow eye in such patients represents a latent form of keratoconus, and as such, has been considered a gold standard for studies aimed at early keratoconus detection. These eyes were also analysed using the Belin-Ambrosio enhanced ectasia display (BAD-D parameter and ART-Max) [20, 24, 82] and the Orbscan SCORE value as described by Saad and Gatinel [28–30].

Table 1 summarizes the diagnosis derived for the fellow eyes using the classification function

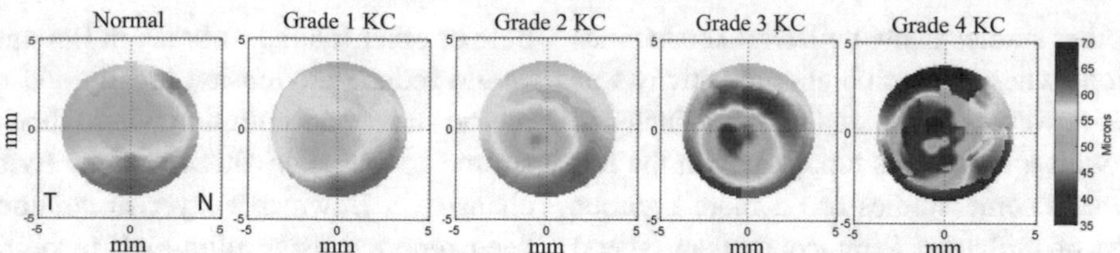

Fig. 13.5 Epithelial thickness maps averaged over all normal corneas and for each keratoconus grade. The departure from the normal epithelial distribution is evident even in grade 1 keratoconus but becomes more obvious with severity. *Reprinted with permission from IOVS: Silverman RH, Urs R, Roychoudhury A, Archer TJ, Gobbe M, Reinstein DZ. Epithelial remodeling as basis for machine-based identification of keratoconus. Invest Ophthalmol Vis Sci. 2014 Mar 13;55(3):1580–7*

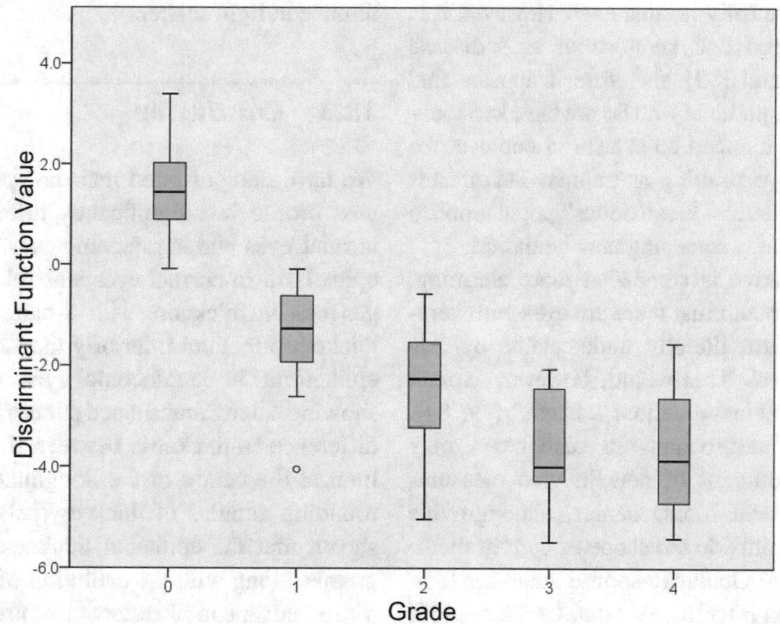

Fig. 13.6 Box and whisker plot of discriminant function value versus keratoconus severity grade. Grade 0 represents normal subjects. Grades 1–4 are based on Krumeich classification. Boxes represent ±1 quartile about median value (*horizontal line*), and whiskers represent full range of values for each group. *Circles* indicate outliers. *Reprinted with permission from IOVS: Silverman RH, Urs R, Roychoudhury A, Archer TJ, Gobbe M, Reinstein DZ. Epithelial remodeling as basis for machine-based identification of keratoconus. Invest Ophthalmol Vis Sci. 2014 Mar 13;55(3):1580–7*

based on epithelial thickness parameters, the classification function combining VHF digital ultrasound (epithelial and stromal thickness) and Pentacam HD parameters, the BAD-D and ART-Max values, and the Orbscan SCORE value. The last column of the table indicates whether the topographic map displayed suspicious features of keratoconus such as inferior steepening and asymmetric bow-tie. The table also shows the percentage of eyes that were classified as keratoconus by each method.

The most interesting finding of this study was that more than 50 % of the fellow eyes were classified as normal by all methods. This was similar to the result reported by Bae et al. [26], who found no difference in the BAD-D or ART-Max values between normal and topographically normal fellow eyes of keratoconus patients. This is in contrast to other studies using unilateral keratoconus populations where a much higher sensitivity was reported; however, these studies often included patients with a suspicious topography in the fellow eye (i.e. some studies use a more rigorous definition of unilateral keratoconus than others) [27]. Therefore, the main conclusion from the study was to put into question the validity of using unilateral keratoconus patients for keratoconus screening studies. The fact that a number of these fellow eyes showed absolutely no indication of keratoconus by any method implies that it is likely that these were truly normal eyes. However, it is generally agreed that keratoconus as a disease must be bilateral [83], therefore it appears that these cases are patients who do not have keratoconus, but have induced an ectasia in one eye, for example by eye rubbing or trauma. This means that using "unilateral keratoconus" populations to study keratoconus screening may be flawed.

The alternative is somewhat more alarming, as this would mean that there are eyes with keratoconus that are literally undetectable by any existing method. This would, however, explain any case of "ectasia without a cause" [79, 84]. Detection of keratoconus in such cases may require development of new in vivo measurements of corneal biomechanics, although this appears to be outside the scope of current methods such as the Ocular Response Analyzer [85–87] and Corvis (Oculus, Wetzlar, Germany) [86, 87] due to the wide scatter in the data acquired. Another factor, as has been described using Brillouin microscopy [88], may be that the biomechanical tensile strength of the cornea may not be different from normal in early keratoconus when measuring the whole cornea globally, but there may only be a difference in the region localized of the cone (or in the location of a future cone). Another potential and final solution would be whether a genotype or other molecular marker for keratoconus could be found [89–91].

Finally, another interpretation of this result is that keratoconus may not necessarily be a disease of abnormal stromal substance. The localization of the reduced corneal biomechanics found in keratoconus suggests that this may be caused by a local defect in Bowman's layer due to eye rubbing or other trauma. A break in Bowman's layer would reduce the tension locally and the asymmetric stress concentration would then cause the stroma to bulge in this location. Evidence for changes in Bowman's layer in keratoconus has been reported using ultra-high resolution OCT; Shousha et al. [92] showed that Bowman's layer was thinner inferiorly in keratoconus and described a Bowman's ectasia index (BEI) to use for keratoconus screening. Yadav et al. [93] also described differences in the thickness of Bowman's layer in keratoconus, as well as a difference in light scatter.

13.8 Conclusion

We have demonstrated that the epithelial thickness profile was significantly different between normal eyes and keratoconic eyes. Whereas the epithelium in normal eyes was relatively homogeneous in thickness with a pattern of slightly thicker epithelium inferiorly than superiorly, the epithelium in keratoconic eyes was irregular showing a doughnut shaped pattern, and a marked difference in thickness between the thin epithelium at the centre of the doughnut and the surrounding annulus of thick epithelium. We have shown that the epithelial thickness profile progresses along with the evolution of keratoconus. More advanced keratoconus produces more irregularity in the epithelial thickness profile. We have found that the distinctive epithelial doughnut pattern associated with keratoconus can be used to confirm or exclude the presence of an underlying stromal surface cone in cases with normal or suspect front surface topography as well as being a "qualifier" for the finding of an eccentric posterior elevation BFS apex.

Knowledge of the differences in epithelial thickness profile between the normal population and the keratoconic population allowed us to identify several features of the epithelial thickness profile that might help to discriminate between normal eyes and keratoconus suspect eyes. We developed an automated classifier based on these features that provides good sensitivity and specificity for keratoconus diagnosis.

Randleman, in his paper assessing risk factors for ectasia reported that ectasia might still occur after uncomplicated surgery in appropriately screened candidates [33]. Mapping of epithelial thickness profiles might provide an explanation for these cases; it could be that a stromal surface cone was masked by epithelial compensation and the front surface topography appeared normal.

Mapping of the epithelial thickness profile may increase sensitivity and specificity of screening for keratoconus compared to current conventional corneal topographic screening alone and may be useful in clinical practice in two very important ways.

Firstly, epithelial thickness mapping can exclude the appropriate patients by detecting keratoconus earlier or confirming keratoconus in cases where topographic changes may be clinically judged as being "within normal limits". Epithelial information allows an earlier diagnosis of keratoconus as epithelial changes will occur before changes on the front surface of the cornea become apparent. Epithelial thinning coincident with an eccentric posterior elevation BFS apex, and in particular if surrounded by an annulus of thicker epithelium is consistent with keratoconus. Excluding early keratoconic patients from laser refractive surgery will reduce and potentially eliminate the risk of iatrogenic ectasia of this aetiology and therefore increase the safety of laser refractive surgery. From our data, 136 eyes out of 1532 consecutive myopic eyes screened for refractive surgery demonstrated abnormal topography suspect of keratoconus. All 136 eyes were screened with Artemis VHF digital ultrasound arc scanning and individual epithelial thickness profiles were mapped. Out of 136 eyes with suspect keratoconus, only 22 eyes (16 %) were confirmed as keratoconus [94].

Second, epithelial thickness profiles may be useful in excluding a diagnosis of keratoconus despite suspect topography. Epithelial thickening over an area of topographic steepening implies that the steepening is not due to an underlying ectatic surface. In such cases, excluding keratoconus using epithelial thickness profiles appears to allow patients who otherwise would have been denied treatment due to suspect topography to be deemed suitable for surgery. From our data, out of the 136 eyes with suspect keratoconus screened with Artemis VHF digital ultrasound arc scanning, 114 eyes (84 %) showed normal epithelial thickness profile and were diagnosed as non-keratoconic and deemed suitable for corneal refractive surgery. One year post-LASIK follow-up data [94] and preliminary 2-years follow-up data [95] on these demonstrated equal stability and refractive outcomes as matched control eyes.

In summary, epithelial thickness mapping appears to be a new and useful tool for aiding in the diagnosis of keratoconus when topographical changes are equivocal.

Compliance with Ethical Requirements Dr. Reinstein is a consultant for Carl Zeiss Meditec (Jena, Germany). Drs Reinstein and Silverman have a proprietary interest in the Artemis technology (ArcScan Inc., Golden, Colorado) and are authors of patents related to VHF digital ultrasound administered by the Center for Technology Licensing at Cornell University, Ithaca, New York. Timothy Archer, Marine Gobbe, and Raksha Urs declare that they have no conflict of interest.

Informed Consent: All procedures followed were in accordance with the ethical standards of the responsible committee on human experimentation (institutional and national) and with the Helsinki Declaration of 1975, as revised in 2000. Informed consent was obtained from all patients for being included in the study.

No animal studies were carried out by the authors for this chapter.

References

1. Ambrosio Jr R, Wilson SE. Complications of laser in situ keratomileusis: etiology, prevention, and treatment. J Refract Surg. 2001;17(3):350–79.
2. Seiler T, Koufala K, Richter G. Iatrogenic keratectasia after laser in situ keratomileusis. J Refract Surg. 1998;14(3):312–7.
3. Krachmer JH, Feder RF, Belin MW. Keratoconus and related non-inflammatory corneal thinning disorders. Surv Ophthalmol. 1984;28:293–322.
4. Wilson SE, Klyce SD. Screening for corneal topographic abnormalities before refractive surgery. Ophthalmology. 1994;101(1):147–52.
5. Klyce SD. Computer-assisted corneal topography. High-resolution graphic presentation and analysis of keratoscopy. Invest Ophthalmol Vis Sci. 1984;25(12):1426–35.
6. Rabinowitz YS, Yang H, Brickman Y, Akkina J, Riley C, Rotter JI, et al. Videokeratography database of normal human corneas. Br J Ophthalmol. 1996;80(7):610–6.

7. Rabinowitz YS, McDonnell PJ. Computer-assisted corneal topography in keratoconus. Refract Corneal Surg. 1989;5(6):400–8.
8. Rabinowitz YS. Videokeratographic indices to aid in screening for keratoconus. J Refract Surg. 1995;11(5):371–9.
9. Rabinowitz YS. Tangential vs sagittal videokeratographs in the "early" detection of keratoconus. Am J Ophthalmol. 1996;122(6):887–9.
10. Rabinowitz YS, Rasheed K. KISA% index: a quantitative videokeratography algorithm embodying minimal topographic criteria for diagnosing keratoconus. J Cataract Refract Surg. 1999;25(10):1327–35.
11. Smolek MK, Klyce SD. Current keratoconus detection methods compared with a neural network approach. Invest Ophthalmol Vis Sci. 1997;38(11):2290–9.
12. Maeda N, Klyce SD, Smolek MK. Comparison of methods for detecting keratoconus using videokeratography. Arch Ophthalmol. 1995;113(7):870–4.
13. Nesburn AB, Bahri S, Salz J, Rabinowitz YS, Maguen E, Hofbauer J, et al. Keratoconus detected by videokeratography in candidates for photorefractive keratectomy. J Refract Surg. 1995;11(3):194–201.
14. Chastang PJ, Borderie VM, Carvajal-Gonzalez S, Rostene W, Laroche L. Automated keratoconus detection using the EyeSys videokeratoscope. J Cataract Refract Surg. 2000;26(5):675–83.
15. Maeda N, Klyce SD, Smolek MK, Thompson HW. Automated keratoconus screening with corneal topography analysis. Invest Ophthalmol Vis Sci. 1994;35(6):2749–57.
16. Kalin NS, Maeda N, Klyce SD, Hargrave S, Wilson SE. Automated topographic screening for keratoconus in refractive surgery candidates. Clao J. 1996; 22(3):164–7.
17. Auffarth GU, Wang L, Volcker HE. Keratoconus evaluation using the Orbscan Topography System. J Cataract Refract Surg. 2000;26(2):222–8.
18. Rao SN, Raviv T, Majmudar PA, Epstein RJ. Role of Orbscan II in screening keratoconus suspects before refractive corneal surgery. Ophthalmology. 2002; 109(9):1642–6.
19. Tomidokoro A, Oshika T, Amano S, Higaki S, Maeda N, Miyata K. Changes in anterior and posterior corneal curvatures in keratoconus. Ophthalmology. 2000;107(7):1328–32.
20. Ambrosio Jr R, Alonso RS, Luz A, Coca Velarde LG. Corneal-thickness spatial profile and corneal-volume distribution: tomographic indices to detect keratoconus. J Cataract Refract Surg. 2006;32(11):1851–9.
21. de Sanctis U, Loiacono C, Richiardi L, Turco D, Mutani B, Grignolo FM. Sensitivity and specificity of posterior corneal elevation measured by Pentacam in discriminating keratoconus/subclinical keratoconus. Ophthalmology. 2008;115(9):1534–9.
22. Saad A, Gatinel D. Evaluation of total and corneal wavefront high order aberrations for the detection of forme fruste keratoconus. Invest Ophthalmol Vis Sci. 2012;53(6):2978–92.
23. Luce DA. Determining in vivo biomechanical properties of the cornea with an ocular response analyzer. J Cataract Refract Surg. 2005;31(1):156–62.
24. Ambrosio Jr R, Caiado AL, Guerra FP, Louzada R, Roy AS, Luz A, et al. Novel pachymetric parameters based on corneal tomography for diagnosing keratoconus. J Refract Surg. 2011;27(10):753–8.
25. Fontes BM, Ambrosio Jr R, Salomao M, Velarde GC, Nose W. Biomechanical and tomographic analysis of unilateral keratoconus. J Refract Surg. 2010;26(9):677–81.
26. Bae GH, Kim JR, Kim CH, Lim DH, Chung ES, Chung TY. Corneal topographic and tomographic analysis of fellow eyes in unilateral keratoconus patients using Pentacam. Am J Ophthalmol. 2014;157(1):103–9. e1.
27. Muftuoglu O, Ayar O, Ozulken K, Ozyol E, Akinci A. Posterior corneal elevation and back difference corneal elevation in diagnosing forme fruste keratoconus in the fellow eyes of unilateral keratoconus patients. J Cataract Refract Surg. 2013;39(9):1348–57.
28. Chan C, Ang M, Saad A, Chua D, Mejia M, Lim L, et al. Validation of an objective scoring system for forme fruste keratoconus detection and post-LASIK ectasia risk assessment in Asian eyes. Cornea. 2015;34(9):996–1004.
29. Saad A, Gatinel D. Validation of a new scoring system for the detection of early forme of keratoconus. Int J Kerat Ect Cor Dis. 2012;1(2):100–8.
30. Saad A, Gatinel D. Topographic and tomographic properties of forme fruste keratoconus corneas. Invest Ophthalmol Vis Sci. 2010;51(11):5546–55.
31. Mahmoud AM, Nunez MX, Blanco C, Koch DD, Wang L, Weikert MP, et al. Expanding the cone location and magnitude index to include corneal thickness and posterior surface information for the detection of keratoconus. Am J Ophthalmol. 2013;156(6):1102–11.
32. Randleman JB, Trattler WB, Stulting RD. Validation of the ectasia risk score system for preoperative laser in situ keratomileusis screening. Am J Ophthalmol. 2008;145(5):813–8.
33. Randleman JB, Woodward M, Lynn MJ, Stulting RD. Risk assessment for ectasia after corneal refractive surgery. Ophthalmology. 2008;115(1):37–50.
34. Seiler T, Quurke AW. Iatrogenic keratectasia after LASIK in a case of forme fruste keratoconus. J Cataract Refract Surg. 1998;24(7):1007–9.
35. Speicher L, Gottinger W. Progressive corneal ectasia after laser in situ keratomileusis (LASIK). Klin Monatsbl Augenheilkd. 1998;213(4):247–51.
36. Geggel HS, Talley AR. Delayed onset keratectasia following laser in situ keratomileusis. J Cataract Refract Surg. 1999;25(4):582–6.
37. Amoils SP, Deist MB, Gous P, Amoils PM. Iatrogenic keratectasia after laser in situ keratomileusis for less than −4.0 to −7.0 diopters of myopia. J Cataract Refract Surg. 2000;26(7):967–77.
38. McLeod SD, Kisla TA, Caro NC, McMahon TT. Iatrogenic keratoconus: corneal ectasia following laser

in situ keratomileusis for myopia. Arch Ophthalmol. 2000;118(2):282–4.
39. Holland SP, Srivannaboon S, Reinstein DZ. Avoiding serious corneal complications of laser assisted in situ keratomileusis and photorefractive keratectomy. Ophthalmology. 2000;107(4):640–52.
40. Schmitt-Bernard CF, Lesage C, Arnaud B. Keratectasia induced by laser in situ keratomileusis in keratoconus. J Refract Surg. 2000;16(3):368–70.
41. Rao SN, Epstein RJ. Early onset ectasia following laser in situ keratomileusus: case report and literature review. J Refract Surg. 2002;18(2):177–84.
42. Malecaze F, Coullet J, Calvas P, Fournie P, Arne JL, Brodaty C. Corneal ectasia after photorefractive keratectomy for low myopia. Ophthalmology. 2006;113(5):742–6.
43. Randleman JB, Russell B, Ward MA, Thompson KP, Stulting RD. Risk factors and prognosis for corneal ectasia after LASIK. Ophthalmology. 2003; 110(2):267–75.
44. Leccisotti A. Corneal ectasia after photorefractive keratectomy. Graefes Arch Clin Exp Ophthalmol. 2007;245(6):869–75.
45. Reinstein DZ, Archer T. Combined Artemis very high-frequency digital ultrasound-assisted transepithelial phototherapeutic keratectomy and wavefront-guided treatment following multiple corneal refractive procedures. J Cataract Refract Surg. 2006;32(11):1870–6.
46. Reinstein DZ, Archer TJ, Gobbe M. Rate of change of curvature of the corneal stromal surface drives epithelial compensatory changes and remodeling. J Refract Surg. 2014;30(12):800–2.
47. Reinstein DZ, Silverman RH, Trokel SL, Coleman DJ. Corneal pachymetric topography. Ophthalmology. 1994;101(3):432–8.
48. Reinstein DZ, Silverman RH, Raevsky T, Simoni GJ, Lloyd HO, Najafi DJ, et al. Arc-scanning very high-frequency digital ultrasound for 3D pachymetric mapping of the corneal epithelium and stroma in laser in situ keratomileusis. J Refract Surg. 2000;16(4):414–30.
49. Reinstein DZ, Archer TJ, Gobbe M, Silverman RH, Coleman DJ. Epithelial thickness in the normal cornea: three-dimensional display with Artemis very high-frequency digital ultrasound. J Refract Surg. 2008;24(6):571–81.
50. Reinstein DZ, Silverman RH, Coleman DJ. High-frequency ultrasound measurement of the thickness of the corneal epithelium. Refract Corneal Surg. 1993;9(5):385–7.
51. Prakash G, Agarwal A, Mazhari AI, Chari M, Kumar DA, Kumar G, et al. Reliability and reproducibility of assessment of corneal epithelial thickness by fourier domain optical coherence tomography. Invest Ophthalmol Vis Sci. 2012;53(6):2580–5.
52. Ge L, Shen M, Tao A, Wang J, Dou G, Lu F. Automatic segmentation of the central epithelium imaged with three optical coherence tomography devices. Eye Contact Lens. 2012;38(3):150–7.
53. Li Y, Tan O, Brass R, Weiss JL, Huang D. Corneal epithelial thickness mapping by Fourier-domain optical coherence tomography in normal and keratoconic eyes. Ophthalmology. 2012;119(12):2425–33.
54. Bentivoglio AR, Bressman SB, Cassetta E, Carretta D, Tonali P, Albanese A. Analysis of blink rate patterns in normal subjects. Mov Disord. 1997;12(6):1028–34.
55. Doane MG. Interactions of eyelids and tears in corneal wetting and the dynamics of the normal human eyeblink. Am J Ophthalmol. 1980;89(4):507–16.
56. Young G, Hunt C, Covey M. Clinical evaluation of factors influencing toric soft contact lens fit. Optom Vis Sci. 2002;79(1):11–9.
57. Reinstein DZ, Gobbe M, Archer TJ, Couch D, Bloom B. Epithelial, stromal, and corneal pachymetry changes during orthokeratology. Optom Vis Sci. 2009;86(8):E1006–14.
58. Scroggs MW, Proia AD. Histopathological variation in keratoconus. Cornea. 1992;11(6):553–9.
59. Haque S, Simpson T, Jones L. Corneal and epithelial thickness in keratoconus: a comparison of ultrasonic pachymetry, Orbscan II, and optical coherence tomography. J Refract Surg. 2006;22(5):486–93.
60. Reinstein DZ, Archer TJ, Gobbe M, Silverman RH, Coleman DJ. Epithelial, stromal and corneal thickness in the keratoconic cornea: three-dimensional display with Artemis very high-frequency digital ultrasound. J Refract Surg. 2010;26(4):259–71.
61. Rocha KM, Perez-Straziota CE, Stulting RD, Randleman JB. SD-OCT analysis of regional epithelial thickness profiles in keratoconus, postoperative corneal ectasia, and normal eyes. J Refract Surg. 2013;29(3):173–9.
62. Kanellopoulos AJ, Aslanides IM, Asimellis G. Correlation between epithelial thickness in normal corneas, untreated ectatic corneas, and ectatic corneas previously treated with CXL; is overall epithelial thickness a very early ectasia prognostic factor? Clin Ophthalmol. 2012;6:789–800.
63. Sandali O, El Sanharawi M, Temstet C, Hamiche T, Galan A, Ghouali W, et al. Fourier-domain optical coherence tomography imaging in keratoconus: a corneal structural classification. Ophthalmology. 2013;120(12):2403–12.
64. Gauthier CA, Holden BA, Epstein D, Tengroth B, Fagerholm P, Hamberg-Nystrom H. Role of epithelial hyperplasia in regression following photorefractive keratectomy. Br J Ophthalmol. 1996;80(6): 545–8.
65. Reinstein DZ, Srivannaboon S, Gobbe M, Archer TJ, Silverman RH, Sutton H, et al. Epithelial thickness profile changes induced by myopic LASIK as measured by Artemis very high-frequency digital ultrasound. J Refract Surg. 2009;25(5):444–50.
66. Reinstein DZ, Archer TJ, Gobbe M. Change in epithelial thickness profile 24 hours and longitudinally for 1 year after myopic LASIK: three-dimensional display with Artemis very high-frequency digital ultrasound. J Refract Surg. 2012;28(3):195–201.
67. Kanellopoulos AJ, Asimellis G. Longitudinal postoperative Lasik epithelial thickness profile changes in correlation with degree of myopia correction. J Refract Surg. 2014;30(3):166–71.

68. Reinstein DZ, Archer TJ, Gobbe M, Silverman RH, Coleman DJ. Epithelial thickness after hyperopic LASIK: three-dimensional display with Artemis very high-frequency digital ultrasound. J Refract Surg. 2010;26(8):555–64.
69. Reinstein DZ, Archer TJ, Gobbe M. Epithelial thickness up to 26 years after radial keratotomy: three-dimensional display with Artemis very high-frequency digital ultrasound. J Refract Surg. 2011;27(8):618–24.
70. Reinstein DZ, Srivannaboon S, Holland SP. Epithelial and stromal changes induced by intacs examined by three-dimensional very high-frequency digital ultrasound. J Refract Surg. 2001;17(3):310–8.
71. Reinstein DZ, Silverman RH, Sutton HF, Coleman DJ. Very high-frequency ultrasound corneal analysis identifies anatomic correlates of optical complications of lamellar refractive surgery: anatomic diagnosis in lamellar surgery. Ophthalmology. 1999;106(3):474–82.
72. Reinstein DZ, Archer TJ, Gobbe M. Refractive and topographic errors in topography-guided ablation produced by epithelial compensation predicted by three-dimensional Artemis very high-frequency digital ultrasound stromal and epithelial thickness mapping. J Refract Surg. 2012;28(9):657–63.
73. Reinstein DZ, Archer TJ, Gobbe M. Improved effectiveness of trans-epithelial phototherapeutic keratectomy versus topography-guided ablation degraded by epithelial compensation on irregular stromal surfaces [plus video]. J Refract Surg. 2013;29(8):526–33.
74. Reinstein DZ, Gobbe M, Archer TJ, Youssefi G, Sutton HF. Stromal surface topography-guided custom ablation as a repair tool for corneal irregular astigmatism. J Refract Surg. 2015;31(1):54–9.
75. Reinstein DZ, Archer TJ, Dickeson ZI, Gobbe M. Trans-epithelial phototherapeutic keratectomy protocol for treating irregular astigmatism based population on epithelial thickness measurements by Artemis very high-frequency digital ultrasound. J Refract Surg. 2014;30(6):380–7.
76. Reinstein DZ, Gobbe M, Archer TJ, Couch · D. Epithelial thickness profile as a method to evaluate the effectiveness of collagen cross-linking treatment after corneal ectasia. J Refract Surg. 2011;27(5):356–63.
77. Vinciguerra P, Roberts CJ, Albe E, Romano MR, Mahmoud A, Trazza S, et al. Corneal curvature gradient map: a new corneal topography map to predict the corneal healing process. J Refract Surg. 2014;30(3):202–7.
78. Reinstein DZ, Archer TJ, Gobbe M. Corneal epithelial thickness profile in the diagnosis of keratoconus. J Refract Surg. 2009;25(7):604–10.
79. Klein SR, Epstein RJ, Randleman JB, Stulting RD. Corneal ectasia after laser in situ keratomileusis in patients without apparent preoperative risk factors. Cornea. 2006;25(4):388–403.
80. Silverman RH, Urs R, Roychoudhury A, Archer TJ, Gobbe M, Reinstein DZ. Epithelial remodeling as basis for machine-based identification of keratoconus. Invest Ophthalmol Vis Sci. 2014;55(3):1580–7.
81. Temstet C, Sandali O, Bouheraoua N, Hamiche T, Galan A, El Sanharawi M, et al. Corneal epithelial thickness mapping using Fourier-domain optical coherence tomography for detection of form fruste keratoconus. J Cataract Refract Surg. 2015;41(4):812–20.
82. Ambrosio Jr R, Faria-Correia F, Ramos I, Valbon BF, Lopes B, Jardim D, et al. Enhanced screening for ectasia susceptibility among refractive candidates: the role of corneal tomography and biomechanics. Curr Ophthalmol Rep. 2013;1(1):28–38.
83. Gomes JA, Tan D, Rapuano CJ, Belin MW, Ambrosio Jr R, Guell JL, et al. Global consensus on keratoconus and ectatic diseases. Cornea. 2015;34(4):359–69.
84. Ambrosio Jr R, Dawson DG, Salomao M, Guerra FP, Caiado AL, Belin MW. Corneal ectasia after LASIK despite low preoperative risk: tomographic and biomechanical findings in the unoperated, stable, fellow eye. J Refract Surg. 2010;26(11):906–11.
85. Reinstein DZ, Gobbe M, Archer TJ. Ocular biomechanics: measurement parameters and terminology. J Refract Surg. 2011;27(6):396–7.
86. Vellara HR, Patel DV. Biomechanical properties of the keratoconic cornea: a review. Clin Exp Optom. 2015;98(1):31–8.
87. Pinero DP, Alcon N. Corneal biomechanics: a review. Clin Exp Optom. 2014;98:107–16.
88. Scarcelli G, Besner S, Pineda R, Yun SH. Biomechanical characterization of keratoconus corneas ex vivo with Brillouin microscopy. Invest Ophthalmol Vis Sci. 2014;55(7):4490–5.
89. Abu-Amero KK, Al-Muammar AM, Kondkar AA. Genetics of keratoconus: where do we stand? J Ophthalmol. 2014;2014:641708.
90. Burdon KP, Vincent AL. Insights into keratoconus from a genetic perspective. Clin Exp Optom. 2013;96(2):146–54.
91. Rabinowitz YS, Dong L, Wistow G. Gene expression profile studies of human keratoconus cornea for NEIBank: a novel cornea-expressed gene and the absence of transcripts for aquaporin 5. Invest Ophthalmol Vis Sci. 2005;46(4):1239–46.
92. Abou Shousha M, Perez VL, Fraga Santini Canto AP, Vaddavalli PK, Sayyad FE, Cabot F, et al. The use of Bowman's layer vertical topographic thickness map in the diagnosis of keratoconus. Ophthalmology. 2014;121(5):988–93.
93. Yadav R, Kottaiyan R, Ahmad K, Yoon G. Epithelium and Bowman's layer thickness and light scatter in keratoconic cornea evaluated using ultrahigh resolution optical coherence tomography. J Biomed Opt. 2012;17(11):116010.
94. Reinstein DZ, Archer TJ, Gobbe M. Stability of LASIK in corneas with topographic suspect keratoconus, with keratoconus excluded by epithelial thickness mapping. J Refract Surg. 2009;25(7):569–77.
95. Reinstein DZ, Archer TJ, Gobbe M. Stability of LASIK in corneas with topographic suspect keratoconus confirmed non-keratoconic by epithelial thickness mapping: 2-years follow-up. San Francisco: AAO; 2009.

14 Brillouin Scanning Microscopy in Keratoconus

Giuliano Scarcelli and Seok Hyun Yun

14.1 Introduction

The mechanical strength of the cornea is thought to play a major role in the onset and progression of keratoconus and ectatic disorders. However, measuring mechanical properties of the cornea in vivo and in situ is currently difficult. Brillouin microscopy may address this need by providing a noninvasive high-resolution tool for biomechanical measurement. Brillouin scattering arises from the interaction between an incident optical wave and spontaneous acoustic waves within a sample and it thus provides information on the local longitudinal elastic modulus of material through an optical spectroscopy measurement. In the cornea, Brillouin microscopy has found depth-dependent variation of stromal stiffness, variation of corneal strength due to keratoconus ex vivo and ex vivo, and stiffening of the cornea following therapeutic procedures such as corneal collagen cross-linking. Brillouin microscopy promises to become a useful clinical tool to diagnose, monitor the development of keratoconus, as well as to assess the response to treatment and drugs.

This chapter briefly describes the principles of Brillouin light scattering and how this phenomenon can provide information on biomechanical properties of the cornea. An overview of current technology for Brillouin imaging of the cornea is given. Finally, results and perspectives of Brillouin microscopy for corneal applications are outlined.

14.2 Corneal Biomechanics and Keratoconus

Keratoconus is the most common corneal degeneration in the US [1] and the leading cause for corneal transplantation [2]. Undetected keratoconus is also responsible for most cases of corneal ectasia after refractive surgery [3, 4]. The clinical presentation of keratoconus is corneal thinning and steepening. However, these morphological features are probably the last stage of the progression of a degenerative disorder. Normal corneas possess the mechanical integrity required to maintain the corneal shape. Corneal stroma has a high content of collagen [5] and a transverse lamellar structure of collagen fibers. The anterior third of the stroma has more collagen interweaving [6–8] and greater numbers of transverse fiber elements [9, 10], and the posterior segment has collagen fibers mostly running parallel to each other.

G. Scarcelli, Ph.D. (✉)
Fischell Department of Bioengineering, University of Maryland, College Park, MD 20742, USA
e-mail: scarc@umd.edu

S.H. Yun, Ph.D.
Wellman Center for Photomedicine, Massachusetts General Hospital, 65 Landsdowne Street, Cambridge, MA 02139, USA

Department of Dermatology, Harvard Medical School, 55 Fruit Street, Boston, MA 02114, USA
e-mail: syun@hms.harvard.edu

J.L. Alió (ed.), *Keratoconus*, Essentials in Ophthalmology, DOI 10.1007/978-3-319-43881-8_14

The link between keratoconus development and degradation of corneal strength is widely accepted although it is mostly based on indirect mechanical evidence. Genetic and biochemical studies have demonstrated that keratoconus patients have upregulated MMP [11], protein inhibitors that favor collagen degradation and downregulated lysyl oxidase (LOX) activity, known to reduce cross-linking [12]. In ex vivo investigations, keratoconic corneal explants (as well as explants from corneas that developed ectasia after refractive surgery) have shown disrupted collagen orientation [13, 14], reduced number of cross-links [15], and decreased mechanical modulus [16, 17]. Other indirect evidence of the role played by mechanics in keratoconus are in the population and manifestation of the disease: the development and severity of the disease is much amplified in young patients and corneal strength generally increases as a function of age [18]; in addition, the inferior cornea where the corneal ectasia manifests most commonly is known to have the lowest mechanical strength [19]. Finally, collagen cross-linking, generally successful at halting keratoconus progression, is an intrinsically biomechanical procedure. CXL induces the formation of covalent bonds between collagen fibers in the corneal stroma by photoactivation of a photosensitizer such as riboflavin. The increased number of the cross-links increases the elastic modulus of the corneal tissue, and the increased stiffness is believed to be the principal reason for stopping the progression of ectasia.

14.3 Assessing Corneal Mechanical Properties

Measuring the mechanical properties of a material in a quantitative and comprehensive manner requires the application of a stress and the measurement of the corresponding strain. The ratio of stress to strain provides the elastic modulus of the sample. This strategy is not viable for biological studies in vivo as it is destructive [20]. Stress–strain methods are the gold standard of material characterization ex vivo. Most of the early ex vivo experiments to measure corneal strength, assess keratoconic corneas decreased modulus and prove the efficacy of the CXL protocols were all based on extracting the cornea and performing stress–strain tests (e.g., extensiometry) on corneal strips.

Recently, a widespread effort to achieve a noninvasive test of corneal mechanical properties has been put forward. The first technology to get to the market was the Ocular Response Analyzer, which uses an air puff to induce a deformation in the cornea while a laser monitors the displacement of the corneal apex [21]. The corneal hysteresis parameter extracted from this measurement is indirectly related to the mechanical properties of the cornea and it has been shown to correlate with advanced keratoconus [22], but it is not clear whether the ORA can be useful for diagnosis and management of keratoconus [23, 24]. A more sophisticated approach to the same principle is also commercially available (Corvis St., Oculus) and combines the same air-puff deformation strategy with corneal Schleimpfug's imaging. Similarly, the air-puff deformation can be combined with other rapid imaging modalities, such as Optical Coherence Tomography (OCT). All these techniques have had success at assessing corneal mechanical properties; for example, different deformation parameters are observed in untreated corneas vs. cross-linked corneas [25]. The major challenge of these approaches remains to extract the mechanical properties of the cornea from the deformation images because the deformation is strongly affected also by other factors such as corneal geometry and intraocular pressure [25, 26]. To address this issue, finite element modeling of the corneal response to the air puff is probably required. Along this same line of research, two new approaches have been put forward recently based on OCT. In one case, micro air puffs are applied to the cornea and their propagation through the corneal tissue is recorded [27]; in another technology, sound waves are sent to the cornea to induce very small mechanical perturbation which are captured by rapid OCT [28, 29]. Brillouin microscopy, the topic of rest of the chapter, is based on different principles and promises high spatial resolution in corneal mechanical mapping.

14.4 Brillouin Microscopy for Corneal Mechanical Analysis

Brillouin microscopy is based on spontaneous Brillouin light scattering, an inelastic scattering phenomenon where the interaction between light and spontaneous acoustic waves due to thermal fluctuations induces a frequency shift in the scattered light [30]. At a microscopic level, the acoustic waves are directly governed by the mechanical properties of material. As a result, the local mechanical properties of material can be extracted by measuring high-resolution optical spectroscopy. Namely, the Brillouin frequency shift Ω is related to the longitudinal viscoelastic modulus $M^* = M' + iM''$ [31]:

$$M' = \frac{\rho\lambda^2\Omega^2}{4n^2} \quad M'' = \frac{\rho\lambda^2\Omega\Delta\Omega^2}{4n^2} \tag{14.1}$$

Here, λ is the optical wavelength, n is the refractive index of the medium, ρ is the mass density. From Eq. (14.1), we get: $\frac{\Delta\Omega}{\Omega} = \frac{1}{2}\frac{\Delta M}{M} + \frac{\Delta n}{n} - \frac{1}{2}\frac{\Delta\rho}{\rho}$. Based on published data[69,70], we estimate ρ/n^2 to range from 0.565 to 0.5635 g/ml, less than 0.3 % within normal corneas. This allows the last two terms to be canceled out in approximation.

Due to the low compressibility of biological material and the high frequency of Brillouin measurements, the Young's or shear moduli of the cornea in the physiological regime are several orders of magnitude smaller than M' measured by Brillouin technology.

To understand the relationship between Brillouin-measured longitudinal modulus and traditional Young's/shear moduli, we used porcine cornea tissue samples. Brillouin depth profiles were acquired on intact porcine corneas and longitudinal modulus values were computed using fixed index/density data taken from the literature. For shear rheometry, cornea tissue samples were cut with a biopsy punch in order to retrieve thin flaps from anterior, central, and posterior portion of the cornea. The shear modulus of the thin flaps was measured at 0.5 Hz frequency with 0.1 % strain amplitude with a stress-controlled rheometer (AR-G2, TA Instruments). For each flap, thickness was accurately measured in order to calculate the corresponding average longitudinal modulus from the Brillouin depth profile. We found a strong correlation between the Brillouin-derived longitudinal modulus and gold standard Young's modulus in a log–log linear trend (R>0.99). The log–log linear relationship allows estimating the sensitivity to elastic modulus changes of our technology:

$$\frac{\Delta M'}{M'} = a\frac{\Delta E'}{E'} \quad or \quad \frac{\Delta M'}{M'} = a\frac{\Delta G'}{G'} \tag{14.2}$$

where $\Delta M'$, $\Delta E'$, and $\Delta G'$ are respective variations. The coefficients "$a - b$" are intrinsic properties of the material under analysis. From our validation on porcine cornea, we estimate our measurement sensitivity of Young's modulus to be in the order of 5 %.

14.5 Brillouin Microscopy Technology

Since the 1970s, Brillouin scattering spectroscopy has been used for material characterization [32] using the spectrometer developed by J. R. Sandercock. The same spectrometer was also used in the biological realm in the 1980s to measure collagen fibers [33, 34], cornea, and crystalline lens [35] ex vivo. However, the acquisition time of a Brillouin spectrum was in the 10 min to hour range, which made the technology difficult to use in vivo.

Brillouin scattered light is very close in color (i.e., frequency or wavelength) to the input light. In most optical systems and biological specimens, residual components of the input light or reflections, diffusions of the samples are orders of magnitude stronger than Brillouin scattered light. Ordinary spectrometers lack both spectral resolution, i.e., the ability to resolve Brillouin signal from input light, and spectral extinction, i.e., the ability to detect Brillouin scattered light in the presence of strong light with similar color. JR Sandercock's spectrometer successfully measured Brillouin light using a multiple-pass scanning Fabry–Perot (FP) interferometers [36, 37]. However, FP interferometers are extremely slow because the spectral scanning is achieved by changing the spacing between the two mirrors forming a FP cavity and because only a particular narrowband spectral component is transmitted at one time while the remainder components of the spectrum are reflected and lost.

In 2008, the throughput of Brillouin spectrometer was greatly enhanced by parallel detection [38] enabled by a diffractive tilted etalon, called virtually imaged phased array (VIPA) [39, 40]. The VIPA spectrometer has fundamentally superior performances to achieve high spectral resolution with high temporal resolution. The spectral selection is given by the interference of multiple reflections at two optical flats thus providing equivalent performances to FP interferometers in terms of resolution. However, the first surface of a VIPA is totally reflective and coated to allow all the light to enter the interferometer. This feature avoids useful light being wasted in a reflected interference pattern. With respect to an equivalent Fabry–Perot spectrometer, the signal strength in a VIPA spectrometer is improved by about two orders of magnitude. This technical improvement has enabled transitioning Brillouin spectroscopy to Brillouin microscopy by combining a laser-scanning confocal microscope with a VIPA-based spectrometer.

VIPA-based Brillouin spectroscopy has been dramatically improved since 2008 in both spectral extinction and efficiency [41–44]. A clinically viable Brillouin microscope and the first Brillouin measurement of the human eye in vivo were reported in 2012. The clinical instrument, sketched in Fig. 14.1, employs low-power laser light at 780 nm scanned across each location of the eye and a Brillouin spectrometer optimized for the infrared wavelength [45].

14.6 Brillouin Microscopy in Keratoconic Corneas

Recent Brillouin measurements for the analysis of keratoconus both ex vivo and in vivo are promising [46, 47]. For ex vivo investigation, normal tissue samples were obtained from donor corneas used in Descemet's stripping endothelial keratoplasty (DSEK) while keratoconic tissue samples were obtained as the discarded tissue of deep anterior lamellar keratoplasty (DALK) procedure in advanced keratoconus patients. For in vivo investigation, patients with advanced keratoconus were measured just before undergoing DALK surgery and their corneal strength was compared to healthy volunteer corneas. The results of ex vivo and in vivo analysis point at several similar features. Overall, keratoconic corneas had lower Brillouin shift, thus lower elastic modulus and decreased mechanical stability. In addition, while the Brillouin shift of the normal corneas was relatively uniform across the central region of the cornea, in keratoconus patients a strong spatial variation was measured with the cone showing the lowest Brillouin shift. The keratoconus cone showed a decrease in longitudinal modulus of ~2–3 % which corresponds to a ~70 % reduction in Young's modulus based on our empirical conversion factor measured with porcine cornea tissue samples. Interestingly, away from the cone, the elastic modulus was very similar to normal cornea in both ex vivo and in vivo investigations (Fig. 14.2).

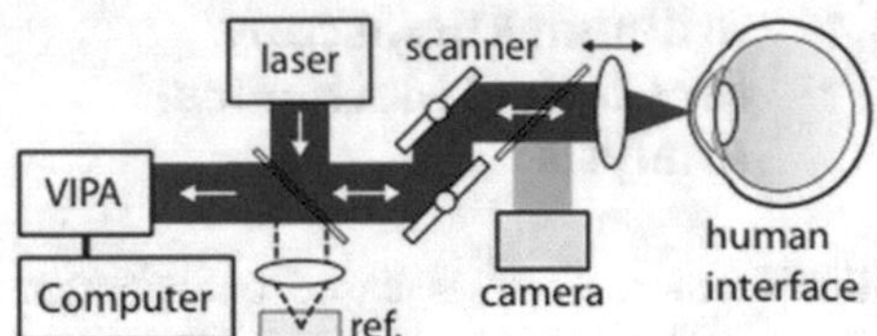

Fig. 14.1 Schematic of the in vivo instrument for Brillouin microscopy

Brillouin microscopy has thus provided the first experimental evidence of a focal weakening or a lack of spatial asymmetry in the distribution of elastic modulus in keratoconic corneas. From a mechanical standpoint, this has important consequences because the focal loss of mechanical strength is thought to represent a critical factor in the progression of keratoconus [48]. From a diagnostic standpoint, this is encouraging because the spatial variation of Brillouin mechanical signatures could be a superior metric to detect the onset and progression of keratoconus. Evaluating the diagnostic and prognostic potential of Brillouin technology will now require the measurement of

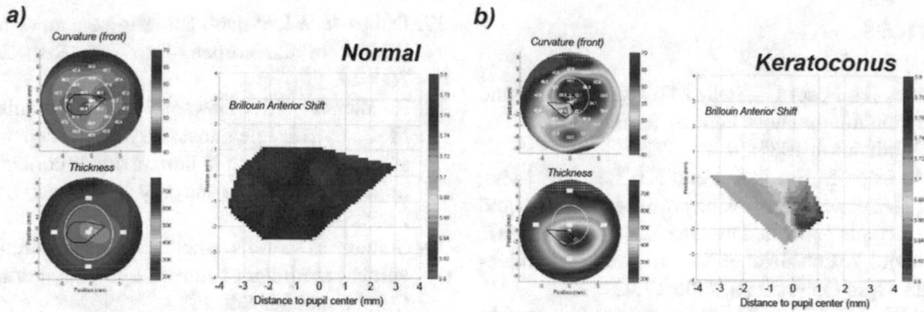

Fig. 14.2 Representative maps of the mean anterior Brillouin shift for (**a**) a healthy subject and (**b**) a patient with advanced keratoconus. The panels on the left report the respective curvature and pachymetry maps with outlined Brillouin scanned areas

nonadvanced keratoconus cases and the comparison with morphological changes (pachymetry and topography).

14.7 Future Directions

Brillouin microscopy has the unique potential of providing high-resolution maps of corneal elasticity. For keratoconus this could have widespread application in both ophthalmic research and in the clinic. Currently, the standard of care is morphological characterization by pachymetry and topography; if properly analyzed, the biomechanical properties of the cornea may become an important indicator of corneal health. Early diagnosis of ectasia and keratoconus could allow patients to receive interventions such as corneal cross-linking (CXL) to halt disease progression. Monitoring CXL mechanical outcome could improve the management of keratoconus progression. The identification of early keratoconus could improve screening procedures for LASIK surgery. Beyond keratoconus, biomechanical measurement of corneal elastic modulus is expected to improve the accuracy of tonometry to estimate the intraocular pressure [49, 50].

In summary, at present Brillouin microscopes are being tested in the clinic to assess the potential to characterize keratoconus and ectasia patients as well as CXL procedures. However, a major component of the future of Brillouin microscopy is tied to its technology development. The difference in Brillouin shift between an advanced keratoconic cornea and a healthy control is not difficult to measure, but earlier stages of keratoconus will probably show much smaller differences in Brillouin shift. At the current level of instrumental sensitivities, about ten separable categories are provided by Brillouin microscopy for the stratification of patients into different disease stages. Improving the sensitivity of mechanical modulus measurement will likely result into higher capability of stratifying patients and detecting early cases. Immediate improvement in speed and sensitivity of the instrument could come by increasing the light power used for the Brillouin measurements as all the clinical tests so far reported have used about 1/8 of the illumination power deemed as safe. Straightforward improvement could also come from engineering efforts aimed at reducing the size, cost, and operation burden of Brillouin instrumentation. Such technological development should improve the availability of Brillouin technology to many medical and research facilities thus accelerating its validation for diagnosis and management of keratoconus.

Conflict of Interest Giuliano Scarcelli and Seok Hyun Yun declare that they have no conflict of interest.

Informed Consent: All procedures followed were in accordance with the ethical standards of the responsible committee on human experimentation (institutional and national) and with the Helsinki Declaration of 1975, as revised in 2000. Informed consent was obtained from all patients for being included in the study.

Animal Studies: No animal studies were carried out by the authors for this article

References

1. Krachmer JH, Feder RS, Belin MW. Keratoconus and related noninflammatory corneal thinning disorders. Surv Ophthalmol. 1984;28:293–322.
2. Jun AS, Cope L, Speck C, Feng XJ, Lee SW, Meng HA, et al. Subnormal cytokine profile in the tear fluid of keratoconus patients. Plos One. 2011;6(1):e16437.
3. Rabinowitz Y. Ectasia after laser in situ keratomileusis. Curr Opin Ophthalmol. 2006;17:421–7.
4. Binder PS, Lindstrom RL, Stulting RD, Donnenfeld E, Wu H, McDonnell P, et al. Keratoconus and corneal ectasia after LASIK. J Refract Surg. 2005;21: 749–52.
5. Maurice DM. The cornea and sclera. In: Davson H, editor. The eye. vol. 1b: Vegetative physiology and biochemistry. Orlando: Academic; 1984. p. 1–158.
6. Komai Y, Ushiki T. The three-dimensional organization of collagen fibrils in the human cornea and sclera. Invest Ophthalmol Vis Sci. 1991;32:2244–58.
7. Polack FM. Morphology of the cornea. I. Study with silver stains. Am J Ophthalmol. 1961;51:1051–6.
8. Smolek MK, McCarey BE. Interlamellar adhesive strength in human eyebank corneas. Invest Ophthalmol Vis Sci. 1990;31:1087–95.
9. Winkler M, Chai D, Kriling S, Nien CJ, Brown DJ, Jester B, et al. Nonlinear optical macroscopic assessment of 3-D corneal collagen organization and axial biomechanics. Invest Ophthalmol Vis Sci. 2011;52: 8818–27.
10. Winkler M, Shoa G, Xie Y, Petsche SJ, Pinsky PM, Juhasz T, et al. Three-dimensional distribution of transverse collagen fibers in the anterior human corneal stroma. Invest Ophthalmol Vis Sci. 2013;54(12):7293–301.
11. Seppala HPS, Maatta M, Rautia M, Mackiewicz Z, Tuisku I, Tervo T, et al. EMMPRIN and MMP-1 in keratoconus. Cornea. 2006;25:325–30.
12. Dudakova L, Liskova P, Trojek T, Palos M, Kalasova S, Jirsova K. Changes in lysyl oxidase (LOX) distribution and its decreased activity in keratoconus corneas. Exp Eye Res. 2012;104:74–81.
13. Meek K, Tuft S, Huang Y, Gill P, Hayes S, Newton R, et al. Changes in collagen orientation and distribution in keratoconus corneas. Invest Ophthalmol Vis Sci. 2005;46:1948–2004.
14. Morishige N, Wahlert A, Kenney M, Brown D, Kawamoto K, Chikama T-I, et al. Second-harmonic imaging microscopy of normal human and keratoconus cornea. Invest Ophthalmol Vis Sci. 2007;48: 1087–181.
15. Zimmermann DR, Fischer RW, Winterhalter KH, Witmer R, Vaughan L. Comparative studies of collagens in normal and keratoconus corneas. Exp Eye Res. 1988;46:431–42.
16. Andreassen TT, Simonsen AH, Oxlund H. Biomechanical properties of keratoconus and normal corneas. Exp Eye Res. 1980;31:435–41.
17. Dupps Jr WJ, Wilson SE. Biomechanics and wound healing in the cornea. Exp Eye Res. 2006;83(4): 709–20.
18. Randleman JB, Dawson DG, Grossniklaus HE, McCarey BE, Edelhauser HF. Depth-dependent cohesive tensile strength in human donor corneas: implications for refractive surgery. J Refract Surg. 2008; 24:S85–9.
19. Smolek MK. Interlamellar cohesive strength in the vertical meridian of human eye bank corneas. Invest Ophthalmol Vis Sci. 1993;34:2962–9.
20. Discher D, Dong C, Fredberg JJ, Guilak F, Ingber D, Janmey P, et al. Biomechanics: cell research and applications for the next decade. Ann Biomed Eng. 2009;37:847–59.
21. Luce DA. Determining in vivo biomechanical properties of the cornea with an ocular response analyzer. J Cataract Refract Surg. 2005;31:156–62.
22. Shah S, Laiquzzaman M, Bhojwani R, Mantry S, Cunliffe I. Assessment of the biomechanical properties of the cornea with the ocular response analyzer in normal and keratoconic eyes. Invest Ophthalmol Vis Sci. 2007;48:3026–31.
23. Fontes BM, Ambrosio Jr R, Velarde GC, Nose W. Ocular response analyzer measurements in keratoconus with normal central corneal thickness compared with matched normal control eyes. J Refract Surg. 2011;27:209–15.
24. Fontes BM, Ambrosio Jr R, Jardim D, Velarde GC, Nose W. Corneal biomechanical metrics and anterior segment parameters in mild keratoconus. Ophthalmology. 2011;117:673–9.
25. Dorronsoro C, Pascual D, Perez-Merino P, Kling S, Marcos S. Dynamic OCT measurement of corneal deformation by an air puff in normal and cross-linked corneas. Biomed Opt Express. 2012;3:473–87.
26. Roberts CJ, Mahmoud AM, Ramos I, Caldas D, da Silva RS, Ambrosio Jr R. Factors influencing corneal deformation and estimation of intraocular pressure. Invest Ophthalmol Vis Sci. 2011;52:4384.
27. Twa M, Li J, Vantipalli S, Singh M, Aglyamov S, Emelianov S, et al. Spatial characterization of corneal biomechanical properties with optical coherence elastography after UV cross-linking. Biomed Opt Express. 2014;5:1419–27.
28. Akca BI, Chang EW, Kling S, Ramier A, Scarcelli G, Marcos S, et al. Observation of sound-induced corneal vibrational modes by optical coherence tomography. Biomed Opt Express. 2015;6:3313–9.
29. Kling S, Akca I, Chang E, Scarcelli G, Bekesi N, Yun S, et al. Numerical model of optical coherence tomographic vibrography imaging to estimate corneal biomechanical properties. J R Soc Interface. 2014;11.
30. Brillouin L. Diffusion de la lumiere et des rayonnes X par un corps transparent homogene; influence del'agitation thermique. Ann Phys. 1922;17:88.
31. Randall J, Vaughan JM. The measurement and interpretation of Brillouin scattering in the lens of the eye. Proc R Soc London Ser B. 1982;214:449–70.

32. Dil JG. Brillouin-scattering in condensed matter. Rep Prog Phys. 1982;45:285–334.
33. Harley R, James D, Miller A, White JW. Phonons and elastic-moduli of collagen and muscle. Nature. 1977;267:285–7.
34. Randall J, Vaughan JM. Brillouin-scattering in systems of biological significance. Philos Trans R Soc London Ser A. 1979;293:341–8.
35. Vaughan JM, Randall JT. Brillouin-scattering, density and elastic properties of the lens and cornea of the eye. Nature. 1980;284:489–91.
36. Sandercock JR. Some recent developments in Brillouin-scattering. RCA Review. 1975;36:89–107.
37. Sandercock JR. Light-scattering from surface acoustic phonons in metals and semiconductors. Solid State Commun. 1978;26:547–51.
38. Scarcelli G, Yun SH. Brillouin confocal microscopy for three dimensional mechanical imaging. Nat Photonics. 2008;2:39–43.
39. Shirasaki M. Large angular dispersion by a virtually imaged phased array and its application to a wavelength demultiplexer. Opt Lett. 1996;21:366–8.
40. Xiao SJ, Weiner AM, Lin C. Experimental and theoretical study of hyperfine WDM demultiplexer performance using the virtually imaged phased-array (VIPA). J Lightwave Technol. 2005;23:1456–67.
41. Scarcelli G, Kim P, Yun SH. Cross-axis cascading of spectral dispersion. Opt Lett. 2008;33:2979–81.
42. Scarcelli G, Yun SH. Multistage VIPA etalons for high-extinction parallel Brillouin spectroscopy. Opt Express. 2011;19:10913–22.
43. Scarcelli G, Polacheck WJ, Nia HT, Patel K, Grodzinsky AJ, Kamm RD, et al. Noncontact three-dimensional mapping of intracellular hydromechanical properties by Brillouin microscopy. Nat Methods. 2015;12(12):1132–4.
44. Berghaus K, Zhang J, Yun S-H, Scarcelli G. High-finesse sub-GHz-resolution spectrometer employing VIPA etalons of different dispersion. Opt Lett. 2015;40(19):4436–9.
45. Scarcelli G, Yun SH. In vivo Brillouin optical microscopy of the human eye. Opt Express. 2012;20:9197.
46. Scarcelli G, Besner S, Pineda R, Yun SH. Biomechanical characterization of keratoconus corneas ex vivo with Brillouin microscopy. Invest Ophthalmol Vis Sci. 2014;55:4490–5.
47. Scarcelli G, Besner S, Pineda R, Kalout P, Yun SH. In vivo biomechanical mapping of normal and keratoconus corneas. JAMA Ophthalmol. 2015;133(4):480–2.
48. Roberts CJ, Dupps Jr WJ. Biomechanics of corneal ectasia and biomechanical treatments. J Cataract Refract Surg. 2014;40:991–8.
49. Liu J, Roberts CJ. Influence of corneal biomechanical properties on intraocular pressure measurement—quantitative analysis. J Cataract Refract Surg. 2005;31:146–55.
50. Pepose JS, Feigenbaum SK, Qazi MA, Sanderson JP, Roberts CJ. Changes in corneal biomechanics and intraocular pressure following LASIK using static, dynamic, and noncontact tonometry. Am J Ophthalmol. 2007;143:39–47.

Part III

The Clinical Profile of Keratoconus

15 Keratoconus Grading and Its Therapeutic Implications

Alfredo Vega Estrada, Pablo Sanz Díez, and Jorge L. Alió

15.1 Introduction

Keratoconus is an ectatic corneal disease characterized by a progressive corneal thinning and irregular astigmatism that negatively impact in the visual function and the optical quality of the patients [1]. Its prevalence has been estimated to be 57/100.000 inhabitants with a prevalence of 4,5/100.000/year in the Caucasian population [2]. It is a disease that usually is diagnosed during the first decade of life in which 73 % of cases are presented before 24 years old and present a faster progressive pattern as earliest age of diagnosis [3]. Nowadays, there are several therapeutic options to treat such a pathological condition, such as contact lens wearing, thermokeratoplasty procedures, corneal collagen cross-linking, intracorneal ring segment implantation, and lamellar or penetrating keratoplasty procedures.

Regarding classification of the disease, keratoconus is a disorder with a wide range of presentation that comes from a mild alteration of the corneal geometry that is only recognizable using corneal topography, until severe tissue distortion that can induce a significant impairment from the optical system of the patient.

The purpose of the following chapter is to describe the main grading keratoconus system that are used in the clinical practice and performed a critical analysis of its limitations when results of some of the therapeutic options are evaluated taking into consideration a classification system based on new diagnosis parameters.

A. Vega Estrada, Ph.D. (✉)
Keratoconus Unit, Vissum Alicante, Alicante, Spain
e-mail: alfredovega@vissum.com

P. Sanz Díez, O.D., M.Sc. • J.L. Alió, M.D., Ph.D.
Keratoconus Unit, Department of Refractive Surgery
Vissum Alicante, Alicante, Spain

Division of Ophthalmology, Miguel Hernández
University, Alicante, Spain
e-mail: pablosanz9143@gmail.com; jlalio@vissum.com

15.2 Anatomical-Based Grading Keratoconus

Keratoconus is a disorder that is included within a group of diseases known as corneal ectatic disorders [4]. From the point of view of its *origin*, keratoconus is a *primary* ectatic disorder unlike than post-LASIK ectasia that will be the main representative of ectatic diseases *secondary* in origin [4].

As previously commented, keratoconus is a corneal disease with a wide spectrum of presentation. On its more benign side, we found the *subclinical keratoconus*, also known by other authors with the name of form fruste keratoconus or keratoconus suspect [4–6]. The main features of this entity are the lack of clinical signs of keratoconus, being the diagnosis of the disease performed just by the changes in the corneal topography and with a corrected visual acuity within normal levels [4–6].

J.L. Alió (ed.), *Keratoconus*, Essentials in Ophthalmology, DOI 10.1007/978-3-319-43881-8_15

On the other hand, keratoconus is characterized by corneal thinning and morphological alterations of the tissue that induce an irregular astigmatism with different degrees of visual impairment on the patients. In contrast to subclinical keratoconus, corneal topography is used in keratoconus patients as a tool to confirm the diagnosis.

Until now, several grading systems have been proposed in order to classify the disease but some of them include just one isolated variable (keratometric readings, pachymetry, morphology), which represents obvious limitations and therefore are not used as routine in the clinical practice. Classifications that are more widespread are those which include more than one variable for characterizing the disease, such as Amsler-Krumeich or Alio-Shabayek grading systems.

Following we describe some of the keratoconus classifications that are more often used in the clinical practice:

- **Buxton classification** [7] based on the magnitude of the keratometric readings:
  - Mild: less than 45 diopters (D)
  - Moderate: between 46 and 52 D.
  - Advance: between 53 and 59 D.
  - Severe: more than 60 D.
- **Morphological classification** [8]:
  - Oval: cone that is affecting one or two quadrants, generally inferior.
  - Globe: cone that is affecting a large area of the cornea.
  - Nipple: cone that is limited in diameter but may reach any degree of conicity.
- **Hom's classification** based on the clinical features of the pathology [7]:
  - Preclinical keratoconus: subclinical keratoconus or keratoconus suspect.
  - Mild keratoconus: absence of scars, good spectacle corrected visual acuity, mild corneal thinning, and scissoring light reflex.
  - Moderate keratoconus: absence of scars, good contact lenses corrected visual acuity.
- **Amsler-Krumeich classification** it is the more extended grading system used in keratoconus. One of the main advantages is that it combines refractive, keratometric, and clinical signs of keratoconus in order to grade the severity of the disease. Table 15.1 presents the main variables included in this classification.

Table 15.1 Amsler-Krumeich classification

Grade I	Grade II
– Eccentric corneal steepening	– Absence of scarring
– Myopia and/or astigmatism <5 D	– Myopia and/or astigmatism 5–8 D
– Mean central K readings ≤48.00 D	– Mean central K readings >48.00 to ≤53 D
	– Minimum corneal thickness >400 μm
Grade III	**Grade IV**
– Absence of scarring	– Central corneal scarring
– Myopia and/or astigmatism 8–10 D	– Not reliable refraction
– Mean central K readings >53.00 to ≤55 D	– Mean central K readings >55 D
– Minimum corneal thickness 300 to 400 μm	– Minimum corneal thickness 200 μm

15.3 Optical-Based Keratoconus Grading

- **Alio-Shabayek classification** [9], this grading system was created taking into account the analysis of the anterior corneal higher order aberrations in patients with keratoconus. By means of evaluation of the corneal wavefront, the authors categorize the severity of the disease assessing the asymmetric aberrations, specifically the coma and its radial orders, which are the more affected in keratoconic patients. Table 15.2 summarizes the main characteristics of this classification.

As we can see, there are several grading systems found in the literature aiming to classify the severity of keratoconus. Nevertheless, many of them are obsolete or are based just in isolated or morphological parameters without taking into considerations other variables closely associated with the optical quality, such as the visual acuity, which additional is related with the quality of life of the patients.

Table 15.2 Alio-Shabayek Classification

Grade I	Grade II
– Absence of scarring	– Absence of scarring
– RMS of coma-like aberration from 1.50 to 2.50 μm	– RMS of coma-like aberration from 2.50 to 3.50 μm
– Mean central K readings ≤48.00 D	– Mean central K readings >48.00 to ≤53 D
	– Minimum corneal thickness >400 μm
Grade III	**Grade IV**
– Absence of scarring	– Central corneal scarring
– RMS of coma-like aberration from 3.50 to 4.50 μm	– RMS of coma-like aberration >4.50 μm
– Mean central K readings >53.00 to ≤55 D	– Mean central K readings >55 D
– Minimum corneal thickness 300 to 400 μm	– Minimum corneal thickness 200 μm

15.4 Visual Function-Based Grading Keratoconus

Recently, our research group developed a grading system based on the analysis of almost 800 cases of keratoconus in which was evaluated the visual, refractive, topographic, aberrometric, and biomechanical variables in order to classify the severity of the disease [10]. The principal features of this grading system are presented in Fig. 15.1.

As shown in Fig. 15.1, this new classification system includes morphological parameters that are directly correlated with functional variables as the visual acuity of the patient. In addition, includes new parameters as the internal astigmatism and corneal asphericity which is also significantly affected in keratoconic patients. Moreover, it also analyses the biomechanical alterations on every case. Even when we do not observe a statistically significant difference on the biomechanical

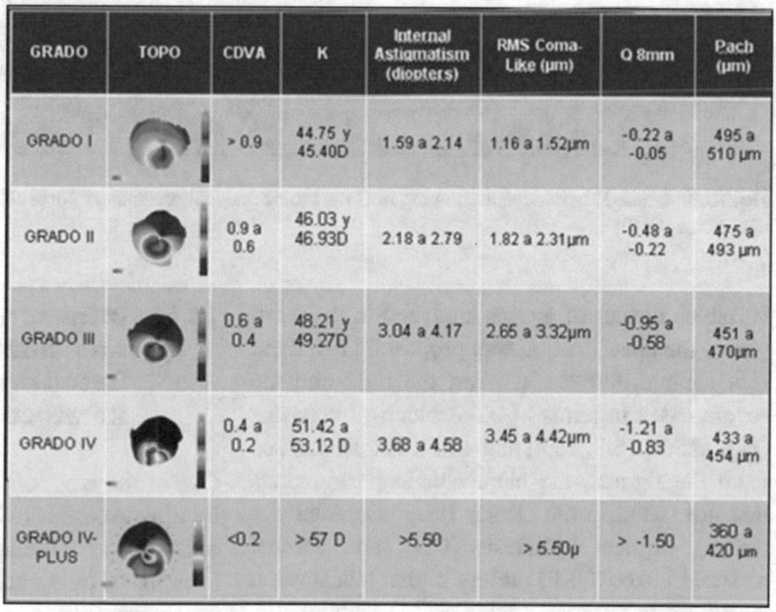

GRADO	TOPO	CDVA	K	Internal Astigmatism (diopters)	RMS Coma-Like (μm)	Q 8mm	Pach (μm)
GRADO I		> 0.9	44.75 y 45.40D	1.59 a 2.14	1.16 a 1.52μm	-0.22 a -0.05	495 a 510 μm
GRADO II		0.9 a 0.6	46.03 y 46.93D	2.18 a 2.79	1.82 a 2.31μm	-0.48 a -0.22	475 a 493 μm
GRADO III		0.6 a 0.4	48.21 y 49.27D	3.04 a 4.17	2.65 a 3.32μm	-0.95 a -0.58	451 a 470μm
GRADO IV		0.4 a 0.2	51.42 a 53.12 D	3.68 a 4.58	3.45 a 4.42μm	-1.21 a -0.83	433 a 454 μm
GRADO IV-PLUS		<0.2	> 57 D	>5.50	> 5.50μ	> -1.50	360 a 420 μm

Fig. 15.1 The principal features of the visual function based grading system

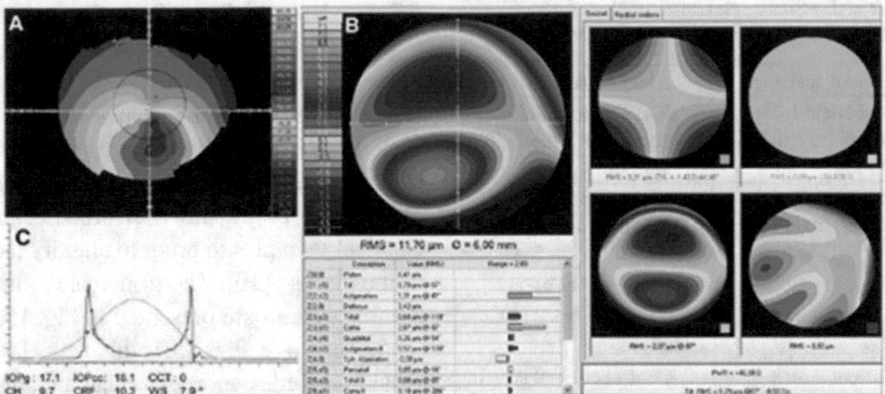

Fig. 15.2 Grade I keratoconus showing in C the biomechanical parameters corneal hysteresis (CH) and corneal resistant factor (CRF). We can also observe the high peaks on the waveform

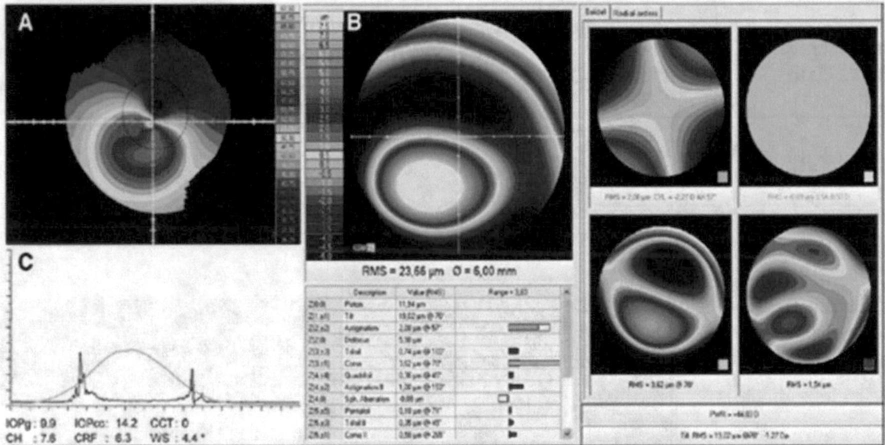

Fig. 15.3 Grade II keratoconus showing in C the biomechanical parameters corneal hysteresis (CH) and corneal resistant factor (CRF)

variables in pair of groups analyzed in the work where the classification was proposed [10], there is a clear difference between the mild and the severe cases in terms of biomechanical behavior (Figs. 15.2, 15.3, 15.4, and 15.5). As we can see from the figures, the biomechanical parameters that are found in the Ocular Response Analyzer (ORA), corneal hysteresis (CH), and corneal resistant factor (CRF) present higher levels when compared to the most severe cases. Additionally, in the severe cases the shape of the waveform is more flat and almost null when compared to the mild cases.

15.5 Intracorneal Ring Segment Implantation Outcomes Based on Our New Keratoconus Classification

One of the main objectives of grading the severity of a disease is to be able to assess the efficacy of the different therapeutic alternatives that exists in order to treat such pathology. As commented in the previous section, one of the main limitations of the grading systems that are used to classify keratoconus is that they are based on morphological variables without taking into

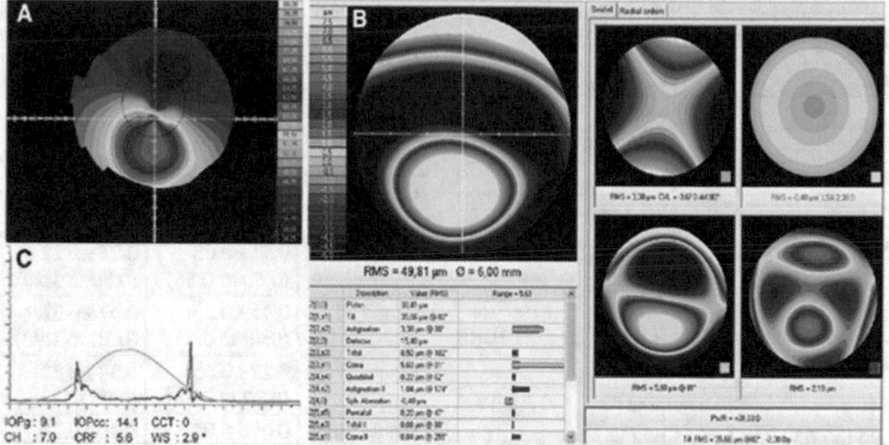

Fig. 15.4 Grade III keratoconus showing in C the biomechanical parameters corneal hysteresis (CH) and corneal-resistant factor (CRF)

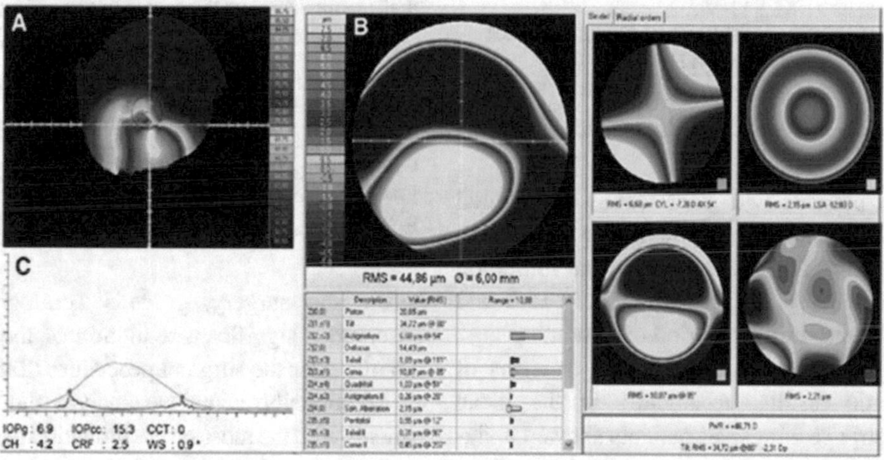

Fig. 15.5 Grade IV keratoconus showing in C the biomechanical parameters corneal hysteresis (CH) and corneal resistant factor (CRF). We can also observe the flat peaks on the waveform

account the visual function of the patients. Therefore, in a recent work developed by the authors, it was assessed the outcomes of intracorneal ring segments (ICRS) implantation to treat keratoconic patients based on a new grading system.

If we revised the published literature, we will find that most of the series reported an improvement in the visual and refractive variables when treating keratoconus with ICRS [11–16]. Nevertheless and as previously commented, the majority of these works are based on grading systems whose pitfalls have been already mentioned. Moreover, most of the authors in those studies do not evaluate the results of the surgical technique independently of the severity of the disease but analyzing the outcomes of all the population under study as a whole.

Therefore, the purpose of our study was to analyze the outcomes of implanting ICRS evaluating the results based on the severity of the disease taking into account the visual limitation of the patients [17]. For that purpose we conducted a multicentric study in which was analyzed more

Table 15.3 Population of ICRS implantation study divided according to visual limitation

Keratoconus	CDVA (decimal scale)
Grade I	≥0.9
Grade II	≥0.6 and <0.9
Grade III	≥0.4 and <0.6
Grade IV	≥0.2 and <0.4
Grade plus	<0.2

Table 15.4 Keratometric readings 6 months after ICRS implantation

Km Pre	Km 6 months	*P* value
44.90 ± 2.96 (35.65 to 54.96)	43.35 ± 1.69 (38.63 to 47.45)	<0.01
46.24 ± 4.13 (34.57 to 59.10)	44.52 ± 4.41 (34.32 to 56.10)	<0.01
48.93 ± 5.67 (36.25 to 78.80)	46.09 ± 5.07 (32.60 to 59.52)	<0.01
51.65 ± 6.06 (32.65 to 72.70)	47.64 ± 4.87 (39.88 to 60.11)	<0.01
54.40 ± 8.00 (38.48 to 82.62)	48.81 ± 4.39 (39.54 to 57.34)	<0.01

than 600 patients with keratoconus and treated with ICRS. The population under study was divided taking into account the visual limitation of the patients as described in Table 15.3 and were followed during a period of 6 months.

In that study, we observed that in terms of topographic results, specifically in the mean keratometric readings, all patients showed a significant reduction of the keratometric readings 6 months after ICRS implantation (Table 15.4).

These results are consistent with the published data reported by most of the authors when analyzing ICRS implantation taking into account other grading systems. Nevertheless, when we analyzed the results related to the visual function of the patient, specifically the visual acuity, we observed that the outcomes are somehow different. For instance, when we assess the changes that were found in the corrected visual acuity (CDVA) 6 months after ICRS implantation basing the analysis on the degree of visual limitation, we observed that most of the grades showed a significant improvement of the CDVA, with the exception of patients classified as grade I. In those patients who had the better visual acuity before the surgery, grade I keratoconus, we observed a significant reduction of the vision 6 months after the surgical procedure (Table 15.5).

Table 15.5 Changes in the corrected visual acuity (CDVA) 6 months after ICRS implantation, based on degree of visual limitation

CDVA (decimal scale)	Pre	6 months	*P* value
Grade I	0.97 ± 0.06 (0.90 to 1.15)	0.86 ± 0.18 (0.40 to 1.20)	<0.01
Grade II	0.71 ± 0.08 (0.60 to 0.86)	0.75 ± 0.22 (0.30 to 1.20)	=0.04
Grade III	0.45 ± 0.53 (0.40 to 0.58)	0.57 ± 0.22 (0.10 to 1.00)	<0.01
Grade IV	0.27 ± 0.05 (0.20 to 0.38)	0.50 ± 0.22 (0.05 to 1.00)	<0.01
Grade plus	0.09 ± 0.05 (0.01 to 0.15)	0.38 ± 0.26 (0.05 to 1.00)	<0.01

Table 15.6 Comparison of patient outcomes after ICRS implantation based on the degree of visual limitation

KCN	Gain ≥ 1 line CDVA (%)	Lost ≥ 1 line CDVA (%)	Lost ≥ 2 lines CDVA (%)
CDVA ≥ 0.6 grade I + II	37.9	36.2	25.8
CDVA ≤ 0.4 grade IV + plus	82.8	10.0	4.2

Additionally, when we analyze the group of patients with the most severe limitation of the visual acuity before the surgery and compare with the ones who had the better levels of vision we found that the best results are achieved in those cases classified of having a serious visual impairment. As described in Table 15.6, patients who have a CDVA better than 0.6 on the decimal scale before ICRS implantation showed almost the same percentage of probability of gaining or losing 1 line of corrected vision after the surgical intervention; we can also see how more than 25 % of the cases in this group of patients were prone to lose 2 or more lines of corrected vision. On the other hand, the majority of cases with a CDVA worst than 0.4 on the decimal scale before the procedure will gain at least 1 line of corrected vision after surgery while just the 4 % of the cases showed loss of 2 or more corrected visual acuity lines after ICRS implantation.

Results from this study clearly demonstrate that if we take into account the visual limitation of the patients with keratoconus those cases that benefit the most of ICRS implantation are the ones with a significant visual impairment before the surgery. Additionally, it also shows that the efficacy of the surgical technique will depend on the classification system that the clinicians use in order to grade the severity of the disease before the procedure.

15.6 Final Considerations

In medicine, to have an appropriate classification system of any particular disease is fundamental in order to perform an accurate diagnosis of the disease, consider the best therapeutic approach, and perform a correct follow-up of the patient. In the specific case of keratoconus, most of the grading systems that are nowadays available in the clinical practice are obsolete or based on isolated or morphological variables. Such is the case, that when we apply a new classification to assess the results of a particularly treatment, such as ICRS implantation, we found that results may be different to those that we see in our routine as we have discussed in the previous section of this chapter. Thus, it is necessary to update the different parameters that we use to classify the disease by including the source of information that is provided by the new instruments and advances in technology that we employed in our daily practice. Moreover, the main objective of any ophthalmic procedure should be aimed in improving and not in deteriorating the visual function of the patient, this way, a keratoconus classification should include variables that directly discriminate the visual limitation, as a grading system will clearly have an implication in the treatment that we chose for our keratoconus patients. The new classification that was proposed by our research team has led us to change the way that we made the diagnosis and decide the treatment of our keratoconus patients. Currently, we are working in the detailed characterization of the different clinical features of the severity of keratoconus taking into account the grading system based on the visual acuity of the patients.

Compliance with Ethical Requirements Alfredo Vega-Estrada, Pablo Sanz Díez, and Jorge L. Alió declare that they have no conflict of interest.

All procedures followed were in accordance with the ethical standards of the responsible committee on human experimentation (Vissum Ethical Committee Board) and with the Helsinki Declaration of 1975, as revised in 2000. Informed consent was obtained from all patients for being included in the study.

No animal studies were carried out by the authors for this chapter.

References

1. Rabinowitz YS. Keratoconus. Surv Ophthalmol. 1998;42:297–319.
2. Pearson AR, Soneji B, Sarvananthan N, Sandford-Smith JH. Does ethnic origin influence the incidence or severity of keratoconus? Eye (Lond). 2000;14 (Pt 4):625–8.
3. Ihalainen A. Clinical and epidemiological features of keratoconus genetic and external factors in the pathogenesis of the disease. Acta Ophthalmol Suppl. 1986;178:1–64.
4. Binder PS, Lindstrom RL, Stulting RD, et al. Keratoconus and corneal ectasia after LASIK. J Refract Surg. 2005;21:749–52.
5. Sonmez B, Doan MP, Hamilton DR. Identification of scanning slit-beam topographic parameters important in distinguishing normal from keratoconic corneal morphologic features. Am J Ophthalmol. 2007;143: 401–8.
6. Waring GO. Nomenclature for keratoconus suspects. Refract Corneal Surg. 1993;9:219–22.
7. de Rojas Silva V. Clasificacion del queratocono. In: Albertazzi R, editor. Queratocono: pautas para su diagnóstico y tratamiento. Buenos Aires: Ediciones cientificas argentinas para la Keratoconus Society; 2010. p. 33–97.
8. Perry HD, Buxton JN, Fine BS. Round and oval cones in keratoconus. Ophthalmology. 1980;87:905–9.
9. Alio JL, Shabayek MH. Corneal higher order aberrations: a method to grade keratoconus. J Refract Surg. 2006;22:539–45.
10. Alio JL, Pinero DP, Aleson A, et al. Keratoconus-integrated characterization considering anterior corneal aberrations, internal astigmatism, and corneal biomechanics. J Cataract Refract Surg. 2011;37: 552–68.
11. Colin J, Cochener B, Savary G, Malet F. Correcting keratoconus with intracorneal rings. J Cataract Refract Surg. 2000;26:1117–22.
12. Alio JL, Shabayek MH, Artola A. Intracorneal ring segments for keratoconus correction: long-term follow-up. J Cataract Refract Surg. 2006;32:978–85.
13. Kwitko S, Severo NS. Ferrara intracorneal ring segments for keratoconus. J Cataract Refract Surg. 2004;30:812–20.
14. Shetty R, Kurian M, Anand D, et al. Intacs in advanced keratoconus. Cornea. 2008;27:1022–9.

15. Boxer Wachler BS, Christie JP, Chandra NS, et al. Intacs for keratoconus. Ophthalmology. 2003;110:1031–40.
16. Pinero DP, Alio JL. Intracorneal ring segments in ectatic corneal disease—a review. Clin Experiment Ophthalmol. 2010;38:154–67.
17. Vega-Estrada A, Alió JL, Brenner LF, 3, et al. Outcome analysis of intracorneal ring segments for the treatment of keratoconus based on visual, refractive, and aberrometric impairment. Am J Ophthalmol. 2013;155:575–84.

Part IV

Therapeutic Tools in Keratoconus

16 Contact Lenses for Keratoconus

Amy Watts and Kathryn Colby

16.1 Contact Lenses for Keratoconus

There are many different contact lens modalities that can be used to improve visual acuity in patients with keratoconus. Corneal topography, including amount and location of ectasia, is the key factor to consider when choosing a lens. However, a patient's lifestyle, dexterity, occupation, and other ocular health conditions are all important factors in choosing the optimal lens.

Patients with mild keratoconus are often able to achieve clear vision with spectacles simply by correcting for the spherical and regular astigmatism components of refractive error. In patients with moderate to severe keratoconus, the inferior decentration and steepness of the corneal apex causes a significant amount of irregular astigmatism and higher order aberrations (HOA), which spectacles cannot optically correct. In order to optimize visual acuity in these instances, contact lenses are used to mask the irregular astigmatism and reduce the higher order aberrations.

16.2 Corneal Rigid Gas Permeable (RGP) Contact Lenses

Corneal RGPs (Fig. 16.1) remain the most popular contact lens modality for improving vision in patients with keratoconus. As the name implies, these lenses are "rigid" and hold their shape when placed on an irregular cornea. The irregular surface between the back of the contact lens and the front of the cornea is filled in with tears and creates what is called a "lacrimal lens." This interaction creates an optically improved surface by masking the regular and irregular astigmatism and reducing the HOA. However HOA can persist, in particular vertical coma, and can prevent patients with more advanced keratoconus from achieving 20/20 vision [1]. When patients have apical scarring in addition to uncorrected HOA, the visual acuity may be poor even with contact lens correction and surgical intervention would be required. According to the Collaborative Longitudinal Evaluation of keratoconus(CLEK) study ($n = 1209$ patient with keratoconus), corneal scarring was found in one or both eyes of 53 % of patients and was associated with decreased high and low contrast visual acuity [2].

An ideal keratoconus corneal RGP fit should center well to provide optimal vision and move

A. Watts, O.D., F.A.A.O. (✉)
Department of Ophthalmology, Massachusetts Eye and Ear, 243 Charles Street, Boston, MA 02114, USA

Instructor in Ophthalmology, Harvard Medical School, Boston, MA, USA
e-mail: Amy_Watts@MEEI.HARVARD.EDU

K. Colby, M.D., Ph.D.
Department of Ophthalmology and Visual Science, University of Chicago, Chicago, IL, USA
e-mail: kcolby@bsd.uchicago.edu

J.L. Alió (ed.), *Keratoconus*, Essentials in Ophthalmology, DOI 10.1007/978-3-319-43881-8_16

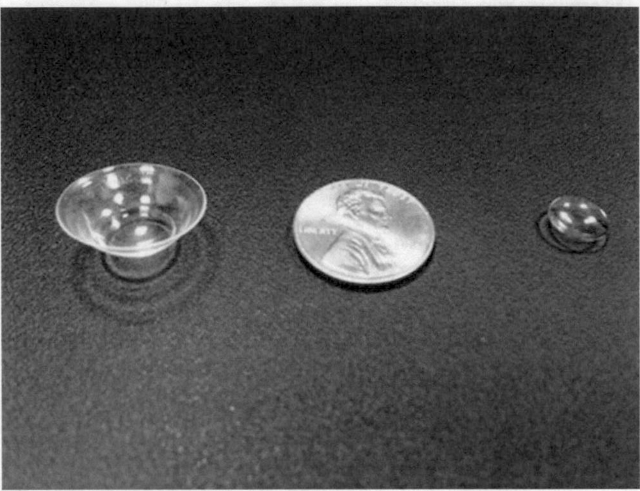

Fig. 16.1 From left to right, a scleral lens of 18.0 mm diameter, a penny for size reference, and a Rose K corneal RGP of 8.3 mm diameter

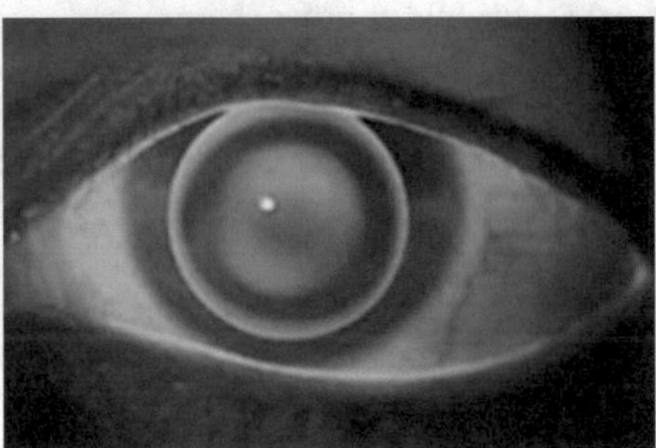

Fig. 16.2 Ideal fluorescein pattern of a corneal gas permeable lens in a patient with keratoconus. Note bulls eye pattern with central light apical touch

approximately 0.5–1.0 mm with blink to allow for oxygen-rich tear exchange beneath the lens. The ideal fluorescein pattern is called "3 point touch" and should show light touch at the apex with surrounding pooling and midperipheral touch with pooling of the 0.5–1.0 mm edge of the lens. The resultant fluorescein pattern is a bull's eye pattern of concentric rings (see Fig. 16.2). The midperipheral touch helps to distribute the weight of the lens across a larger area rather than placing the full burden on the apex of the cone. Patients are able to see well in flat fitted lenses that push on the apex of the cone since the reshaping causes a reduction in HOA [3]. In 1982, Korb et al. published a paper describing apical scarring as a result of apical fit, flat lenses [4]. The much larger CLEK study also reviewed the effect of RGP wear and corneal scarring and found that the risk of scarring in keratoconic patient was two times more likely in contact lens wearers compared to noncontact wearers. However, patients with more severe ectasia were more likely to wear contact lenses than patients with milder ectasia so a causal relationship could not be established [5]. Due to this ongoing debate, many practitioners do not fit apically flat lenses. In instances where three-point touch is not achievable, the corneal epithelium cannot tolerate the lens, or lens retention is a problem, another lens modality should be chosen.

There are many different RGP manufacturers that design and produce corneal RGP lenses specifically for keratoconus. For example, Acculens makes the Accukone®, Blanchard makes the CentraCone®, and Lens Dynamics makes the Dyna Cone®. In addition to the different designs that are specific to each manufacturer, many will carry the Rose K®, Rose K2®, and Rose K2 IC® lenses that were designed by an optometrist from New Zealand named Paul Rose. The line of Rose K lenses is widely available and is currently distributed in over 88 countries [6]. The Rose K and Rose K2 designs can be used for mild to severe keratoconus with base curves available between 4.30 and 8.60 and diameters between 7.9 and 10.4 mm. The Rose K2 differs from the previous Rose K design in that the Rose K2 has aspheric curves to reduce HOA and a larger optic zone to improve acuity in low light. Additionally, Rose K and Rose K2 are now available with Asymmetric

Cornea Technology (ACT). This allows the inferior quadrant of the lens to be steeper in order to correspond to the steepest portion of the cornea.

The Rose K2 IC design is a larger diameter corneal RGP that works well for mild to moderate keratoconus. It is available in base curves between 5.70 and 9.3 and diameters between 9.4 and 12.0 mm [7]. New wearers may adapt more easily to this design for two reasons. The first is that a large diameter lens often centers well on the cornea and a well-centered lens causes less lens awareness than a decentered lens. Also, large diameter lenses tend to move less than smaller diameter lenses and less movement allows for less lens awareness. The challenge with this design in more advanced keratoconus is that as the central base curve needs to be adjusted steeper, the sagittal depth increases significantly due to the large diameter and the lens may suction, or adhere, to the cornea. An adhered corneal RGP is always considered an unacceptable fit as the epithelium cannot tolerate the pressure of the lens or the reduced oxygen levels that occur when there is no longer oxygen-rich tear exchange beneath the lens. Additionally, while this design works well for mild to moderate keratoconus, it does not work well for nipple cones. Due to the large diameter, this lens creates more pressure on the cornea than smaller diameter lenses. A broad cone can disperse this pressure over a larger area and the epithelium will be able to tolerate it. A nipple cone disperses the pressure over the much smaller area of ectasia and epithelial erosions can occur at the apex. Nipple cones can be fit successfully with small diameter cornea RGPs or one of the other modalities discussed later.

Keratoconus designs can be carved from a variety of gas permeable material buttons. Most labs make these designs from common RGP materials such as Bausch and Lomb's Boston ES, EO, XO, or XO2® or Menicon's Menicon Z®. These materials vary in their composition, wetting angle, and oxygen permeability (Dk) (Table 16.1). The wetting angle quantifies the wettability of a solid surface by a liquid. The closer the wetting angle is to zero, the more hydrophilic the surface of the lens. Dk refers to oxygen permeability of the material and the higher the number, the more oxygen permeable. Both Dk and wetting angle improved as Boston ES® evolved to EO®, then XO®. RGP lenses for keratoconus are now commonly made with XO2® and Menicon Z®.

Table 16.1 Common rigid gas permeable materials

Name	Material	Dk	Wetting angle
Boston ES®	Enflufocon A	18	52
Boston EO®	Enflufocon B	58	49
Boston XO®	Hexafocon A	100	49
Boston XO2®	Hexafocon B	141	38
Menicon Z®	Tisilfocon A	163	24

The advantages to the corneal RGP lenses are that they are fairly simple to fit and are well tolerated by the cornea due to the high Dk materials available. They are also easy to insert, remove, and clean and are relatively inexpensive compared to other options. The natural deposit resistance of the RGP materials is also preferred over the soft lens materials for atopic patients. Some insurance companies will cover corneal RGP lenses for patients with keratoconus.

This lens modality has limited success when the apex of the cone is decentered unusually inferior. The lens will tend to center over the apex of the cone, which can cause the visual axis to be outside the optic zone of the lens. This results in poor acuity and glare complaints. An inferiorly decentered lens is also difficult for a patient to adapt to since the upper lid will hit the edge of the lens with each blink and push the lens into the cornea.

These lenses may also fail in cases of extreme ectasia where lenses tend to have poor stability and are poorly retained. They are also not ideal for patients that work in dusty environments (i.e., construction, landscaping, farming), since debris can get under the lens causing cornea abrasion and discomfort.

16.3 Piggyback Lens

In some instances, a patient's corneal epithelium may not tolerate the RGP lens touch at the apex of the cone and dense superficial punctate keratitis may occur. Patients with subepithelial nodules may also be unable to tolerate even the light touch of a well-fitted RGP lens. To improve patient comfort and increase lens wear time, some practitioners may place a soft contact lens beneath the RGP, called piggybacking. A daily disposable, 2 week, or monthly hydrogel or silicone hydrogel lens can be used on a daily wear basis. For optimal oxygen transmissibility, a silicone hydrogel should be chosen. X-Cel's "Flexlens Piggyback®" is a soft hydrogel lens designed specifically to be used with an RGP and may be helpful if the RGP continues to decenter with a normal soft lens. The Flexlens Piggyback is designed with a central cutout depression, which keeps the RGP centered on the cornea to optimize acuity and comfort. For some patients piggybacking works well, but others need to be refit to a different lens modality that does not touch the cornea, called a scleral lens.

16.4 Scleral Lenses

Scleral lenses are large diameter RGP lenses that rest completely on the insensitive sclera and vault over the cornea without touching it (Image 1). The lenses are designed with a central optic zone, an area of limbal clearance, and the edge of the lens, called the haptic. The haptic is fitted to the sclera and supports the weight of the lens. The sclera has significant toricity in the majority of patients and this often requires a specific design of the haptic.

Patients fill the lens with nonpreserved saline solution before lens insertion, which creates the lacrimal lens between the scleral lens and cornea to mask the regular and irregular astigmatism optically just like the corneal RGP does with tears.

Just like corneal RGP lenses, many manufacturers have their own scleral lens design (Table 16.2).

Advantages of scleral lenses are numerous.

- Since the lens vaults over the irregular surface of the cornea, these lenses can be used even in severe cases of ectasia that cannot be fit with other modalities.

Table 16.2 Currently available scleral lens designs

Lab	Scleral design
Blanchard	MSD® and ONEFIT®
Advanced Visionary Optics	AVT Scleral Lens® and ALC Scleral Lens®
Art Optical	SO2 Clear Corneal Scleral Design®
Essilor	Jupiter®
AccuLens	Maxim®
Valley Contax	Custom Stable®
Alden	ZenLens®
X-Cel	Atlantis®
Lens Dynamics	Dyna Scleral Lens®
Visionary Optics	Europa® and Jupiter®
TruForm Optics	DigiForm

- Excellent for patients with nodules at the apex of the cone who cannot tolerate other corneal lens designs
- Work well in patients with concurrent ocular surface disease such as Sjogrens Syndrome and ocular Graft Versus Host Disease (GVHD)
- Can be made from high Dk materials for optimal corneal tolerance
- Due to the large diameter, centration is usually excellent which provides clearer vision through the optic zone
- The lenses tend to be comfortable for three reasons:
  - The lens sits on the insensitive sclera and does not touch the cornea
  - The large diameter causes the lens to have minimal detectable movement to the patient
  - The large diameter allows for minimal lid interaction since the edge of the lens sits beyond the palpebral aperture

Disadvantages are that fitting appointments can be numerous and lengthy. These lenses can be complicated to fit properly and require a provider with experience in fitting this type of lens. If improperly fitted, the complications can be significant. The two most common and significant mistakes are as follows: (1) If the sagittal depth is too low and the back of the lens comes in contact with the cornea, a serious corneal abrasion may occur in the area of touch. (2) If the haptic is too tight and the patient is experiencing conjunctival compression and impingement at the edge of the lens, corneal neovascularization and conjunctival hypertrophy can occur.

Due to the large size and that the lenses must be inserted with saline solution, some patients are unable to easily insert and remove them. In many patients, the vision becomes cloudy after a few hours of wear and the patient must remove, rinse, and reinsert the lenses during the day. This has been termed "mid day fogging" (MDF) and occurs as the natural tears and metabolic waste from the tear film exchanges with the clear saline in the reservoir of the lens causing reservoir turbidity. This is only significant with scleral lenses since the thickness of the lacrimal lens layer (average 200–250 μm) is much greater than with any other modality.

These lenses are usually contraindicated in patients with a glaucoma drainage device since the haptic can press on the device causing IOP to increase. The lenses may also be contraindicated in patients with endothelial compromise (endothelial cell count less than 1000 cells/mm^2) as corneal edema may occur [8].

Finally, these lenses are expensive to fit and replace and insurance does not provide coverage in some instances.

16.5 BostonSight® PROSE Treatment

Prosthetic Replacement of the Ocular Surface Ecosystem (PROSE) is a scleral lens device designed by the Boston Foundation For Sight. It is called PROSE since it is frequently used for various ocular surface diseases in addition to keratoconus. Patients who are fit failures with commercially available scleral lenses can benefit from a PROSE trial. The advantage of PROSE lenses is that they can be customized for each patient in terms of diameter, toricity of the haptic, and sagittal depth. Sagittal depth and base curve can be specified independently which is not possible with most commercial designs and can be a valuable distinction. The downside to these lenses is that there are limited centers that have the ability to fit them: 12 centers in the U.S., 3 centers in India, and 1 in Japan. Additionally, the fees associated with the extensive fitting may be cost prohibitive to some patients. Insurance will cover PROSE devices in some instances and low-income patients may also be eligible for care at reduced or no cost.

16.6 Hybrid Lenses

Hybrid lenses have an RGP center and a soft silicone hydrogel or hydrogel surrounding skirt (see Images 3 and 4). Currently, the sole company that makes these lenses is called SynergEyes®. Lenses are 14.5 mm in overall diameter with 8.5 mm central RGP. The original line of lenses, called the "Legacy Lenses," have a low Dk hydrogel skirt and a high Dk central RGP and include the "SynergEyes KC®" and "Clearkone®" designs. The newest SynergEyes line has a high Dk silicone hydrogel skirt with a high Dk central RGP and includes the "Duette®" and "Ultrahealth®" designs.

In patients with mild keratoconus or in cases of pellucid marginal degeneration, corneal RGP lenses tend to decenter onto the inferior portion of the cornea. This causes discomfort and poor patient adaptation. The advantage to the hybrid lens is that due to the soft skirt, the lenses tend to center well, are well retained, and often have superior comfort. Compared to corneal RGP's, patients may also experience an improvement in visual acuity due to the excellent centration of this lens. These lenses also perform well in dusty environments similar to scleral lenses.

The disadvantages are as follows:

- Limited parameters and cannot fit patients with severe ectasia
- Insertion is more challenging than with a corneal RGP since the lens has to be filled with saline prior to insertion
- The new line of lenses can be challenging for patients to remove. The silicone hydrogel skirt can be difficult for patients with poor dexterity to grip
- Costly since only made by one company and often not covered by insurance
- Can tear at the junction of the soft skirt and RGP center necessitating replacement
- Patients may develop neovascularization with the "Legacy Lenses" due to the low Dk skirt

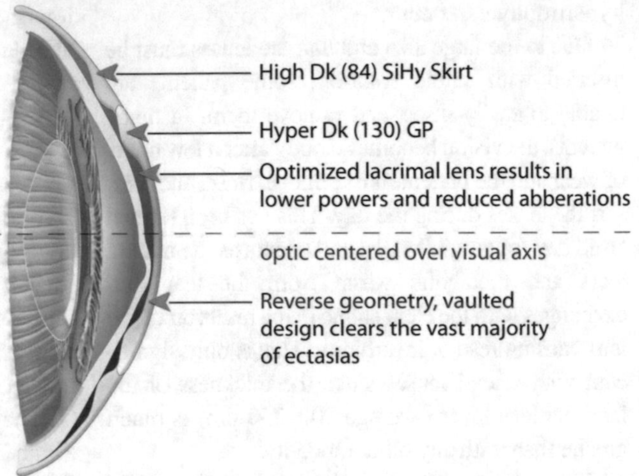

Fig. 16.3 The lacrimal lens created by the RGP center. Image courtesy of SynergEyes

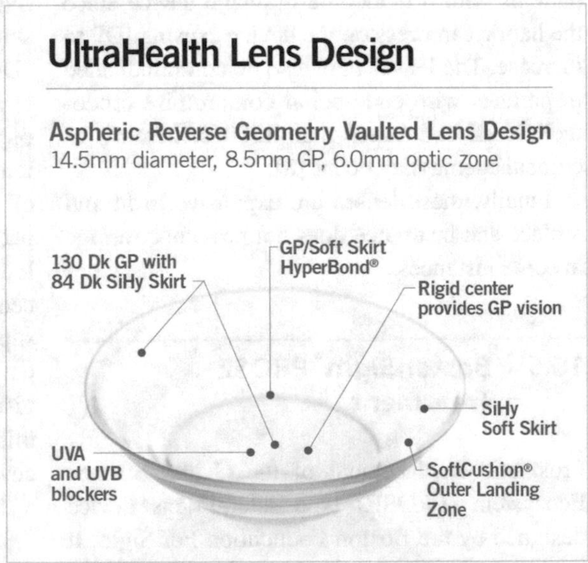

Fig. 16.4 Shows the RGP center in blue with a clear soft skirt. Image courtesy of SynergEyes

Figure 16.3 shows the lacrimal lens created by the RGP center.

Figure 16.4 shows the RGP center in blue with a clear soft skirt.

16.7 Soft Toric: Kerasoft, Novakone, Flexlens

Patients with keratoconus are usually unable to achieve an improvement in vision with soft lenses since the lens tends to drape over the cornea and not create the needed lacrimal lens to reduce the irregular astigmatism and HOA. Bausch and Lomb's Kerasoft®, Alden's Novakone® and X-Cel's Flexlens® are all higher modulus soft toric lenses that can correct myopia, high regular astigmatism, and some irregular astigmatism. Modulus refers to the stiffness or rigidity of the lens where a high modulus lens will have slight rigidity and ability to hold its shape over an irregular corneal surface. The advantage of these lenses is that patients report excellent comfort and they work well in dusty

Table 16.3 Different contact lens modalities and their advantages and disadvantages

Lens modality	Ease of care/ handling	Vision	Corneal health	Stability	Comfort	Cost
Corneal RGP	a	a	a	b	b	$
Piggyback	b	b	b	b	b	$$
Legacy hybrid	c	a	b	a	a	$$$
New hybrids	c	a	a	a	a	$$$
Commercial scleral	c	a	a	a	a	$$$–$$$$
PROSE	c	a	a	a	a	$$$$
KC soft toric	a	c	b	a	a	$$

$ $200–$500 per year, *$$* $400–$600 per year, *$$$* $800–$1100 per year, *$$$$* $1200 per year and up
[a]Best choice
[b]better choice
[c]good choice

environments. These lenses work well for mild keratoconus or in instances when all other modalities have failed due to comfort. The disadvantages are that the patient may find vision unacceptable, the Dk and/or thickness of lens reduces oxygen to the cornea, and they are often not covered by insurance.

16.8 Conclusions

There are many lens modalities for patients with keratoconus with advantages and disadvantages to each. The best corrected vision with a corneal RGP, scleral lens, piggyback, or hybrid lens would be essentially the same since all use the same approach of a rigid surface and lacrimal lens. Kerasoft®, Novakone®, and Flexlens® produce an improvement in vision compared to other soft lenses, but cannot optimize acuity in moderate or severe keratoconus. Lens type should be chosen based on a variety of factors including not just topography, but also manual dexterity, hobbies/occupation, history of atopy, history of ocular surface disease/dry eye, history of glaucoma with drainage device, and cost (Table 16.3).

It is important to note that contact lenses have no therapeutic effect on corneal ectasia. Patients should be advised that wearing contact lenses does not prevent the progression of keratoconus and should be worn only when vision with spectacles is poor compared to vision with contact lenses.

Table 16.4 Contact lens modality chosen depends on severity of ectasia

Lens modality	Early KC	Mild KC	Moderate KC	Severe KC
Corneal RGP	✓	✓	✓	✓
Piggyback		✓	✓	
Hybrid	✓	✓	✓	
Commercial scleral			✓	✓
PROSE			✓	✓
KC soft toric	✓	✓		

Patients and providers must both realize that the contact lens fitting for patients with keratoconus may require multiple lengthy visits. Lens modality may need to change as the patient's ectasia progresses (Table 16.4). Reevaluation should occur every 6–12 months in unstable keratoconus and every 12 months in stable keratoconus. If all lens modalities fail, surgical intervention may be required.

In summary, there are many contact lens modalities used to improve vision in patients with keratoconus. The most common and successful remains the corneal RGP with other designs gaining in popularity. Understanding the various options will result in a successful contact lens fitting for the patient.

Acknowledgements Thank you to Shannon Bligdon, O.D. and Brittney Mazza, O.D. for reviewing this chapter.

Compliance with Ethical Requirements: Amy Watts and Kathryn Colby declare that they have no conflict of interest. No human or animal studies were carried out by the authors for this chapter.

References

1. Koasaki R, Maeda N, Bessho K, et al. Magnitude and orientation of Zernike terms in patients with keratoconus. Invest Ophthalmol Vis Sci. 2007;48(7):3062–8.
2. Szczotka LB, Barr JT, Zadnik K. A summary of the findings from the collaborative longitudinal evaluation of keratoconus (CLEK) study. CLEK Study Group. Optometry. 2001;72(9):574–84.
3. Jinabhai A, Radhakrishnan H, O'Donnell C. Visual acuity and ocular aberrations with different rigid gas permeable lens fittings in keratoconus. Eye Contact Lens. 2010;36(4):233–7.
4. Korb DR, Finnermore VM, Herman JP. Apical changes and scarring in keratoconus as related to contact lens fitting techniques. J Am Optom Assoc. 1982;53(3):199–205.
5. Wagner H, Barr JT, Zadnik K, et al. Collaborative longitudinal evaluation of keratoconus (CLEK) study: methods and findings to date. Contact Lens Anterior Eye. 2007;30(4):223–32.
6. http://www.roseklens.com/about/.
7. Tyler's Quarterly, Inc. Editor T.T. Tyler Thompson, OD. No author is listed. Copyright June 2015 by T.T. Tyler Thompson OD. www.tylersq.com
8. van der Worp E. A guide to scleral lens fitting, version 2.0 [monograph online]. Forest Grove, OR: Pacific University; 2015, 58p. http://commons.pacificu.edu/mono/10/.

17 Intracorneal Ring Segments: Types, Indications and Outcomes

Aylin Kılıç, Jorge L. Alió del Barrio, and Alfredo Vega Estrada

17.1 Introduction

Keratoconus is a progressive corneal ectatic disorder characterized by alterations in the morphology of the corneal stromal tissue that will negatively impact in the visual function and the optical quality of the patients by the generation of a progressive and severe irregular astigmatism that cannot be corrected with spectacles [1]. Nowadays, there are several therapeutic options in order to manage this pathological condition, such as thermokeratoplasty procedures (currently abandoned), corneal collagen crosslinking (CXL), intracorneal ring segment (ICRS) implantation, lamellar keratoplasty and penetrating keratoplasty [2–6]. Nevertheless, rigid gas permeable contact lenses are still the gold standard for the visual rehabilitation of these patients as this non-invasive option provides the best visual performance and they can be adjusted to further changes in the corneal shape of the patient. However, they have the inherent risks related to any contact lens wear such us infective or non-infective keratitis, and the challenge raises for those patients that become intolerant to the use of either rigid, hybrid or scleral lenses or when the cornea is too steep that the contact lens becomes unstable.

Intracorneal ring segments (ICRS) are small devices made of synthetic materials (PMMA) that are implanted within the corneal stroma in order to induce a change in the geometry and in the refractive power of the tissue. Prof. Joseph Colin proposed the use of such medical device for the treatment of keratoconus for first time in the year 2000 [4]. Nevertheless, the idea of implanting a corneal ring into the cornea was introduced by Reynolds in 1978, being the first design a complete full ring of 360° [7]. This design led to several postoperative complications like wound healing-related problems in the incision site, which was the main reason to abandon the full ring design and change it for the ring segments that we know today. During the 1980s and in the beginning of the 1990s, the ring segment design was extensively investigated as an alternative for the correction of refractive errors, specifically myopia. In spite of the success of ICRS for the correction of such refractive error, this technology was overcome by the good results and popularity of corneal excimer laser procedures.

A. Kılıç, M.D. (✉)
Department of Cataract and Refractive Surgery, Istanbul Göz Hastanesi, İstanbul, Turkey
e-mail: aylinkilicdr@gmail.com

J.L. Alió del Barrio, M.D., Ph.D.
Keratoconus Unit, Department of Refractive Surgery Vissum Alicante, Alicante, Spain

Division of Ophthalmology, Miguel Hernández University, Alicante, Spain
e-mail: jorge_alio@hotmail.com

A. Vega Estrada, Ph.D.
Keratoconus Unit, Vissum Alicante, Alicante, Spain
e-mail: alfredovega@vissum.com

J.L. Alió (ed.), *Keratoconus*, Essentials in Ophthalmology, DOI 10.1007/978-3-319-43881-8_17

By this time, Colin and his co-workers observed that ICRS were able to flatten the central cornea and regularize the asymmetry of the tissue, thus leading to a reduction in the keratometric readings and improving the refraction and vision of keratoconus patients. Since then, several authors have reported the benefit of using ICRS in keratoconic eyes with the added value of delaying or avoiding more complex interventions like keratoplasty procedures.

17.2 Mechanism of Action of the ICRS

ICRS will act as spacer elements between the collagen fibres of the corneal tissue [8]. Thus, ICRS induce an arc shortening effect of the corneal geometry that in consequence flattens the central area of the corneal tissue. For the correction of astigmatism, the end point of each segment may produce a traction force on the surface, inducing an additional flattening on this reference axis. Some theoretical models based on finite element analysis have proven that the flattening observed after ICRS implantation is directly proportional to the thickness of the segment and inversely proportional to the corneal diameter where it is implanted. This means that the thicker and the smallest the diameter, the higher the flattening effect that will be induced by the segment [9]. Nevertheless, these theoretical analyses apply just to normal corneas where there is an orthogonal arrangement of the collagen fibres. As we know, in patients with keratoconus this special disposition of the fibres is lost, which leads to a more unpredictable outcome in this type of corneas [10]. Another theory that may explain the mechanism of action of the ICRS is the "thickness law" proposed by Barraquer which quote that when tissue is added to the periphery of the cornea or tissue is removed from the centre a flattening of the cornea will be achieved and vice versa [11]. However, there is not enough scientific data published in the literature that supports this theory.

17.3 Indications

Selecting the adequate patient for ICRS represents an important challenge for the clinician when are facing the therapeutic approach of a keratoconic patient. A full ophthalmic examination should be performed including the following: (1) *corrected and uncorrected visual acuity*; (2) *corneal topography including corneal aberrometry*: the majority of patients with keratoconus wear contact lenses, so discontinuing them must be advised for at least 1 week prior to the examination in those cases where soft contact lenses are used and 2 weeks in those cases wearing rigid contact lenses, in order to increase the reliability of the examination. Although a longer period of rigid contact lens discontinuation may be advisable, it is often unacceptable for the patient as many of them are functionally blind without them; (3) *corneal pachymetry*, preferably a corneal pachymetric map aiming to assess the appropriate thickness in the area where the ICRS would be implanted; (4) *corneal biomechanics*, either Ocular Response Analyser (ORA) or Corvis ST.

Before the implantation of any intracorneal segment, we must take into account a number of preoperative indications in order to increase the likelihood of attaining the best possible postoperative outcome for the patient [12]:

- Corrected distance visual acuity <0.9 in the decimal scale.
- Internal astigmatism <3 D.
- Alignment of refractive and keratometric axes. The flattest meridian of the cornea (K1) should be aligned with the refractive cylinder axis (expressed as a negative value). When the meridian and the axis form an angle of between 0 and 15° they are considered properly aligned.
- Corneal pachymetry >250/300 μm in the site of the corneal tunnel (depending on the thickness of ICRS to be implanted).
- Absence of central corneal scarring.

17.4 Types of Intracorneal Ring Segments

Nowadays, there are different types of ICRS that are commercially available, but the ones that are commonly used in the clinical practice are the *Keraring* (Mediphacos) (Fig. 17.1), the *Intacs* (Addition technologies) (Fig. 17.2) and the *Ferrara* segments (AJL Ophthalmic). Table 17.1 summarizes the main characteristics of these ICRS. Triangular designs generate a prismatic effect of the light coming through the implant, being reflected, thus reducing incidence of glare and halos. In addition, there are two other types of ICRS that because of their smaller diameter and different design have more flattening capabilities and are reserved for those keratoconic eyes that present high myopic refractive errors: the *Intacs SK* (Addition technologies), and the *Myoring* (Dioptex) (Fig. 17.3). The features of these two types of ICRS are shown in Table 17.2:

- *Intacs SK* (SK means severe keratoconus) are designed with rounded edges to potentially reduce the incidence of visual symptoms since SK segments are placed closer to patient's visual axis than the standard Intacs segments. They are indicated for the treatment of moderate to severe keratoconus (SK) with steep keratometric values >55.00 dioptres. Intacs SK segments seem to offer a compromise between the standard Intacs with 7 mm diameter and the Ferrara or Kerarings which are 5 mm in diameter, because diameter is inversely proportional to effectivity.
- *The Myoring* is the only one with a full ring (360°) design with published clinical data, and it is implanted within a corneal stromal pocket. They have a greater capacity to flatten and reduce the spherical equivalent than the segments, but do not usually significantly reduce astigmatism and therefore their use is limited to cases in which patients have a high spherical error and low astigmatism. Daxer et al. support that, while ICRS and incomplete rings are biomechanically neutral, MyoRing strengthens and stabilizes the cornea considerably and subsequently it is no longer necessary to combine it with CXL in progressive keratoconus [13]. This statement still requires long-term studies before its confirmation.

17.5 Surgical Procedure

In order to implant the ICRS into the deep cornea, we need to perform channels within the stroma where the rings will be implanted. For this purpose there are two different surgical options: mechanical and femtosecond laser-assisted technique.

In the mechanical or manual technique, the surgeon must mark the centre of the pupil in order to use it as a reference point during the procedure. Then a calibrated diamond knife is used to create an incision at a depth of 70 % of the cor-

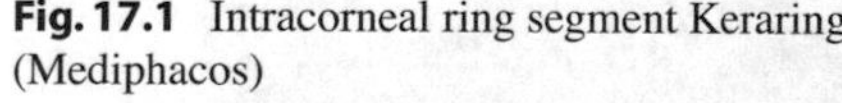
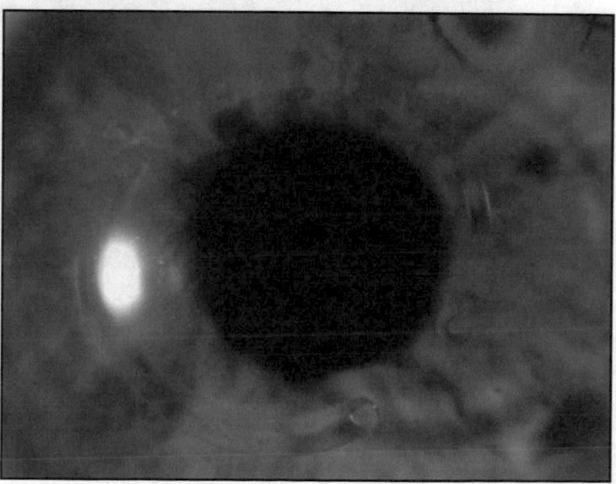

Fig. 17.1 Intracorneal ring segment Keraring (Mediphacos)

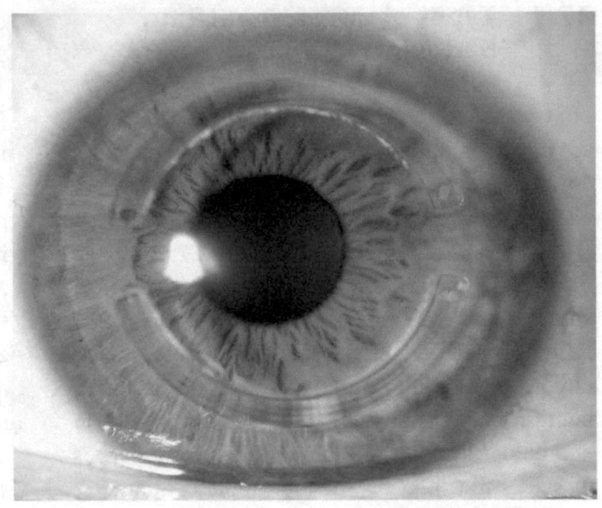

Fig. 17.2 Intracorneal ring segment Intacs (addition technologies)

Table 17.1 Main characteristics of the intracorneal ring segments most commonly used in the clinical practice

Design	Intacs	Kerarings	Ferrara
Arc length (degrees)	150°	90°–210°	90°–210°
Cross section	Hexagonal	Triangular	Triangular
Thickness (mm)	0.25–0.35	0.15–0.35	0.15–0.30
Inner diameter (mm)	6.77	6.00	4.8
Outer diameter (mm)	8.10	7.00	5.4

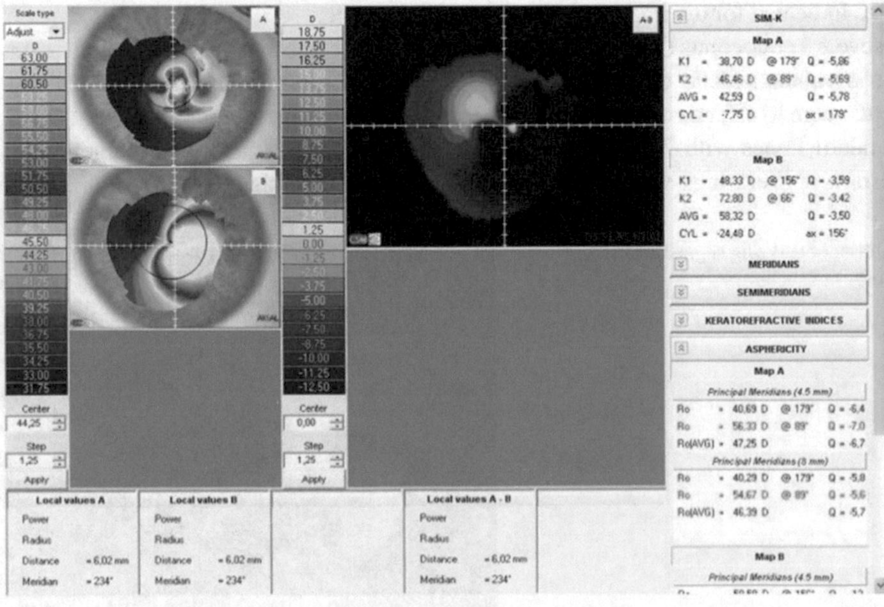

Fig. 17.3 Topography of a patient implanted with a Myoring (Dioptex) showing the significant flattening that is observed in the postoperative period. Map A: postoperative topography showing an average SimK of 42.59 D; Map B: preoperative topography showing an average SimK of 58.32 D

Table 17.2 Main characteristics of the intracorneal ring segments with higher flattening capabilities, reserved for those eyes with high myopic refractive errors

Design	Intacs SK	Myoring
Arc length (degrees)	150°	360°
Cross section	Oval	Triangular
Thickness (mm)	0.40–0.45	0.15–0.35
Inner diameter (mm)	6.00	5.00–8.00
Outer diameter (mm)	7.00	5.00–8.00

neal pachymetry at the incision point. A suction ring is placed around the corneal limbus in order to fixate the eye during the dissection of the corneal stroma. Then, two semi-circular dissectors are placed through the incision and advanced into the deep stroma in a clockwise and counterclockwise movement aiming to perform the tunnel.

With the femtosecond laser-assisted technique, a disposable suction ring is placed and centred. Afterwards, the cornea is flattened with a disposable aplannation cone, which allows a precise focus of the laser beam thus creating the dissection on the desire depth. Then the tunnel is created at approximately 70 or 80 % of the corneal pachymetry without direct manipulation of the eye. Finally, ICRS are inserted in the created tunnels.

Femtosecond laser produces a more precise and controlled stromal dissection than the manual technique. However, if we are talking about visual and refractive outcomes, most studies that have been conducted concur that both techniques produce similar results in cases of ICRS implantation for keratoconus. On the other hand, femtosecond laser makes the process faster, easier (especially for inexperienced surgeons) and more comfortable for the patient [14–17]. Apart from the safety and efficacy differences between both techniques, Alió and co-workers found that intrastromal segment implantation using femtosecond laser is a method that produces a greater reduction in corneal high order aberrations in eyes with coma aberration >3.0 μm [14, 15].

17.6 Implantation Nomograms

Regardless of the technique used to make the tunnels in the corneal stroma, the number, thickness, position and arc length of the segments are determined based on the manufacturer's nomograms. Likewise, rings are chosen from the nomogram taking into account the refractive error and the topographic map of the disease. It should also be noted that the incision guiding implantation of the segments in the tunnel is located on the axis of the steepest meridian of the corneal topography.

It is important to consider that although several authors have reported good results implanting ICRS in keratoconic eyes, the main limitations that nomograms have is that most of them are based in anecdotic clinical data, or variables that are very subjective in patients with keratoconus, such as sphero-cylindrical refraction and topographic pattern of the cone. For instance, it was found that based on the topographic pattern of the keratoconus the best choice was to implant one segment in those cases of inferior steepening and two segments in central cones [18].

Other works published in the literature support that the best location to implant the segments is by placing the corneal incision in the temporal site of the cornea [19–22] or in the steepest meridian of the cornea [23, 24]. There are other works that have reported good results when implanting the ICRS guided by the comatic axis [25]. Recently, Alió and co-workers published a scientific work in which we concluded that the best outcomes for implanting ICRS were observed in those cases where the refractive and topographic cylinder did not differ in more than 15° [12].

As we can see, there are different approaches regarding the guidelines to be used when implanting ICRS. Nevertheless, today the most widespread nomograms that are used in the clinical practice are those developed by the main manufacturers of ICRS:

17.6.1 Keraring Implant

Three types of nomograms (A, B and C) are used based on the type of corneal asymmetry (Fig. 17.4), on keratometric values and on corrected distance visual acuity (CDVA). The corneal asymmetry type is determined by studying the distribution of corneal irregularity (red) relative to the reference meridian. Accordingly, each case is classified according to Fig. 17.4:

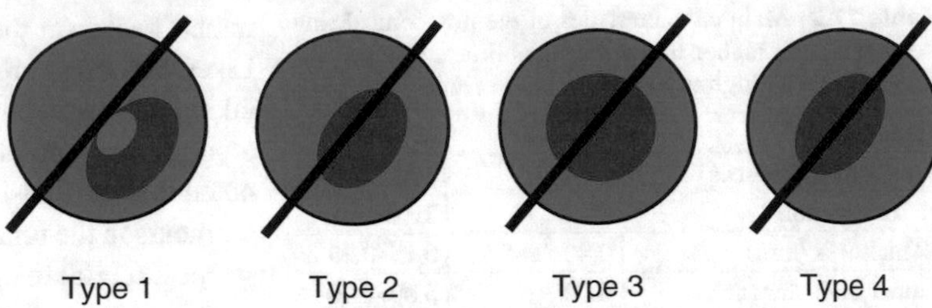

Fig. 17.4 Corneal asymmetry classification according to the area where the corneal irregularity (*red*) is found relative to the reference meridian (*black line*)

Type 1: 100 % of the steep area is located on one side of the reference meridian.
Type 2: The distribution of the steep area is approximately 20/80 %.
Type 3: The distribution of the steep area is approximately 40/60 %.
Type 4: The distribution of the steep area is approximately 50/50 %.

For type 1 and type 2 nomogram A is applied. Nomogram B for type 3 and nomogram C for type 4 (Fig. 17.5). These nomograms should be considered and used as a general guideline only and they should be customised by the surgeon depending on each patient particularities and the results obtained.

The steps and measures to be taken for ICRS implantation are as follows:

1. Obtain manifest subjective refraction.
2. Perform corneal topography (axial map).
3. Take pachymetric map. Determine the minimum corneal thickness at 5.5 and 6.5 mm optical zones.
4. Determine the steepest corneal meridian (SIM-K). If the refractive axis and the steepest topographic axis do not match, select the topographic meridian.
5. Compare the thickness of the proposed segment according to the selected nomogram with the minimal corneal thickness obtained in the 6 mm optical zone. The thickness of the segment should not exceed 60 % of the minimal corneal thickness. If it does, a segment with less thickness should be selected (Table 17.3).

Then we move on to select the reference meridian: If the CDVA > 0.5, we select the steepest meridian. If the CDVA < 0.5, select the total coma aberration axis or the steepest meridian by topography (SIM-K). Then draw a line along the reference meridian selected.

To determine the treatment strategy: If the CDVA > 0.4, program the treatment based on refractive sphere and cylinder obtained by manifest refraction. If the CDVA < 0.3 or if the manifest refraction is not very reliable, program the treatment based on kerometric values.

When it comes to implantation, when the nomogram suggests using two segments, the nomogram data appearing in the top line of the box should be used for the segment implanted in the area where the ectasia is smaller (flatter meridian), and the data on the lower line shall be for the segment implanted on the steepest meridian. When the nomogram suggests only one segment, this should be implanted on the steepest meridian, where the ectatic area is greater.

17.6.2 Ferrara Implant

Similar tasks must be performed before implanting these segments (Tables 17.4 and 17.5). From topographic astigmatism, the thickness of the ring is defined (Tables 17.6, 17.7 and 17.8). However, in the case of nipple keratoconus, this measurement is not used and the spherical equivalent is used to define the thickness of the ring, which it should be a 210° arc ring (exclusive for this type of keratoconus) (Table 17.9).

17.6.3 Intacs Implant

The recommendation is to select between symmetric or asymmetric segments depending on the ectatic area and spherical and cylindrical refractive power.

- Use *symmetric* segments when the ectatic area is within the 3–5 mm central optical zone and

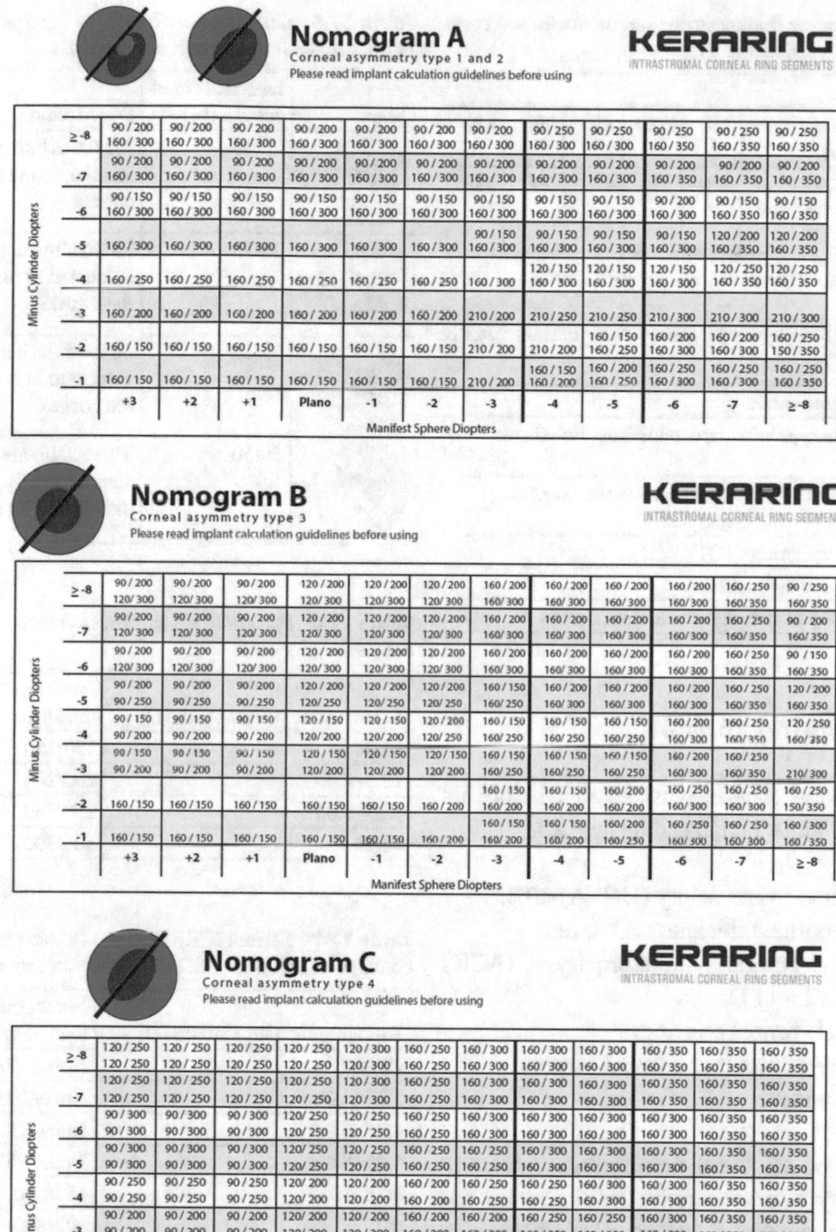

Minus Cylinder Diopters	+3	+2	+1	Plano	-1	-2	-3	-4	-5	-6	-7	≥ -8
≥ -8	90 / 200 160 / 300	90 / 200 160 / 300	90 / 200 160 / 300	90 / 200 160 / 300	90 / 200 160 / 300	90 / 200 160 / 300	90 / 200 160 / 300	90 / 250 160 / 300	90 / 250 160 / 300	90 / 250 160 / 350	90 / 250 160 / 350	90 / 250 160 / 350
-7	90 / 200 160 / 300	90 / 200 160 / 300	90 / 200 160 / 300	90 / 200 160 / 300	90 / 200 160 / 300	90 / 200 160 / 300	90 / 200 160 / 300	90 / 200 160 / 300	90 / 200 160 / 300	90 / 200 160 / 350	90 / 200 160 / 350	90 / 200 160 / 350
-6	90 / 150 160 / 300	90 / 150 160 / 300	90 / 150 160 / 300	90 / 150 160 / 300	90 / 150 160 / 300	90 / 150 160 / 300	90 / 150 160 / 300	90 / 150 160 / 300	90 / 150 160 / 300	90 / 200 160 / 300	90 / 150 160 / 350	90 / 150 160 / 350
-5	160 / 300	160 / 300	160 / 300	160 / 300	160 / 300	160 / 300	90 / 150 160 / 300	90 / 150 160 / 300	90 / 150 160 / 300	90 / 150 160 / 300	120 / 200 160 / 350	120 / 200 160 / 350
-4	160 / 250	160 / 250	160 / 250	160 / 250	160 / 250	160 / 250	160 / 300	120 / 150 160 / 300	120 / 150 160 / 300	120 / 150 160 / 300	120 / 250 160 / 350	120 / 250 160 / 350
-3	160 / 200	160 / 200	160 / 200	160 / 200	160 / 200	160 / 200	210 / 200	210 / 250	210 / 250	210 / 300	210 / 300	210 / 300
-2	160 / 150	160 / 150	160 / 150	160 / 150	160 / 150	160 / 150	210 / 200	210 / 200	160 / 150 160 / 250	160 / 200 160 / 300	160 / 200 160 / 300	160 / 250 150 / 350
-1	160 / 150	160 / 150	160 / 150	160 / 150	160 / 150	160 / 150	210 / 200	160 / 150 160 / 200	160 / 200 160 / 250	160 / 250 160 / 300	160 / 250 160 / 300	160 / 250 160 / 350

Manifest Sphere Diopters

Minus Cylinder Diopters	+3	+2	+1	Plano	-1	-2	-3	-4	-5	-6	-7	≥ -8
≥ -8	90 / 200 120/ 300	90 / 200 120/ 300	90 / 200 120/ 300	120 / 200 120/ 300	120 / 200 120/ 300	120 / 200 120/ 300	160 / 200 160/ 300	160 / 200 160/ 300	160 / 200 160/ 300	160 / 200 160/ 300	160 / 250 160/ 350	90 / 250 160/ 350
-7	90 / 200 120/ 300	90 / 200 120/ 300	90 / 200 120/ 300	120 / 200 120/ 300	120 / 200 120/ 300	120 / 200 120/ 300	160 / 200 160/ 300	160 / 200 160/ 300	160 / 200 160/ 300	160 / 200 160/ 300	160 / 250 160/ 350	90 / 200 160/ 350
-6	90 / 200 120/ 300	90 / 200 120/ 300	90 / 200 120/ 300	120 / 200 120/ 300	120 / 200 120/ 300	120 / 200 120/ 300	160 / 200 160/ 300	160 / 200 160/ 300	160 / 200 160/ 300	160 / 200 160/ 300	160 / 250 160/ 350	90 / 150 160/ 350
-5	90 / 200 90 / 250	90 / 200 90 / 250	90 / 200 90 / 250	120 / 200 120/ 250	120 / 200 120/ 250	120 / 200 120/ 250	160 / 150 160/ 250	160 / 200 160/ 300	160 / 200 160/ 300	160 / 200 160/ 300	160 / 250 160/ 350	120 / 200 160/ 350
-4	90 / 150 90 / 200	90 / 150 90 / 200	90 / 150 90 / 200	120 / 150 120/ 200	120 / 150 120/ 200	120 / 200 120/ 250	160 / 150 160/ 250	160 / 150 160/ 250	160 / 150 160/ 250	160 / 200 160/ 300	160 / 250 160/ 350	120 / 250 160/ 350
-3	90 / 150 90 / 200	90 / 150 90 / 200	90 / 150 90 / 200	120 / 150 120/ 200	120 / 150 120/ 200	120 / 150 120/ 200	160 / 150 160/ 250	160 / 150 160/ 250	160 / 150 160/ 250	160 / 200 160/ 300	160 / 250 160/ 350	210/ 300
-2	160 / 150	160 / 150	160 / 150	160 / 150	160 / 150	160 / 200	160 / 150 160/ 200	160 / 150 160/ 200	160/ 200 160/ 200	160 / 250 160/ 300	160 / 250 160/ 300	160 / 250 150/ 350
-1	160 / 150	160 / 150	160 / 150	160 / 150	160 / 150	160 / 200	160 / 150 160/ 200	160 / 150 160/ 200	160/ 200 160/ 250	160 / 250 160/ 300	160 / 250 160/ 300	160 / 300 160 / 350

Manifest Sphere Diopters

Minus Cylinder Diopters	+3	+2	+1	Plano	-1	-2	-3	-4	-5	-6	-7	≥ -8
≥ -8	120 / 250 120 / 250	120 / 250 120 / 250	120 / 250 120 / 250	120 / 250 120 / 250	120 / 300 120 / 300	160 / 250 160 / 250	160 / 300 160 / 300	160 / 300 160 / 300	160 / 300 160 / 300	160 / 350 160 / 350	160 / 350 160 / 350	160 / 350 160 / 350
-7	120 / 250 120 / 250	120 / 250 120 / 250	120 / 250 120 / 250	120 / 250 120 / 250	120 / 300 120 / 300	160 / 250 160 / 250	160 / 300 160 / 300	160 / 300 160 / 300	160 / 300 160 / 300	160 / 350 160 / 350	160 / 350 160 / 350	160 / 350 160 / 350
-6	90 / 300 90 / 300	90 / 300 90 / 300	90 / 300 90 / 300	120/ 250 120/ 250	120 / 250 120 / 250	160 / 250 160 / 250	160 / 300 160 / 300	160 / 300 160 / 300	160 / 300 160 / 300	160 / 300 160 / 300	160 / 350 160 / 350	160 / 350 160 / 350
-5	90 / 300 90 / 300	90 / 300 90 / 300	90 / 300 90 / 300	120/ 250 120/ 250	120 / 250 120 / 250	160 / 250 160 / 250	160 / 250 160 / 250	160 / 300 160 / 300	160 / 300 160 / 300	160 / 300 160 / 300	160 / 350 160 / 350	160 / 350 160 / 350
-4	90 / 250 90 / 250	90 / 250 90 / 250	90 / 250 90 / 250	120/ 200 120/ 200	120 / 200 120 / 200	160 / 200 160 / 200	160 / 250 160 / 250	160 / 250 160 / 250	160 / 300 160 / 300	160 / 300 160 / 300	160 / 350 160 / 350	160 / 350 160 / 350
-3	90 / 200 90 / 200	90 / 200 90 / 200	90 / 200 90 / 200	120/ 200 120/ 200	120 / 200 120 / 200	160 / 200 160 / 200	160 / 200 160 / 200	160 / 250 160 / 250	160 / 250 160 / 250	160 / 300 160 / 300	160 / 350 160 / 350	160 / 350 160 / 350
-2	90 / 150 90 / 150	90 / 150 90 / 150	90 / 150 90 / 150	120/ 150 120/ 150	120 / 150 120 / 150	160 / 150 160 / 150	160 / 200 160 / 200	160 / 200 160 / 200	160 / 250 160 / 250	160 / 250 160 / 250	160 /300 160 /300	160 / 300 160 / 300
-1	90 / 150 90 / 150	90 / 150 90 / 150	90 / 150 90 / 150	120/ 150 120/ 150	120 / 150 120 / 150	160 / 150 160 / 150	160 / 150 160 / 150	160 / 200 160 / 200	160 / 250 160 / 250	160 / 250 160 / 250	160 /300 160 /300	160 / 300 160 / 300

Manifest Sphere Diopters

Fig. 17.5 Keraring implantation nomograms

when, in the manifest refraction with the positive cylinder, the spherical power is greater than the cylindrical power (Table 17.10).

- Use *asymmetric* segments when the ectatic area is outside the 3 mm geometric centre and when, in the manifest refraction with the positive cylinder, the cylindrical power is greater than the spherical power (Table 17.11).

Table 17.3 Safety thickness measurements for selection of intracorneal ring segments

Safety limits					
Proposed segment thickness (μm)	150	200	250	300	350
Minimal corneal thickness required for implant (μm)	250	335	420	500	580

Table 17.4 Step-by-step tasks for Ferrara ICRS implantation

Ferrara ring nomogram
1. Define the type of keratoconus: sag, bowtie or nipple
2. Distribution of the ectatic area in the cornea: 0/100, 25/75, 33/66 and 50/50
3. Corneal asphericity (Q)
4. Topographic astigmatism
5. Pachymetry at incision site and ring track

17.6.4 Myoring Implant

Some inclusion criteria must be met before its nomogram (Table 17.12) can be applied:

- Uncorrected visual acuity (UCVA) < 0.3.
- Minimal corneal thickness >360 μm.
- Average central keratometry (ACK) (K1 + K2)/2 > 44 D.
- No central corneal scarring.
- No history of previous corneal surgery.
- Age <50 years.

In spite of all these nomograms, complete predictability in postoperative results is still not possible due to changes in corneal biomechanics in keratoconic eyes [26]. It has been found a significant correlation between the corneal resistance factor (CRF), measured using an ocular response analyser (ORA; Reichert) and the magnitude of the corneal spherical-like aberrations [27]. Also it has been shown that the visual outcomes post-ICRS implantation correlated inversely with the magnitude of some corneal higher order aberrations. It should therefore be considered that larger amounts of corneal higher

Table 17.5 Distribution of area of corneal ectasia for Ferrara ICRS implantation nomogram

Map	Distribution of ectasia (%)	Description
	0/100	All the ectatic area is located at one side of the cornea
	25/75	75 % of the ectatic area is located at one side of the cornea
	33/66	66 % of the ectatic area is located at one side of the cornea
	50/50	The ectatic area is symmetrically distributed on the cornea

Table 17.6 Ferrara ICRS thickness choice in symmetric bowtie keratoconus

Topographic astigmatism (D)	Intracorneal segment thickness
<2.00	150/150
2.25–4.00	200/200
4.25–6.00	250/250
>6.25	300/300

Table 17.7 Ferrara ICRS thickness choice in sag keratoconus with 0/100 % and 25/75 % asymmetry index

Topographic astigmatism (D)	Intracorneal segment thickness
<2.00	None/150
2.25–4.00	None/200
4.25–6.00	None/250
6.25–8.00	None/300
8.25–10.00	150/250
>10	200/300

Table 17.8 Ferrara ICRS thickness choice in sag keratoconus with 33/66 % asymmetry index

Topographic astigmatism (D)	Intracorneal segment thickness
<2.00	None/150
4.25–6.00	200/250
<2.00	None/150
4.25–6.00	200/250

Table 17.9 Ferrara ICRS thickness choice in nipple keratoconus (210 arc ring)

Spherical equivalent (D)	Intracorneal segment thickness
>2.00	150
2.25–4.00	200
4.25–6.00	250
>6.25	300

Table 17.10 Intacs nomogram for symmetric segments

Symmetric		
Spherical power	Inferior Intacs (mm)	Superior Intacs (mm)
−0.00 to −1.00 D	0.210	0.210
−1.00 to −1.75 D	0.250	0.250
−2.00 to −2.75 D	0.300	0.300
−3.00 to −3.75 D	0.350	0.350
−4.00 to −4.75 D	0.400	0.400
>−5.00 D	0.450	0.450

Table 17.11 Intacs nomogram for asymmetric segments

Asymmetric		
Cylindrical power	Inferior Intacs (mm)	Superior Intacs (mm)
2.00–3.00 D	0.350	0.210
3.00–4.00 D	0.400	0.210
4.00 and higher	0.450	0.210

Table 17.12 Myoring implantation nomogram

Average central keratometry (D)	Implant diameter (mm)	Implant thickness (μm)
ACK < 44	7	280
44 < ACK < 48	6	240
48 < ACK < 52	6	280
52 < ACK < 55	5	280
55 < ACK	5	320

order aberrations are an important factor especially in advanced keratoconic corneas where biomechanical alteration would be more pronounced. Therefore, the predictability models could be improved if high order corneal aberrations were included. In other words, the introduction of the aberrometric factor could be an indirect manner of considering part of the biomechanical corneal factor. In any case, this indirect contribution of aberrometry to corneal biomechanics is limited, and it does not account for the total biomechanical effect. The analysis of the corneal biomechanical properties of the cornea in vivo is not an easy task in clinical practice and we also have to remember that the exact contributions of the elastic and viscous components to the magnitude of these parameters are not yet fully understood.

17.7 ICRS Outcomes

Since Colin reported for first time the results of ICRS implantation for the treatment of keratoconus in the year 2000 [4] several authors have demonstrated the efficacy of this surgical technique in reducing the spherical equivalent and keratometric readings in patients with keratoconus [28–32]. Most of these studies report an improvement in the uncorrected and corrected visual acuity, as well in the spherical equivalent and cylinder. The majority of the authors observed a central flattening of the cornea that was consistent with a mean reduction of the keratometric readings that goes between 3 and 5 dioptres [28–32]. Additionally, studies that have assessed the optical quality by analysing the changes in anterior corneal higher order aberrations have found a reduction in these variables after ICRS implantation, specifically in the asymmetric aberrations (coma and coma like). These changes observed in the aberrometric coefficient are expected to occur due to the capability of the implants in regularizing the geometry of the corneal tissue [14, 32, 33].

In a recent multicentric study performed by Alió and co-workers it was found that the efficacy of ICRS implantation is related to the visual impairment of the patients at the moment of the surgery [32]. In the aforementioned investigation, the outcomes of the surgical procedure were analysed based on a grading system that takes into account the visual acuity of the patients (RETICS classification) [34]. We observed that those patients with good visual function at the moment of the surgery were more prone to lose

Table 17.13 ICRS results in CDVA according to the RETICS classification [32]

CDVA	Pre	6 months	*p* value
STAGE I	0.97±0.06 (0.90–1.15)	0.86±0.18 (0.40–1.20)	<0.01
STAGE II	0.71±0.08 (0.60–0.86)	0.75±0.22 (0.30–1.20)	=0.04
STAGE III	0.45±0.53 (0.40–0.58)	0.57±0.22 (0.10–1.00)	<0.01
STAGE IV	0.27±0.05 (0.20–0.38)	0.50±0.22 (0.05–1.00)	<0.01
STAGE PLUS	0.09±0.05 (0.01–0.15)	0.38±0.26 (0.05–1.00)	<0.01

Table 17.14 Comparison of success and failure rates according to the degree of visual impairment [32]

Visual acuity	Gain ≥ 1 line CDVA (%)	Lost ≥ 1 line CDVA (%)	Lost ≥ 2 lines CDVA (%)
CDVA ≥ 0.6 GRADE I+II	37.90	36.29	25.80
CDVA ≤ 0.4 GRADE IV+PLUS	82.85	10.00	4.28

lines of vision after the procedure; on the other hand, those cases with a severe visual impairment before the procedure were the ones that benefit the most from ICRS implantation [32] (Tables 17.13 and 17.14).

This study also analysed topographical changes after ICRS implantation according to the visual impairment of patients with keratoconus. Table 17.15 summarizes the topographical results found in this study. Although they were able to demonstrate a significant reduction in all keratometry measurements in all groups ($p<0.01$), the greatest reduction was in patients classified as Stage Plus, i.e. those with the most severe form of the disease. These findings lead us to the consideration that ICRS implantation in cases with keratoconus and good vision should be undertaken with extreme caution because of the risk of losing vision in this group of patients who have “little to gain and much to lose”.

Long-term outcomes of ICRS implantation for the treatment of keratoconus have been always a topic of debate. There are some studies published in the literature that hypothesized that due to the distribution of the forces along the stroma that is observed after the implant this may help in reducing the stress on a specific point of the tissue thus leading to a more biomechanical stability of the cornea [35]. Nevertheless, these observations have not been proven in the clinical practice. Even when there are some long-term studies that have reported the stability of the surgical procedure [23, 33, 36] there is a clear limitation in most of these reports as they do not specify if the type of patients that they are evaluating within their cohort belong to cases with the progressive or stable form of the disease. In a recent study was observed that long-term stability of ICRS implantation depends on the progression pattern of the keratoconus at the moment of the surgical technique. Thus, in those cases with the stable form of the disease, ICRS implantation remains without significant changes after long period of follow up [33]. Nevertheless, in those cases that show clinical signs of progression, the benefit achieved immediately after the procedure is expected to be lost after long period of time. From that work, we conclude that stability of the disease should be confirmed before suggesting ICRS implantation in keratoconic patients [37], as in those progressive cases ICRS implantation should be combined with corneal collagen crosslinking in order to halt the progression of the disease and keep the response obtained with the ICRS in the long term.

It is important to take into account that ICRS have the advantage that they can be removed in the event of failure and can be combined with other techniques such as corneal collagen crosslinking, PRK and phakic intraocular lenses. They can also be exchanged for segments with different characteristics, being possible to improve the results when these prove unfavourable [38].

17.8 A Glance at the Future

Further changes in the ICRS design may enhance their results. Our investigation team is currently developing a new type of ICRS, the VR technology, which is not yet commercially available and combines an asymmetric design in an almost

Table 17.15 ICRS topographic results according to the RETICS classification [32]

	K1 Pre	K1 6 months	*p* value	K2 Pre	K2 6 months	*p* value	Km Pre	Km 6 months	*p* value
STAGE I	43.75 ± 2.95 (36.22–49.10)	41.95 ± 2.13 (35.50–46.10)	<0.01	45.91 ± 3.87 (36.00–58.82)	44.71 ± 2.20 (41.56–49.38)	<0.01	44.90 ± 2.96 (35.65–54.96)	43.35 ± 1.69 (38.63–47.45)	<0.01
STAGE II	45.09 ± 4.44 (34.07–56.00)	43.17 ± 4.47 (33.46–53.94)	<0.01	47.41 ± 5.42 (34.10–65.09)	46.08 ± 5.25 (34.10–59.23)	<0.01	46.24 ± 4.13 (34.57–59.10)	44.52 ± 4.41 (34.32–56.10)	<0.01
STAGE III	48.10 ± 6.00 (33.37–74.69)	44.56 ± 4.90 (32.45–54.49)	<0.01	49.88 ± 6.71 (37.25–83.67)	47.68 ± 5.68 (32.75–64.06)	<0.01	48.93 ± 5.67 (36.25–78.80)	46.09 ± 5.07 (32.60–59.52)	<0.01
STAGE IV	51.41 ± 6.69 (31.50–69.40)	45.94 ± 4.62 (38.00–58.02)	<0.01	51.89 ± 6.69 (33.80–74.48)	49.34 ± 5.74 (41.76–62.20)	<0.01	51.65 ± 6.06 (32.65–72.70)	47.64 ± 4.87 (39.88–60.11)	<0.01
STAGE PLUS	53.13 ± 8.10 (32.20–79.08)	47.73 ± 4.97 (35.37–59.10)	<0.01	55.68 ± 9.15 (38.10–85.51)	50.24 ± 5.11 (40.40–61.93)	<0.01	54.40 ± 8.00 (38.48–82.62)	48.81 ± 4.39 (39.54–57.34)	<0.01

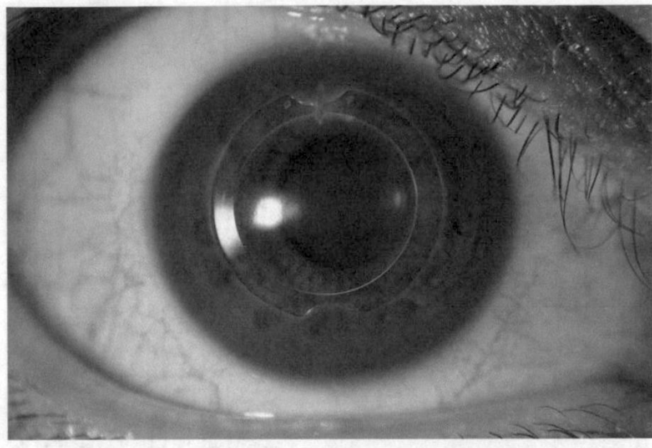

Fig. 17.6 VR Technology

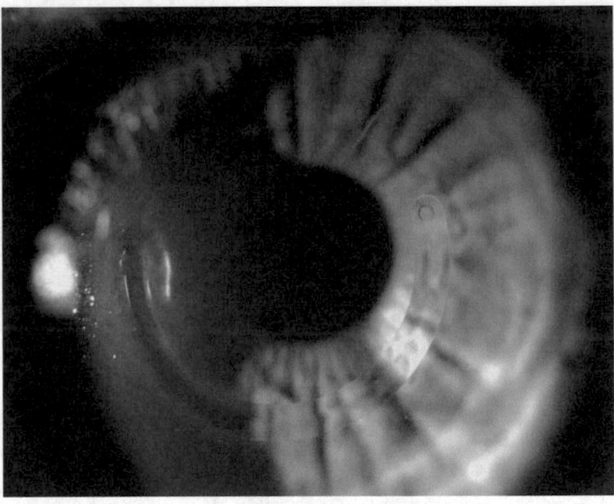

Fig. 17.7 Keraring 210° in a patient with pellucid marginal degeneration (courtesy of Efekan Coskunseven, Dunya Eye Hospital, Istanbul)

complete full ring of 350° of arc length (Fig. 17.6). The potential advantages of this design is that it may achieve both, the reduction of the asymmetry of the cornea that is observed with the segments and the significant flattening that is induced by the full ring devices (like Myoring). Also, as it is an incomplete ring, its implantation will be possible through a single incision in the cornea, avoiding then a stromal pocket.

Dr. Efekan Coskunseven (Dunya Eye Hospital, Istanbul, Turkey) is currently analysing the results obtained with the new 210° Keraring for the treatment of pellucid marginal degeneration (PMD), reporting encouraging results. Despite larger number of patients are still required before considering the introduction of this segment in the clinical practise, the initial results show an improvement of 1 or more lines of unaided vision in 55.5 % of patients with PMD, and a recovery of 1 or more lines of best corrected visual acuity (BCVA) in 77.7 % of the cases (Fig. 17.7).

ICRS are a powerful and useful therapeutic option for patients with corneal ectatic disorders, including keratoconus. Nevertheless, it's critical to understand their limitations and to discuss with the patient the impossibility of an accurate and predictable postoperative result, being often necessary their combination with other treatment options like crosslinking, PRK or phakic intraocular lenses. Subsequently it is necessary to expand our knowledge in corneal biomechanics and the changes induced by ICRS on it in order to be able to perform mathematical models that could predict better our results.

Compliance with Ethical Requirements Ayilin Kılıç, Jorge L. Alió del Barrio and Alfredo Vega-Estrada declare that they have no conflict of interest.

All procedures followed were in accordance with the ethical standards of the responsible committee on human experimentation (institutional and national) and with the Helsinki Declaration of 1975, as revised in 2000. Informed consent was obtained from all patients for being included in the study.

No animal studies were carried out by the authors for this chapter.

References

1. Rabinowitz YS. Keratoconus. Surv Ophthalmol. 1998;42:297 319.
2. Barnett M, Mannis MJ. Contact lenses in the management of keratoconus. Cornea. 2011;30:1510–6.
3. Vega-Estrada A, Alió JL, Plaza Puche AB, et al. Outcomes of a new microwave procedure followed by accelerated cross-linking for the treatment of keratoconus: a pilot study. J Refract Surg. 2012;28:787–93.
4. Colin J, Cochener B, Savary G, et al. Correcting keratoconus with intracorneal rings. J Cataract Refract Surg. 2000;26:1117–22.
5. Snibson GR. Collagen cross-linking: a new treatment paradigm in corneal disease—a review. Clin Experiment Ophthalmol. 2010;38:141–53.
6. Busin M, Scorcia V, Zambianchi L, et al. Outcomes from a modified microkeratome-assisted lamellar keratoplasty for keratoconus. Arch Ophthalmol. 2012;130:776–82.
7. Burris TE. Intrastromal corneal ring technology: results and indications. Curr Opin Ophthalmol. 1998;9:9–14.
8. Silvestrini T, Mathis M, Loomas B, et al. A geometric model to predict the change in corneal curvature from the intrastromal corneal ring (ICR). Invest Ophthalmol Vis Sci. 1994;35:2023.
9. Burris TE, Baker PC, Ayer CT, et al. Flattening of central corneal curvature with intrastromal corneal rings of increasing thickness: an eye-bank eye study. J Cataract Refract Surg. 1993;19:182–7.
10. Daxer A, Fratzl P. Collagen orientation in the human corneal stroma and its implication in keratoconus. Invest Ophthalmol Vis Sci. 1997;38:121–9.
11. Albertazzi R. Tratamiento del queratocono con segmentos intracorneales. In: Albertazzi R, editor. Queratocono: pautas para su diagnóstico y tratamiento. Buenos Aires: Ediciones cientificas argentina para la keratoconus society; 2010. p. 205–68.
12. Peña-García P, Alió JL, Vega-Estrada A, et al. Internal, corneal and refractive astigmatism as prognostic factor for ICRS implantation in mild to moderate keratoconus. J Cataract Refract Surg. 2014;40:1633–44.
13. Daxer A. Biomechanics of corneal ring implants. Cornea. 2015;34:1493 8.
14. Shabayek MH, Alió JL. Intrastromal corneal ring segment implantation by femtosecond laser for keratoconus correction. Ophthalmology. 2007;114:1643–52.
15. Alió JL, Piñero DP, Daxer A. Clinical outcomes after complete ring implantation in corneal ectasia using the femtosecond technology: a pilot study. Ophthalmology. 2011;118:1282–90.
16. Rabinowitz YS. Intacs for keratoconus. Int Ophthalmol Clin. 2006;46:91–103.
17. Ertan A, Kamburoglu G, Akgun U. Comparison of outcomes of 2 channel sizes for intrastromal ring segment implantation with a femtosecond laser in eyes with keratoconus. J Cataract Refract Surg. 2007;33:648–53.
18. Alió JL, Artola A, Hassanein A, et al. One or two Intacs segments for the correction of keratoconus. J Cataract Refract Surg. 2005;31:943–53.
19. Colin J, Cochener B, Savary G, et al. Intacs inserts for treating keratoconus. One-year results. Ophthalmology. 2001;108:1409–14.
20. Hellstedt T, Mäkelä J, Uusitalo R, et al. Treating keratoconus with Intacs corneal ring segments. J Refract Surg. 2005;21:236–46.
21. Kanellopoulos AJ, Pe LH, Perry HD, et al. Modified intracorneal ring segment implantations (Intacs) for the management of moderate to advanced keratoconus. Efficacy and complications. Cornea. 2006;25:29–33.
22. Kwitko S, Severo NS. Ferrara intracorneal ring segments for keratoconus. J Cataract Refract Surg. 2004;30:812–20.
23. Alió JL, Shabayek MH, Artola A. Intracorneal ring segments for keratoconus correction: long-term follow-up. J Cataract Refract Surg. 2006;32:978–85.
24. Shetty R, Kurian M, Anand D, et al. Intacs in advanced keratoconus. Cornea. 2008;27:1022–9.
25. Alfonso JF, Lisa C, Merayo-Lloves J, et al. Intrastromal corneal ring segment implantation in paracentral keratoconus with coincident topographic and coma axis. J Cataract Refract Surg. 2012;38:1576–82.
26. Piñero DP, Alió JL, Teus MA, et al. Modeling the intracorneal ring segment effect in keratoconus using refractive, keratometric, and corneal aberrometric data. Invest Ophthalmol Vis Sci. 2010;51:5583–91.
27. Piñero DP, Alió JL, Barraquer RI, et al. Corneal biomechanics, refraction and corneal aberrometry in keratoconus: an integrated study. Invest Ophthalmol Vis Sci. 2010;51:1948–55.
28. Piñero DP, Alio JL. Intracorneal ring segments in ectatic corneal disease—a review. Clin Experiment Ophthalmol. 2010;38:154–67.
29. Siganos D, Ferrara P, Chatzinikolas K, et al. Ferrara intrastromal corneal rings for the correction of keratoconus. J Cataract Refract Surg. 2002;28:1947–51.
30. Coskunseven E, Kymionis GD, Tsiklis NS, et al. One-year results of intrastromal corneal ring segment implantation (KeraRing) using femtosecond laser in patients with keratoconus. Am J Ophthalmol. 2008;145:775–9.
31. Alió JL, Shabayek MH, Belda JI, et al. Analysis of results related to good and bad outcomes of Intacs

implantation for keratoconus correction. J Cataract Refract Surg. 2006;32:756–61.
32. Vega-Estrada A, Alio JL, Brenner LF, et al. Outcome analysis of intracorneal ring segments for the treatment of keratoconus based on visual, refractive, and aberrometric impairment. Am J Ophthalmol. 2013;155:575–84.
33. Vega-Estrada A, Alió JL, Brenner LF, et al. Outcomes of intrastromal corneal ring segments for treatment of keratoconus: five-year follow-up analysis. J Cataract Refract Surg. 2013;39:1234–40.
34. Alió JL, Piñero DP, Alesón A, et al. Keratoconus-integrated characterization considering anterior corneal aberrations, internal astigmatism, and corneal biomechanics. J Cataract Refract Surg. 2011;37:552–68.
35. Roberts CJ. Chapter 10: Biomecanics of INTACS in keratoconus. In: Ertan A, Colin J, editors. Intracorneal ring segments and alternative treatment for corneal ectatic diseases. Ankara, Turkey: Kudret Eye Hospital; 2007. p. 157–66.
36. Torquetti L, Berbel RF, Ferrara P. Long-term follow-up of intrastromal corneal ring segments in keratoconus. J Cataract Refract Surg. 2009;35:1768–73.
37. Vega-Estrada A, Alió JL, Plaza-Puche A. Keratoconus progression following intrastromal corneal ring segments in young patients: five-year follow-up. J Cataract Refract Surg. 2015;41:1145–52.
38. Alió JL, Piñero DP, Söğütlü E, et al. Implantation of new intracorneal ring segments after segment explanation for unsuccessful outcomes in eyes with keratoconus. J Cataract Refract Surg. 2010;36:1303–10.

Intracorneal Ring Segments: Complications

18

Aylin Kılıç and Jorge L. Alió del Barrio

18.1 Introduction

Intrastromal corneal ring segments (ICRS) are a promising and reversible refractive procedure for keratoconus management [1]. There have been reported multiple associated complications, however ICRS explantation is rarely necessary. Ferrer et al. evaluated the main causes of ICRS-related serious complications [2]. The most frequent serious complication was extrusion (48.3 %), followed by refractive failure (37.9 %), keratitis (6.9 %), and corneal melting (5.2 %). One case (1.7 %) of corneal perforation was observed. This study could not find differences in the complication rate between the manual and femtosecond laser-assisted techniques.

It has been reported that the use of femtosecond laser to create the corneal tunnels makes ICRS implantation safer and significantly reduces the complication rate due to the precise depth of implantation [3-5]. Femtosecond laser-assisted technique is easier for the surgeon, more comfortable for the patient, and ensures an accurate depth of implantation, which cannot be guaranteed with the manual technique [6]. Many corneal surgeons, who had abandoned the surgical technique with the mechanical spreader due to technical difficulties experienced with the device supplied by the manufacturer, have now once again started carrying out this procedure using the femtosecond laser to create the channels, due to the high degree of certainty of the depth of placement of the rings [7]. Ertan et al. reported that femtosecond laser provides precise tunnels depth, width, and location (rarely requiring suture placement); minimal channel haze or edema; an uniform 360° channel; minimum risk for epithelial defects; low risk of infectious keratitis due to the absence of a foreign element placed in the cornea; and a completion within seconds without manipulation of the cornea [1].

Piñero et al. reported an ICRS extrusion rate of 8.33 % for the mechanical technique and 10.52 % for the femtosecond laser technique, while the explantation rate was 20.83 % and 10.53 %, respectively [8].

Kanellopoulos et al. reported the highest postoperative complication rate (35 %, n:20) [9].

A. Kılıç, M.D. (✉)
Department of Cataract and Refractive Surgery, İstanbul Göz Hastanesi, İstanbul, Turkey
e-mail: aylinkilicdr@gmail.com

J.L. Alió del Barrio, M.D., Ph.D.
Keratoconus Unit, Department of Refractive Surgery Vissum Alicante Alicante, Spain

Division of Ophthalmology, Miguel Hernández University, Alicante, Spain
e-mail: jorge_alio@hotmail.com

J.L. Alió (ed.), *Keratoconus*, Essentials in Ophthalmology, DOI 10.1007/978-3-319-43881-8_18

18.2 Early Complications

18.2.1 Epithelial Defects

ICRS patients will usually experience a minor foreign body sensation for the first 24 h. Without any special intervention, these defects will generally heal within 24–72 h. A large epithelial defect is best managed with a bandage contact lens.

18.2.2 Corneal Edema

Postoperative corneal edema is usually mild and its resolution is expected quickly. Rare cases of persistent, focal edema of the stroma adjacent to the segments have been reported. Always be aware of the possibility of an infection and observe these eyes carefully (Fig. 18.1).

18.2.3 Filamentary Keratitis

Filament formation around the incision site can be treated with debridement.

18.2.4 Stromal Thinning and Segment Extrusion

The extrusion of the segment is one of the most common postoperative complications and requires its explantation. Explantation rate varies among studies ranging from 0.98 to 30 % [1]. Colin et al. reported explantation of the segment in 12 % of eyes implanted with Intacs, due to dissatisfaction and visual symptoms [10].

Ideally, an intrastromal implant should not affect the normal physiology of the cornea, as an impermeable implant has the potential to impede fluid and nutrients movement within the cornea. A nutritional deficiency of the stroma anterior to the inlay can result in anterior stromal edema and melting with corneal ulceration and implant extrusion [11].

By determining the stromal depth of the segment during slit lamp evaluation, the surgeon can identify those cases where stromal thinning and extrusion are more likely. Deep implantations allow an adequate nutrition of the overlying stroma and there is less risk of extrusion. The first sign of stromal thinning is usually punctate epithelial staining over the ring. Ultimately the epithelium breaks down, the stroma melts, and the segment extrudes (Fig. 18.2).

The extrusion or removal rate for Intacs SK has been reported at 19.3 %, greater than the one reported for regular Intacs. Nevertheless, Kwitko and Severo et al. reported an extrusion rate for Ferrara rings of 19.6 % [12].

Ferrer et al. evaluated the main causes of intrastromal ring segment extrusion over a 9-year period and its relationship with microscopic findings on the ICRS surface [2]. Intrastromal segments were explanted with a rate of 22.8 %. The main cause was extrusion (48.2 % of explanted segments), followed by unsatisfying refractive outcome (37.9 %) and keratitis (6.8 %).

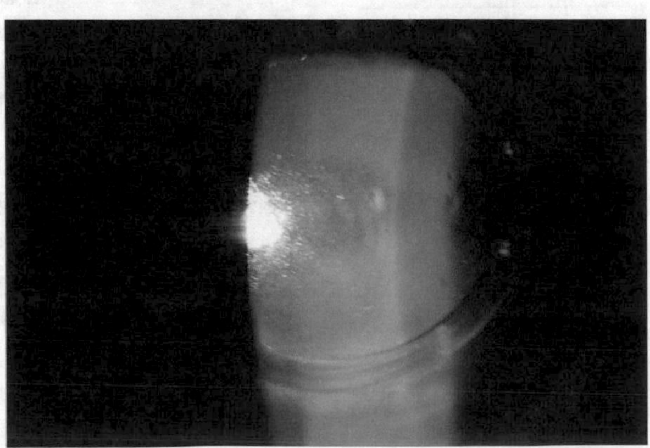

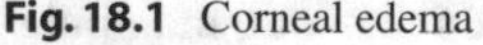

Fig. 18.1 Corneal edema

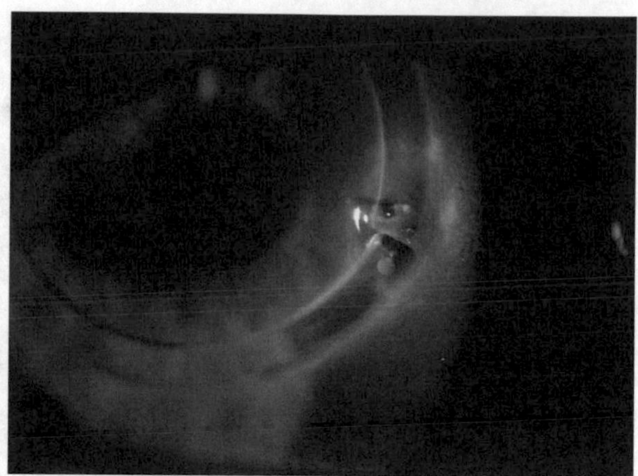

Fig. 18.2 Ring extrusion

Shallow implantation is one of the main risk factors of extrusion as it has been associated with ring superficialization, stromal thinning, and epithelial breakdown [13]. Khan et al. suggested as risk factors for extrusion a thin cornea and a history of atopy with eye rubbing [14].

Lai et al. performed an optical coherence tomography (OCT) between 7 and 43 days after ICRS implantation to study their final stromal depth. They observed that the distal and inferior portions of the segments tended to be placed at a shallower depth. They suggested that a shallower placement of the segments may result in more complications, such as epithelial–stromal breakdown and extrusion, because of the greater anterior stromal tensile strain [15].

Kamburoğlu et al. used Pentacam to assess the depth of Intacs implanted by femtosecond laser, and reported a decreased depth at the end of the first postoperative year in all measured points, being these differences statistically significant at the superior, inferior, and temporal sides of the Intacs [16].

Toroquetti and Ferrara identified two major causes of ICRS extrusion: superficial implantation and the placement of a segment close to the incision [17]. They claimed that, as a general rule, the thickness of the implanted ICRS should not be more than 50 % of the corneal thickness in the ring track. Deeply located ICRS produce better results and also leave a greater amount of corneal stroma between the ICRS and the corneal epithelium, what should theoretically protect from extrusion.

18.2.5 Segment Migration

When segment migration brings the end of the implant adjacent to the incision, this represents an unacceptable risk for wound melt. In this scenario, the segment should be repositioned as soon as possible. This can be easily accomplished with a Sinskey hook placed into the corneal tunnel through the entry wound. If after an initial repositioning, the segment continues to migrate to the incision, it will be necessary to remove it (Fig. 18.3).

18.2.6 Infection

Infectious keratitis after ICRS implantation is very rare, and culture-proven infections were less than 1 % in several large clinical series [13, 18]. According to the literature, the incidence of infectious keratitis after Intacs implantation for the treatment of myopia is low, ranging from 0.2 to 0.63 % [13].

Bourcier et al. reported a case of late bacterial keratitis after ICRS implantation. Cultures were positive for *Clostridium perfringens* and *Staphylococcus epidermidis*, showing the risk of microbial keratitis even months after the implantation [18].

Bilateral infections after uncomplicated ICRS implantation have also been described [19]. An early recognition of the infection, aggressive treatment with antibiotics and, in many cases, removal of the ICRS are critical to prevent serious sight-threatening complications.

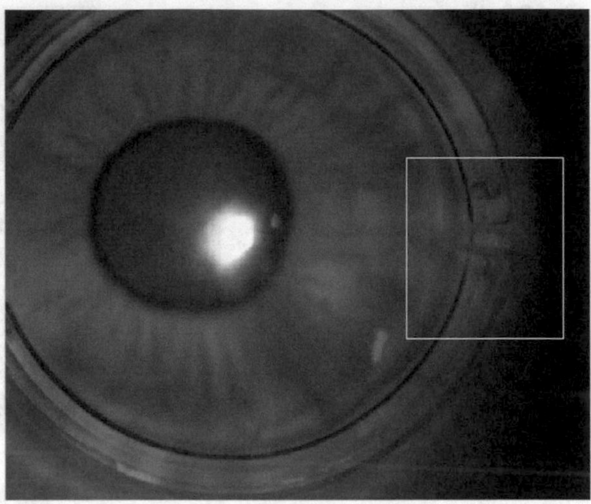

Fig. 18.3 Segment migration

Traumatic shattering of intrastromal segments due to blunt trauma is possible [20]. Sharp edges of the shattered segments may compromise the anterior or posterior stroma, so their removal should be assessed in order to avoid the risk of corneal erosions and a subsequent infection.

European multicenter study of Intacs reported 1 case of channel infection that was observed 3 weeks after the implantation [13]. No microorganisms were identified in that case, and the infection resolved with high dose topical antibiotics without requiring the explant of the ICRS. Results of phase II and III of US Food and Drug Administration trials reported 1 case of infectious keratitis among 499 eyes with Intacs [21]. Infectious keratitis should be differentiated from simple deposits of extracellular substance, which accumulates in the lamellar channel around the segments [22].

Several mechanisms can help to explain the presentation of channel infection after ICRS: the incisional keratotomy to create the channel puts the wound perpendicular to the corneal plane, which tends to heal slowly. Also, the presence of an intrastromal foreign body carries an additional risk of postoperative infection because of the possible adhesion of cells, proteins, or microorganisms onto the surface of the biomaterial.

Infectious keratitis has been reported with either implantation technique (manual or femtosecond laser assisted) [23].

If a patient complains of photophobia or aching pain after the surgery an examination to rule out infection should be performed as soon as possible. Signs of infection include edema or an infiltrate involving the stroma adjacent to the segment (Fig. 18.4). A minimal infiltrate may initially be treated with hourly broad-spectrum antibiotic drops. If the infiltrate worsens or the initial stromal reaction is more advanced, removal of the ICRS should be considered.

18.2.7 Reduction of Corneal Sensitivity

In all forms of keratorefractive surgery, transitory reduction of corneal sensitivity may occur. With corneal ring segments, all these findings are minor. In most of the cases, in 2–3 months period, corneal sensitivity returns to the preoperative baseline values, without any neurotrophic effects [24].

18.2.8 Epithelial Ingrowth

Minor epithelial cysts or plugs should be considered normal. Very large plugs may indicate excessive wound gape and can induce against-the-rule astigmatism.

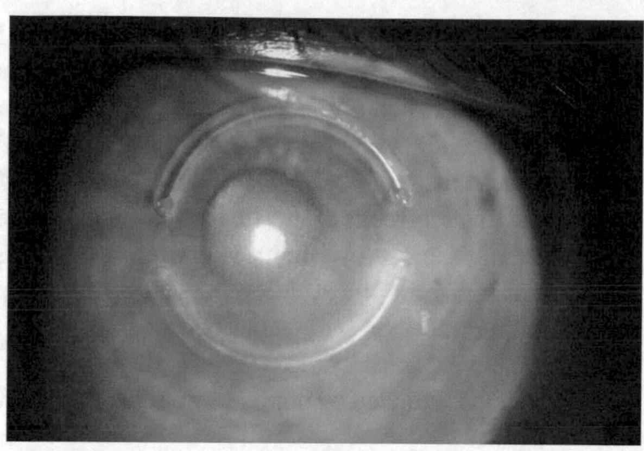

Fig. 18.4 Infection after ring implantation

18.2.9 Astigmatism Induction After ICRS and Other Visual Complications

An unsutured radial corneal incision alone (without segment implantation) has specific effects on the corneal topography [25, 26]. Flattening of the incised meridian with steepening of the perpendicular meridian is seen. A wound which is too long or too traumatized is prone to excessive gap, and a 12 o'clock wound which gapes too much may induce an against-the-rule (ATR) astigmatism. Nevertheless, as the wound contracts, these effects will resolve by themselves. On the other hand, a tight 12 o'clock wound can be associated with a with-the-rule (WTR) astigmatism. Thus, an overly tight suture will induce steepening in the incised meridian, although due to the coupling created by the presence of the segments there will not be a compensatory flattening of the meridian 90° away, resulting in a WTR cylinder and a myopic shift. Early removal of the tight suture may relax the steep meridian and may allow a shift of the spherical equivalent toward emmetropia.

Patients may complaint of short-term glare or halos. As the tunnels are dissected, the lamellae split and this creates temporary tunnel haze just central to the inner aspect of each implanted segment. This haze will resolve after 30–60 days but may induce glare for a few months in a minority of patients. Patients with large pupils are more prone to develop these visual symptoms.

A small percentage of patients may experience diurnal visual fluctuations, what is observed more frequently with thicker segments [27, 28]. Keratoconus patients experience a morning hyperopic shift and an evening myopic shift. Thus, undercorrected patients see better in the mornings than in the evenings, except emmetropic and overcorrected patients (induced hyperopia) who experience an increase in visual acuity during the day. The reason of the drift is unknown, although it should be related to the effects of the nighttime lid closure, causing metabolic alterations by oxygen deprivation.

As we have already discussed in the previous chapter, due to the abnormal corneal biomechanical response, the precise outcome of an ICRS implantation in a keratoconic eye is not possible to accurately predict, and this should be informed to the patient during the preoperative evaluation [29, 30]. However, the refractive effect of an ICRS is reversible, so a worsened refractive defect after ring implantation may be improved to the preoperative values by simple explantation of the device [31].

Alternatively, ICRS adjustment surgery may be attempted: this adjustment surgery is defined as any combination of removal, exchange, addition, or shifting an ICRS to improve its refractive effect over the cornea. Actually, Alió et al. reported a significant visual and refractive improvement by implanting a new ICRS combination after previous unsuccessful ICRS, which were explanted due to either poor visual results or extrusion [32]. Pokroy et al. reported that approximately 10 % of keratoconic eyes managed with ICRS may require an adjustment surgery, which often has a good outcome [33]. In this study, the indications for ICRS adjustment were increased astigmatism in four eyes, induced hyperopia (overcorrection) in three eyes, and undercorrection in one eye. Induced astigmatism and hyperopia were most often managed by removing the superior segment. The undercorrected eye, having initially received a single inferior segment, was treated by implanting a superior segment.

18.2.10 Sterile Infiltrates

These infiltrates commonly occur during the second week after surgery and they are usually asymptomatic. If the physician feels that the stromal reaction may be infectious (based on timing, appearance, and clinical presentation), it should be treated immediately with antibiotic drops as we have already seen.

18.3 Late Complications

18.3.1 Anterior Stromal Necrosis

Bourges et al. reported an anterior stromal aseptic necrosis 5 years after ICRS implantation [34]. A progressive idiopathic paracentral keratolysis associated with increased quantities of matrix metalloproteinases (MMPs) has been described [35].

Samimi et al. evaluated the histopathological changes induced by ICRS in keratoconic corneas [36]. They observed hypoplasia of the epithelium immediately surrounding the channel, no evidence of any inflammatory response or foreign body reaction, keratocyte density decreased above and below the tunnel, and synthesis of collagen IV in the scar area. Several reports have demonstrated that the refractive and topographic changes induced by ICRS are reversible after their explantation, and this study demonstrated that the histological changes are as well reversible after insert removal.

Fabre et al. reported that this chronic epithelial injury induces apoptosis via interleukin 1, and they hypothesized that these keratocyte apoptosis with release of degradative enzymes (as MMPs) and other components, induced by ICRS, would damage the area next to the tunnel explaining these cases of progressive keratolysis after ICRS implantation [37].

18.3.2 Chronic Pain

Randleman et al. reported persistent discomfort that did not improve with topical medications or a bandage contact lens [38]. Confocal biomicroscopy demonstrated a corneal nerve in direct contact with the inferior segment. Both segments were removed and the patient reported complete resolution of the pain. In patients with keratoconus and ectasia post-LASIK, where corneal thinning has occurred and corneal nerves may be found in abnormal locations, there may be a greater chance that ICRS segments and corneal nerves end up in contact, resulting in chronic pain.

18.3.3 Intrastromal Tunnel Deposits

One of the findings that are more frequently observed is white deposits around the segment inside the tunnel (Fig. 18.5). Histopathological analysis has demonstrated that these deposits correspond to fatty acids and do not interfere with the visual function of the patient [22]. The accumulation of this substance is self-limited and nonprogressive: deposits start to accumulate around the third postoperative month, and they tend to increase until the 6th–12th month, when finally come to a steady state. They remain confined to the intrastromal tunnel without central or peripheral expansion.

Ruckhofer et al. reported that the incidence of these intrastromal deposits (intracellular lipids) in the corneal tunnel can be as high as 60 % [22]. They performed confocal microscopy on a total of 21 eyes concluding that the central corneal zone appears unchanged, but the corneal stroma adjacent to the ICRS displays a slight but distinct activation

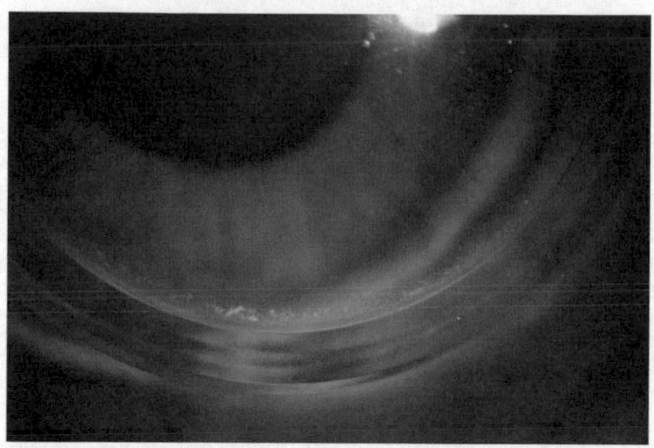

Fig. 18.5 Intrastromal tunnel deposits

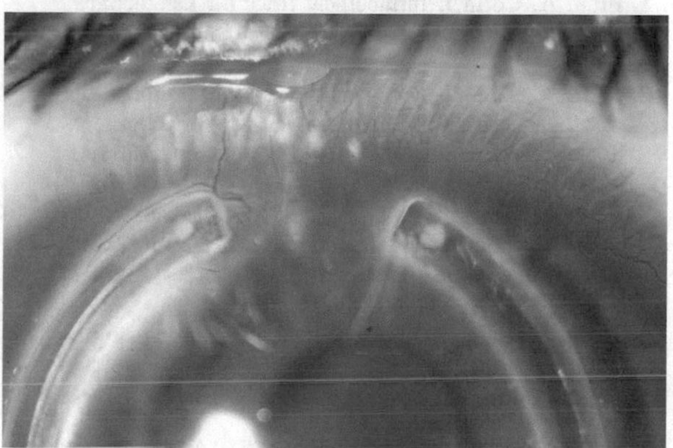

Fig. 18.6 Neovascularization of the stromal tunnel

of wound healing with mild fibrosis. Epithelial cells with highly reflective nuclei were seen as well in this region, what may be an indicator of increased biologic stress caused by the device [39].

18.3.4 Corneal Neovascularization

Neovascularization of the tunnel is uncommon (Fig. 18.6). Superficial neovascularization has usually little clinical concern, but deep neovascularization can occur at the wound site and treatment should include topical steroids. Unresponsive, severe, and progressive cases may require segment explantation. Risk factors for corneal neovascularization include previous contact lens wear, corneal sutures, and wound trauma during surgery.

18.3.5 Epithelization of the Stromal Tunnel

ICRS related epithelial ingrowth never shows an aggressive behavior. It occurs very rarely and is nonprogressive.

18.3.6 Late Dislocation of Ring Segment into the Anterior Chamber

Dislocation of a segment into the anterior chamber can occur intraoperatively, but Park et al. reported a case who presented with a dislocated ICRS in the anterior chamber 3 weeks postop [40]. They identified eye rubbing (due to patient eczema) as a possible etiology.

Compliance with Ethical Requirements Ayilin Kılıç and Jorge L. Alió del Barrio declare that they have no conflict of interest.

All procedures followed were in accordance with the ethical standards of the responsible committee on human experimentation (institutional and national) and with the Helsinki Declaration of 1975, as revised in 2000. Informed consent was obtained from all patients for being included in the study.

No animal studies were carried out by the authors for this article.

References

1. Ertan A, Colin J. Intracorneal rings for keratoconus and keratectasia. J Cataract Refract Surg. 2007;33:1303–14.
2. Ferrer C, Alio JL, Montanes AU, Perez-Santonja JJ, et al. Causes of intrastromal corneal ring segment explantation: Clinicopathologic correlation analysis. J Cataract Refract Surg. 2010;36:970–7.
3. Ertan A, Kamburoğlu G, Bahadır M. Intacs insertion with the femtosecond laser for the management of keratoconus; one-year results. J Cataract Refract Surg. 2006;32:2039–42.
4. Ertan A, Kamburoğlu G. Intacs implantation using a femtosecond laser for management of keratoconus: comparison of 306 cases in different stages. J Cataract Refract Surg. 2008;34:1521–6.
5. Coşkunseven E, Kymionis GD, Tsiklis NS, Atun S, Arslan E, Jankov MR, Pallikaris IG. One-year results of intrastromal ring segment implantation (KeraRing) using femtosecond laser in patient with keratoconus. Am J Ophthalmol. 2008;145:775–9.
6. Rabinowitz YS, Li X, Ignacio TS, et al. INTACS inserts using the femtosecond laser compared to the mechanical spreader in the treatment of keratoconus. J Refract Surg. 2006;22:764–71.
7. Rabinowitz YS. Intacs for keratoconus. Int Ophthalmol Clin. 2010;50(3):63–76.
8. Pinero DP, Alio JL, El Kandy B, Coskunseven E, Morbelli H, Uceda-Montanes A, Maldonado MJ, Cuevas D, Pascual I. Refractive and aberrometric outcomes of intracorneal ring segments for keratoconus: mechanical versus femtosecond assited procedures. Ophthalmology. 2009;116:1675–87.
9. Kanellopoulos AJ, Pe LH, Perry HD, Donnenfeld ED. Modified intracorneal ring segment implantations (INTACS) for the management of moderate to advanced keratoconus: efficacy and complications. Cornea. 2006;25:29–33.
10. Colin J. European clinical evaluation: use of Intacs prescription inserts for the treatment of keratoconus. J Cataract Refract Surg. 2006;32:747–55.
11. Lovisolo CF, Fleming JF, Pesando PM. Corneal biomechanics and astigmatism management after intrastromal intrastromal inserts. In: Lovisolo CF, Fleming JF, Pesando PM, editors. Intrastromal corneal ring segments. Canelli: Fabiano Ed; 2002. p. 35–47.
12. Kwitko S, Severo NS. Ferrara intracorneal ring segments for keratoconus. J Cataract Refract Surg. 2004;30:812–20.
13. Ruckhofer J, Stoiber J, Alzner E, Grabner G. One year results of European Multicenter Study of intrastromal ring sements. Part 2: complications, visual symptoms, and patient satisfaction. J Cataract Refract Surg. 2001;27:287–96.
14. Khan MI, Injarie A, Muhtaseb M. Intracorneal ring segments for advanced keratoconus and cases with high keratometric asymmetry. J Cataract Refract Surg. 2012;38:129–36.
15. Lai MM, Tang M, Andrade EM, Li Y, Khurana RN, Song JC. Optical coherence tomography to assess intrastromal ring segment depth in keratoconic eyes. J Cataract Refract Surg. 2006;32(11):1860–5.
16. Kamburoğlu G, Ertan A, Saraçbaşı O. Measurement of depth of Intacs implanted via femtosecond laser using pentacam. J Refract Surg. 2009;25:377–82.
17. Toroquetti L, Ferrara P. Reasons for intrastromal corneal ring segment explantation. J Cataract Refract Surg. 2010;36:2014.
18. Bourcier T, Borderie V, Laroche L. Late bacterial keratitis after implantation of intrastromal corneal ring segments. J Cataract Refract Surg. 2003;29:407–9.
19. Chaudhry IA, Al-Ghamdi AA, Kirat O, Al-Swelmi F, Al-Rashed W, Shamsi FA. Bilateral infectious keratitis after implantation of intrastromal ring segments. Cornea. 2010;29:339–41.
20. Liu A, Manche EE. Traumatic shattering of intrastromal corneal ring segments. J Cataract Refract Surg. 2010;36:1042–4.
21. Schanzlin DJ, Abbott RL, Asbell PA, et al. Two-year outcomes of intrastromal corneal ring segments for the correction of myopia. Ophthalmology. 2001;108:1688–94.
22. Ruckhofer J, Twa MD, Schanzlin DJ. Clinical characteristics of lamellar channel deposits after implantation of Intacs. J Cataract Refract Surg. 2000;26:1473–9.
23. Mulet ME, Perez-Santonja JJ, Ferrer C, Alio JL. Microbial keratitis after intrastromal corneal ring segment implantation. J Refract Surg. 2010;20:780–4.
24. Lovisolo CF, Fleming JF, Pesando PM. Postoperative course and complication management. In: Lovisolo CF, Fleming JF, Pesando PM, editors. Intrastromal corneal ring segments. Canelli: Fabiano Ed; 2002. p. 81–95.
25. Serdaroviç O. Keratoplasty, contact lenses preferred for keratoconus: complications and long term success. Br J Ophthalmol. 1991;75:142–6.
26. Thornton SP. Astigmatic keratotomy: a review of basic concepts with case reports. J Cataract Refract Surg. 1990;16:430–5.
27. Baikof G, et al. Diurinal variations in keratometry and refraction with intracorneal ring segments. J Cataract Refract Surg. 1999;25:1056–61.

28. Baikof G, Maia N, Poulhalec D, Fontaine A, Giusiono B. Diurinal variations of refraction and keratometry after intracorneal rings. J Fr Ophthalmol. 1999;22:169–75.
29. Colin J, Cochener B, Savary G, Malet F. Correcting keratoconus with intracorneal rings. J Cataract Refract Surg. 2000;26:1117–22.
30. Tunç Z, Deveci N, Sener B, Bahcecioglu H. Anneaux intracorneens (Intacs) pour le traitement de l'astigmatisme asymetrique du keratocone: recul de plus de deuxans. J Fr Ophthalmol. 2003;26:824–30.
31. Alió JL, Artola A, Ruiz-Moreno JM, et al. Changes in keratoconic corneas after intracorneal ring segment explantation and reimplantation. Ophthalmology. 2004;111:747–51.
32. Alio JL, Pinero DP, Söğütlü E, Kubaloğlu A. Implantation of new intracorneal ring segments after segment explantation for unsuccesfull outcomes in eyes with keratoconus. J Cataract Refract Surg. 2010;36:1303–10.
33. Pokroy R, Levinger S. Intacs adjustment surgery for keratoconus. J Cataract Refract Surg. 2006;32:986–92.
34. Bourges JL, Trong TT, Ellies P, Briat B, Renard G. Intrastromal corneal ring segments and corneal anterior stromal necrosis. J Cataract Refract Surg. 2003;29:1228–30.
35. Hagen KB, Waring III GO, Johnson-Wint B. Progressive nonulcerative paracentral keratolysis associated with elevated corneal metalloproteinases. Cornea. 1997;16:486–92.
36. Samimi S, Leger F, Touboul D, Colin D. Histopathological findings after ring segment implantation in keratoconic human corneas. J Cataract Refract Surg. 2007;33:247–53.
37. Fabre EJ, Bureau J, Pouliquen Y, Lorans G. Binding sites for human interleukin 1α, gamma interferon and tumor necrosis factor on cultured fibroblasts of normal corneal and keratoconus. Curr Eye Res. 1991;10:585–92.
38. Randleman JR, Dawson DG, Larson PM, Russel B, Edelhauser HE. Chronic pain after Intacs implantation. J Cataract Refract Surg. 2006;32:875–8.
39. Ruckhofer J, Böhnke M, Alzner E, Grabner G. Confocal microscopy after implantation of intrastromal corneal ring segments. Ophthalmology. 2000;107:2144–51.
40. Park S, Ramamurthi S, Ramaesh K. Late dislocation of intrastromal ring segment into the anterior chamber. J Cataract Refract Surg. 2010;36:2003–5.

19 Corneal Collagen Cross-Linking for Corneal Ectasias

David O'Brart

19.1 Corneal Ectatic Disorders

19.1.1 Keratoconus

Keratoconus is a disorder of undetermined aetiology characterized by paracentral/central corneal thinning with secondary conical ectasia. The consequent irregular astigmatism causes visual impairment, ghosting and polyopia [1–3]. It is almost always bilateral but frequently asymmetrical in disease severity. Typically presentation is during adolescence with progression continuing for two decades when the condition often stabilizes. It is the commonest reported corneal dystrophy, occurring in approximately 1 in 1750 individuals [1–3]. Studies of quality-of-life analysis demonstrate that that its degree of public health impact is disproportionate to its prevalence, with scores of life impairment being equivalent to grade 3–4 age-related macular degeneration [4].

The aetiology of Keratoconus has not been fully elucidated. It involves the interaction of genetic, mechanical and biochemical factors. With a range of clinical presentations, it is likely that keratoconus is the final manifestation for several different conditions. It often presents as an isolated condition, but is also associated with some ophthalmic and systemic pathologies, including conjunctival vernal disease, blue sclera, retinitis pigmentosa, atopy, magnesium deficiency, Down's syndrome, Turners' syndrome and connective tissue disorders such as Marfans and Ehlers–Danlos syndrome, osteogenesis imperfecta and pseudoxanthoma elasticuma [1, 2]. It is associated with repeated mild ocular surface trauma such as hard contact lens wear, allergic eye disease and eye rubbing [1, 2]. Genetic factors are undoubtedly relevant with up to 10–20 % of affected individuals reporting a positive family history [5]. Increased activity of proteinase enzymes and reduced activity of proteinase inhibitors has been documented in affected corneas [6], with the consequent amplified stromal protein digestion possibly resulting in thinning and secondary corneal biomechanical instability [7].

19.1.2 Iatrogenic Kerectasia

Kerectasia following corneal refractive surgery is an infrequent but potentially visually devastating complication. Seiler was first to document its occurrence after Laser in situ keratomileusis (LASIK) almost 20 years ago [8]. Its reported incidence is between 0.04 and 0.6 % [9, 10], with

D. O'Brart, M.D., F.R.C.S., F.R.C.O.phth. (✉)
Department of Ophthalmology, Guy's and St. Thomas' NHS Foundation Trust, St. Thomas' Hospital, London SE1 7EH, UK

King's College London, London, UK
e-mail: davidobrart@aol.com

J.L. Alió (ed.), *Keratoconus*, Essentials in Ophthalmology, DOI 10.1007/978-3-319-43881-8_19

one survey in 2004 showing that more than 50 % of responding surgeons had documented its occurrence in at least one patient under their care [11]. Onset ranges from 1 to 45 months with half of all cases presenting within 12 months after LASIK [12, 13]. Frequently it causes significant visual impairment, with a study in the early 2000s, prior to the introduction of corneal collagen cross-linking (CXL), reporting that 35 % of cases eventually required corneal transplantation [12]. As well as LASIK it has been documented after Photorefractive Keratectomy (PRK) [12, 13] and incisional kerato-refractive surgical procedures such as Radial Keratotomy [14]. Meticulous pre-operative tomographic screening is essential to reduce its occurrence as known risk factors for its potential development include pre-existing keratoconus and PMD, including forme fruste cases. These conditions are a contraindication to kerato-refractive surgery. Patients with thin corneas, high myopic corrections and young age at time of surgery are also at risk. Most refractive surgeons now avoid leaving residual stromal beds of less than 300 micrometers (μm) [12, 13, 15]. However, ectasia can still occasionally occur in individuals without currently identifiable risk factors [12, 13, 15].

19.1.3 Pellucid Marginal Degeneration

Pellucid marginal degeneration (PMD) occurs much less frequently than keratoconus. It involves the inferior peripheral, rather than the paracentral, cornea in approximately 85 % and the superior peripheral cornea in 15 % of presentations. It arises in a crescentic fashion usually between the 5 and 7 o'clock locations [16, 17]. It is more frequent in men, with a male-to-female ratio of 3:1 [17]. It is normally bilateral and affects all ethnicities [16, 17]. Usually it presents later in life than keratoconus, typically between the second and fifth decades [16, 17]. Its aetiology remains unknown. Typically it manifests with progressive against-the-rule astigmatism often with good spectacle corrected acuity until the late stages of the disease. Hydrops and spontaneous perforation have been reported [16, 17]. Corneal topography typically demonstrates a "lobster-claw pattern" but this is not exclusive to PMD and may occasionally arise in keratoconus [18]. There is some overlap between keratoconus and PMD, as well as with keratoglobus [16–18].

19.1.4 Overview of the Management of Corneal Ectasia

Management of corneal ectasia depends on the severity of the condition and the degree of irregular astigmatism. Mild cases may be simply correctable with astigmatic spectacles and/or soft toric contact lenses. With disease progression, the cornea becomes increasingly irregular and rigid contact lenses are then needed for adequate visual rehabilitation [19]. In up to 20 % of cases with keratoconus, keratoplasty is necessary because of contact lens intolerance/fitting problems and corneal scarring [20]. None of these treatment modalities treat the underlying pathophysiology and prevent disease progression. Only with the advent of CXL, can we now hope to delay arrest or even to a certain extent reverse keratoconus [20–22].

19.1.5 Corneal Collagen Cross-Linking: Laboratory Studies

The concept of treating ectatic corneal disorders with Riboflavin (vitamin B_2)/ultraviolet A (UVA) (370 nm) CXL was first postulated at the University of Dresden by Spoerl and Seiler [21–24]. Cross-linking occurs in tissues physiologically with ageing via enzymatic pathways such as Transglutaminase and Lysyl Oxidase. Spoerl and Seiler hypothesized that photochemical CXL of collagen within the corneal stroma could be achieved by utilizing the interaction between Riboflavin and UVA to create free radicals (oxygen singlets) which then activate the normal physiological Lysyl Oxidase pathway [24]. As well as acting as a photosensitizer, Riboflavin is thought to prevent injury to internal ocular structures, i.e. the endothelium, lens and retina, by absorbing the potentially mutagenic and cytotoxic UVA within the superficial corneal tissues [24]. The central role of singlet oxygen creation for the Riboflavin/UVA CXL process has been confirmed and in the absence of oxygen CXL does not occur [25]. However, the oxygen free radicals are now considered not to initiate CXL by the Lysyl Oxidase pathway but by three other potential mechanisms: imidazolone production, which can link to molecules, such as histidine, to form novel covalent bonds; the activation of endogenous populations of carbonyl groups in the ECM (allysine, hydroxyallysine) to create cross-links, and/or the degradation of Riboflavin itself, releasing 2,3-butanedione, which interacts with the endogenous carbonyl groups of the stromal proteins [25]. The exact location of the cross-links at the molecular level is unknown as these bonds cannot be seen microscopically. Cross-links cannot be formed between the collagen fibrils themselves, as the distance between the fibrils is too great for any intramolecular bond to be possible. In a series of experiments to investigate stromal ultrastructure utilizing X-ray scattering, hydrodynamic behaviour and enzyme digestion in ex vivo ungulate and rabbit eyes, Hayes et al. [26] postulated that it was probable that the cross-links were occurring on the outside of the collagen fibrils, rather than within them, and in the protein network surrounding the collagen [26].

Whilst the cross-links between the proteins within the stroma cannot be visualized and their existence directly corroborated, ex vivo laboratory studies have reported several changes in the mechanical and chemical properties of the stroma consistent with their existence. Stress–strain measurements of stromal tissue are increased appreciably [23, 24, 27], both immediately as well as several months following CXL [28], with such changes being shown to take place predominantly in the anterior 200 μm of the corneal stroma where the most of UVA absorption occurs [29]. In addition, after CXL a greater thermal shrinkage temperature has been reported in the stroma with a superior effect being documented anteriorly [30], while increased resistance of stromal tissue to enzymatic digestion has been confirmed, with a dose response in relation to UVA irradiation intensity [31]. Similarly an augmented resistance to matrix metalloproteinase (MMP) degradation of collagen, in particular sub-types MMP-1, 2, 9 and 13, and small leucine-rich proteoglycans following CXL has been reported [32]. This increased resistance of collagen and proteoglycans from MMP degradation is liable to be important in the potential of CXL in averting disease progression in corneal ectasias, where increased activity of collagenases has been recognized [18]. Other biophysical changes documented in cross-linked corneas include an increase in collagen fibre diameter in Rabbit corneas [33] and a reduction in hydration behaviour [34] both of which occur to a greater extent in the anterior compared to the posterior stroma. The increased resistance to hydration has led to the proposal that CXL might have a role in the management of corneal decompensation. However, recent investigators have suggested that such changes in hydration behaviour are probably just short-term alterations due to a consequence of the effects of the osmolarity of the dextran-containing Riboflavin solutions used rather than the actual effects of cross-linking and unlikely to be long-term alterations [26, 35]. Finally, there appear to be modifications in the electrophoretic pattern of corneal collagen type I following CXL, with the occurrence of an extra concentrated polymer band, with a molecular size of approximately 1000 kDa, resistant to mercaptoethanol, heat and pepsin [36].

Whilst, the investigations described earlier confirm the expected improvements in biomechanical and biochemical properties of corneas following CXL, it must be remembered that UVA is cytotoxic. It has been shown to cause keratocyte apoptosis and corneal endothelial cell damage/death as well as possible lens and even retinal injury [37–40]. Cell cultures studies of keratocytes have demonstrated an enhanced cytotoxic irradiance point with UVA irradiation combined with photosensitizing Riboflavin [37]. In the clinical setting this occurs in human corneas to a depth of 300 μm [37]. In relation to irreversible endothelial cell damage, cell culture studies have shown a cytotoxic threshold level with irradiation levels greater than 0.35 mW/cm^2 [38]. This cytotoxic level should not be achieved, with the standard CXL UVA dosage of 3mWcm^2 for 30 min (total dosage 5.4 J/cm^2), with corneal thickness greater than 400 μm [38]. In vivo studies have substantiated these laboratory findings and confirmed that with the standard dosage more than 85 % of the UVA radiation is absorbed by the Riboflavin in the anterior 400 μm of the stroma [39, 40]. The resultant irradiance at the level of the endothelium is less than 0.18 mW/cm^2, which is half the cytotoxic level [40–49]. This is similar for the lens and retina, where the level of UVA radiation reaching these tissues is less than 3 % of the cytotoxic limit [40].

19.2 Clinical Studies (Epithelium-Off CXL)

19.2.1 Prospective Cohort Case Series

The first published clinical application of Riboflavin/UVA CXL was not to treat keratoconus, but to address corneal ulceration/melt and was reported to successfully arrest corneal melting in a series of 3 out of 4 eyes [41]. The first investigation of its utilization in keratoconus was published in 2003 [24]. Wollensak et al. in a cases series of 23 eyes with keratoconus who underwent an epithelium-off CXL technique, reported stabilization of ectasia, with up to 5 years follow-up in some eyes. In 70 % an improvement in ectasia was documented, with an average reduction in refractive error of 1D and maximal keratometry (K_{max}) of 2 dioptres (D). Endothelial counts were unchanged and no loss of transparency of the cornea or lens was documented [24]. Since this seminal publication, other research groups have published multiple prospective, cohort case series of epithelium-off CXL with up to 24 months follow-up [41–52], including case series of paediatric patients [54, 55] and advanced keratoconus [56]. These studies have corroborated the preliminary results of Wollensak, with stabilization of keratoconus in the vast majority of treated eyes with few complications and significant improvements in vision, keratometry, corneal shape and higher order aberrations [42–58]. Similarly, prospective case series of epithelium-off CXL to treat iatrogenic post-laser refractive surgery ectasia have documented stability of topographic parameters and improvements in vision with more than 2 years follow-up [57–59] and up to 5 years follow-up in one reported case series [60]. In addition, encouraging results have been seen in case reports of CXL in eyes with PMD [61–63].

19.2.2 Randomized Controlled Studies

While results of prospective cohort case series studies have been supportive of the technique, there a relative paucity of randomized, prospective clinical studies of CXL. O'Brart el al in a randomized, prospective, bilateral study in 22 patients with documented keratoconic progression, in which one eye was treated with an epithelium-off CXL technique and the other left untreated to serve as a control, reported stabilization in all treated eyes with statistically significant improvements in corrected distance visual acuity (CDVA), keratometry, apex power measurements and higher order aberrations, with progression in 14 % of untreated eyes over an 18-month follow-up period [64]. Similarly, Wittig-Silva et al. in a study incorporating 48 untreated control eyes and 46 treated eyes with 3-year follow-up documented a significant increase in K_{max} and refractive cylinder with a reduction in uncorrected visual acuity (UCVA) in control eyes, while treated eyes showed a significant reduction in K_{max} and improvement in UCVA and CDVA [65, 66]. Hersh et al., Greenstein et al., and Chang et al. in a randomized trial reported significant improvements in UCVA, CDVA, higher order aberrations and topographic indices in 66 eyes with keratoconus and 38 with iatrogenic ectasia with 12-month follow-up and found better results in more severely affected eyes [53, 67, 68]. More recently, Lang et al. documented a significant difference between treated and control eyes in terms of changes in corneal

Table 19.1 Visual, refractive and keratometric changes after epithelium-off Riboflavin UVA CXL in prospective case series in which all eyes have a reported follow-up of 24 months or more

Lead author	Year	Number (eyes)	Follow-up (months)	UDVA change (LogMar)	CDVA change (LogMar)	MSE change (D)	K max change (D)	Pachymetry change (μm)	Failure (%)
Raiskup	2008	33	>36		−0.15		−2.57		6
Caporossi A	2010	44	48	−0.37	−0.14	+2.15	−2.26	+0.6	0
Kampik D	2011	46	24		−0.05		−1.23	−21.6	
Vinciguerra A	2012	40	24	−0.21	−0.19	+1.57	−1.27	+14.0	
Goldich Y	2012	14	24		−0.08		−2.40		0
O'Brart D	2013	30	>48	−0.01	−0.1	+0.8	−1.06	+2.0	0
Theuring A Raiskup F	2015	34	120		−0.13		−3.64	−46.0	6
Poli M	2015	36	72	−0.08	−0.14		+0.11	−16.4	11
O'Brart D	2015	36	78	−0.14	−0.13	+0.78	−0.9	−3.0	0

refractive power which reduced in treated eyes and increased in untreated cases over a 3-year follow-up period [69], while Seyedian et al. in a bilateral randomized study found a significant difference in K_{max} and CDVA at 12 months, which improved in treated and worsened in contralateral control eyes [70]. Most recently, Sharma et al. in a randomized trial with a sham treatment (Riboflavin administration with no UVA exposure) in control eyes showed an improvement in 23 treated eyes in terms of UDVA, refractive cylindrical correction and K_{max} while the sham control group of 20 eyes showed no such changes [71]. These randomized, controlled studies while relatively few in number and limited in subjects treated, continue to provide a growing body of evidence to support the efficacy of Riboflavin/UVA epithelium-off CXL to prevent disease progression and improve corneal shape in corneal ectasias.

19.2.3 Long-Term Follow-Up

While prospective cohort and randomized, controlled clinical studies of epithelium-off CXL certainly support its mid-term efficacy and safety, there is scarcity of long-term data. Keratoconus characteristically progresses at an unpredictable rate for about two decades following presentation and then becomes stable, probably as a consequence of physiological age-related cross-linking [1–3]. The rate of molecular turnover of collagen and the extracellular matrix (ECM) within the cornea is as yet undetermined. Given such considerations, the duration of effectiveness of CXL and the necessity to repeat the procedure is unclear. Outcomes from a number of published case series with follow-up of greater than 24 months are shown in Table 19.1. Raiskup-Wolf et al. in 33 eyes with over 3-year follow-up reported stabilization of keratoconus with reduction of keratometry and improvements in vision with time [72]. Caporossi documented stability of ectasia in 44 eyes after 48 months, with a reduction in keratometry and coma and improvements in vision [73]. O'Brart in 29 eyes found stabilization in all cases, with improvements in refraction, vision, keratometry and higher order aberrations at 12 months which showed statistically significant continued enhancement at 4–6 years [74]. Hashemi demonstrated stabilization in 40 eyes of 32 patients with progressive keratoconus with continued improvement in corneal elevation measurements over 5 years of follow-up [75]. Few studies have reported follow-up over 5 years. Poli et al. in 36 eyes of 25 patients reported no evidence of keratoconic progression 6 years after CXL with a significant improvement in CDVA and no sight-threatening complication [76]. Theuring and Raiskup in 34 eyes of 24 patients at 10 years documented significant improvements in vision and keratometry at 10 years, with progression in only 6 % of cases and no change in transparency of the cornea or lens [77, 78]. O'Brart et al. in a series of 36 eyes of 36 patients reported no progression in any eyes at a mean follow-up of 7 years with significant improvements in visual, topographic and corneal wave-front parameters. These parameters continued to improve between 1 and 5 years after surgery with stabilization thereafter, although CDVA continued to improve even between 5 and 7 years [79]. No sight-threatening complications were documented in this series although during the 7-year follow-up 24 % of untreated fellow eyes had an increase in K_{max} of over 1.0 dioptre (D) and underwent CXL [79]. This documented progression in fellow untreated eyes, seen in this and other studies indicate that the improvements in measured visual and topographic parameters in treated eyes with long-term follow-up are unlikely to be due to any physiological age-related changes but to the CXL treatment itself. Such findings from different investigators further support the efficacy and safety of epithelium-off CXL with up to a decade of follow-up. Further follow-up will determine the nature of longer term efficacy and the need if any to repeat the procedure and will elucidate how long and to what degree eyes might continue with improvement in visual and topographic parameters even years after CXL. The recurrence of keratoconus following keratoplasty, which classically, albeit rarely, occurs 10 to 20 years following surgery [80], suggests that turnover of corneal collagen and ECM may be measured in decades and that CXL might be effective for at least this length of time if not longer given physiological cross-linking changes with age.

19.2.4 Description of the Standard Epithelium-Off CXL Procedure

As described earlier, all long-term data over 5 years, together with the vast majority of prospective cohort case series with reported follow-up between 12 and 24 months and most published randomized prospective studies are with epithelium-off CXL using the standard UVA exposure of 3 mw/cm^2 for 30 min (total UV dosage 5.4 J/cm^2). As more has been published and is known about this particular CXL methodology and as its efficacy and safety is supported by the current scientific literature it must be regarded as the gold standard technique. The following section describes this operative technique.

Prior to CXL, it is typically necessary to obtain documented evidence of progression of ectasia. The precise and best parameters to define progression are not agreed and remain undefined and indeed undetermined. However, many studies and surgeons define progression as an increase in K_{max}/average keratometry and/or refractive astigmatism of over 1.0D and/or decrease in pachymetry greater than 10 % over the preceding 12–18 months [64, 74, 79]. In addition, many surgeons will offer CXL in all adolescent and paediatric keratoconus patients and all with iatrogenic ectasia, even in the absence of documented progression, because of the high risk of worsening of ectasia in such eyes and the improvements in corneal shape and vision documented in most eyes after CXL with time.

To minimize the risk of endothelial damage and corneal decompensation it should be ensured that prior to surgery the corneal thickness is greater than 450 micrometers (μm) (400 μm with the epithelium off) at its thinnest point [38–40]. Following fully informed consent, CXL is typically performed under topical anaesthesia. In the standard epithelium-off technique the central 9 millimetre (mm) of the corneal epithelium is debrided to enable adequate stromal Riboflavin absorption [24, 42–79]. Following epithelial debridement, Riboflavin 0.1 % is applied every 2–3 min for at least 30 min to allow sufficient and homogeneous stromal uptake prior to UVA exposure [81]. In the initial studies the Riboflavin was suspended in a 20 % dextran solution. Whilst this is still used, many formulations now used clinically are isotonic to avoid stromal dehydration and inadvertent corneal thinning during the procedure and contain hydroxypropyl methylcellulose instead of dextran [82]. Intraoperative pachymetry is advocated by many surgeons to monitor corneal thickness prior to UVA exposure and to administer hypotonic Riboflavin drops if the cornea thins excessively (below 400 μm) during Riboflavin administration. The central 8 to 9 mm of the cornea is then irradiated with UVA at 3 mW/cm^2 for 30 min. During this time, Riboflavin 0.1 % drops are applied to the stromal surface every 3–5 min during the 30-min irradiation period. Following irradiation, topical antibiotics and corticosteroids are prescribed until corneal re-epithelialization. Systemic analgesic and bandage soft contact lenses can be used for pain management. Topical anaesthetics in limited dosage, no more than 2 hourly and only for 48 h may also be of benefit [83]. Significant ocular pain is typically experienced for the first 24–48 h following surgery and vision is blurred for 1–2 weeks. Patients need to be carefully counselled concerning the expected occurrence of post-operative pain and slow visual recovery in the early post-operative period to avoid unnecessary distress. Contact lens wear can be resumed once the epithelium has fully healed, typically at about 3 weeks.

19.2.4.1 Wound Healing Changes and Confocal Microscopy During the First 12 Months After CXL

Studies using confocal microscopy have identified oedema, superficial nerve loss, rarefaction of keratocytes in the anterior and mid-stroma and isolated endothelial damage in the immediate post-operative period [84–86]. During the first 3 months after surgery there is keratocyte re-population, which is usually complete by 6 months. An increased density of the extracellular matrix occurs to a depth of 300–350 µm, which forms the so-called demarcation line which can be observed on slit lamp examination [87]. Regeneration of nerve fibres, with re-establishment of the sub-epithelial plexus occurs usually within 12 months with return of full corneal sensitivity. Confocal investigations have confirmed the lack of endothelial damage, with no alterations of cell density changes or hexagonality [84–86]. These in vivo confocal microscopic changes after epithelium-off CXL have been confirmed by histological examination of corneal buttons after keratoplasty [87–90] and corroborate keratocyte loss and damage, which can be prolonged [87], with an increase in collagen fibril diameter [87–90].

19.2.4.2 Epithelium-On Versus Epithelium-Off Techniques

Riboflavin is a hydrophilic and is unable to pass through the tight junctions of the intact corneal epithelial barrier. Spoerl et al. confirmed the requirement for full central epithelial debridement to allow sufficient stromal uptake of Riboflavin. They found no modifications in the biomechanical properties of corneal tissue where the CXL was performed with the epithelium intact [22, 23]. These findings were confirmed by a series of ex vivo laboratory investigations, utilizing photospectrophotometry to indirectly measure stromal Riboflavin concentration, which demonstrated the necessity with standard 0.1 % solutions to completely remove all layers of epithelium to achieve adequate stromal Riboflavin concentrations [91–93]. Superficial epithelial trauma, pre-operative, multiple administration of topical Tetracaine 1 %, application of 20 % Alcohol solution, grid pattern epithelial removal were all found to be insufficient to attain significant and/or homogeneous Riboflavin stromal absorption [91–93]. On the basis of such studies, the epithelium was debrided prior to Riboflavin administration in the first clinical investigations and became the gold standard CXL methodology as described earlier [24, 42–79]. In an attempt to reduce post-operative pain, speed visual recovery, reduce risks of infection, reduce corneal scarring (by decreasing epithelial/stromal cytokine interaction) and limit potential endothelial damage (by having a greater overall corneal thickness and preventing perioperative stromal dehydration and thinning), some investigators postulated performing CXL with the epithelium on. Research has been directed at methodologies to enhance epithelial permeability by using multiple applications of topical anaesthesia [94], the addition of chemical additives to the Riboflavin solution such as trometamol (Tris-(hydroxymethyl)aminomethane) [96], Sodium Ethylenediaminetetraacetic acid (EDTA) [95], Benzalkonium Chloride (BAC) and Sodium Chloride [96], partial mechanical disruption [97], iontophoresis [98], increased Riboflavin concentrations, reduced solution osmolarity [99] and/or increased application times.

19.3 Partial Mechanical Epithelial Disruption

Partial Mechanical Epithelial Disruption may be achieved using superficial scratches or specially designed surgical instruments [100]. Rechichi used a corneal disruptor to create pockmarks in the epithelium in 28 patients and reported an improvement in vision and to a certain extent in refraction and corneal topography at 12 months [100]. Similarly, Hashemi in 40 eyes using a technique with 3–4 vertical strips of complete debridement with intact islands of epithelium in-between, reported significant improvements in CDVA and anterior and posterior corneal elevation at 5 years but no changes in K_{max}, refraction or pachymetry [75]. However, whilst these two studies show some efficacy, two comparative studies, Hashemi in a retrospective study of 80 eyes in 65 patients [101] and Razmjoo in a randomized controlled study in 44 eyes of 22 patients [102], suggested that while visual outcomes in terms of CDVA may be better with partial disruption, improvement in topographic indices are superior with complete epithelial debridement [101, 102]. Clearly, long-term comparative studies are needed to compare these two approaches in terms of stability of outcomes and cessation of progression of ectasia, before partial disruption can be considered as efficacious as the gold standard epithelium-off technique.

19.4 Epithelium-On CXL: Chemical Enhancers

The use of Trometamol and EDTA in Riboflavin solutions to enhance transepithelial CXL is equivocal. Filippello in a prospective case series reported rapid visual recovery, little post-operative pain and outcomes in terms of reduction in K_{max} comparable to epithelium-off CXL albeit with a shallower demarcation line [96]. Such results were also seen in 22 eyes of paediatric cases by Salman, who observed a 2.0D decrease in keratometry, improved vision and no progression at 12 months with a worsening of topographic parameters in untreated control eyes [103] and by Magli in a retrospective comparative study who found little difference between epithelial-on and epithelial-off CXL [104]. However, Buzonetti in 13 eyes treated with epithelium-on CXL with solutions containing Trometamol and EDTA, reported that although CDVA had improved, keratometry and higher order aberrations were worse at 12 months [105]. Similarly, Caporossi documented failure of treatment and had to retreat 50 % of his cases with epithelium-off CXL at 24 months, suggesting little efficacy with the use of these chemical "enhancers" [106].

Correspondingly, the use of BAC and multiple administration of topical anaesthetics has shown limited efficacy, despite some encouraging results in ex vivo pre-clinical studies [96]. Leccisotti and Islam in a prospective, paired-eye study in 51 patients, with the eye with more severe keratoconus being treated and the fellow acting as a control, showed an improvement in CDVA, refraction and keratometry in treated compared to control eyes, but with less effect than that reported with epithelium-off CXL [107], while Koppen in 53 similarly treated eyes of 38 patients showed an improvement in CDVA at 12 months, but with progression of K_{max} and pachymetry [108]. In an as yet unpublished study (Gatzioufas, personal communication) reported a high failure rate in epithelium-on treated eyes using Riboflavin 0.25 % with BAC. Not only did 24 % of eyes progress with an increase in K_{max} greater than 1.0D at 12 months but almost 50 % of eyes had epithelial defects on the first day following surgery due to epithelial toxicity from prolonged BAC application. Such findings are consistent with those of Yuksel et al., who found higher pain scores on day 1 and longer epithelialization with epithelium-on treatments [109].

In terms of comparative studies of epithelium-on CXL, with chemical enhancers and solution modification, with epithelium-off treatment, results are equivocal. Whilst a few showed little difference between techniques some clearly indicate better results with epithelial debridement. Rossi in a limited randomized prospective study of 20 eyes (10 per treatment group) utilizing an epithelium-on technique with EDTA and

Trometamol reported no differences between the two treatments at 12 months [110]. Likewise Nawaz et al. in a non-randomized study of 40 patients using an isotonic Riboflavin solution found no differences in outcomes between epithelium-off or on CXL at 6 months [111]. However, Al Fayez et al. in a randomized study of 70 patients with 3-year follow-up reported better results with epithelium-off CXL with no progression and an average reduction of K_{max} of 2.4D, while 55 % of eyes with epithelium-on CXL showed progression and an average increase of K_{max} by 1.1D [112]. Similarly, Soeters in a randomized study of 51 eyes documented better reduction of K_{max} with epithelium-off CXL, with progression being reported in 23 % of epithelium-on treated eyes, utilizing EDTA and Trometamol, at 12 months, although improvement in CDVA with epithelium-on CXL was better and complications were less [113]. Finally, Kocak in a retrospective study in 36 eyes with 12-month follow-up showed a greater reduction in cone apex power with epithelium-off CXL, while there was progression in 65 % of epithelium-on treatments [114].

It therefore appears that there still remains a great deal of uncertainty concerning the efficacy of current commercially available epithelium-on CXL methodologies using Riboflavin solution modifications and the addition of chemical enhancers, with many studies reporting high rates of treatment failure. This is probably due to limited stromal Riboflavin penetration through the intact hydrophobic epithelial barrier as seen in photospectrometry studies [91–93] and confirmed recently by a series of published investigations conducted with 2-photon fluorescence microscopy to more directly measure Riboflavin concentration within the stroma [115, 116]. These studies by Gore et al. show very limited uptake with the use of epithelium-on CXL with chemical enhancers with at best only 20–50 % of the Riboflavin concentrations achieved with the standard epithelium-off technique within the first 100 μm of stroma, which falls further at increasing depths [116]. In addition with BAC-containing compounds, significant epithelial damage was observed after 30 min of solution application time and there appeared to be considerable loading of the epithelium with Riboflavin with all solutions that must cause shielding of the stroma from UVA during irradiation [116]. This shielding of UVA reaching the stroma is likely to further limit the efficacy of epithelium-on treatments.

19.5 Iontophoretic Epithelium-On CXL

In addition to the novel formulations discussed earlier, laboratory investigations have shown enhanced transepithelial Riboflavin absorption using iontophoretic delivery [117–121]. Riboflavin is an effective molecule for iontophoretic transfer as it is small, negatively charged at physiological pH and is easily soluble in water. Cassagne using 0.1 % Riboflavin and 1 mA current for 5 min reported 50 % of the stromal concentration seen with epithelium-off CXL in a Rabbit eye model with similar enhancements in extensiometry and collagenase digestion [117]. In a rabbit eye and human cadaver model, Vinciguerra et al. reported better Riboflavin uptake and increased extensiometry changes with iontophoresis compared to epithelium-on CXL without iontophoresis but less than epithelium-off treatments [118]. Mastropasqua et al. documented increased stiffening of human cadaver corneas following iontophoretic CXL using a noncontact air pulse tonometer [119] and Lombardo found comparable stiffness to that seen with epithelium-off CXL using an inflation methodology of ex vivo human globes [120].

Published clinical studies of iontophoretic CXL are limited but encouraging. Bikbova and Bikbov treated 22 eyes using Riboflavin 0.1 % and 1 mA for 10 min and reported a mean reduction of K_{max} of 2.0D at 12 months [121]. Vinciguerra treated 20 eyes, using Riboflavin 0.1 % and 1 mA for 5 min and showed an improvement in CDVA and stable keratometry, higher order aberrations, pachymetry and endothelial counts at 12 months [122]. Similarly, Li using Riboflavin 0.1 % and 1 mA for 5 min in 15 eyes, documented improvement in visual and topographic parameters, with a demarcation line with an average depth of 288 μm at 6 months [123], while Buzzonetti et al. in 14 paediatric cases showed an improvement in CDVA, stability of refraction and topography at 15 months but with an average demarcation line depth of 180 μm [124].

These results are encouraging, but at present there are no published comparative studies with epithelium-off CXL so this technique must be regarded as investigative at present. In addition, iontophoresis is currently being utilized to provide reduced application times of 5–10 min, instead of the usual 30 min epithelium-off application time. In a series of laboratory investigation, O'Brart and colleagues have shown that by increasing Riboflavin concentration, iontophoresis application times and allowing short periods of time for the Riboflavin, which is initially deposited only into the epithelium and anterior stroma by the iontophoresis, to diffuse deeper into the stroma, concentrations of up to 60–80 % of that achieved with epithelium-off application with a homogeneous distribution throughout the stroma can be achieved [125, 126]. With such improved transepithelial Riboflavin penetration it is hoped that results similar to epithelium-off CXL may be achieved. Randomized, prospective, comparative studies are currently being undertaken (O'Brart, personal communication, ISRCT No: 04451470).

19.5.1 Epithelium-on CXL Other Methodologies

As well as iontophoresis, other methodologies currently under pre-clinical investigation to facilitate transepithelial Riboflavin stromal absorption include the use of ultrasound [127], nano-emulsion systems [128], other epithelial permeation enhancers such as d-Alpha-tocopheryl poly(ethylene glycol) 1000 succinate (Vitamin E-TPGS) [129] and the creation of femto second laser intrastromal pockets [130]. At present there are no large case series or comparative studies of these techniques which are only at an investigational stage but might hold promise in the future.

19.5.2 Rapid (Accelerated/High-Fluence) CXL Techniques

Current protocols utilize UVA energies of 3 mW/cm^2 and require 30 min of UVA exposure to achieve the desired clinical effect [24, 42–79]. It has been hypothesized that by increasing the UVA fluence while simultaneously reducing the exposure time (the Bunsen–Roscoe law of reciprocity), the same sub-threshold cytotoxic corneal endothelial UVA dosage can be delivered (5.4 J/cm^2), thereby maintaining efficacy and safety, but with a reduced treatment time. Reduced treatment time as well as improving case throughput and surgeon convenience may offer improved patient comfort as well as shortened keratocyte exposure time, which it has been postulated may result in less keratocyte damage and apoptosis.

Preclinical ex vivo studies were encouraging, with similar biomechanical changes as measured by scanning acoustic microscopy and extensiometry, seen between the standard UVA exposure of 3 mw/cm^2 for 30 min (SCXL) compared with higher fluencies with shorter exposure times [131–133], albeit with a sudden decrease in efficacy with very high intensity UV light greater than 45 mW/cm^2 [133]. This decrease in efficacy with higher fluencies is not understood but might be related to oxygen consumption and availability, which has been shown to limit the photochemical cross-linking process [25].

Published clinical studies at present are limited. Cinar et al. in a study of 23 eyes showed that accelerated CXL (ACXL) produced a significant reduction in topographic keratometry values and an improvement in corrected distance acuity with a limited follow-up of 6 months [134]. Shetty et al. in 30 eyes of 14 paediatric cases with a UVA dosage 9 mW/cm^2 for 10 min documented an improvement in vision and refractive cylinder at 24 months [135], while using the same accelerated protocol, Marino in 40 eyes with post-LASIK ectasia reported stabilization in all eyes at 2 years [136] and Elbaz et al. documented stability in 16 keratoconic eyes at 12 month with an improvement in UDVA [137].

Comparative studies of ACXL and SCXL have been conflicting. Ng in a comparative study of 26 eyes found a greater reduction in K_{max} and K_{mean} with SCXL at 6–18 months compared to ACXL (9 mW/cm^2 for 10 min) [138], while Brittingham in 131 eyes found a reduction of K_{max} in SCXL but not ACXL at 12 months, with a similar high fluence protocol [139]. In contrast, Kanellopoulos in a randomized, bilateral study of 21 eyes using a UVA power of 7 mW/cm^2 for 15 min demonstrated similar results to SCXL at 18–56 months [140]. Similarly, comparable results between ACXL and SCXL were reported by Hashemian et al. in 153 eyes of 153 patients with 15-month follow-up [141], Hashemi in 62 eyes with 6-month follow-up, and an ACXL of 18 mW/cm^2 for 5 min [142], Shetty et al. in 138 eyes of 138 patients with 12-month follow-up, who found ACXL protocols of 9 mW/cm^2 for 10 min and 18 mW/cm^2 for 5 min had similar outcomes to SCXL but 30mWcm^2 for 3 min was not as efficacious [143], and Sherif who in 25 eyes of 18 patients comparing 30 mW/cm^2 for a 4 min 20 s (to give an 33 % increased total UVA dose of 7.2 J/cm^2) found comparative results at 12 months with SCXL [144]. Such outcomes are somewhat confusing but do cast some doubt on ACXL protocols especially with fluencies greater than 18 mw/cm^2. The reasons for this possibly reduced efficacy seen in some studies with ACXL are uncertain but may, as discussed earlier, be related to excessive oxygen consumption with higher fluencies of UVA and subsequent reduced oxygen availability, which has been shown to be central to the CXL process [25]. Certainly recently published ex vivo pepsin digestion studies have suggested reduced CXL efficacy with increasing UVA fluencies despite the total UVA dosage remaining unchanged at 5.4 J/cm^2 [145].

This uncertain efficacy has led some investigators to postulate the need to increase UVA exposure time by 30–40 % [144, 146] or employ fractionated/pulsed treatments [147, 148]. Thus far, there is little clinical data but as discussed earlier Sherif found comparable results with SCXL by increasing exposure time by one-third with 30 mW/cm^2 exposure [144] and Kymionis found the same depth of demarcation line by increasing exposure time by 40 % from 10 to 14 min with the 9 mW/cm^2 protocol [146]. Mazotta et al. in a comparative non-randomized study of 20 eyes found a greater reduction in keratometry with pulsed treatment compared to non-pulsed with a UVA fluence of 30 mW/cm^2 at 12 months [147], while Moramarco et al. found significantly deeper demarcation lines with pulsed treatments using the same protocol. Whilst interesting these studies with differing ACXL protocols are at an investigational stage at present and the efficacy uncertain further randomized controlled, long-term studies are clearly indicated to ascertain their efficacy to the gold-standard SCXL.

19.5.3 Treatment of Thin Corneas

Due to potential UVA endothelial toxicity, CXL using the standard protocol is contraindicated for individuals with corneas thinner than 400 μm. However, it is not uncommon in the clinical setting to see eyes which meet the criteria for cross-linking in terms of progression and good visual rehabilitation with contact lenses whose corneas are less than 400 μm at their thinnest points. This has led investigators to develop a number of protocols to treat such eyes. In a number of studies, hypo-osmolar Riboflavin solutions have been used to swell the cornea intraoperatively to over 400 μm and enable CXL to be undertaken. Raiskup and Spoerl in a series of 32 eyes with corneas thinner than 400 μm showed stability of vision and keratometry with no adverse events at 12 months [149], whilst Nassaralla et al. in 18 eyes demonstrated swelling of the cornea with the intraoperative administration of hypo-osmolar 0.1 % Riboflavin with no post-operative complications [150]. However, in one study of CXL in thin corneas endothelial counts were shown to be somewhat reduced, although vision and keratometry were improved [151] and in one case report, progression continued after CXL in an eye with a central thickness of less than 330 μm [151]. In addition to the use of hypo-osmolar Riboflavin, Spadea and

Mencucci demonstrated efficacy with no endothelial damage with transepithelial CXL in corneas as thin as 331–389 μm [152, 153]. Other proposed techniques for CXL in thin corneas include the use of Riboflavin-soaked, non-UVA filtering bandage contact lenses to be placed on the cornea during UVA irradiation [154] and the avoidance of epithelial debridement over the corneal thinnest point [155]. As yet all these published case series of novel CXL techniques in thin corneas contain small number of treated eyes with limited follow up. Undoubtedly, there is a need to cross-link such eyes and larger clinical series with further long-term follow-up are required to establish if these procedures in thin corneas are as effective and safe as standard CXL in corneas with thicknesses greater than 400 μm.

19.5.4 CXL in Combination with Other Treatment Modalities

As well as an isolated treatment, CXL has been used in combination with other treatment modalities to optimize visual outcomes in keratoconic and post-laser ectasia. Excimer laser epithelial removal has been postulated as a more efficacious methodology than mechanical epithelial debridement in standard epithelium-off CXL. Reinstein et al. using high resolution ultrasonic mapping, showed the epithelium to some extent masks the severity of any ectasia by showing hypoplasia/thinning over the cone apex and hyperplasia/thickening around the cone base [156]. Hence phototherapeutic laser removal could theoretically improve outcomes as the cone would be slightly flattened due to superficial stromal tissue removal over its apex during laser ablation. Kapasi et al. in a comparative study of 34 patients comparing excimer laser with mechanical debridement demonstrated better improvement in refractive error and astigmatism with laser removal [157]. Similarly, superior visual and refractive outcomes with laser removal were reported in a comparative study by Kymionis in 38 eyes [158]. Kymionis et al. also published long-term follow-up utilizing this technique of up to 4 years with an average reduction in K_{max} of 3.4D in 23 eyes [159]. This technique shows promise and randomized, prospective studies to compare mechanical and excimer laser removal as well as long-term studies to ensure that progression rates are not increased by stromal tissue removal in these already biomechanically unstable eyes are indicated.

Combined CXL and limited topography-guided PRK in selected eyes with moderate ectasia and adequate corneal thicknesses has been shown to be effective with marked improvements in visual, refractive and topographic parameters and stabilization of the ectatic process in the vast majority of eyes [160–165]. Such treatments have been shown to be associated with significant improvements in quality of life scores [166]. Follow-up in these studies, however, is limited to only 3 years so that long-term biomechanical stability has not been fully elucidated [167] and progression of ectasia has been reported (T. Seiler, personal communication). In addition, significant corneal haze/scarring has been reported following these combined treatments [168, 169]. Undoubtedly, further follow-up studies, beyond 5 years in large patient series and comparative studies would be of great interest to establish this combined procedure.

CXL has also been used after intracorneal ring segment (ICRS) insertion and even in a three-step procedure with both PRK and ICRS insertion [170]. Some studies have suggested that CXL may have an additive effect with intracorneal ring segments [171], although this has not been demonstrated in all studies [172]. The sequencing of the two treatments is as yet undetermined with a single small randomized study suggesting that better results could be obtained with simultaneous treatment rather than sequential [173].

Limited high fluence CXL has also been used in conjunction with keratorefractive procedures such as PRK and LASIK in an attempt to improve long-term stability and reduce the possible occurrence of post-surgery ectasia [174, 175]. As yet, such studies are limited in terms of numbers treated and long-term follow-up. However, results are encouraging, with a contra-lateral eye study by Kanellopoulos of CXL after hyperopic

LASIK in 23 eyes demonstrating less regression of correction over a mean follow-up of 23 months [176] and a comparative study by the same author of high myopic LASIK corrections combined with CXL reporting better visual outcomes [177]. Whilst such studies are of great interest, it should be noted that long-term studies of CXL have demonstrated continued flattening of the cornea and continued hyperopic refractive shift in some eyes for up to 5 years follow-up [77–79] and whilst adjunctive CXL may be useful in LASIK longer follow-up over 5 years and randomized, prospective comparative studies are indicated.

19.6 New Methodologies

Whilst Riboflavin/UVA CXL has been shown to be effective, other methodologies which are potentially more rapid and less invasive are currently under investigation. Rocha et al. reported a flash-linking process with UVA and Polyvinyl pyrrolidone may have the potential to photochemically cross-link the cornea in only 30 s [178]. Paik et al. have investigated the topical application of short-chain Aliphatic beta-nitro alcohols [179] and Cherfan et al. demonstrated an almost fourfold increase in corneal stiffness with no reduction in keratocyte viability with Rose Bengal 0.1 % administration and green light application and a less than 5 min total treatment time [180]. Undoubtedly other methodologies and applications will become available over the several next years due to the vast interest in this area of research.

19.7 Complications of Corneal Collagen Cross-Linking

To be discussed in separate chapter.

19.8 Summary

Clinical studies of CXL have shown great promise in stabilizing keratoconus and post-refractive surgery ectasia. Whilst further randomized, prospective and long-term follow up studies are necessary, it is very likely that in the future corneal ectasia can be halted at an early stage and perhaps the need for rigid contact lenses and keratoplasty avoided. Future refinement in techniques may allow for safer and more rapid procedure with less patient discomfort but require further investigation. Combined treatment with other methodologies to treat ectasia shows promise but also requires further investigative and long-term studies.

Compliance with Ethical Requirements David P.S. O'Brart declares that he has no conflict of interest. He holds a non-commercial grant from Alcon Inc for research into Femto-second laser assisted cataract surgery. No human or animal studies were carried out by the author for this review.

References

1. Krachmer JH, Feder RS, Belin MW. Keratoconus and related non-inflammatory corneal thinning disorders. Surv Ophthalmol. 1984;28:293–322.
2. Rabinowitz YS. Keratoconus. Surv Ophthalmol. 1998;42(4):297–319.
3. Kennedy RH, Bourne WM, Dyer JA. A 48-year clinical and epidemiological study of keratoconus. Am J Ophthalmol. 1986;101(3):267–73.
4. Kymes SM, Walline JJ, Zadnik K, Sterling J, Gordon MO. Changes in the quality of life of people with keratoconus. Am J Ophthalmol. 2004;138:527.
5. Hammerstein W. Zur genetic des keratoconus. Albrecht Von Graefes Arch Klin Exp Ophthalmol. 1974;190:293–308.
6. Zhou L, Sawaguchi S, Twining SS, Sugar J, Feder RS, Yue BY. Expression of degradative enzymes and protease inhibitors in corneas with keratoconus. Invest Ophthalmol Vis Sci. 1998;39:1117–24.
7. Andreassen T, Simonsen AH, Oxlund H. Biomechanical properties of keratoconus and normal corneas. Exp Eye Res. 1980;31(4):435–41.
8. Seiler T, Quurke AW. Iatrogenic keratectasia after LASIK in a case of forme fruste keratoconus. J Cataract Refract Surg. 1998;24(7):1007–9.
9. Randleman JB, Russell B, Ward MA, Thompson KP, Stulting RD. Risk factors and prognosis for corneal ectasia after LASIK. Ophthalmology. 2003; 110(2):267–75.
10. Pallikaris IG, Kymionis GD, Astyrakakis NI. Corneal ectasia induced by laser in situ keratomileusis. J Cataract Refract Surg. 2001;27(11):1796–802.
11. Duffey RJ, Leaming D. US trends in refractive surgery: 2004 ISRS/AAO survey. J Refract Surg. 2005;21(6):742–8.

12. Twa MD, Nichols JJ, Joslin CE, Kollbaum PS, Edrington TB, Bullimore MA, Mitchell GL, Cruickshanks KJ, Schanzlin DJ. Characteristics of corneal ectasia after LASIK for myopia. Cornea. 2004;23(5):447–57.
13. Randleman JB, Woodward M, Lynn MJ, Stulting RD. Risk assessment for ectasia after corneal refractive surgery. Ophthalmology. 2008;115(1):37–50.
14. Shaikh S, Shaikh NM, Manche E. Iatrogenic keratoconus as a complication of radial keratotomy. J Cataract Refract Surg. 2002;28(3):553–5.
15. Rabinowitz YS. Ectasia after laser in situ keratomileusis. Curr Opin Ophthalmol. 2006;17(5):421–6.
16. Jinabhai A, Radhakrishnan H, O'Donnell C. Pellucid corneal marginal degeneration: a review. Cont Lens Anterior Eye. 2011;34(2):56–63.
17. Sridhar MS, Mahesh S, Bansal AK, Nutheti R, Rao GN. Pellucid marginal corneal degeneration. Ophthalmology. 2004;111(6):1102–7.
18. Lee BW, Jurkunas UV, Harissi-Dagher M, Poothullil AM, Tobaigy FM, Azar DT. Ectatic disorders associated with a claw-shaped pattern on corneal topography. Am J Ophthalmol. 2007;144(1):154–6.
19. Mandell RB. Keratoconus. In: Mandell RB, editor. Contact lens practice. 4th ed. Springfield: Charles C. Thomas; 1988. p. 824–49.
20. Kirkness CM, Ficker LA, Steele AD, Rice NS. The success of penetrating keratoplasty for keratoconus. Eye. 1990;4:673–88.
21. Spoerl E, Huhle M, Seiler T. Erhohung der Festigkeit der Horn haut durch Vernetzung. Ophthalmologe. 1997;94(12):902–6.
22. Spoerl E, Huhle M, Seiler T. Induction of cross-links in corneal tissue. Exp Eye Res. 1998;66(1):97–103.
23. Spoerl E, Schreiber J, Hellmund K, et al. Untersuchungen zur Verfestigung der Hornhaut am kaninchen. Ophthalmologe. 2000;97(3):203–6.
24. Wollensak G, Spoerl E, Seiler T. Riboflavin/ultraviolet-a-induced collagen cross-linking for the treatment of keratoconus. Am J Ophthalmol. 2003;135(5):620–7.
25. McCall AS, Kraft S, Edelhauser HF, et al. Mechanisms of corneal tissue cross-linking in response to treatment with topical riboflavin and long-wavelength ultraviolet radiation (UVA). Invest Ophthalmol Vis Sci. 2010;51(1):129–38.
26. Hayes S, Kamma-Lorger CS, Boote C, Young RD, Quantock AJ, Rost A, Khatib Y, Harris J, Yagi N, Terrill N, Meek KM. The effect of riboflavin/UVA collagen cross-linking therapy on the structure and hydrodynamic behaviour of the ungulate and rabbit corneal stroma. PLoS One. 2013;8(1), e52860.
27. Wollensak G, Spoerl E, Seiler T. Stress-strain measurements of human and porcine cornea after riboflavin/ultraviolet-a-induced crosslinking. J Cataract Refract Surg. 2003;29:1780–5.
28. Wollensak G, Iomdina E. Long-term biomechanical properties of rabbit cornea after photodynamic collagen crosslinking. Acta Ophthalmol. 2009;87: 48–51.
29. Kohlhaas M, Spoerl E, Schilde T, Unger G, Wittig C, Pillunat LE. Biomechanical evidence of the distribution of cross-links in corneas treated with riboflavin and ultraviolet A light. J Cataract Refract Surg. 2006;3292:279–83.
30. Spoerl E, Wollensak G, Dittert DD, Seiler T. Thermomechanical behavior of collagen-cross-linked porcine cornea. Ophthalmologica. 2004; 218(2):136–40.
31. Spoerl E, Wollensak G, Seiler T. Increased resistance of cross linked cornea against enzymatic digestion. Curr Eye Res. 2004;29(1):35–40.
32. Zhang Y, Mao X, Schwend T, Littlechild S, Conrad GW. Resistance of corneal RFUVA–cross-linked collagens and small leucine-rich proteoglycans to degradation by matrix metalloproteinases. Invest Ophthalmol Vis Sci. 2013;54(2):1014–25. doi:10.1167/iovs.12-11277.
33. Wollensak G, Wilsch M, Spoerl E, Seiler T. Collagen fiber diameter after riboflavin/UVA induced collagen-crosslinking in the rabbit cornea. Cornea. 2004;23(5):503–7.
34. Wollensak G, Aurich H, Pham DT, Wirbelauer C. Hydration behavior of porcine cornea crosslinked with riboflavin and ultraviolet A. J Cataract Refract Surg. 2007;33(3):516–21.
35. Hayes S, Boote C, Kamma-Lorger CS, Rajan MS, Harris J, Dooley E, Hawksworth N, Hiller J, Terill NJ, Hafezi F, Brahma AK, Quantock AJ, Meek KM. Riboflavin/UVA collagen cross-linking-induced changes in normal and keratoconus corneal stroma. PLoS One. 2011;6(8), e22405.
36. Wollensak G, Redl B. Gel electrophoretic analysis of corneal collagen after photodynamic cross-linking treatment. Cornea. 2008;27(3):353–6.
37. Wollensak G, Spoerl E, Reber F, Seiler T. Keratocyte cytotoxicity of Riboflavin/UVA-treatment in vitro. Eye. 2004;18(7):718–22.
38. Wollensak G, Sporl E, Reber F, Pillunat L, Funk R. Corneal endothelial cytotoxicity of riboflavin/UVA treatment in vitro. Ophthalmic Res. 2003;35(6):324–8.
39. Wollensak G, Spoerl E, Wilsch M, Seiler T. Endothelial damage after riboflavin-ultraviolet-A treatment in the rabbit. J Cataract Refract Surg. 2003;29(9):1786–90.
40. Spoerl E, Mrochen M, Sliney D, et al. Safety of UVA riboflavin cross-linking of the cornea. Cornea. 2007;26(4):385–9.
41. Scnitzler E, Sporl E, Seiler T. Crosslinking of the corneal collagen by UV radiation with riboflavin for the mode of treatment melting ulcer of the cornea, first results of four patients. Klin Monbl Augenheilkd. 2000;217(3):190–3.
42. Caporossi A, Baiocchi S, Mazzotta C, et al. Parasurgical therapy for keratoconus by riboflavin-ultraviolet type A rays induced cross-linking of the corneal collagen; preliminary refractive results in an Italian study. J Cataract Refract Surg. 2006;32(5): 837–45.

43. Vinciguerra P, Albe E, Trazza S, et al. Refractive, topographic, tomographic, and abberometric analysis of keratoconic eyes undergoing corneal cross-linking. Ophthalmology. 2009;116(3):369–78.
44. Coskunseven E, Jankov 2nd MR, Hafezi F. Contralateral eye study of corneal collagen cross-linking with riboflavin and UVA radiation in patients with keratoconus. J Refract Surg. 2009;25(4):371–6.
45. Agrawal VB. Corneal collagen cross-linking with riboflavin and ultraviolet—a light for keratoconus: results in Indian eyes. Indian J Ophthalmol. 2009;57(2):111–4.
46. Arbelaez MC, Sekito MB, Vidal C, Choudhury SR. Collagen cross-linking with riboflavin and ultraviolet-a light in keratoconus: one-year results. Oman J Ophthalmol. 2009;2(1):33–8.
47. Vinciguerra P, Albè E, Trazza S, Seiler T, Epstein D. Intraoperative and postoperative effects of corneal collagen cross-linking on progressive keratoconus. Arch Ophthalmol. 2009;127(10):1258–65.
48. Fournié P, Galiacy S, Arné JL, Malecaze F. [Corneal collagen cross-linking with ultraviolet-A light and riboflavin for the treatment of progressive keratoconus]. J Fr Ophtalmol. 2009;32(1):1–7.
49. Henriquez MA, Izquierdo Jr L, Bernilla C, Zakrzewski PA, Mannis M. Riboflavin/Ultraviolet A corneal collagen cross-linking for the treatment of keratoconus: visual outcomes and Scheimpflug analysis. Cornea. 2011;30(3):281–6.
50. Kampik D, Koch M, Kampik K, Geerling G. Corneal riboflavin/UV-A collagen cross-linking (CXL) in keratoconus: two-year results. Klin Monbl Augenheilkd. 2011;228(6):525–30.
51. Goldich Y, Marcovich AL, Barkana Y, Mandel Y, Hirsh A, Morad Y, Avni I, Zadok D. Clinical and corneal biomechanical changes after collagen cross-linking with riboflavin and UV irradiation in patients with progressive keratoconus: results after 2 years of follow-up. Cornea. 2012;31(6):609–14.
52. Asri D, Touboul D, Fournié P, Malet F, Garra C, Gallois A, Malecaze F, Colin J. Corneal collagen crosslinking in progressive keratoconus: multicenter results from the French National Reference Center for Keratoconus. J Cataract Refract Surg. 2011;37(12):2137–43.
53. Hersh PS, Greenstein SA, Fry KL. Corneal collagen crosslinking for keratoconus and corneal ectasia: one-year results. J Cataract Refract Surg. 2011;37(1):149–60.
54. Arora R, Gupta D, Goyal JL, Jain P. Results of corneal collagen cross-linking in pediatric patients. J Refract Surg. 2012;28(11):759–62.
55. Vinciguerra P, Albé E, Frueh BE, Trazza S, Epstein D. Two-year corneal cross-linking results in patients younger than 18 years with documented progressive keratoconus. Am J Ophthalmol. 2012;154(3):520–6.
56. Ivarsen A, Hjortdal J. Collagen cross-linking for advanced progressive keratoconus. Cornea. 2013;32(7):903–6.
57. Hafezi F, Kanellopoulos J, Wiltfang R, Seiler T. Corneal collagen crosslinking with riboflavin and ultraviolet A to treat induced keratectasia after laser in situ keratomileusis. J Cataract Refract Surg. 2007;33(12):2035–40.
58. Vinciguerra P, Camesasca FI, Albè E, Trazza S. Corneal collagen cross-linking for ectasia after excimer laser refractive surgery: 1-year results. J Refract Surg. 2010;26(7):486–97.
59. Salgado JP, Khoramnia R, Lohmann CP, Winkler von Mohrenfels C. Corneal collagen crosslinking in post-LASIK keratectasia. Br J Ophthalmol. 2011;95(4):493–7.
60. Richoz O, Mavrakanas N, Pajic B, Hafezi F. Corneal collagen cross-linking for ectasia after LASIK and photorefractive keratectomy: long-term results. Ophthalmology. 2013;120(7):1354–9.
61. Spadea L. Corneal collagen cross-linking with riboflavin and UVA irradiation in pellucid marginal degeneration. J Refract Surg. 2010;26(5):375–7.
62. Hassan Z, Nemeth G, Modis L, Szalai E, Berta A. Collagen cross-linking in the treatment of pellucid marginal degeneration. Indian J Ophthalmol. 2013;10.
63. Bayraktar S, Cebeci Z, Oray M, Alparslan N. Corneal collagen cross-linking in pellucid marginal degeneration: 2 patients, 4 eyes. Case Rep Ophthalmol Med. 2015;2015:840687.
64. O'Brart DP, Chan E, Samaras K, Patel P, Shah SP. A randomised, prospective study to investigate the efficacy of riboflavin/ultraviolet A (370 nm) corneal collagen cross-linkage to halt the progression of keratoconus. Br J Ophthalmol. 2011;95(11):1519–24.
65. Wittig-Silva C. A randomized controlled trial of corneal collagen cross-linking in progressive keratoconus; preliminary results. J Refract Surg. 2008;24(7):S720–5.
66. Wittig-Silva C, Chan E, Islam FM, Wu T, Whiting M, Snibson GR. A randomized, controlled trial of corneal collagen cross-linking in progressive keratoconus: three-year results. Ophthalmology. 2014;121(4):812–21.
67. Chang CY, Hersh PS. Corneal collagen cross-linking: a review of 1-year outcomes. Eye Contact Lens. 2014;40(6):345–52.
68. Greenstein SA, Fry KL, Hersh PS. Corneal topography indices after corneal collagen crosslinking for keratoconus and corneal ectasia: one-year results. J Cataract Refract Surg. 2011;37(7):1282–90.
69. Lang SJ, Messmer EM, Geerling G, Mackert MJ, Brunner T, Dollak S, Kutchoukov B, Böhringer D, Reinhard T, Maier P. Prospective, randomized, double-blind trial to investigate the efficacy and safety of corneal cross-linking to halt the progression of keratoconus. BMC Ophthalmol. 2015;15:78.
70. Seyedian MA, Aliakbari S, Miraftab M, Hashemi H, Asgari S, Khabazkhoob M. Corneal collagen cross-linking in the treatment of progressive keratoconus: a randomized controlled contralateral eye study. Middle East Afr J Ophthalmol. 2015;22(3):340–5.

71. Sharma N, Suri K, Sehra SV, Titiyal JS, Sinha R, Tandon R, Vajpayee RB. Collagen cross-linking in keratoconus in Asian eyes: visual, refractive and confocal microscopy outcomes in a prospective randomized controlled trial. Int Ophthalmol. 2015;35(6):827–32.
72. Raiskup-Wolf F, Hoyer A, Spoerl E, Pillunat LE. Collagen cross-linking with riboflavin and ultraviolet A light in keratoconus: long term results. J Cataract Refract Surg. 2008;34(5):796–801.
73. Caporossi A, Mazzotta C, Baiocchi S, Caporossi T. Long-term results of riboflavin ultraviolet a corneal collagen cross-linking for keratoconus in Italy: the Siena eye cross study. Am J Ophthalmol. 2010;149(4):585–93.
74. O'Brart DP, Kwong TQ, Patel P, McDonald RJ, O'Brart NA. Long-term follow-up of riboflavin/ultraviolet A (370 nm) corneal collagen cross-linking to halt the progression of keratoconus. Br J Ophthalmol. 2013;97(4):433–7.
75. Hashemi H, Seyedian MA, Miraftab M, Fotouhi A, Asgari S. Corneal collagen cross-linking with riboflavin and ultraviolet A irradiation for keratoconus: long-term results. Ophthalmology. 2013;120(8):1515–20.
76. Poli M, Lefevre A, Auxenfans C, Burillon C. Corneal collagen cross-linking for the treatment of progressive corneal ectasia: 6-year prospective outcome in a French population. Am J Ophthalmol. 2015;160(4):654–62.
77. Theuring A, Spoerl E, Pillunat LE, Raiskup F. Corneal collagen cross-linking with riboflavin and ultraviolet-A light in progressive keratoconus. Results after 10-year follow-up. Ophthalmologe. 2015;112(2):140–7.
78. Raiskup F, Theuring A, Pillunat LE, Spoerl E. Corneal collagen crosslinking with riboflavin and ultraviolet-A light in progressive keratoconus: ten-year results. J Cataract Refract Surg. 2015;41(1):41–6.
79. O'Brart DP, Patel P, Lascaratos G, Wagh VK, Tam C, Lee J, O'Brart NA. Corneal cross-linking to halt the progression of keratoconus and corneal ectasia: seven-year follow-up. Am J Ophthalmol. 2015;160(6):1154–63.
80. Javadi MA, Motlagh BF, Jafarinasab MR, et al. Outcomes of penetrating keratoplasty in keratoconus. Cornea. 2005;24:941–6.
81. Gore D, Margineanu A, French P, O'Brart D, Dunsby C, Allan D. Two-photon fluorescence microscopy of corneal riboflavin absorption. Invest Ophthamol Vis Sci. 2014;55(4):2476–81.
82. Jain V, Gazali Z, Bidayi R. Isotonic riboflavin and HPMC with accelerated cross-linking protocol. Cornea. 2014;33(9):910–3.
83. Verma S, Corbett MC, Marshall J. A prospective, randomized, double-masked trial to evaluate the role of topical anesthetics in controlling pain after photorefractive keratectomy. Ophthalmology. 1995;102(12):1918–24.
84. Croxatto JO, Tytiun AE, Argento CJ. Sequential in vivo confocal microscopy study of corneal wound healing after cross-linking in patients with keratoconus. J Refract Surg. 2009;24:1–8.
85. Mazzotta C, Balestrazzi A, Traversi C, et al. Treatment of progressive keratoconus by riboflavin UVA induced cross linking of corneal collagen: ultrastructural analysis by Heidelberg retinal tomography II in vivo confocal microscopy in humans. Cornea. 2007;26(4):390–7.
86. Mazzotta C, Balestrazzi A, Baiocchi S. Stromal haze after combined riboflavin-UVA corneal collagen cross-linking in keratoconus: in vivo confocal microscopic evaluation. Clin Exp Ophthalmol. 2007;35(6):580–2.
87. Seiler T, Hafezi F. Corneal cross-linking induced stromal demarcation line. Cornea. 2006;25(9):1057–9.
88. Mencucci R, Marini M, Paladini I, Sarchielli E, Sgambati E, Menchini U, Vannelli GB. Effects of riboflavin/UVA corneal cross-linking on keratocytes and collagen fibres in human cornea. Clin Experiment Ophthalmol. 2010;38(1):49–56.
89. Akhtar S, Almubrad T, Paladini I, Mencucci R. Keratoconus corneal architecture after riboflavin/ultraviolet A cross-linking: ultrastructural studies. Mol Vis. 2013;19:1526–37.
90. Messmer EM, Meyer P, Herwig MC, Loeffler KU, Schirra F, Seitz B, Thiel M, Reinhard T, Kampik A, Auw-Haedrich C. Morphological and immunohistochemical changes after corneal cross-linking. Cornea. 2013;32(2):111–7.
91. Hayes S, O'Brart DP, Lamdin LS, Doutch J, Samaras K, Meek KM, Marshall J. An investigation into the importance of complete epithelial debridement prior to riboflavin/ultraviolet A (UVA) corneal collagen crosslinkage therapy. J Cat Ref Surg. 2008;34:557–61.
92. Samaras K, O'Brart DPS, Doutch J, Hayes S, Marshall J, Meek K. Effect of epithelial retention and removal on riboflavin absorption in porcine corneas. J Refract Surg. 2009;25(9):771–5.
93. Tariq AA, O'Brart DPS, O'Brart AL, Meek KM. An investigation of trans-epithelial stromal Riboflavin absorption with Ricrolin TE ® (Riboflavin 0.1% with trometamol and sodium EDTA) using spectrophotometry. J Cat Ref Surg. 2012;38:884–9.
94. Chan C, Sharma M, Wachler B. Effect of inferior segment Intacs with and without C3-R on keratoconus. J Cataract Refract Surg. 2007;33(1):75–80.
95. Filippello M, Stagni E, O'Brart D. Trans-epithelial corneal collagen cross-linking: a bilateral, prospective study. J Cat Ref Surg. 2012;38(2):283–91.
96. Kissner A, Spoerl E, Jung R, Spekl K, Pillunat LE, Raiskup F. Pharmacological modification of the epithelial permeability by benzalkonium chloride in UVA/Riboflavin corneal collagen cross-linking. Curr Eye Res. 2010;35(8):715–21.
97. Samaras KE, Lake DB. Corneal collagen cross linking: a review. Int Ophthalmol Clin. 2010; 50(3):89–100.
98. Vinciguerra R, Spoerl E, Romano MR, Rosetta P, Vinciguerra P. Comparative stress strain measure-

ments of human corneas after Transepithelial UV-A induced cross-linking: impregnation with iontophoresis, different riboflavin solutions and irradiance power. Invest Ophthalmol Vis Sci. 2012;53:1518 [ARVO 2012 Abstract].

99. Raiskup F, Pinelli R, Spoerl E. Riboflavin osmolar modification for transepithelial corneal cross-linking. Curr Eye Res. 2012;37(3):234–8.
100. Rechichi M, Daya S, Scorcia V, Meduri A, Scorcia G. Epithelial-disruption collagen crosslinking for keratoconus: one-year results. J Cataract Refract Surg. 2013;39(8):1171–8.
101. Hashemi H, Miraftab M, Hafezi F, Asgari S. Matched comparison study of total and partial epithelium removal in corneal cross-linking. J Refract Surg. 2015;31(2):110–5.
102. Razmjoo H, Rahimi B, Kharraji M, Koosha N, Peyman A. Corneal haze and visual outcome after collagen crosslinking for keratoconus: a comparison between total epithelium off and partial epithelial removal methods. Adv Biomed Res. 2014;3:221.
103. Salman AG. Transepithelial corneal collagen cross-linking for progressive keratoconus in a pediatric age group. J Cataract Refract Surg. 2013;39(8):1164–70.
104. Magli A, Forte R, Tortori A, Capasso L, Marsico G, Piozzi E. Epithelium-off corneal collagen cross-linking versus transepithelial cross-linking for pediatric keratoconus. Cornea. 2013;32(5):597–601.
105. Buzzonetti L, Petrocelli G. Transepithelial corneal cross-linking in pediatric patients: early results. J Refract Surg. 2012;28(11):763–7.
106. Caporossi A, Mazzotta C, Paradiso AL, Baiocchi S, Marigliani D, Caporossi T. Transepithelial corneal collagen crosslinking for progressive keratoconus: 24-month clinical results. J Cataract Refract Surg. 2013;39(8):1157–63.
107. Leccisotti A, Islam T. Transepithelial corneal collagen cross-linking in keratoconus. J Refract Surg. 2010;26(12):942–8.
108. Koppen C, Wouters K, Mathysen D, Rozema J, Tassignon MJ. Refractive and topographic results of benzalkonium chloride-assisted transepithelial cross-linking. J Cataract Refract Surg. 2012;38(6):1000–5.
109. Yuksel E, Novruzlu S, Ozmen MC, Bilgihan K. A study comparing standard and transepithelial collagen cross-linking riboflavin solutions: epithelial findings and pain scores. J Ocul Pharmacol Ther. 2015;31(5):296–302.
110. Rossi S, Orrico A, Santamaria C, Romano V, De Rosa L, Simonelli F, De Rosa G. Standard versus trans-epithelial collagen cross-linking in keratoconus patients suitable for standard collagen cross-linking. Clin Ophthalmol. 2015;9:503–9. doi:10.2147/OPTH.S73991 [eCollection 2015].
111. Nawaz S, Gupta S, Gogia V, Sasikala NK, Panda A. Trans-epithelial versus conventional corneal collagen crosslinking: a randomized trial in keratoconus. Oman J Ophthalmol. 2015;8(1):9–13.
112. Al Fayez MF, Alfayez S, Alfayez Y. Transepithelial versus epithelium-Off corneal collagen cross-linking for progressive keratoconus: a prospective randomized controlled trial. Cornea. 2015;34 Suppl 10:S53–6.
113. Soeters N, Wisse RP, Godefrooij DA, Imhof SM, Tahzib NG. Transepithelial versus epithelium-off corneal cross-linking for the treatment of progressive keratoconus: a randomized controlled trial. Am J Ophthalmol. 2015;159(5):821–8.
114. Kocak I, Aydin A, Kaya F, Koc H. Comparison of transepithelial corneal collagen crosslinking with epithelium-off crosslinking in progressive keratoconus. J Fr Ophtalmol. 2014;37(5):371–6.
115. Gore DM, French P, O'Brart D, Dunsby C, Allan BD. Two-photon fluorescence microscopy of corneal riboflavin absorption through an intact epithelium. Invest Ophthamol Vis Sci. 2015;56(2): 1191–2.
116. Gore DM, O'Brart D, Dunsby C, French P, Allan BD. Transepithelial riboflavin absorption in an ex-vivo rabbit corneal model. Invest Ophthamol Vis Sci. 2015;56(8):5006–11.
117. Cassagne M, Laurent C, Rodrigues M, Galinier A, Spoerl E, Galiacy SD, Soler V, Fournié P, Malecaze F. Iontophoresis transcorneal delivery technique for transepithelial corneal collagen crosslinking with riboflavin in a rabbit model. Invest Ophthalmol Vis Sci. 2016;57:594–603. doi:10.1167/iovs.13-12595 [Epub ahead of print].
118. Vinciguerra P, Mencucci R, Romano V, Spoerl E, Camesasca FI, Favuzza E, Azzolini C, Mastropasqua R, Vinciguerra R. Imaging mass spectrometry by matrix-assisted laser desorption/ionization and stress-strain measurements in iontophoresis transepithelial corneal collagen cross-linking. Biomed Res Int. 2014;2014:404587. doi:10.1155/2014/404587 [Epub 2014 Sep 2].
119. Mastropasqua L, Lanzini M, Curcio C, Calienno R, Mastropasqua R, Colasante M, Mastropasqua A, Nubile M. Structural modifications and tissue response after standard epi-off and iontophoretic corneal cross-linking with different irradiation procedures. Invest Ophthalmol Vis Sci. 2014;55(4):2526–33.
120. Lombardo M, Serrao S, Rosati M, Ducoli P, Lombardo G. Biomechanical changes in the human cornea after transepithelial corneal crosslinking using iontophoresis. J Cataract Refract Surg. 2014;40(10):1706–15.
121. Bikbova G, Bikbov M. Transepithelial corneal collagen cross-linking by iontophoresis of riboflavin. Acta Ophthalmol. 2014;92(1):e30–4.
122. Vinciguerra P, Randleman JB, Romano V, Legrottaglie EF, Rosetta P, Camesasca FI, Piscopo R, Azzolini C, Vinciguerra R. Transepithelial iontophoresis corneal collagen cross-linking for progressive keratoconus: initial clinical outcomes. J Refract Surg. 2014;30(11):746–53.
123. Li N, Fan Z, Peng X, Pang X, Tian C. Clinical observation of transepithelial corneal collagen cross-linking by lontophoresis of riboflavin in treatment of keratoconus. Eye Sci. 2014;29(3):160–4.

124. Buzzonetti L, Petrocelli G, Valente P, Iarossi G, Ardia R, Petroni S. Iontophoretic transepithelial corneal cross-linking to halt keratoconus in pediatric cases: 15-month follow-up. Cornea. 2015;34(5):512–5.
125. Hayes S, Morgan S, O'Brart D P, O'Brart N, Meek KM. A study of stromal riboflavin absorption using new and existing delivery protocols for corneal cross-linking. Acta Ophthalmol. 2016 Mar;94(2): e109–17.
126. Gore DM, O'Brart D, Dunsby C, French P, Allan BD. A comparison of different corneal iontophoresis protocols for promoting transepithelial riboflavin penetration. Invest Ophthalmol Vis Sci. 2015;56(13):7908–14.
127. Lamy R, Chan E, Zhang H, Salgaonkar VA, Good SD, Porco TC, Diederich CJ, Stewart JM. Ultrasound-enhanced penetration of topical riboflavin into the corneal stroma. Invest Ophthalmol Vis Sci. 2013;54(8):5908–12.
128. Bottos KM, Oliveira AG, Bersanetti PA, Nogueira RF, Lima-Filho AA, Cardillo JA, Schor P, Chamon W. Corneal absorption of a new riboflavin-nanostructured system for transepithelial collagen cross-linking. PLoS One. 2013;8(6), e66408.
129. Ostacolo C, Caruso C, Tronino D, Troisi S, Laneri S, Pacente L, Del Prete A, Sacchi A. Enhancement of corneal permeation of riboflavin-5'-phosphate through vitamin E TPGS: a promising approach in corneal trans-epithelial cross linking treatment. Int J Pharm. 2013;440(2):148–53.
130. Kanellopoulos AJ. Collagen cross-linking in early keratoconus with riboflavin in a femtosecond laser-created pocket: initial clinical results. J Refract Surg. 2009;25(11):1034–7.
131. Beshtawi IM, Akhtar R, Hillarby MC, O'Donnell C, Zhao X, Brahma A, Carley F, Derby B, Radhakrishnan H. Biomechanical properties of human corneas following low- and high-intensity collagen cross-linking determined with scanning acoustic microscopy. Invest Ophthalmol Vis Sci. 2013;54(8):5273–80.
132. Schumacher S, Oeftiger L, Mrochen M. Equivalence of biomechanical changes induced by rapid and standard corneal cross-linking, using riboflavin and ultraviolet radiation. Invest Ophthalmol Vis Sci. 2011;52(12):9048–52.
133. Wernli J, Schumacher S, Spoerl E, Mrochen M. The efficacy of corneal cross-linking shows a sudden decrease with very high intensity UV light and short treatment time. Invest Ophthalmol Vis Sci. 2013;54(2):1176–80.
134. Cınar Y, Cingü AK, Turkcu FM, Yüksel H, Sahin A, Yıldırım A, Caca I, Cınar T. Accelerated corneal collagen cross-linking for progressive keratoconus. Cutan Ocul Toxicol. 2014;33(2):168–71.
135. Shetty R, Nagaraja H, Jayadev C, Pahuja NK, Kurian Kummelil M, Nuijts RM. Accelerated corneal collagen cross-linking in pediatric patients: two-year follow-up results. Biomed Res Int. 2014;2014:894095.
136. Marino GK, Torricelli AA, Giacomin N, Santhiago MR, Espindola R, Netto MV. Accelerated corneal collagen cross-linking for postoperative LASIK ectasia: two-year outcomes. J Refract Surg. 2015;31(6):380–4.
137. Elbaz U, Shen C, Lichtinger A, Zauberman NA, Goldich Y, Chan CC, Slomovic AR, Rootman DS. Accelerated (9-mW/cm2) corneal collagen crosslinking for keratoconus-A 1-year follow-up. Cornea. 2014;33(8):769–73.
138. Ng AL, Chan TC, Cheng AC. Conventional versus accelerated corneal collagen cross-linking in the treatment of keratoconus. Clin Experiment Ophthalmol. 2015. doi:10.1111/ceo.12571 [Epub ahead of print].
139. Brittingham S, Tappeiner C, Frueh BE. Corneal cross-linking in keratoconus using the standard and rapid treatment protocol: differences in demarcation line and 12-month outcomes. Invest Ophthalmol Vis Sci. 2014;55(12):8371–6.
140. Kanellopoulos AJ. Long term results of a prospective randomized bilateral eye comparison trial of higher fluence, shorter duration ultraviolet A radiation, and riboflavin collagen cross linking for progressive keratoconus. Clin Ophthalmol. 2012;6: 97–101.
141. Hashemian H, Jabbarvand M, Khodaparast M, Ameli K. Evaluation of corneal changes after conventional versus accelerated corneal cross-linking: a randomized controlled trial. J Refract Surg. 2014;30(12):837–42.
142. Hashemi H, Fotouhi A, Miraftab M, Bahrmandy H, Seyedian MA, Amanzadeh K, Heidarian S, Nikbin H, Asgari S. Short-term comparison of accelerated and standard methods of corneal collagen crosslinking. J Cataract Refract Surg. 2015;41(3):533–40.
143. Shetty R, Pahuja NK, Nuijts RM, Ajani A, Jayadev C, Sharma C, Nagaraja H. Current protocols of corneal collagen cross-linking: visual, refractive, and tomographic outcomes. Am J Ophthalmol. 2015;160(2):243–9.
144. Sherif AM. Accelerated versus conventional corneal collagen cross-linking in the treatment of mild keratoconus: a comparative study. Clin Ophthalmol. 2014;8:1435–40.
145. Nada H, Aldahlawi AH, Hayes S, O'Brart DPS, Meek KM. Standard versus accelerated riboflavin/ultraviolet corneal cross-linking: resistance against enzymatic digestion. J Cataract Refract Surg. 2015;41(9):1989–96.
146. Kymionis GD, Tsoulnaras KI, Grentzelos MA, Liakopoulos DA, Tsakalis NG, Blazaki SV, Paraskevopoulos TA, Tsilimbaris MK. Evaluation of corneal stromal demarcation line depth following standard and a modified-accelerated collagen cross-linking protocol. Am J Ophthalmol. 2014;158(4):671–5.
147. Mazzotta C, Traversi C, Paradiso AL, Latronico ME, Rechichi M. Pulsed light accelerated crosslinking versus continuous light accelerated crosslinking: One-year results. J Ophthalmol. 2014;2014:604731.

148. Moramarco A, Iovieno A, Sartori A, Fontana L. Corneal stromal demarcation line after accelerated crosslinking using continuous and pulsed light. J Cataract Refract Surg. 2015;41(11):2546–51.
149. Raiskup F, Spoerl E. Corneal cross-linking with hypo-osmolar riboflavin solution in thin keratoconic corneas. Am J Ophthalmol. 2011;152(1):28–32.
150. Nassaralla BA, Vieira DM, Machado ML, Figueiredo MN, Nassaralla Jr JJ. Corneal thickness changes during corneal collagen cross-linking with UV-A irradiation and hypo-osmolar riboflavin in thin corneas. Arq Bras Oftalmol. 2013;76(3):155–8.
151. Kymionis GD, Portaliou DM, Diakonis VF, Kounis GA, Panagopoulou SI, Grentzelos MA. Corneal collagen cross-linking with riboflavin and ultraviolet-A irradiation in patients with thin corneas. Am J Ophthalmol. 2012;153(1):24–8.
152. Hafezi F. Limitation of collagen cross-linking with hypoosmolar riboflavin solution: failure in an extremely thin cornea. Cornea. 2011;30(8):917–9.
153. Spadea L, Mencucci R. Transepithelial corneal collagen cross-linking in ultrathin keratoconic corneas. Clin Ophthalmol. 2012;6:1785–92. doi:10.2147/OPTH.S37335 [Epub 2012 Nov 2].
154. Jacob S, Kumar DA, Agarwal A, Basu S, Sinha P, Agarwal A. Contact lens-assisted collagen cross-linking (CACXL): a new technique for cross-linking thin corneas. J Refract Surg. 2014;30(6):366–72.
155. Mazzotta C, Ramovecchi V. Customized epithelial debridement for thin ectatic corneas undergoing corneal cross-linking: epithelial island cross-linking technique. Clin Ophthalmol. 2014;8:1337–43.
156. Reinstein DZ, Gobbe M, Archer TJ, Silverman RH, Coleman DJ. Epithelial, stromal, and total corneal thickness in keratoconus: three-dimensional display with artemis very-high frequency digital ultrasound. J Refract Surg. 2010;26(4):259–71.
157. Kapasi M, Baath J, Mintsioulis G, Jackson WB, Baig K. Phototherapeutic keratectomy versus mechanical epithelial removal followed by corneal collagen crosslinking for keratoconus. Can J Ophthalmol. 2012;47(4):344–7.
158. Kymionis GD, Grentzelos MA, Kounis GA, Diakonis VF, Limnopoulou AN, Panagopoulou SI. Combined transepithelial phototherapeutic keratectomy and corneal collagen cross-linking for progressive keratoconus. Ophthalmology. 2012;119(9):1777–84.
159. Kymionis GD, Grentzelos MA, Kankariya VP, Liakopoulos DA, Karavitaki AE, Portaliou DM, Tsoulnaras KI, Pallikaris IG. Long-term results of combined transepithelial phototherapeutic keratectomy and corneal collagen crosslinking for keratoconus: Cretan protocol. J Cataract Refract Surg. 2014;40(9):1439–45.
160. Kanellopoulos AJ, Binder PS. Management of corneal ectasia after LASIK with combined, same-day, topography-guided partial transepithelial PRK and collagen cross-linking: the athens protocol. J Refract Surg. 2011;27(5):323–31.
161. Kymionis GD, Portaliou DM, Diakonis VF, Karavitaki AE, Panagopoulou SI, Jankov Ii MR, Coskunseven E. Management of post laser in situ keratomileusis ectasia with simultaneous topography guided photorefractive keratectomy and collagen cross-linking. Open Ophthalmol J. 2011;5:11–3.
162. Krueger RR, Kanellopoulos AJ. Stability of simultaneous topography-guided photorefractive keratectomy and riboflavin/UVA cross-linking for progressive keratoconus: case reports. J Refract Surg. 2010;26(10):S827–32.
163. Alessio G, L'abbate M, Sborgia C, La Tegola MG. Photorefractive keratectomy followed by cross-linking versus cross-linking alone for management of progressive keratoconus: two-year follow-up. Am J Ophthalmol. 2013;155(1):54–65.
164. Lin DT, Holland S, Tan JC, Moloney G. Clinical results of topography-based customized ablations in highly aberrated eyes and keratoconus/ectasia with cross-linking. J Refract Surg. 2012;28(11 Suppl):S841–8.
165. Sakla H, Altroudi W, Muñoz G, Albarrán-Diego C. Simultaneous topography-guided partial photorefractive keratectomy and corneal collagen crosslinking for keratoconus. J Cataract Refract Surg. 2014;40(9):1430–8.
166. Labiris G, Giarmoukakis A, Sideroudi H, Gkika M, Fanariotis M, Kozobolis V. Impact of keratoconus, cross-linking and cross-linking combined with photorefractive keratectomy on self-reported quality of life. Cornea. 2012;31(7):734–9.
167. Kanellopoulos AJ, Asimellis G. Keratoconus management: long-term stability of topography-guided normalization combined with high-fluence CXL stabilization (the Athens Protocol). J Refract Surg. 2014;30(2):88–93.
168. Kymionis GD, Portaliou DM, Diakonis VF, Kontadakis GA, Krasia MS, Papadiamantis AG, Coskunseven E, Pallikaris AI. Posterior linear stromal haze formation after simultaneous photorefractive keratectomy followed by corneal collagen cross-linking. Invest Ophthalmol Vis Sci. 2010;51(10):5030–3.
169. Güell JL, Verdaguer P, Elies D, Gris O, Manero F. Late onset of a persistent, deep stromal scarring after PRK and corneal cross-linking in a patient with forme fruste keratoconus. J Refract Surg. 2014;30(4):286–8.
170. Coskunseven E, Jankov 2nd MR, Grentzelos MA, Plaka AD, Limnopoulou AN, Kymionis GD. Topography-guided transepithelial PRK after intracorneal ring segments implantation and corneal collagen CXL in a three-step procedure for keratoconus. J Refract Surg. 2013;29(1):54–8.
171. Ertan A, Karacal H, Kamburoğlu G. Refractive and topographic results of transepithelial cross-linking treatment in eyes with intacs. Cornea. 2009;28(7):719–23.

172. Renesto Ada C, Melo Jr LA, Sartori Mde F, Campos M. Sequential topical riboflavin with or without ultraviolet a radiation with delayed intracorneal ring segment insertion for keratoconus. Am J Ophthalmol. 2012;153(5):982–93.
173. El-Raggal TM. Sequential versus concurrent KERARINGS insertion and corneal collagen cross-linking for keratoconus. Br J Ophthalmol. 2011; 95(1):37–41.
174. Kanellopoulos AJ. Long-term safety and efficacy follow-up of prophylactic higher fluence collagen cross-linking in high myopic laser-assisted in situ keratomileusis. Clin Ophthalmol. 2012;6: 1125–30.
175. Celik HU, Alagöz N, Yildirim Y, Agca A, Marshall J, Demirok A, Yilmaz OF. Accelerated corneal cross-linking concurrent with laser in situ keratomileusis. J Cataract Refract Surg. 2012;38(8):1424–31.
176. Kanellopoulos AJ, Kahn J. Topography-guided hyperopic LASIK with and without high irradiance collagen cross-linking: initial comparative clinical findings in a contralateral eye study of 34 consecutive patients. J Refract Surg. 2012;28(11 Suppl):S837–40.
177. Kanellopoulos AJ, Asimellis G. Combined laser in situ keratomileusis and prophylactic high-fluence corneal collagen crosslinking for high myopia: two-year safety and efficacy. J Cataract Refract Surg. 2015;41(7):1426–33.
178. Rocha KM, Ramos-Esteban JC, Qian Y, et al. Comparative study of riboflavin-UVA cross-linking and "flash-linking" using wave elastometry. J Refract Surg. 2008;24(7):S748–51.
179. Paik D, Wen Q, Braunstein RE, et al. Initial studies using ali phatic ß-nitro alcohols for therapeutic corneal cross linking. Invest Ophthalmol Vis Sci. 2009;50(3):1098–105.
180. Cherfan D, Verter EE, Melki S, Gisel TE, Doyle Jr FJ, Scarcelli G, Yun SH, Redmond RW, Kochevar IE. Collagen cross-linking using rose bengal and green light to increase corneal stiffness. Invest Ophthalmol Vis Sci. 2013;54(5): 3426–33.

20 Complications of Corneal Collagen Cross-Linking

David O'Brart

20.1 Introduction

Riboflavin/Ultraviolet A (UVA) corneal collagen cross-linking (CXL) is the first treatment modality that may halt the progression of keratoconus and other corneal ectatic disorders. Within the scientific literature there are multiple published prospective case series [1–12] and randomised controlled trials [13–15] with up to 36-month follow-up supporting its efficacy in keratoconus, including paediatric [16, 17] and advanced cases [18], pellucid marginal degeneration [19, 20] and iatrogenic ectasia [21–23]. In addition to cessation of progression, most investigators have also reported consistent improvements in visual, keratometric and topographic parameters with time [1–23].

Its precise mechanism of action at a molecular level is as yet not fully determined. At present follow-up is limited to 7–10 years but suggests continued stability and improvement in corneal shape with time [24, 25]. Most published data is with epithelium-off techniques [1 25]. Epithelium-on studies suggest some efficacy but less than with the epithelium-off procedures and long-term data are not currently available [26–28]. The use of Riboflavin/UVA CXL for in management of infectious and non-infectious keratitis appears very promising [29–32]. Its use in the management of bullous keratopathy is equivocal [33–35].

20.2 Adverse Effects of CXL

Whilst clinical studies indicate that it is a safe procedure with few sight-threatening complications, adverse events can occur. Complications attributable to CXL include corneal haze and scarring, infectious and non-infectious keratitis, endothelial failure, treatment failure with progression of ectasia, excessive corneal flattening with associated hyperopic shift and possible limbal stem cell changes.

20.3 Anterior Corneal Haze (the "Demarcation" Line)

An anterior, mid-stromal haze occurs in the majority of eyes after CXL, typically appearing at 2–6 weeks and clearing by 9–12 months (Fig. 20.1). It appears to be the result of an increased "density of extracellular" matrix and arises at a depth of 300–350 μm [36, 37]. It forms the so-called

D. O'Brart, M.D., F.R.C.S., F.R.C.O.phth. (✉)
Department of Ophthalmology, Guy's and St. Thomas' NHS Foundation Trust, St. Thomas' Hospital, London SE1 7EH, UK

King's College London, London, UK
e-mail: davidobrart@aol.com

J.L. Alió (ed.), *Keratoconus*, Essentials in Ophthalmology, DOI 10.1007/978-3-319-43881-8_20

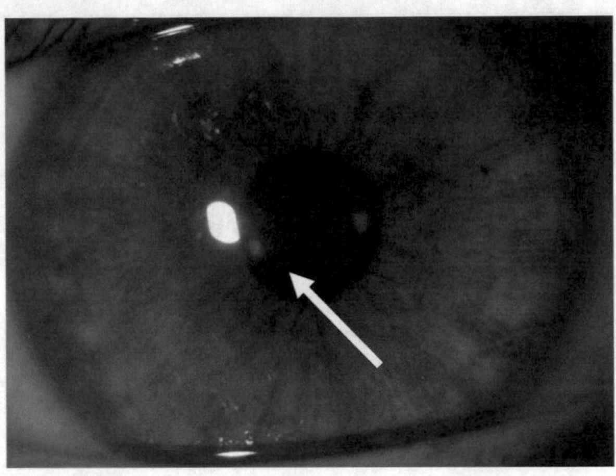

Fig. 20.1 Self- limiting stromal haze (*white arrow*) 3 months after CXL

"demarcation line" which can be easily seen on slit lamp examination [38]. As this change is self-limiting, topical cortical steroids are not indicated. The "demarcation line" has been shown to be shallower with accelerated, high fluence CXL [39] and with epithelium-on treatments [40]. It has been postulated that it represents the demarcation between cross-linked and non-cross-linked tissue and has been used by some investigators as a means of quantifying the efficacy of CXL [39]. However, it has be shown to be shallower in older patients and eyes with more advanced keratoconus receiving the same technique, with the depth of the line not being correlated to visual or keratometric changes at 6 months [41]. It is generally thicker centrally and more shallow in the para-central treated cornea [42, 43], with a deeper depth of the line centrally being found in one study to be related to a larger decrease in corneal thickness within the first 12 months after surgery [44]. Therefore while CXL is undoubtedly associated with the development of an anterior/mid-stromal haze during the first year after surgery, there is a yet no absolute evidence that it is the true delineation between cross-linked and uncross-linked tissue and may only represent a natural wound healing response. Until more evidence is forthcoming it would be unwise to consider in depth as an accurate way to assess the efficacy of any particular CXL technique [45].

20.4 Corneal Scarring

Persistent loss of corneal transparency (scarring) over the axial cornea/cone apex rather than transient changes may occur after CXL (Fig. 20.2). Raiskup et al. reported stromal scarring in 14 (8.6 %) of a series of 163 eyes at 12 months [46]. Compared to eyes without such changes, affected eyes had a higher pre-operative apex power (average power 72.0 dioptres (D)), higher 3.00 mm keratometry (average 54.75D) and thinner central pachymetry (average 420 micrometers (μm)) compared to unaffected eyes. On the basis of these findings, Raiskup et al. advised caution and careful patient counselling before CXL is undertaken in patients with advanced keratoconus [46]. However, scarring with associated impairment of post-operative visual performance has been reported in mild cases of keratoconus after CXL [47]. Therefore, all patients need to be carefully counselled pre-operatively as to this possible occurrence. Stromal scarring may also be more prevalent in eyes receiving simultaneous photorefractive keratectomy (PRK) followed by CXL. Kymoinis et al. documented the occurrence of posterior linear haze formation persistent at 12 months in a series of 13 (46 %) of 26 such treated eyes [48], while Guell reported late onset deep stromal scarring in a similarly treated patient that reoccurred after 2 years [49].

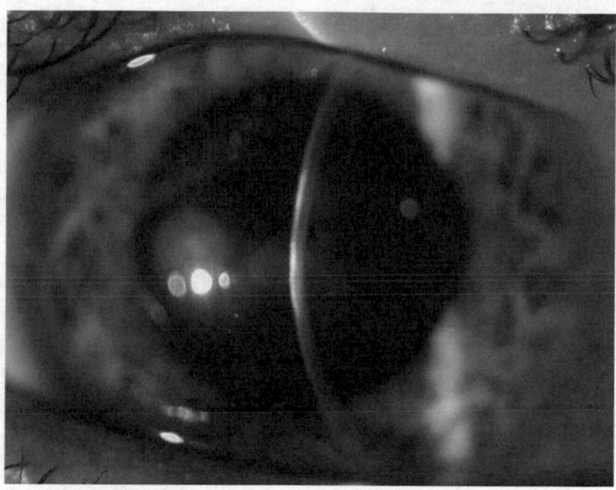

Fig. 20.2 Corneal scarring following keratitis after CXL (courtesy of Dr. Carina Koppen)

20.5 Failure of Treatment: Progression

With the standard epithelium-off technique, utilising Riboflavin 0.1 % and UVA at 3 mw/cm^2 for 30 min, the vast majority of patient achieving a follow-up of over 5 years demonstrate no progression of ectasia [24, 25, 50, 51]. Raskup-Wolf et al. in a series of 241 eyes with a follow-up of over 6 months documented progression in only 2 cases (0.8 %), which subsequently underwent re-treatment [52]. Koller et al. in their series of 117 eyes, all of which reached 12-month follow-up, reported progression of ectasia in 9 eyes (7.6 %) [53], while Ivarsen in 28 eyes with advanced keratoconus, all with a maximum keratometry greater than 55.0D and a mean follow-up of 22 months, documented progression in only one eye (3.5 %) [18]. Similarly, Sloot in a series of 53 eyes with 12-month follow-up, documented progression in only 5 (8 %), with little difference between advanced and mild keratoconic cases [54]. Such results are very encouraging and offer great hope for the control of this often visually debilitating disease [55]. Indeed although published follow-up is still limited at present in the 102 eyes reported in the long-term follow-up studies of Theuring, O'Brart and Poli, progression was evident in only 8 % of cases at 5–10 years [25, 50, 51].

20.6 Sterile Infiltrates

Sterile infiltrates occurring during the early post-operative period are not infrequent (Fig. 20.3). They typically present within the first days/weeks after CXL and resolve after within a month with topical corticosteroid medication. Koller et al. reported sterile infiltrates in 8 eyes (7.6 %) in a series of 117 cases, which resolved within 4 weeks with topical dexamethasone 0.1 % treatment [53]. Lam et al. reported a cluster of 4 cases of sterile keratitis and compared them retrospectively to 144 eyes their group treated with no such problem. They found eyes with sterile infiltrates generally had advanced keratoconus with maximum keratometry values greater than 60.0D and central corneal thicknesses less than 425 μm [56].

20.7 Non-infectious Keratitis

Whilst transient, non-sight threatening, sterile infiltrates are not uncommon, serious cases of non-infectious keratitis following CXL with significant visual loss have been occasionally reported. Koppen et al. published four cases occurring within 4 days of CXL. Two of their patients were atopic, two had permanent visual loss and one eye underwent penetrating keratoplasty [57]. Eberwein reported a single case of corneal melting associated with activation of

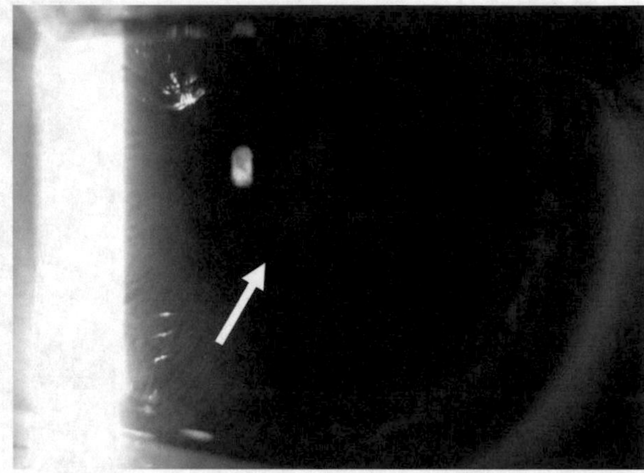

Fig. 20.3 Sterile infiltrates occurring within 1 week of CXL (*white arrow*), which gradually cleared by 6 weeks

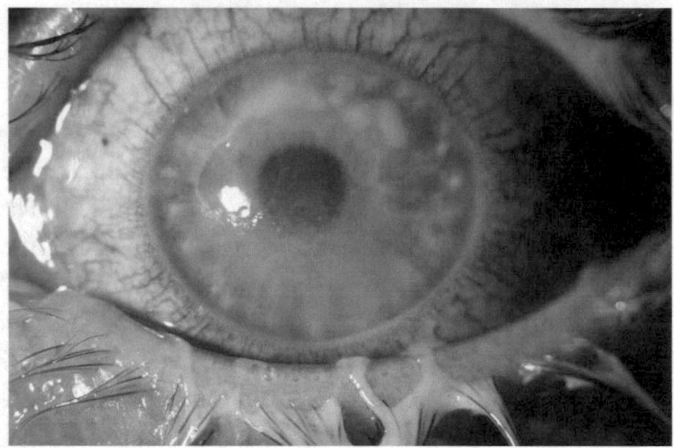

Fig. 20.4 Infectious keratitis after CXL (courtesy of Dr. Carina Koppen)

herpes simplex keratitis, which necessitated penetrating keratoplasty [58]. Whilst such episodes are rare, it is necessary to counsel patients pre-operatively of such serious sight-threatening adverse events. It is also prudent to control atopic eye disease prior to CXL, with topical and if indicated systemic medication, and to give prophylactic systemic Acyclovir to patients with a history of previous Herpetic Eye disease.

20.8 Infectious Keratitis

Infectious keratitis following CXL has been reported (Fig. 20.4). This is to be expected as debriding the corneal epithelium can expose the corneal stroma to microbial infection, during the operative and early healing phases. Most case reports of microbial infection have been bacterial in nature. Infections with *Staphylococcus epidermidis*, *Escherichia coli*, *Pseudomonas aeruginosa* and Coagulase-negative Staphylococcus have been published with resultant documented permanent visual loss [59–62]. A number of these cases have been associated with post-operative bandage contact lens use and misuse and it is necessary to inform patients not to replace, remove or try to clean these lenses themselves.

The precise incidence of microbial keratitis is as yet undetermined. It would be expected to have a much rarer occurrence than other operative procedures involving corneal epithelial debridement given the potential role of CXL in the management of corneal microbial infections [30, 63]. Shetty et al. reported four cases of infectious keratitis following CXL in a series of 2350 patients (1715 epithelium-off CXL, 310 epithelium-on CXL), giving an overall incidence of 0.0017 %

[64]. Similar to previously published reports all their cases were treated with an epithelium-off technique. All were due to Methicillin-resistant Staphylococcus Aureus (MRSA) and all had atopic dermatitis and conjunctivitis [64]. Similar to Shetty, Facciani and Rana reported post-CXL microbial keratitis due to MRSA, with an association with atopic dermatitis in one case [65] and perforation in two eyes [66]. Such reports, while anecdotal re-enforce the need to control atopic dermatitis and conjunctivitis prior to CXL and to counsel patients pre-operatively of such rare sight-threatening complications.

In addition to bacterial keratitis, other microbial pathogens have been implicated. Rama reported a case of acanthamoeba keratitis in a patient that had rinsed his bandage contact lens in tap water post-operatively and then replaced it [67]. Al-Qarni reported two cases of dendritic ulceration occurring with 2 weeks after CXL in patients with no previous history of herpetic keratitis, that responded well to topical antiviral therapy [68].

These case reports, whilst few in number compared to the hundreds of thousands of eyes that have undergone CXL worldwide, highlight the possible rare occurrence of this sight-threatening complication and the need to inform patients to immediately report and seek urgent medical advice if there is any increasing pain and redness after the initial 12–24 h period post-operatively or the occurrence of purulent discharge, so that if infectious keratitis if present it can be promptly and appropriately managed.

20.9 Endothelial Failure

Endothelial failure has been reported very occasionally after CXL resulting in corneal oedema post-operatively. Sharma et al. in a retrospective series of 350 patients treated with a standard epithelium-off protocol in eyes with corneal thicknesses greater than 400 μm after epithelial removal reported persistent problems in five patients (1.4 %), 2 of whom (0.6 %) required penetrating keratoplasty [69]. Bagga et al. reported a single case with keratouveitis and endothelial failure that required keratoplasty [70]. Whilst such complications are rare, they highlight the need to warn patients pre-operatively of severe sight-threatening complications and the very occasional need for keratoplasty after CXL. The aetiology of such problems has not been fully elucidated but endothelial damage after CXL may occur even in corneas with adequate thickness perhaps due to severe stromal thinning intra-operatively due to the use of hyper- and iso-osmolar Riboflavin solutions and/or lack of homogenicity with hot spots in the UV beams associated with the use of diodes and limited focusing/alignment systems.

20.10 Excessive Axial Flattening and Hyperopic Shift

O'Brart et al. in a long-term study of 36 eyes who underwent a standard epithelium-off technique and followed up for 7 years demonstrated continued statistically significant flattening of corneal topographic parameters between 1 and 5 years [24]. At 7 years this continued corneal flattening had resulted in a mean hyperopic shift of almost +0.8D. Eight (22 %) of the 36 eyes of the 36 patients (with a mean age less than 28 years) examined in this study experienced a hyperopic shift of over +2.0D compared to pre-operative refractive status and 4 eyes (11 %) had more than +3.0D of hyperopic refractive change [24] (Fig. 20.5). Such refractive changes with time need to be taken into consideration in the already hyperopic patient. In addition, the use of CXL has been postulated in the non-ectatic routine refractive surgery patient to improve post-operative refractive and corneal biomechanical stability in the so-called LASIK Extra procedure [71, 72]. CXL in these eyes might result in late and progressive corneal flattening and unwelcome long-term hyperopic refractive outcomes. Caution needs to be adopted with such treatments and potential patients counselled pre-operatively concerning these possible changes with time.

Indeed, occasionally corneal flattening can be very excessive. Santhiago reported two cases, one a 28-year-old woman with flattening of greater

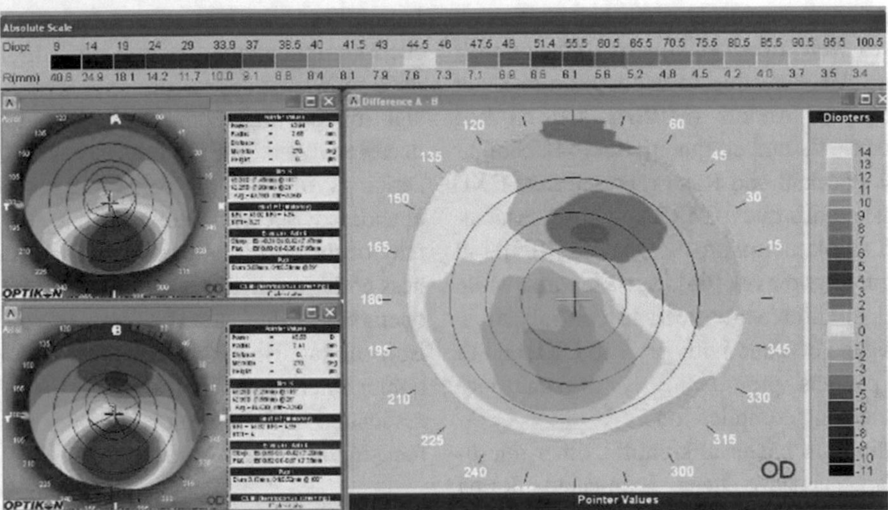

Fig. 20.5 Comparison map pre-operative and 8 years showing almost 4.0 dioptres of corneal flattening with a 28-year-old patient with a +3.0 dioptre hyperopic shift

than 14.0D and the other a 14-year-old boy with flattening of 7.0D at 12 months [73], while Kymionis reported a 23-year-old woman with over 11.0D of corneal flattening, with associated corneal thinning of over 220 μm during a 5-year follow-up period [74]. The pathophysiology of such changes is at yet unclear. Santhiago postulated that such cases may be more apparent with a central cone location and more advanced disease resulting in a greater CXL and wound healing effect. However, in their cases there was no excessive corneal thinning while in that reported by Kymionis this occurred, suggesting perhaps differing mechanisms for this occurrence.

20.11 Potential Limbal Stem Cell Damage

CXL is typically undertaken on young individuals. UVA radiation is known to have potential mutagenic and toxic cellular effects. Corneal limbal stem cells could theoretically be adversely affected by UVA radiation, with potential damage not being clinically evident for years/decades following CXL. Moore et al. exposed cultured corneal epithelial cells and ex vivo corneal tissue to the standard clinical cross-linking protocol and found evidence of oxidative nuclear DNA damage in corneal limbal epithelial cells [75]. Vimalin et al. subjected cadaveric eyes to CXL and demonstrated damage to limbal epithelial cells with a drop in viable cells [76]. Both investigators demonstrated that such changes could be easily avoided by avoiding UVA limbal irradiation/shielding the limbus at the time of CXL.

As yet long-term clinical studies have shown no evidence of limbal stem cell dysfunction with up to 7–10 year follow-up [24, 25]. However, such changes may take decades to occur. In a single case report, Krumeich described a patient who presented with conjunctival intraepithelial neoplasia 2 years after CXL and deep anterior lamellar keratoplasty [77]. While causation between CXL and the development of CIN cannot be established with a single case report, it seems entirely prudent to protect the limbus and avoid its irradiation during CXL.

20.12 Summary

CXL offer great promise for the corneal ectatic disorders. Whilst it is a relatively simple outpatient procedure with good efficacy and an excellent safety profile, sight-threatening complications can occur albeit rarely. Patients need to be counselled pre-operatively of these potential adverse events. Conjunctival atopy, if present, needs to be adequately controlled pre-operatively and it is advised to give systemic prophylaxis if there is a previous history of ocular Herpes simplex. Patients need to be fully informed not to abuse post-operative contact lens wear and return if any symptoms of infectious keratitis occur. It is advisable to avoid UVA irradiation of the limbus during the procedure.

Compliance with Ethical Requirements David P.S. O'Brart declares that he has no conflict of interest. He holds a non-commercial grant from Alcon, Inc. for research into Femtosecond laser assisted cataract surgery. No human or animal studies were carried out by the author for this review.

References

1. Wollensak G, Spoerl E, Seiler T. Riboflavin/ultraviolet-A-induced collagen cross-linking for the treatment of kertatoconus. Am J Ophthalmol. 2003;135(5):620–7.
2. Caporossi A, Baiocchi S, Mazzotta C, et al. Parasurgical therapy for keratoconus by riboflavin-ultraviolet type A rays induced cross-linking of the corneal collagen; preliminary refractive results in an Italian study. J Cataract Refract Surg. 2006;32(5): 837–45.
3. Vinciguerra P, Albe E, Trazza S, et al. Refractive, topographic, tomographic, and abberometric analysis of keratoconic eyes undergoing corneal cross-linking. Ophthalmology. 2009;116(3):369–78.
4. Coskunseven E, Jankov 2nd MR, Hafezi F. Contralateral eye study of corneal collagen cross-linking with riboflavin and UVA radiation in patients with keratoconus. J Refract Surg. 2009;25(4):371–6.
5. Agrawal VB. Corneal collagen cross-linking with riboflavin and ultraviolet—a light for keratoconus: results in Indian eyes. Indian J Ophthalmol. 2009;57(2):111–4.
6. Arbelaez MC, Sekito MB, Vidal C, Choudhury SR. Collagen cross-linking with riboflavin and ultraviolet-A light in keratoconus: one-year results. Oman J Ophthalmol. 2009;2(1):33–8.
7. Vinciguerra P, Albè E, Trazza S, Seiler T, Epstein D. Intraoperative and postoperative effects of corneal collagen cross-linking on progressive keratoconus. Arch Ophthalmol. 2009;127(10):1258–65.
8. Fournié P, Galiacy S, Arné JL, Malecaze F. Corneal collagen cross-linking with ultraviolet-A light and riboflavin for the treatment of progressive keratoconus. J Fr Ophtalmol. 2009;32(1):1–7.
9. Henriquez MA, Izquierdo Jr L, Bernilla C, Zakrzewski PA, Mannis M. Riboflavin/ultraviolet A corneal collagen cross-linking for the treatment of keratoconus: visual outcomes and Scheimpflug analysis. Cornea. 2011;30(3):281–6.
10. Kampik D, Koch M, Kampik K, Geerling G. Corneal riboflavin/UV-A collagen cross-linking (CXL) in keratoconus: two-year results. Klin Monbl Augenheilkd. 2011;228(6):525–30.
11. Goldich Y, Marcovich AL, Barkana Y, Mandel Y, Hirsh A, Morad Y, Avni I, Zadok D. Clinical and corneal biomechanical changes after collagen cross-linking with riboflavin and UV irradiation in patients with progressive keratoconus: results after 2 years of follow-up. Cornea. 2012;31(6):609–14.
12. Asri D, Touboul D, Fournié P, Malet F, Garra C, Gallois A, Malecaze F, Colin J. Corneal collagen crosslinking in progressive keratoconus: multicenter results from the French National Reference Center for Keratoconus. J Cataract Refract Surg. 2011;37(12): 2137–43.
13. Hersh PS, Greenstein SA, Fry KL. Corneal collagen crosslinking for keratoconus and corneal ectasia: one-year results. J Cataract Refract Surg. 2011;37(1): 149–60.
14. O'Brart DP, Chan E, Samaras K, Patel P, Shah SP. A randomised, prospective study to investigate the efficacy of riboflavin/ultraviolet A (370 nm) corneal collagen cross-linkage to halt the progression of keratoconus. Br J Ophthalmol. 2011;95(11):1519–24.
15. Wittig-Silva C, Chan E, Islam FM, Wu T, Whiting M, Snibson GR. A randomized, controlled trial of corneal collagen cross-linking in progressive keratoconus: three-year results. Ophthalmology. 2014;121(4):812–21. doi:10.1016/j.ophtha.2013.10.028 [Epub 2014 Jan 6].
16. Arora R, Gupta D, Goyal JL, Jain P. Results of corneal collagen cross-linking in pediatric patients. J Refract Surg. 2012;28(11):759–62.
17. Vinciguerra P, Albé E, Frueh BE, Trazza S, Epstein D. Two-year corneal cross-linking results in patients younger than 18 years with documented progressive keratoconus. Am J Ophthalmol. 2012;154(3):520–6.
18. Ivarsen A, Hjortdal J. Collagen cross-linking for advanced progressive keratoconus. Cornea. 2013;32(7):903–6.
19. Spadea L. Corneal collagen cross-linking with riboflavin and UVA irradiation in pellucid marginal degeneration. J Refract Surg. 2010;26(5):375–7.
20. Hassan Z, Nemeth G, Modis L, Szalai E, Berta A. Collagen cross-linking in the treatment of pellucid marginal degeneration. Indian J Ophthalmol. 2014;62(3):367–70.
21. Hafezi F, Kanellopoulos J, Wiltfang R, Seiler T. Corneal collagen crosslinking with riboflavin and ultraviolet A to treat induced keratectasia after laser in situ keratomileusis. J Cataract Refract Surg. 2007;33(12):2035–40.
22. Vinciguerra P, Camesasca FI, Albè E, Trazza S. Corneal collagen cross-linking for ectasia after excimer laser refractive surgery: 1-year results. J Refract Surg. 2010;26(7):486–97.

23. Salgado JP, Khoramnia R, Lohmann CP, Winkler von Mohrenfels C. Corneal collagen crosslinking in post-LASIK keratectasia. Br J Ophthalmol. 2011;95(4):493–7.
24. O'Brart DP, Patel P, Lascaratos G, Wagh VK, Tam C, Lee J, O'Brart NA. Corneal cross-linking to halt the progression of keratoconus and corneal ectasia: seven-year follow-up. Am J Ophthalmol. 2015;160(6):1154–63. doi:10.1016/j.ajo.2015.08.023 [Epub 2015 Aug 22].
25. Raiskup F, Theuring A, Pillunat LE, Spoerl E. Corneal collagen crosslinking with riboflavin and ultraviolet-A light in progressive keratoconus: ten-year results. J Cataract Refract Surg. 2015;41(1):41–6. doi:10.1016/j.jcrs.2014.09.033.
26. Shalchi Z, Wang X, Nanavaty MA. Safety and efficacy of epithelium removal and transepithelial corneal collagen crosslinking for keratoconus. Eye (Lond). 2015;29(1):15–29. doi:10.1038/eye.2014.230 [Epub 2014 Oct 3].
27. Soeters N, Wisse RP, Godefrooij DA, Imhof SM, Tahzib NG. Transepithelial versus epithelium-off corneal cross-linking for the treatment of progressive keratoconus: a randomized controlled trial. Am J Ophthalmol. 2015;159(5):821-8.e3. doi:10.1016/j.ajo.2015.02.005 [Epub 2015 Feb 19].
28. Al Fayez MF, Alfayez S, Alfayez Y. Transepithelial versus epithelium-Off corneal collagen cross-linking for progressive keratoconus: a prospective randomized controlled trial. Cornea. 2015;34 Suppl 10:S53–6. doi:10.1097/ICO.0000000000000547.
29. Makdoumi K, Mortensen J, Crafoord S. Infectious keratitis treated with corneal crosslinking. Cornea. 2010;29:1353–8.
30. Alio JL, Abbouda A, Valle DD, Del Castillo JM, Fernandez JA. Corneal cross linking and infectious keratitis: a systematic review with a meta-analysis of reported cases. J Ophthalmic Inflamm Infect. 2013;3(1):47.
31. Famose F. Evaluation of accelerated collagen cross-linking for the treatment of melting keratitis in eight dogs. Vet Ophthalmol. 2014;17(5):358–67. doi:10.1111/vop.12085.
32. Hellander-Edman A, Makdoumi K, Mortensen J, Ekesten B. Corneal cross-linking in 9 horses with ulcerative keratitis. BMC Vet Res. 2013;9:128.
33. Krueger RR, Ramos-Esteban JC, Kanellopoulos AJ. Staged intrastromal delivery of riboflavin with UVA cross-linking in advanced bullous keratopathy: laboratory investigation and first clinical case. J Refract Surg. 2008;24(7):S730–6.
34. Wollensak G, Aurich H, Wirbelauer C, Pham DT. Potential use of riboflavin/UVA cross-linking in bullous keratopathy. Ophthalmic Res. 2009;41(2):114–7.
35. Ghanem RC, Santhiago MR, Berti TB, Thomaz S, Netto MV. Collagen crosslinking with riboflavin and ultraviolet-A in eyes with pseudophakic bullous keratopathy. J Cat Ref Surg. 2010;36:273–6.
36. Mazzotta C, Balestrazzi A, Traversi C, et al. Treatment of progressive keratoconus by riboflavin UVA induced cross linking of corneal collagen: ultrastructural analysis by Heidelberg retinal tomography II in vivo confocal microscopy in humans. Cornea. 2007;26(4):390–7.
37. Mazzotta C, Balestrazzi A, Baiocchi S. Stromal haze after combined riboflavin-UVA corneal collagen cross-linking in keratoconus: in vivo confocal microscopic evaluation. Clin Exp Ophthalmol. 2007;35(6):580–2.
38. Seiler T, Hafezi F. Corneal cross-linking induced stromal demarcation line. Cornea. 2006;25(9):1057–9.
39. Touboul D, Efron N, Smadja D, Praud D, Malet F, Colin J. Corneal confocal microscopy following conventional, transepithelial, and accelerated corneal collagen cross-linking procedures for keratoconus. J Refract Surg. 2012;28(11):769–76.
40. Filippello M, Stagni E, O'Brart D. Transepithelial corneal collagen crosslinking: bilateral study. J Cataract Refract Surg. 2012;38(2):283–91.
41. Yam JC, Chan CW, Cheng AC. Corneal collagen cross-linking demarcation line depth assessed by Visante OCT After CXL for keratoconus and corneal ectasia. J Refract Surg. 2012;28(7):475–81.
42. Yam JC, Cheng AC. Reduced cross-linking demarcation line depth at the peripheral cornea after corneal collagen cross-linking. J Refract Surg. 2013;29(1):49–53.
43. Kymionis GD, Grentzelos MA, Plaka AD, Stojanovic N, Tsoulnaras KI, Mikropoulos DG, Rallis KI, Kankariya VP. Evaluation of the corneal collagen cross-linking demarcation line profile using anterior segment optical coherence tomography. Cornea. 2013;32(7):907–10.
44. Doors M, Tahzib NG, Eggink FA, Berendschot TT, Webers CA, Nuijts RM. Use of anterior segment optical coherence tomography to study corneal changes after collagen cross-linking. Am J Ophthalmol. 2009;148(6):844–51.
45. O'Brart DP. Is accelerated corneal cross-linking for keratoconus the way forward? Yes or No. Eye (Lond). 2015;29(2):293. doi:10.1038/eye.2014.274 [Epub 2014 Nov 14].
46. Raiskup F, Hoyer A, Spoerl E. Permanent corneal haze after riboflavin-UVA-induced cross-linking in keratoconus. J Refract Surg. 2009;25(9):S824–8.
47. Lim LS, Beuerman R, Lim L, Tan DT. Late-onset deep stromal scarring after riboflavin-UV-A corneal collagen cross-linking for mild keratoconus. Arch Ophthalmol. 2011;129(3):360–2.
48. Kymionis GD, Portaliou DM, Diakonis VF, Kontadakis GA, Krasia MS, Papadiamantis AG, Coskunseven E, Pallikaris AI. Posterior linear stromal haze formation after simultaneous photorefractive keratectomy followed by corneal collagen cross-linking. Invest Ophthalmol Vis Sci. 2010;51(10):5030–3.
49. Güell JL, Verdaguer P, Elies D, Gris O, Manero F. Late onset of a persistent, deep stromal scarring after PRK and corneal cross-linking in a patient with forme fruste keratoconus. J Refract Surg. 2014;30(4):286–8.

50. Poli M, Lefevre A, Auxenfans C, Burillon C. Corneal collagen cross-linking for the treatment of progressive corneal ectasia: 6-year prospective outcome in a French population. Am J Ophthalmol. 2015;160(4):654–62.
51. Theuring A, Spoerl E, Pillunat LE, Raiskup F. Corneal collagen cross-linking with riboflavin and ultraviolet-A light in progressive keratoconus. Results after 10-year follow-up. Ophthalmologe. 2015;112(2):140–7.
52. Raiskup-Wolf F, Hoyer A, Spoerl E, Pillunat LE. Collagen crosslinking with riboflavin and ultraviolet-A light in keratoconus: long-term results. J Cataract Refract Surg. 2008;34(5):796–801.
53. Koller T, Mrochen M, Seiler T. Complication and failure rates after corneal crosslinking. J Cataract Refract Surg. 2009;35(8):1358–62.
54. Sloot F, Soeters N, van der Valk R, Tahzib NG. Effective corneal collagen crosslinking in advanced cases of progressive keratoconus. J Cataract Refract Surg. 2013;39(8):1141–5.
55. Kymes SM, Walline JJ, Zadnik K, Sterling J, Gordon MO. Changes in the quality of life of people with keratoconus. Am J Ophthalmol. 2004;138:527–35.
56. Lam FC, Georgoudis P, Nanavaty MA, Khan S, Lake D. Sterile keratitis after combined riboflavin-UVA corneal collagen cross-linking for keratoconus. Eye (Lond). 2014;28(11):1297–303.
57. Koppen C, Vryghem JC, Gobin L, Tassignon MJ. Keratitis and corneal scarring after UVA/riboflavin cross-linking for keratoconus. J Refract Surg. 2009;25(9):S819–23.
58. Eberwein P, Auw-Hädrich C, Birnbaum F, Maier PC, Reinhard T. Corneal melting after cross-linking and deep lamellar keratoplasty in a keratoconus patient. Klin Monbl Augenheilkd. 2008;225(1):96–8. doi:10.1055/s-2008-1027128.
59. Pollhammer M, Cursiefen C. Bacterial keratitis early after corneal crosslinking with riboflavin and ultraviolet A. J Cataract Refract Surg. 2009;35(3):588–9.
60. Perez Santonja J, Artola A, Javaloy J, et al. Microbial keratitis after corneal collagen crosslinking. J Cataract Refract Surg. 2009;35(6):1138–40.
61. Sharma N, Maharana P, Singh G, Titiyal JS. Pseudomonas keratitis after collagen crosslinking for keratoconus: case report and review of literature. J Cataract Refract Surg. 2010;36(3):517–20.
62. Zamora KV, Males JJ. Polymicrobial keratitis after a collagen cross-linking procedure with postoperative use of a contact lens: a case report. Cornea. 2009;28(4):474–6.
63. Papaioannou L, Miligkos M, Papathanassiou M. Corneal collagen cross-linking for infectious keratitis: a systematic review and meta-analysis. Cornea. 2015;35(1):62–71.
64. Shetty R, Kaweri L, Nuijts RM, Nagaraja H, Arora V, Kumar RS. Profile of microbial keratitis after corneal collagen cross-linking. Biomed Res Int. 2014;2014:340509 [Epub 2014 Sep 11].
65. Fasciani R, Agresta A, Caristia A, Mosca L, Scupola A, Caporossi A. Methicillin-resistant Staphylococcus aureus ocular infection after corneal cross-linking for keratoconus: potential association with atopic dermatitis. Case Rep Ophthalmol Med. 2015;2015:613273 [Epub 2015 Mar 18].
66. Rana M, Lau A, Aralikatti A, Shah S. Severe microbial keratitis and associated perforation after corneal crosslinking for keratoconus. Cont Lens Anterior Eye. 2015;38(2):134–7.
67. Rama P, Di Matteo F, Matuska S, et al. Acanthamoeba keratitis with perforation after corneal crosslinking and bandage contact lens use. J Cataract Refract Surg. 2009;35(4):788–91.
68. Al-Qarni A, AlHarbi M. Herpetic keratitis after corneal collagen cross-linking with riboflavin and ultraviolet-A for keratoconus. Middle East Afr J Ophthalmol. 2015;22(3):389–92.
69. Sharma A, Nottage JM, Mirchia K, Sharma R, Mohan K, Nirankari VS. Persistent corneal edema after collagen cross-linking for keratoconus. Am J Ophthalmol. 2012;154(6):922–6.
70. Kanellopoulos AJ, Asimellis G. Combined laser in situ keratomileusis and prophylactic high-fluence corneal collagen crosslinking for high myopia: two-year safety and efficacy. J Cataract Refract Surg. 2015;41(7):1426–33.
71. Tan J, Lytle GE, Marshall J. Consecutive laser in situ keratomileusis and accelerated corneal crosslinking in highly myopic patients: preliminary results. Eur J Ophthalmol. 2014 [Epub ahead of print].
72. Bagga B, Pahuja S, Murthy S, Sangwan VS. Endothelial failure after collagen cross-linking with riboflavin and UV-A: case report with literature review. Cornea. 2012;31(10):1197–200.
73. Santhiago MR, Giacomin NT, Medeiros CS, Smadja D, Bechara SJ. Intense early flattening after corneal collagen cross-linking. J Refract Surg. 2015;31(6):419–22.
74. Kymionis GD, Tsoulnaras KI, Liakopoulos DA, Paraskevopoulos TA, Kouroupaki AI, Tsilimbaris MK. Excessive corneal flattening and thinning after corneal cross-linking: single-case report with 5-year follow-up. Cornea. 2015;34(6):704–6.
75. Moore JE, Atkinson SD, Azar DT, Worthington J, Downes CS, Courtney DG, Moore CB. Protection of corneal epithelial stem cells prevents ultraviolet A damage during corneal collagen cross-linking treatment for keratoconus. Br J Ophthalmol. 2014;98(2):270–4.
76. Vimalin J, Gupta N, Jambulingam M, Padmanabhan P, Madhavan HN. The effect of riboflavin-UV-A treatment on corneal limbal epithelial cells—a study on human cadaver eyes. Cornea. 2012;31(9):1052–9.
77. Krumeich JH, Brand-Saberi B, Chankiewitz V, Chankiewitz E, Guthoff R. Induction of neoplasia after deep anterior lamellar keratoplasty in a CXL-treated cornea. Cornea. 2014;33(3):313–6.

Pediatric Corneal Cross-Linking

21

Sabine Kling and Farhad Hafezi

21.1 Keratoconus and CXL Efficacy in Children

Keratoconus is a degrading corneal disease and typically manifests in adolescence or early adulthood. While pediatric keratoconus is rare, it is difficult to manage due to its fast progression and often advanced state at the time of diagnosis. Also, children rub their eyes more frequently, which favors comorbidities such as vernal keratoconjunctivitis [1] but also keratoconus progression [2].

The natural degree of collagen cross-linking and hence the stiffness of the cornea increases with age [3]. Keratoconus progression therefore often stops in patients over 40 years. However, pediatric patients do not benefit from the age-related stiffness increase, which may explain the faster keratoconus progression in children.

Visual function in children is important for development, education, and leisure activities. Often subjective suffering is higher in these patients. Until recently keratoplasty [4] was the sole indication for pediatric keratoconus. However, the limited graft durability makes it a nonoptimal solution. Corneal cross-linking by riboflavin and UV-A is an emerging alternative, which has been successfully applied to treat adult keratoconus for nearly 15 years [5]. Standard corneal cross-linking (CXL) according to the Dresden protocol involves de-epithelialization, instillation of 0.1 % riboflavin for 30 min, followed by UV-A irradiation at 3 mW/cm^2 for 30 min.

While CXL reliably stops keratoconus progression in approximately 97 % of adults, different success rates have been reported in children: While studies with follow-up times of up to 24 months report a similar efficacy in children as in adults [6–10], keratoconus progression was observed at a follow-up time of 36 months [11]. Chatzis and Hafezi speculated that keratoconus in children may be slowed down but not completely stopped by CXL. While still more studies are needed to confirm this hypothesis, it demonstrates the need for continuous follow-up examination in pediatric patients. Kankariya et al. [12] reviewed the success of CXL in pediatric patients in more detail.

S. Kling, Ph.D.
Center for Applied Biotechnology and Molecular Medicine (CABMM), University of Zurich, Zurich, Switzerland
e-mail: kling.sabine@gmail.com

F. Hafezi, M.D., Ph.D. (✉)
Center for Applied Biotechnology and Molecular Medicine (CABMM), University of Zurich, Zurich, Switzerland

ELZA Institute, Dietikon, Zurich, Switzerland

University of Southern California, Los Angeles, CA, USA

University of Geneva, Geneva, Switzerland
e-mail: farhad@hafezi.ch

J.L. Alió (ed.), *Keratoconus*, Essentials in Ophthalmology, DOI 10.1007/978-3-319-43881-8_21

21.2 Indication for CXL in Children

In adults the indication for CXL is given when keratoconus progression has been documented during at least 6 months. Although the rate of keratoconus progression is similar in children (79 % [13] to 88 % [11]) as in adults [13], pediatric keratoconus is often advised to be treated immediately as it advances faster and therefore is often diagnosed in a late stage. CXL treatment is only possible in a limited time frame: On the one hand, CXL is most effective in an early stage. On the other hand, as soon as the residual stromal thickness is below 400 μm CXL is considered unsecure with respect to UV damage at the endothelium [14]. A consensus on CXL treatment in children does not exist yet. Similar to adult keratoconus different CXL protocols are under investigation. While standard CXL using 3 mW/cm^2 for 30 min is the most efficient [15] up to date, it requires a long treatment session and significant postsurgical pain. Modified CXL protocols avoid de-epithelialization, reduce the riboflavin soaking, and UV irradiation time. These treatment modalities aim especially at children or patients with reduced compliance.

21.3 Complications with Pediatric CXL: The GENEVA Protocol

Generally, the complication rate after CXL is similar in children as in adults. However, eye rubbing is a potential risk factor that favors infections and postsurgical complications. Down patients have an elevated risk due to their lack of postoperative compliance [16]. The incidence rate of keratoconus is this patient group is also significantly higher (1:64) compared to the general population (1:1250). Therefore, the Light for Sight foundation has established the Geneva protocol (personal communication Prof. F. Hafezi), which recommends different CXL protocols dependent on patient compliance (Fig. 21.1). For normal compliance, epi-off CXL under topical anesthesia is recommended. The patient is expected to tolerate manipulations at the cornea and to look straight into the light. Postoperatively, the patient must abstain from rubbing or touching the eye. For reduced compliance, epi-on CXL with slow irradiation (30 min) under topical anesthesia is recommended. As healing is faster, these patients experience less pain and inadvertent eye rubbing is less severe. Infections are less probable as the epithelium acts as a barrier. For patients

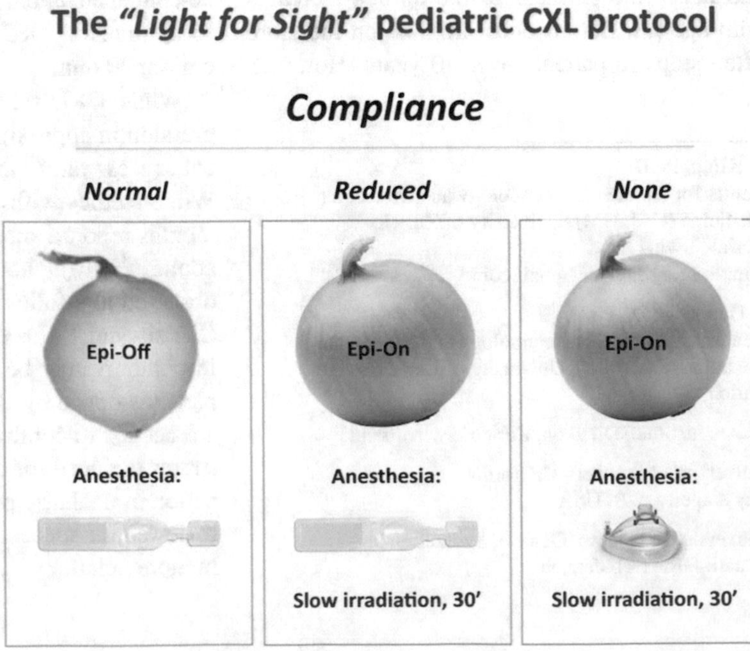

Fig. 21.1 The Geneva protocol for corneal cross-linking (CXL) in pediatric patients

with strongly reduced or no compliance, epi-on CXL with slow irradiation (30 min) under general anesthesia is recommended. While the surgery can be performed without problem, attention needs to be paid to prevent eye rubbing and infection postoperatively.

21.4 Patient Comfort Versus CXL Efficacy

Recently, new and less invasive protocols for CXL treatment have been proposed. Accelerated CXL uses higher irradiances (9 or 18 mW/cm^2) and is applied to reduce the irradiation time (10 or 5 min, respectively). Transepithelial CXL [17] does not require de-epithelialization due to the aggregation of benzalconium chloride or ethylenediaminetetraacetic acid (EDTA) to the riboflavin solution. Additionally, the riboflavin diffusion speed into the corneal stroma can be increased by iontophoresis [18]. Transepithelial treatment is less painful and increases the speed of postoperative wound healing. There are several studies that suggest accelerated CXL [19, 20], transepithelial CXL without [21, 22] or with iontophoresis [23] is effective in pediatric patients. Others in contrast reported that transepithelial CXL did not stop pediatric keratoconus progression [24]. There is ongoing research performed to develop faster and more comfortable treatment protocols. However, current laboratory studies suggest that standard CXL is most effective in terms of biomechanical stiffness increase [15]. Therefore, the authors suggest to use the Geneva protocol as a tool in the decision-making process for cross-linking procedures.

Compliance with Ethical Requirements Farhad Hafezi is co-founder of the Light for Sight Foundation. Sabine Kling has no conflict of interest. No human or animal studies were carried out by the authors for this article.

References

1. Butrus SI, Tabbara KF. Vernal keratoconjunctivitis and keratoconus. Am J Ophthalmol. 1983;95:704–5.
2. Karseras A, Ruben M. Actiology of keratoconus. Br J Ophthalmol. 1976;60:522–5.
3. Malik NS, Moss SJ, Ahmed N, Furth AJ, Wall RS, Meek KM. Ageing of the human corneal stroma: structural and biochemical changes. Biochim Biophys Acta (BBA) Mol Basis Dis. 1992;1138:222–8.
4. Patel H, Ormonde S, Brookes N, Moffatt L, Mcghee C. The indications and outcome of paediatric corneal transplantation in New Zealand: 1991–2003. Br J Ophthalmol. 2005;89:404–8.
5. Wollensak G, Spörl E, Seiler T. Treatment of keratoconus by collagen cross linking. Ophthalmologe: Zeitschrift der Deutschen Ophthalmologischen Gesellschaft. 2003;100:44–9.
6. Arora R, Gupta D, Lal Goyal J, Jain P. Results of corneal collagen cross-linking in pediatric patients. J Refract Surg. 2012;28:759–62.
7. Caporossi A, Mazzotta C, Baiocchi S, Caporossi T, Denaro R, Balestrazzi A. Riboflavin-UVA-induced corneal collagen cross-linking in pediatric patients. Cornea. 2012;31:227–31.
8. Soeters N, van der Valk R, Tahzib NG. Corneal cross-linking for treatment of progressive keratoconus in various age groups. J Refract Surg. 2014;30:454–60.
9. Vinciguerra P, Albe E, Frueh BE, Trazza S, Epstein D. Two-year corneal cross-linking results in patients younger than 18 years with documented progressive keratoconus. Am J Ophthalmol. 2012;154:520–6.
10. Zotta PG, Moschou KA, Diakonis VF, Kymionis GD, Almaliotis DD, Karamitsos AP, Karampatakis VE. Corneal collagen cross-linking for progressive keratoconus in pediatric patients: a feasibility study. J Refract Surg. 2012;28:793–9.
11. Chatzis N, Hafezi F. Progression of keratoconus and efficacy of corneal collagen cross-linking in children and adolescents. J Refract Surg. 2012;28:753–8.
12. Kankariya VP, Kymionis GD, Diakonis VF, Yoo SH. Management of pediatric keratoconus—evolving role of corneal collagen cross-linking: an update. Indian J Ophthalmol. 2013;61:435–40.
13. Léoni-Mesplié S, Mortemousque B, Touboul D, Malet F, Praud D, Mesplié N, Colin J. Scalability and severity of keratoconus in children. Am J Ophthalmol. 2012;154:56-62.e1.
14. Spoerl E, Mrochen M, Sliney D, Trokel S, Seiler T. Safety of UVA-riboflavin cross-linking of the cornea. Cornea. 2007;26:385–9.
15. Hammer A, Richoz O, Mosquera SA, Tabibian D, Hoogewoud F, Hafezi F. Corneal biomechanical properties at different corneal cross-linking (CXL) irradiances. Invest Ophthalmol Vis Sci. 2014;55:2881–4.
16. Koppen C, Leysen I, Tassignon MJ. Riboflavin/UVA cross-linking for keratoconus in down syndrome. J Refract Surg. 2010;26:623–4.
17. Leccisotti A, Islam T. Transepithelial corneal collagen cross-linking in keratoconus. J Refract Surg. 2010;26:942.
18. Bikbova G, Bikbov M. Transepithelial corneal collagen cross-linking by iontophoresis of riboflavin. Acta Ophthalmol. 2014;92:e30–4.
19. Ozgurhan EB, Kara N, Cankaya KI, Kurt T, Demirok A. Accelerated corneal cross-linking in pediatric

patients with keratoconus: 24-month outcomes. J Refract Surg. 2014;30:843–9.
20. Shetty R, Nagaraja H, Jayadev C, Pahuja NK, Kurian Kummelil M, Nuijts RM. Accelerated corneal collagen cross-linking in pediatric patients: two-year follow-up results. Biomed Res Int. 2014;2014:894095.
21. Magli A, Forte R, Tortori A, Capasso L, Marsico G, Piozzi E. Epithelium-off corneal collagen cross-linking versus transepithelial cross-linking for pediatric keratoconus. Cornea. 2013;32:597–601.
22. Salman AG. Transepithelial corneal collagen cross-linking for progressive keratoconus in a pediatric age group. J Cataract Refract Surg. 2013;39:1164–70.
23. Buzzonetti L, Petrocelli G, Valente P, Iarossi G, Ardia R, Petroni S. Iontophoretic transepithelial corneal cross-linking to halt keratoconus in pediatric cases: 15-month follow-up. Cornea. 2015;34:512–5.
24. Buzzonetti L, Petrocelli G. Transepithelial corneal cross-linking in pediatric patients: early results. J Refract Surg. 2012;28:763–7.

Carbon Nanomaterials: An Upcoming Therapy for Corneal Biomechanic Enhancement

22

Alfredo Vega Estrada, Jorge L. Alió, and Joaquin Silvestre-Albero

22.1 Introduction

Corneal debilitating disorders are characterized by progressive changes of the geometry of the tissue that leads to an irregular astigmatism that negatively impacts in the visual system of the patients. The mechanism responsible for the corneal weakening that induces the aforementioned geometrical abnormalities is the biomechanical alterations of the collagen fibers within the corneal stroma [1–3]. Until the date, riboflavin/UV light exposure corneal collagen cross-linking is the only treatment option that has proved to stop the progressive nature of the corneal ecstatic disorders [4]. However, it is a long and uncomfortable surgical procedure for both the patient and the surgeon and it is also a technique not exempt of complications.

Carbon nanostructures, mainly carbon nanotubes (CNTs) and graphene, have attracted great attention in the last few years due to their small size and their extraordinary physicochemical properties (they are the stiffest and strongest materials known). Whereas graphene is a flat monolayer of carbon atoms tightly packed into a two-dimensional (2D) honeycomb lattice, carbon nanotubes can be visualized as rolled sheets of graphene built from sp2 carbon units. Previous studies described in the literature have shown that carbon nanomaterials offer potential as structural reinforcement in biomolecules and are used in regenerative medicine due to their high mechanical strength and good biocompatibility [5–7].

The purpose of the present chapter is to present an innovative application of carbon nanomaterials in ophthalmology. Furthermore, we will present a summary of the main results that our research group has obtained in the application of this new technology in the reinforcement of the ocular tissues.

22.2 Corneal Biomechanics

The term biomechanics is used to describe the study of the different mechanical structures that compound the living beings. This scientific discipline is based on different biomedical science and utilizes the knowledge from mechanics, engineering, anatomy, physiology, and other disciplines to analyze the different structures of the human body and how they behave in a given situation.

A. Vega Estrada, Ph.D. (✉)
Keratoconus Unit, Vissum Alicante, Alicante, Spain
e-mail: alfredovega@vissum.com

J.L. Alió, M.D., Ph.D., F.E.B.O.
Keratoconus Unit, Department of Refractive Surgery, Vissum Alicante, Alicante, Spain

Division of Ophthalmology, Miguel Hernández University, Alicante, Spain
e-mail: jlalio@vissum.com

J. Silvestre-Albero, Ph.D.
Inorganic Chemical Department, Universidad de Alicante, Alicante, Spain
e-mail: joaquin.silvestre@ua.es

J.L. Alió (ed.), *Keratoconus*, Essentials in Ophthalmology, DOI 10.1007/978-3-319-43881-8_22

In the specific case of ophthalmology, corneal ectatic disorders are characterized for an alteration in the mechanical properties of the main components of the corneal tissue, the collagen fibers. The mechanical stability of the cornea is determined by the structure of the collagen fibers and their disposition within the stroma. The corneal stroma is composed basically of type I collagen arranged in approx. 200 lamellae in the human cornea [1]. Orientation of the collagen fibers follows an orthogonal orientation in the normal subjects which is one of the main responsible factors for its stability. On contrast, this special arrangement is lost in patients with corneal ectatic disorders which negatively impact in the biomechanical stability of the tissue. Furthermore, biochemical studies have shown that these pathological corneas have an increasing amount of collagen degradation mediated by collagenolysis, loss of keratocytes, and reduced cross-links binding among the collagen fibers also representing an additional factor related in the biomechanical instability of the stroma [8].

Determining in vivo biomechanical behavior of the cornea has become a significant challenge and a topic of important research in ophthalmology mainly as a tool in characterizing corneal ectatic disorders. Nowadays, there are two systems commercially available that can be used in the clinical practice in order to determine the biomechanical behavior of the cornea, the Ocular Response Analyzer (ORA) (Reichert, Inc. Depew, New York, USA) (Fig. 22.1) and the CorVis ST (Oculus Optikgerate GmbH, Wetzlar, Germany) (Fig. 22.2).

Both instruments work in a similar manner and are by analyzing the deformation of the cornea an air pulse. The ORA system provides two biomechanical parameters, the corneal hysteresis and corneal resistant factor, which have shown to be reproducible in normal patients and be altered in eyes with corneal ectatic disorders [9]. On the other hand, the CorVis utilizes a Scheimpflug camera which is able to assess more than 4000 frames per second aiming to evaluate the dynamic behavior of the cornea during the deformation process [10].

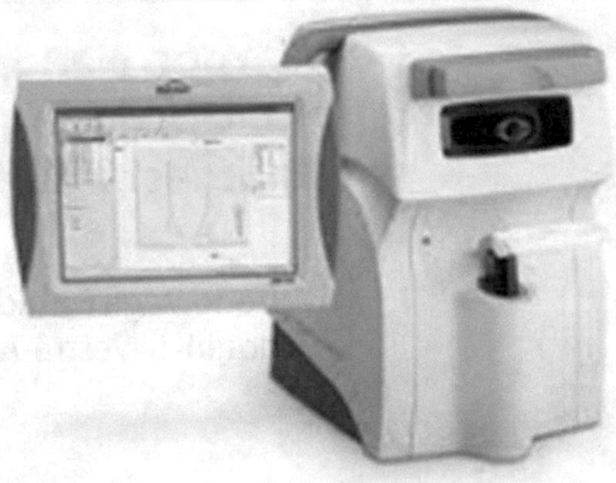

Fig. 22.1 The Ocular Response Analyzer (ORA) (Reichert, Inc. Depew, New York, USA)

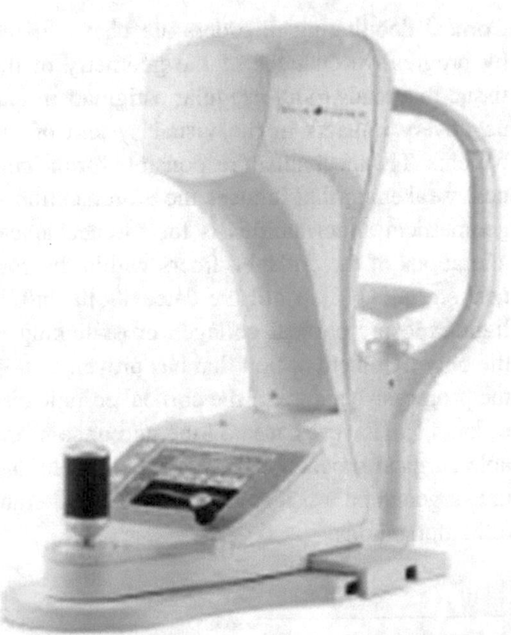

Fig. 22.2 The CorVis ST (Oculus Optikgerate GmbH, Wetzlar, Germany)

Corneal biomechanical behavior can also be evaluated by using ex vivo techniques. One of the most widespread procedures used for that purpose is by means of the analysis of the modulus of elasticity of the corneal tissue. For this technique, stress–strain measurements are determined performing extensiometry experiments. In this type of experiments, a strip of corneal tissue is clamped into a mechanical press which pulls the ends of the corneal strip. Then, by means of strain control, samples undergo deformation in a ramp with a constant speed. The equipment registers the force that is necessary to perform this deformation and the stress–strain graphics are plotted. This way, the elastic modulus of the sample can be determined and denotes the relationship between the stress and the strain of the sample. Corneas with a higher elastic modulus are supposed to be stiffer and able to bear a bigger amount of load in comparison to those with a lower elastic modulus and therefore more weak from the biomechanical point of view.

22.3 Carbon Nanomaterials: Structure and Properties

Nanomaterials have emerged in the last two decades as highly versatile platforms with unparalleled properties compared to systems with the same composition in the bulk phase. The excellent properties of materials are based in their precise engineering at the nanometer length scale (ultra-small size, large surface area-to-mass ratio, and high reactivity), thus providing exciting properties not only in traditional fields such as engineering and electronics, but also in new research branches such as therapeutics (e.g., drug delivery, cancer treatment), tissue engineering, and so on. These carefully designed nanoscale agents provide more efficient systems in applications such as drug delivery, with controlled release, lower therapeutic toxicity, and reduced healthcare costs. Taking into account the vast scope of materials for biomedicine (polymers, nanoparticles, etc.), in this section we will briefly focus on carbon nanostructures and their biomedical application.

Although activated carbon materials (activated charcoal) have been widely used in medicine since many decades (for instance, to reduce intestinal gas, treat poisoning, lower cholesterol levels, etc.), it was not until the 90s, when a large revolution started thanks to the discovery of new fibrous carbon nanostructures (e.g., mainly carbon nanotubes and carbon nanofibers), followed by the isolation of a single graphene in 2010. These carbon materials together with graphene oxide nanoribbons and nanodiamonds have made a significant impact in science and technology, from enhancing the mechanical properties of composite materials, to miniaturizing electronics, providing more efficient energy storage and facilitating the early detection and treatment of diseases [11–16]. It is the versatility of the carbon nanostructures that makes them attractive and versatile for various applications. They are nanoscopic in size, have high length-to-width and surface-to-volume ratio, can have hollow core and are chemically inert to many reagents but can be easily modified to possess different surface chemistry. Among them, carbon nanotubes (CNTs), discovered by Japanese scientist Iijima in 1991, have being postulated as the most attractive carbon nanomaterials due to their intrinsic properties such as impressive structural, mechanical, and electronic properties (they have conducting or semiconducting properties) and their unique optical properties [14–16]. These nanomaterials are allotropes of carbon, made of graphene, and they can be described as a rolled up graphene sheet with sp2 carbons giving rise to cylindrical tubes with nanometer scale in diameter and several millimeters in length [17, 18]. Depending on the number of cylindrical graphene layers, CNTs can be classified as single-wall carbon nanotubes (SWCNTs) or multiwalled carbon nanotubes (MWCNTs). SWCNTs consist of a single graphene cylinder with diameter between 0.4 and 2 nm, whereas MWCNTs consist of two to several coaxial cylinders, with an outer diameter ranging from 2 to 100 nm.

Figure 22.3 shows TEM images and schematic drawing of carbon nanotubes: single-walled carbon nanotube (SWCNT) and a multiwalled nanotube (MWCNT) [14].

CNTs exhibit high tensile strength, stiffness, and ductility [19]. In fact, the tensile strength of SWCNTs is 100 times that of steel, making them the strongest material ever known [16]. Concerning the electrical properties, SWCNTs can be metallic or semiconducting depending on their helicity, whereas MWCNTs exhibit a range of electronic behavior (metallic, semiconducting, and semimetallic) [20].

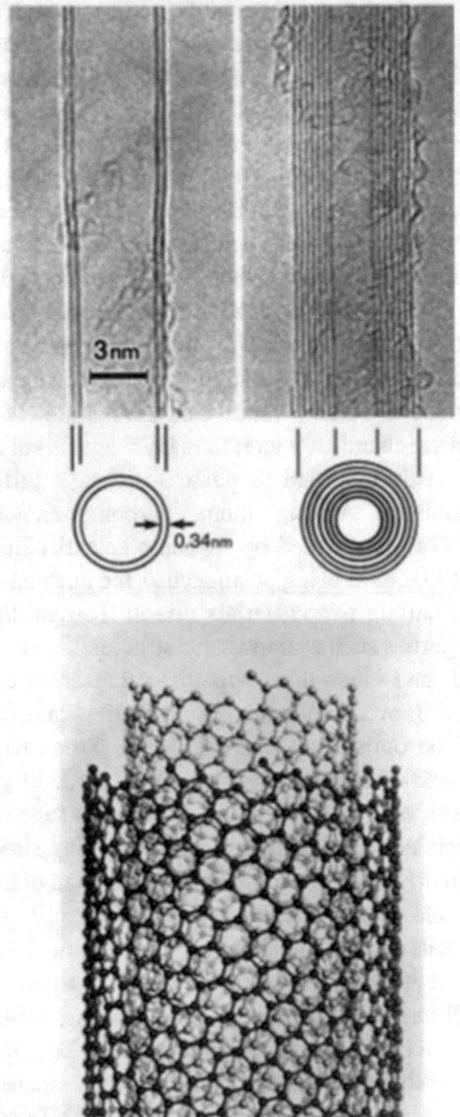

Fig. 22.3 TEM images and schematic drawing of carbon nanotubes: single-walled carbon nanotube (SWCNT) and a multiwalled nanotube (MWCNT). Reprinted from S. Iijima, "Carbon nanotubes: past, present and future", Physica B 323 (2002) 1–5 [14], with permission of Elsevier

However, the reactivity of carbon surfaces varies greatly with surface microstructure, cleanliness, and functional groups [21].

As described earlier, although carbon nanotubes were first used as additives to improve the performance of structural materials for electronics, optics, plastics, etc., since the beginning of the twenty-first century they have been introduced in pharmacy and medicine for drug delivery systems in therapeutics. Nowadays they are used as excellent drug vehicles for drug delivery by penetration into the cells while keeping the drug intact without metabolism during transport in the body [15–18]. When bonded to CNTs, these drugs are delivered more effectively and safely into cells as compared to other conventional methods. CNTs have also being applied to bind antineoplastic and antibiotic drugs for cancer and infection treatments, respectively. Similar linkages of biomolecules (genes, proteins, DNA, antibodies, vaccines, biosensors, cells, etc.) have also been assayed for gene therapy, immunotherapy, tissue regeneration, and diagnosis of different ailments [22–24]. Therefore, the applications of CNTs are very wide and very exciting in a wide variety of disciplines.

CNTs of various diameters, lengths, and structure can be fabricated using a variety of methods from arc discharge method (using arc vaporization of two carbon rods), laser ablation method (using graphite), catalytic chemical vapor deposition (C-CVD), using hydrocarbon sources such as CO, methane, ethylene, etc., plasma enhanced chemical vapor deposition (C-PECVD), and template-based CVD. After preparation, CNTs usually contain amorphous carbon, fullerenes, and catalytic metal particles (e.g., Co or Ni) as impurities that must be carefully removed before any further processing. Usually the purification process involves several steps from an initial oxidation upon heating to ~350 °C in air, to remove amorphous carbon, followed by a nonoxidizing acid refluxing to remove the metal nanoparticles and a final annealing at temperatures in excess of 1000 °C in vacuum to remove all the defects created in early steps [25].

22.4 Carbon Nanomaterials in Biomedical Applications

One of the most important concerns after the preparation of the purified carbon nanomaterials and before their application in any biomedical application concerns their functionalization. The introduction of surface functional groups in the open or defect carbon sites (principally oxygen surface groups) allows increasing their solubility in aqueous solutions, and in addition improves the biocompatibility and reduces the toxicity for their medical application [26]. The incorporation of functional groups can be performed by covalent attachment (e.g., incorporation of carboxyl (-COOH) groups to the carbon atoms at edges or defect sites of the nanotubes via an oxidation treatment with strong acids), or by noncovalent attachment (e.g., physisorption of large macromolecules via noncovalent interactions with the aromatic surface of the nanotubes), depending on the final application. Upon functionalization, carbon nanotubes become more hydrophilic and consequently, their solubility in physiological media is highly improved. Furthermore, the presence of functional groups improves the anchoring of drugs and biomolecules (e.g., enzymes, biosensors, proteins, DNA, etc.).

Figure 22.4 shows the chemical modification of carbon nanotubes through thermal oxidation using strong acids, followed by a subsequent esterification or amidization of the carboxyl groups [27].

The main applications of carbon nanomaterials in medicine and pharmacy are based on their unique structural, electronic, and mechanical properties. These applications include electrochemical sensors, biosensors, drug deliver to organs or cells, vaccine vehicles, tissue engineering, etc.

Due to the high ratio of surface area to volume, CNT-based electrodes exhibit a significant increase in the signal-to-noise ratio compared to other electrochemical sensors with the corresponding increase in the detection sensitivity. For instance, Huang et al. used ferrocene functionalized SWCNTs noncovalent film to detect L-glutamate [28]. The unique interdigitated structure of the ferrocene/SWCNT film provided a high catalytic efficiency, a high sensitivity, and a fast response during the detection at low concentrations. Similar electrochemical sensors were developed by Lin et al. for selective detection of glucose. Glucose oxidase was covalently immobilized on CNTs surface through the EDC/sulfo-NHS linker moieties [29]. Experimental results show that the biosensor effectively performs a selective electrochemical analysis of glucose in the presence of common interferents (e.g., acetaminophen, uric and ascorbic acid).

SWCNT and MWCNT-based field effect transistors can also be used as sensors for detection of gases and vapors with high sensitivity based on the variations in their electrical resistance with

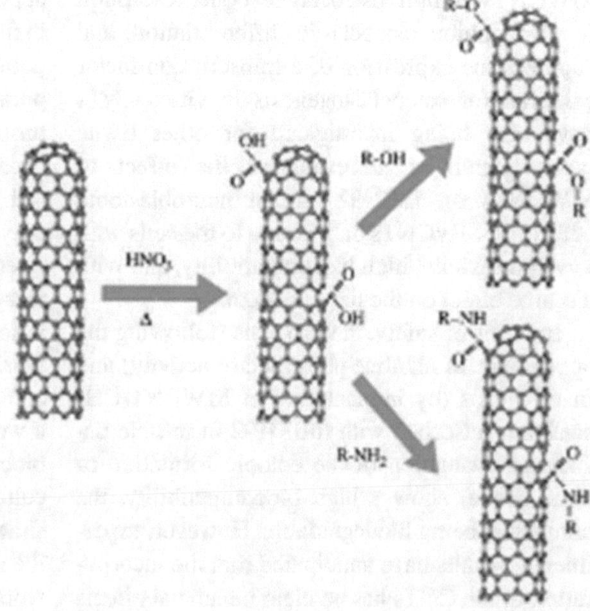

Fig. 22.4 Chemical modification of carbon nanotubes through thermal oxidation using strong acids, followed by a subsequent esterification or amidization of the carboxyl groups. Reprinted from K. Balasubramanian, M. Burghard, "Chemically functionalized carbon nanotubes", Small, 1, 180–192 (2005) [27], with permission of John Wiley and Sons

changes in the environment (e.g., when molecules adsorb on the surface). Compared to other solid-state sensors at room temperature, CNTs sensors exhibit a faster response and a substantially higher sensitivity. These studies include detection of small molecules such as nitrogen dioxide, ammonia, and oxygen, as well as larger odor molecules such as trimethylamine, dinitrotoluene, and dimethylphosphonate [30, 31]. The application of CNTs as a sensor has been extended to larger macromolecules. For instance, researchers of the NASA Ames research center have used CNTs to detect ribonucleic acid (RNA), DNA, and DNA polymerase chain reaction (PCR) amplicons in the solution [32, 33].

Another application of CNTs concerns its use in bone regeneration. Mwenifumbo et al. evaluated the growing of human osteoblastic cells (SaOs-2) on MWCNT constructs and compared to a control based on flat highly ordered pyrolytic graphite (HOPG) surfaces to investigate cellular attachment, cell metabolic activity, and construct cytocompatibility [34]. Experimental results demonstrate that cells attach and survive on the MWCNT constructs, with higher metabolic activity compared to control surfaces and metabolic activity negatively correlating with nanotube diameter. Usui et al. showed that MWCNTs are highly biocompatible [35]. Furthermore, MWCNTs inhibit osteoclastic bone resorption in vivo, inhibit osteoclastic differentiation, and suppress the expression of a transcription factor essential for osteoclastogenesis in vitro. CNTs have also being investigated for other tissue types. Hanui et al. evaluated the effect of MWCNTs on IMR-32 human neuroblastoma cells [36]. MWCNTs only bound to the cells with low cytotoxicity, high biocompatibility, and with a scarce effect on the nerve system.

In terms of safety, in vitro tests (following the appearance of alkaline phosphatase activity) and in vivo tests (by implantation of MWCNT/CHI scaffolds adsorbed with rhBMP-2 in muscle tissue and evaluation of the ectopic formation of bone tissue) show a high biocompatibility, the composite being biodegradable. However, experimental results have anticipated that the incorporation of the CNTs has no clear beneficial effects compared to the base biomaterials, whereas the safety remains an important drawback. Due to the biopersistent character of CNTs and their accumulation in the cells, the CNTs excretion or biodegradation after absorption in the body remains a safety issue before scaffold biomaterials can be applied in human bodies. In despite of this result, other authors that have also analyzed the biocompatibility of such nanomaterials have demonstrated their safety. In the work performed by Zhao et al. the authors observed that CNTs did not interfere with metabolic activity of the cell types that were under study [37]. In the same line, low toxicity and inert biological response have also been reported in another study that investigated the behavior of such nanomaterials in peripheral blood of experimental animals [38]. Nowadays, there are other several investigators that have reported in the scientific literature that carbon nanomaterials are biologically compatible, they are not toxic for the tissues, and that also cleared from circulation when injected intravenously [39–43].

22.5 Carbon Nanomaterials and Biomechanics

In the field of biomedicine, CNTs have also being applied as reinforcement materials for scaffolds in tissue regeneration, i.e., as a reinforce for weak points of existing scaffolds. For instance, incorporation of CNTs to a collagen scaffold has demonstrated an improved mechanical behavior because of the favorable properties of CNTs [44, 45]. Zhang et al. reported that a composite of poly(L-lactide) and MWCNT showed increased direct current conductivity, crystallization, plasticization of the polymer matrix, and growth inhibition of fibroblast cells [46]. Abarrategi et al. fabricated MWCNT-chitosan (CHI) scaffolds composed of MWCNT (up to 89 wt%) and with a well-defined microchannel porous structure as biocompatible and biodegradable supports for culture growth [47]. Other authors have also shown that CNTs may lead to an improvement in the mechanical properties of the collagen. In the work conducted by Cao et al., the authors found an increase of the static tensile modulus and strength of the collagen when adding CNTs to their samples [44]. In the same line of investigation, Tosun also observed a significant enhancement in the rigidity of the collagen gels treated with CNTs [48].

As we can see, CNTs are able to improve the mechanical properties of different materials and biomolecules. In the specific case of the collagen, the enhancement of the mechanical properties is mediated by chemical and physical interaction between the CNTs and the collagen. Some theoretical models have demonstrated the quantum interaction that is present between carbon-based nanostructures and collagen-like peptides [49]. By means of scanning electron microscopy (SEM) and spectrometry, other authors have also showed that there is a chemical interaction and adsorption between carbon nanomaterials and collagen [44, 48, 50].

22.6 Carbon Nanomaterials and Ophthalmology

Based on the aforementioned state of the art, our research group conducted an experimental investigation with the purpose of assessing if carbon nanomaterials were safe within the corneal tissue and also to evaluate the corneal biomechanical properties after its application. To the best of our knowledge that is the first investigation aiming to evaluate how carbon nanomaterials behave in the ocular tissues [51]. In that study, we developed a dissolution containing CNTs that was applied in a pocket created in the middle of the corneal stroma of New Zealand white rabbits. The animals were kept under observation during a period of 3 months and then enucleation of the eyes was performed. Afterward, histopathology evaluation was done in order to assess the biocompatibility of the dissolution and in addition biomechanical assessment by means of stress–strain measurements.

Histopathology using blue Alcian and Masson trichrome staining showed that there were no signs of active inflammation and no fibrous scaring of the corneal stroma after application of the CNTs.

Figure 22.5 shows a histopathology image of the corneal stroma treated with carbon nanotubes (CNTs). Black dots correspond to the CNTs in the area of the corneal stroma where the pocket was created.

For corneal biomechanics assessment, we dissect a strip of corneal stroma of 15 mm in length and 5 mm in width that was clamped into a biomechanical press and then the modulus of elasticity (Young's modulus) was evaluated by means of extensiometry analysis as explained before in the corneal biomechanics section of the current chapter. It was observed that those samples treated with the solution containing the carbon nanomaterials showed an increase in the mechanical properties when they were compared with

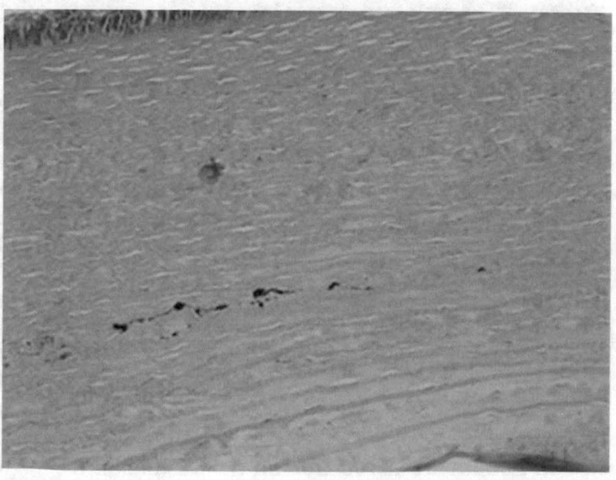

Fig. 22.5 Histopathology image of the corneal stroma treated with carbon nanotubes (CNTs). Black dots correspond to the CNTs in the area of the corneal stroma where the pocket was created

Table 22.1 Biomechanical analysis of the corneal stroma treated with carbon nanotubes (CNTs)

Group	Young's modulus (MPa)
Control	12.1 ± 2.5
Pocket	12.0 ± 4.2
CNTs	13.0 ± 3.9

MPa Megapascals

those untreated samples or with those in which we just performed the corneal pocket but without adding any dissolution (Table 22.1).

It is worth to mention that even when we found a trend toward stiffer corneal stroma after applying the CNTs dissolution, these changes were not statistically significant. It is our hypothesis that a higher enhancement of the mechanical properties of the cornea may be achieved if we are able to obtain a better distribution of the CNTs along the corneal stroma. As we can see previously in the photo of histopathology evaluation, Fig. 22.3, CNTs are just present in the area of the cornea corresponding to the place where the corneal pocket was created. Thus, if we come upon with a technique that allows us to find a better distribution of the carbon nanomaterials within the corneal tissue we believe that a more rigidity of the tissue will also be observed. Currently, we are working in a new research in which enhancement of the dissolution and together with other carbon nanomaterials will lead to an increase in the biomechanical properties of the collagen fibers of the corneal stroma.

22.7 Final Considerations

In summary, the unique physical and chemical properties of carbon nanomaterials make them excellent candidates for the development of new therapeutic applications in the field of medicine. There is enough scientific evidence published in the literature that demonstrate that they are able to improve the mechanical properties of different biomolecules and that they are also biocompatible with different tissues. However, despite the excellent achievements of CNTs in different fields of medicine, the consequences of large exposure to carbon nanomaterials in human health remain a critical issue. In the specific case of ophthalmic research, our investigation group is pioneer in this new technology. We have observed that there is a potential for carbon nanomaterials for the reinforcement of ocular tissues and as a therapeutic agent in different ophthalmic pathologies. Nevertheless and because of its novelty, there is still plenty of investigation to be performed in order to better understand the implications of this new technology in the field of ophthalmology.

Compliance with Ethical Requirements Alfredo Vega-Estrada, Jorge L. Alió, and Joaquin Silvestre have a patent related to the materials discussed in the manuscript. All institutional and national guidelines for the care and use of laboratory animals were followed. No human studies were performed by the authors for this chapter.

References

1. Daxer A, Fratzl P. Collagen fibril orientation in the human corneal stroma and its implication in keratoconus. Invest Ophthalmol Vis Sci. 1997;38(1):121–9.
2. Nash IS, Greene PR, Foster CS. Comparison of mechanical properties of keratoconus and normal corneas. Exp Eye Res. 1982;35:413–24.
3. Andreassen TT, Simonsen AH, Oxlund H. Biomechanical properties of keratoconus and normal corneas. Exp Eye Res. 1980;31:435–41.
4. Meek KM, Hayes S. Corneal cross-linking—a review. Ophthalmic Physiol Opt. 2013;33:78–9.
5. Chen Y, Bilgen B, Pareta RA, Myles AJ, Fenniri H, Ciombor DM, Aaron RK, et al. Self assembled rosette nanotube/hydrogel composites for cartilage tissue engineering. Tissue Eng Part C. 2010;16:1233–44.
6. Song YS. A passive microfluid valve fabricated from a hydrogel filled with carbon nanotubes. Carbon. 2012;50:1417–21.
7. Rodrigues AA, Batista NA, Bavaresco VP, Baranauskas V, Ceragioli HJ, Peterlevitz AC, Santos Jr AR, Belangero WD. Polyvinyl alcohol associated with carbon nanotube scaffolds for osteogenic differentiation of rat bone mesenchymal stem cells. Carbon. 2012;50:450–9.
8. Roy AS, Shetty R, Kummelil MK. Keratoconus: a biomechanical perspective on loss of corneal stiffness. Indian J Ophthalmol. 2013;61(8):392–3.
9. Moreno-Montanes J, Maldonado MJ, Garcia N, et al. Reproducibility and clinical relevance of the ocular response analyzer in nonoperated eyes: corneal biomechanical and tonometric implications. Invest Ophthalmol Vis Sci. 2008;49:968–74.
10. Nemeth G, Hassan Z, Csutak A, et al. Repeatability of ocular biomechanical data measurements with a Scheimpflug-based noncontact device on normal córneas. J Refract Surg. 2013;29:558–63.

11. Gogotsi Y, Presser V, editors. Carbon nanomaterials. Boca Raton: CRC Press; 2014.
12. Li XD, Gao JY, Yang Y, et al. Nanomaterials in the application of tumor vaccines: advantages and disadvantages. OncoTargets and Ther. 2013;6:629–34.
13. Kaur R, Badea I. Nanodiamonds as novel nanomaterials for biomedical applications: drug delivery and imaging systems. Int J Nanomedicine. 2013;8: 203–20.
14. Iijima S. Carbon nanotubes: past, present and future. Physica B. 2002;323:1–5.
15. Hirlekar R, Yamagar M, Garse H, Vij M, Kadam V. Carbon nanotubes and its applications. A review. Asian J Pharm Clin Res. 2009;2:17–27.
16. Singh BGP, Baburao C, Pispati V, et al. Carbon nanotubes. A novel drug delivery system. Int J Res Pharm Chem. 2012;2:523–32.
17. Usui Y, Haniu H, Tsuruoka S, Saito N. Carbon nanotubes innovate on medical technology. Med Chem. 2012;2:1–6.
18. Zhang Y, Bai Y, Yan B. Functionalized carbon nanotubes for potential medicinal applications. Drug Discov Today. 2010;15:428–35.
19. Ruoff RS, Qian D, Liu WK. Mechanical properties of carbon nanotubes: theoretical predictions and experimental measurements. Comptes Rendus Phys. 2003;4:993–1008.
20. Ajayan PM. Nanotubes from carbon. Chem Rev. 1999;99:1787–99.
21. Chen PH, McCreery RL. Control of electron transfer kinetics at glassy carbon electrodes by specific surface modification. Anal Chem. 1996;68:3958–65.
22. Kateb B, Yamamoto V, Alizadeh D, et al. Multi-walled carbon nanotube (MWCNT) synthesis, preparation, labeling and functionalization. Methods Mol Biol. 2010;651:307–17.
23. Liu Z, Sun X, Nakayama-Ratchfold N, Dai H. Supramolecular chemistry on water-soluble carbon nanotubes for drug loading and delivery. ACS Nano. 2007;1:50–6.
24. Zhang W, Zhang Z, Zhang Y. The application of carbon nanotubes in target drug delivery systems for cancer therapies. Nanoscale Res Lett. 2011;6:555–77.
25. Digge MS, Moon RS, Gattani SG. Applications of carbon nanotubes in drug delivery: a review. Int J PharmTech Res. 2012;4:839–47.
26. Lui Z, Tabakman S, Welsher K, Dai H. Carbon nanotubes in biology and medicine: in vitro and in vivo detection, imaging and drug delivery. Nano Res. 2009;2:85–120.
27. Balasubramanian K, Burghard M. Chemically functionalized carbon nanotubes. Small. 2005;1:180–92.
28. Huang X-J, Im H-S, Lee D-H, Kim H-S, Choi Y-K. Ferrocene functionalized single-walled carbon nanotube bundles. Hybrid interdigitated construction film for L-glutamate detection. J Phys Chem C. 2007;111:1200–6.
29. Lin Y, Lu F, Tu Y, Ren Z. Glucose biosensors based on carbon nanotube nanoelectrode ensembles. Nano Lett. 2004;4:191–5.
30. Kong J, Franklin NR, Zhou C, Chaplin MG, Peng S, Cho K, Dai H. Nanotube molecular wires as chemical sensors. Science. 2000;287:622–5.
31. Staii C, Johson AT, Chen M, Gelperin A. DNA-decorated carbon nanotubes for chemical sensing. Nano Lett. 2005;5:1774–8.
32. Nguyen CV, Delzeit L, Cassell AM, Li J, Han J, Meyyappan M. Preparation of nucleic acid functionalized carbon nanotube arrays. Nano Lett. 2002;2: 1079–81.
33. Kochne J, Chen H, Li J, Cassell AM, Ye Q, Ng HT, Han J, Meyyappan M. Ultrasensitive label free DNA analysis using an electronic chip based on carbon nanotube nanoelectrode arrays. Nanotechnology. 2003;14:1239–45.
34. Mwenifumbo S, Shaffer MS, Stevens MM. Exploring cellular behavior with multi-walled carbon nanotube constructs. J Mater Chem. 2007;17:1894–902.
35. Usui Y, Aoki K, Narita N, et al. Carbon nanotubes with high bone-tissue compatibility and bone-formation accelaration effects. Small. 2008;4:240–6.
36. Haniu H, Saito N, Matsuda Y, et al. Elucidation mechanism of different biological responses to multi-walled carbon nanotubes using four cell lines. Int J Nanomedicine. 2011;6:3487–97.
37. Zhao ML, Li DJ, Yuan L, et al. Differences in cytocompatibility and hemocompatibility between carbon nanotubes and nitrogen-doped carbon nanotubes. Carbon. 2011;49:3125–33.
38. Koyama S, Haniu H, Osaka K, Koyama H, Kuroiwa N, Endo M, Kim YA, Hayashi T. Medical application of carbon-nanotube-filled nanocomposites: the microcatheter. Small. 2006;2(12):1406–11.
39. Garibaldi S, Brunelli C, Bavastrello V, Ghigliotti G, Nicolini C. Carbon nanotube biocompatibility with cardiac muscle cells. Nanotechnology. 2006;17:391–7.
40. Aoki N, Yokoyama A, Nodasaka Y, Akasaka T, Uo M, Sato Y, Tohji K, Watari F. Strikingly extended morphology of cells grown on carbon nanotubes. Chem Lett. 2006;35:508–9.
41. Zhang LW, Zeng L, Barron AR, Monteiro-Riviere NA. Biological interactions of functionalized single-wall carbon nanotubes in human epidermal keratinocytes. Int J Toxicol. 2007;26:103–13.
42. Bianco A, Kostarelos K, Prato M. Applications of carbon nanotubes in drug delivery. Curr Opin Chem Biol. 2005;9(6):674–9.
43. Davoren M, Herzog E, Casey A, Cottineau B, Chambers G, Byrne HJ, Lyng FM. In vitro toxicity evaluation of single walled carbon nanotubes on human A549 lung cells. Toxicol In Vitro. 2007;21:438–48.
44. Cao Y, Zhou YM, Shan Y, Ju HX, Xue XJ. Preparation and characterization of grafted collagen-mutiwalled carbon nanotubes composites. J Nanosci Nanotechnol. 2007;7:447–51.
45. MacDonald RA, Laurenzi BF, Viswanathan G, Ajayan PM, Stegemann JP. Collagen-carbon nanotube composite materials as scaffolds in tissue engineering. J Biomed Mater Res A. 2005;74:489–96.

46. Zhang D, Kandadai MA, Cech J, Roth S, Curran SA. Poly(L-lactide) (PLLA)/multiwalled carbon nanotube (MWCNT) composite: characterization and biocompatibility evaluation. J Phys Chem B. 2006;110:12910–5.
47. Abarrategi A, Gutiérrez MC, Moreno-Vicente C, et al. Multiwall carbon nanotube scaffolds for tissue engineering purposes. Biomaterials. 2008;29(1):94–102.
48. Tosun Z, McFetridge PS. A composite SWNT-collagen matrix: characterization and preliminary assessment as a conductive peripheral nerve regeneration matrix. J Neural Eng. 2010;7(6):066002.
49. Cazorla C, Rovira C. Unraveling the quantum interactions of collagen-like peptides with carbon-based nanostructures in aqueous media. In: Science and supercomputing in Europe—research highlights. 2010.
50. Akasaka T, Nakata K, Uo M, Watari F. Modification of the dentin surface by using carbon nanotubes. Biomed Mater Eng. 2009;19(2–3):179–85.
51. Vega-Estrada A, Silvestre-Albero J, Rodriguez A, et al. Carbon nanostructures for ocular tissue reinforcement. Presented as a free paper at European Society of Cataract and Refractive Surgeons (ESCRS), Amsterdam, The Netherlands, 2013.

Part V

Surgery of Keratoconus

23 Surgical Correction of Keratoconus: Different Modalities of Keratoplasty and Their Clinical Outcomes

Jorge L. Alió del Barrio, Francisco Arnalich Montiel, and Jorge L. Alió

23.1 Introduction

Surgical treatment of keratoconus has received considerable attention and a formidable number and variety of surgical procedures, before keratoplasty was even considered the most suitable procedure [1]. Surgical options that have been proposed include intraocular operations such as paracentesis of the anterior chamber, lens extraction or needling, or deviation of the pupil by incarcerating the iris in a corneal incision to achieve a stenopeic slit-like pupil; cone excision procedures; or flattening techniques by scar formation, brought by cauterization of the conus with chemicals, electrocautery, high frequency current, or by splitting of Descemet membrane [1].

Before keratoplasty became an option, Alfred Appelbaum in 1936 [2] stated concerning the surgical treatment of keratoconus "surgical intervention aims to produce flattening of the cornea in order to improve eyesight. When no degree of useful vision is obtained with the use of contact glasses, operative intervention may be considered-but no sooner. Only in cases of advanced or nearly hopeless conditions should the patient undergo operation. Most ophthalmologists agree with this. Too much cannot be expected of surgical treatment. At best, it gives a result far from ideal and none too lasting. The unsightliness which inevitably follows must be anticipated, and the appearance of the eye is always marred to some extent."

Castroviejo a Spanish ophthalmologist born in Logroño, Spain, performed the first penetrating keratoplasty (PKP) for keratoconus in 1936 [1] in the Columbia Presbyterian Medical Center in New York. Several years later in an article about keratoplasty for the treatment of keratoconus he concluded that keratoplasty was the only surgical procedure that fulfilled the two essential requirements for treating keratoconus: surgery had to be limited to the cornea, and the whole corneal protrusion had to be removed and replaced with normal tissue of normal curvature and thickness, leaving the pupillary area free of scarring. Based on his experience, when a suitable technique was used, the percentage of permanently, greatly improved vision was from 75 to 90 % [1].

Lamellar keratoplasty (LKP) was described earlier than penetrating keratoplasty. However, although Arthur von Hippel performed the first

J.L. Alió del Barrio, M.D., Ph.D.
J.L. Alió, M.D., Ph.D., F.E.B.O. (✉)
Keratoconus Unit, Department of Refractive Surgery, Vissum Alicante, Alicante, Spain

Division of Ophthalmology, Miguel Hernández University, Alicante, Spain
e-mail: jorge_alio@hotmail.com

F. Arnalich Montiel, M.D., Ph.D.
Ophthalmology Department, IRYCIS, Ramón y Cajal University Hospital, Madrid, Spain

Cornea Unit, Hospital Vissum Madrid, Madrid, Spain

J.L. Alió (ed.), *Keratoconus*, Essentials in Ophthalmology, DOI 10.1007/978-3-319-43881-8_23

successful LKP in man in 1888 [3], decades earlier than the first successful human PKP by Edward Zinn, this technique was abandoned in 1914 for PKP, and was not reintroduced until the1940s [4]. However, the concept of deep lamellar keratoplasty extending down to Descemet membrane is relatively new. Gasset reported a series of keratoconus patients in the late 1970s who received full-thickness grafts stripped of Descemet's membrane transplanted into relatively deep lamellar beds and enjoyed good surgical results with 80 % of cases achieving 20/30 or better vision [5]. Dissection of host tissue 'close to' the Descemet's membrane and the term 'deep lamellar keratoplasty' (DLKP) in the conventional sense were first introduced by Archilla in 1984, who also showed the use of intrastromal air injection to opacify the corneas a method to facilitate removal of host tissue [6]. Sugita and Kondo reported the first extensive study on the results of DLKP compared with PKP in 1997 [7]. They showed that postoperative visual acuity was similar between DLKP and PKP, with no episodes of immunological rejection in over 100 eyes followed. Despite the clear benefits of DLKP, the classical technique of removing stroma layer by layer was at that stage time consuming and was greatly dependent on surgical experience. Only in the last two decades DLKP has gained momentum thanks to improvement in surgical techniques and the availability of new surgical instruments and devices. Probably the two most relevant papers on techniques were those from Melles and Anwar.

In 1999, Melles described a technique to visualize the corneal thickness and the dissection depth during surgery creating an optical interface at the posterior corneal surface by filling the anterior chamber with air completely [8]. In 2002, Anwar described his popular "big-bubble" technique in baring Descemet Membrane by injecting air into the deep stroma to create a large bubble between the stroma and the Descemet's membrane [9].

Approximately about 12–20 % of the keratoconus patients may require a corneal transplantation [10]. The Australian Graft Report of 2012 shows that keratoconus, with almost 1/3 of the corneal grafts performed, was the first reason for keratoplasty, followed by bullous keratoplasty and failed previous grafts. The 2012 Eye Banking statistical Report published by the Eye Banking Associations of America finds that keratoconus was the reason for penetrating keratoplasty in 18 % of the cases, and in 40 % of the DALK cases. Surprisingly penetrating keratoplasty represented almost 80 % of the total grafts, while DALK only accounted for 3 % of the total keratoplasties done, meaning that time consuming and surgical experience are still a factor reducing the popularity of DALK in the United States of America. Increasingly, however, DALK is becoming the preferred surgical option, largely thanks to improvements in operative technique, and now representing 10–20 % of all transplants for KC and 30 % when eyes with previous hydrops are excluded [11]. In the UK, the percentage of transplants for keratoconus in which DALK was used increased from 10 % in 1999–2000 to 35 % in 2007–2008 [12].

While the scope of this article is mainly corneal grafting as treatment of keratoconus, it is important to point out that the main goal of treatment of keratoconus has changed over the last few years from that aiming to improve visual acuity with keratoplasty to a number of relatively new procedures focused on the prevention of the progression of the disease or to restore or support contact lens tolerance by making wear more comfortable. These include ultraviolet crosslinking (UV-CXL), intracorneal ring segments (ICRS), and a newly proposed type of "corneal transplant" known as Bowman Layer (BL) transplantation described by Gerrit Melles [13].

23.2 Indications of Corneal Graft in Keratoconus

Corneal graft is the traditional recourse for advanced keratoconus. There are many different grading schemes for keratoconus from scales based on outdated indices such as the Amsler-Krumeich scale, to scales using a variety of detailed metrics of corneal structure provided by anterior segment optical coherence tomography and Pentacam imaging. Other scales (RETICS classification) include functional parameters (corrected distance visual acuity—CDVA) in order to assess the severity of the disease. All these different scales do not always correlate well with disease impact. While there are eyes with milder disease that may exhibit contact lens (CL) intolerances, there are other eyes with severe disease that obtain good functional vision with contact lenses.

Therefore, although there is no precise definition for advanced disease, most specialists would agree that a keratoconus patient is eligible for corneal transplant, when spectacle correction is insufficient, continued CL wear is intolerable, and visual acuity has fallen to unacceptable levels [11]. Nevertheless, there has been a strong push to extend other treatment modalities such UV-CXL and ICRS, both of which were originally meant for mild to moderate disease, to treat advanced disease. In 2014, BL transplantation was also described for advanced KC with extreme thinning/steepening [13]. These less troublesome therapeutic alternatives will seek to arrest disease progression, reenable comfortable contact lens, or improve visual acuity to some extent, although rarely do the visual gains exceed one or two lines in advanced disease. These techniques would permit PK or DALK to be postponed or avoided entirely [11].

Nowadays, despite the excellent outcomes of PK, DALK may be preferred in patients with keratoconus because of the absence of risk of endothelial rejection, earlier tapering of steroids, decreased risk of secondary glaucoma, and increased wound strength [14]. The advantage of DALK is even more evident in patients with mental retardation in which PK has a higher incidence of postoperative complications such as globe rupture, corneal ulceration, and graft rejection; in phakic patients; and in corneas with significant peripheral thinning [11].

PK would be considered more suitable in cases in which endothelial dysfunction is present, or when deep corneal scarring affects severely the visual axis up to the Descemet membrane level (such as in previous hydrops). It is not unusual for KC to coexist with endothelial dysfunction that might be underestimated as stromal thinning of KC may mask the corneal edema. Fuchs endothelial dystrophy is the most common of such disorders, but also includes posterior polymorphous dystrophy a peculiar condition of endothelial depletion and guttae excrescences that may be the product of the KC itself rather than a distinct entity [15]. If central deep corneal scarring is present PK will provide a better visual acuity than DALK, but with a higher risk. In some instances, safety of DALK can outbalance the better visual acuity of PK. In fact, when corneal scars arise from previous hydrops, PK outcomes tend to be worse as the risk of graft rejection is higher [11]. In these cases, manual lamellar dissection for DALK is a good choice as Anwar big bubble technique is contraindicated owing to the high risk of perforation during surgery.

23.3 Penetrating Keratoplasty in Keratoconus

Penetrating keratoplasty (PKP/PK) has traditionally been the surgery of choice for keratoconus, but nowadays lamellar techniques are the gold standard for patients with mild to moderate disease. Currently, an elective PK is reserved for those advanced cases where the Descemet membrane (DM) and endothelium appear splitted due to a previous corneal hydrops. Frequently a previous hydrops is not clearly reported by the patient but, in absence of an obvious endothelial split, deep stromal scars involving the DM are observed. In such cases, a lamellar technique can still be attempted, mainly if these scars are not affecting the visual axis, but as the integrity of the DM is not intact anymore this layer has a great tendency to rupture through the area of the scar (mainly if a Big Bubble technique is used) and the surgery will require to be converted into a PK intraoperatively if a big tear is observed (longer than 2–3 clock hours).

Penetrating keratoplasty technique for keratoconus does not differ significantly from the technique used for other etiologies, but some considerations should be taken into account:

23.3.1 Donor Size

A 7.5–8.5 mm host trephine (in relation with the corneal horizontal diameter) is often used and centered with the optical axis. However, in keratoconus the cone is often inferiorly displaced and should be fully removed to avoid residual or recurrent disease [16]. Therefore, the extent of the cone should be well known before surgery and thinning mapped out by slit lamp examination, as this will be difficult to discern with the operating microscope. Fleischer iron ring formation, which usually circumscribes the cone, may assist on its delineation. Corneal topography is not reliable in advanced scarred conus and should not be considered for surgical planning. Donor size will have then to be adjusted in relation with the host limbal white-to-white measurement and conus extension, so larger grafts than 8.5 mm may occasionally be needed in severe conus, as well as its partial decentration respecting the optical axis in cases of very advanced conus with a severe thinning up to the perilimbal area. On the other hand, the risk of rejection increases with grafts larger than 8.5 mm in diameter and as the graft–host junction moves closer to the limbus, so this should be considered into the postoperative treatment and management [17, 18]. Decentered grafts can as well induce a significant irregular astigmatism into the visual axis, requiring rigid lenses for the visual rehabilitation of the patient and occasionally a second centered graft for visual purposes.

The donor tissue trephine is routinely sized 0.25 mm larger than the host trephine because, using current techniques, donor corneal tissue cut with a trephine from the endothelial surface measures approximately 0.25 mm less in diameter than host corneal tissue cut with the same diameter trephine from the epithelial surface [19]. Keratoconus patients may benefit from using same-diameter trephines for both donor and host tissue, which in effect undersizes the donor button and helps to reduce postoperative myopia (reducing donor size by 0.25 mm causes the mean postoperative refractive error to shift toward hyperopia by approximately 2 D) [20, 21], but the surgeon should be aware that obtaining watertight wound closure with an undersized donor tissue can be challenging and may require additional sutures. Moreover, a flattened corneal contour could complicate contact lens fitting in the anisometropic patient and also laser excimer ablation for correction of a significant residual hyperopia after PK may not be possible as it is not as predictable and efficient as it is with residual myopia, thus requiring phakic or pseudophakic piggyback intraocular lenses for patients who are intolerant of spectacles and contact lenses, always once suture removal has been completed [22]. Considering this, despite undersizing the donor cornea may provide better visual outcome in patients with keratoconus, it should be selected carefully in PK. Axial length can be an important factor in the refractive error outcome following PK [23]. Ultrasound axial length measured from the anterior lens capsule to retina reveals a broad range in length from 18.77 to 25.65 mm. Reducing donor size, in a relatively short eye, could result in significant postoperative hyperopia, so same-size donor and host corneal buttons should not be used when the anterior lens-to-retina length is less than 20.19 mm, the mean length for nonkeratoconic individuals with emmetropia.

The degree of postoperative myopia is determined by both corneal curvature and axial length. Lanier et al. [23] found a mean and range of axial length in keratoconic eyes to be fairly close to those observed in emmetropic eyes. Mean corneal curvature and anterior chamber depth, however, are consistently greater than in other eyes [20, 24]. As keratoconic corneas are steeper, with an increased anterior chamber depth, trephination leaves a peripheral corneal rim that is longer (ellipsoid shape) and steeper than normal (mainly if the base of the cone is not completely excised). Thus, placement of a normally sized donor results in a steep cornea and deeper anterior chamber, reasons for part of the postoperative myopia and astigmatism. Placement of a relatively small diameter donor can counteract this by rotating the peripheral rim downwards, reducing the final keratometry and anterior chamber depth, and so, the postoperative myopia. However, if the steepening is asymmetric, which commonly is the case in keratoconus, the length and steepness of the peripheral rim vary around its circumference. Therefore, the bed is not round, and placement of a round donor, even if undersized, will not result in a spherical cornea, leaving significant irregular astigmatism in spite of reducing the postoperative myopia.

A suggested alternative to reduce the postoperative astigmatism as well as the myopia after PK in patients with keratoconus is to cauterize the vertex of the recipient cornea [25]. Cauterization of the cornea (thermokeratoplasty) of patients with keratoconus was introduced by Gasset and Kaufman [26] in the 1970s with the purpose of flattening the cone by shrinking the surrounding corneal tissue. The effect of this procedure, although often remarkable, was limited in time and the technique was abandoned. In 1998 Busin et al. recovered this technique with the theory that this induced corneal shrinkage could flatten the keratoconus and "regularize" the corneal shape of the recipient rim before trephination during PK surgery [25]. They superficially cauterized a central area of 6 mm in diameter with bipolar forceps until whitening and shrinkage of corneal tissue was observed. Their results show a significant decrease in the postoperative spherical equivalent and keratometric astigmatism before and after suture removal compared with the control group, subsequently improving the postoperative uncorrected and best-corrected visual acuity results. The cauterization of the apex should be avoided during DALK as it will induce a severe adherence of the DM to the overlying stroma as well as the damage or perforation of the endothelium, compromising severely any attempt of lamellar keratoplasty.

23.3.2 Suturing Technique

Once the four cardinal 10-0 nylon sutures have been placed the surgeon can use the preferred suture technique: interrupted sutures (IS), combined continuous and interrupted sutures (CCIS), single continuous suture (SCS), or double continuous suture (DCS). IS should be always the closure method of choice in cases where a partial or complete suture removal in one region of the graft is likely to be necessary at some point during the postoperative period: pediatric keratoplasty (as sutures become loose quickly); vascularization in the host cornea (occasionally seen after a hydrops episode or contact lens-related keratitis); multiple previous rejections, or other inflammatory concomitant conditions that may predispose to localized vascularization, rejection, or ulceration of the donor tissue. Also large and decentered grafts that are placed close to the limbal area present, as already discussed, an increased risk of rejection, being necessary the use of IS for its closure.

However, most of the keratoconic eyes do not present any additional risk for graft rejection or infection, so a SCS or DCS are generally preferred by most surgeons. The advantages of a continuous suture are ease of placement, the ease with which the suture can be removed at a later date, and the potential for suture adjustment intra- (with an intraoperative keratometer) and postoperatively to reduce astigmatism. With DCS a 12-bite 10-0 nylon suture placed with bites at approximately 90 % depth and a second continuous suture (10-0 or 11-0 nylon) placed with bites alternating between each of the original suture's bites for 360° at approximately 50–60 % corneal depth are used. The second suture is tied with only enough tension to take up slack in the suture. The second suture permits early removal or adjustment of the 10-0 nylon first suture for astigmatism control in 2–3 months; the second suture acts as a safety net if the deep suture breaks during the adjustment and is generally left in place for 12–18 months postoperatively (Fig. 23.1).

Interrupted sutures, CCIS, and a single continuous suture (SCS) have shown comparable postoperative astigmatism [27]. In addition, a comparison of astigmatism in keratoconus patients utilizing a single continuous versus a double continuous suture showed that after suture removal, astigmatism was comparable (DCS −4.6 D, SCS −5.2 D) between the two groups [28]. Therefore, it is apparent that all methods of suture closure can work well. The ultimate choice rests with the surgeon.

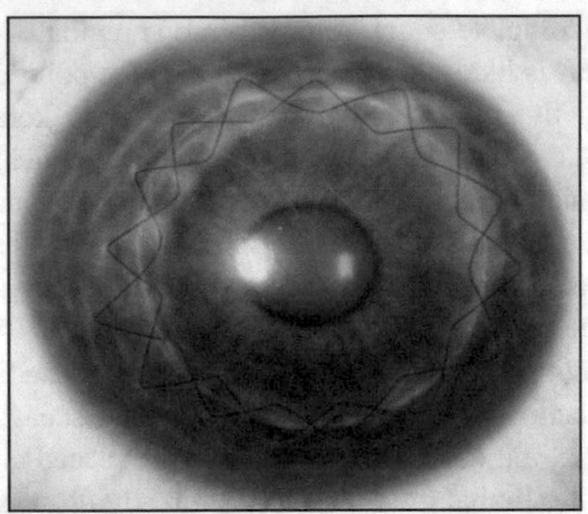

Fig. 23.1 Clinical picture of a keratoconic eye after penetrating keratoplasty with a double continuous 10/0 Nylon suture

Regardless of the preferred method, it is very important to have clear concepts of each suture technique. As a basic idea for standard graft suturing, the needle is passed 90 % depth through the donor cornea and then through the host cornea. The ideal bite is as close to Descemet's membrane as possible, and there should be an equal amount of tissue purchased in the donor and host cornea in order to approximate Bowman's layer in both the donor and host. Discrepancies frequently exist in the thickness of the donor and host cornea if donor corneas are thick due to the hyperosmolar glycosaminoglycans in the preservation medium, or fresh donor tissue is used in patients with severe corneal edema. In keratoconic eyes this scenario is frequent, where the graft is sutured to a relatively thin host cornea. Closing Bowman's layer to Bowman's layer should always be attempted to avoid steps in the graft–host junction and subsequent exposed sutures, so in areas where the recipient cornea presents thin (assessed preoperatively by slit lamp examination) partial thickness bites (50–70 % depth) in the donor tissue should be in relation with deep bites (95 % depth) in the host thin stroma (Fig. 23.2).

The postoperative astigmatism management and elective suture adjustment/removal for PK in

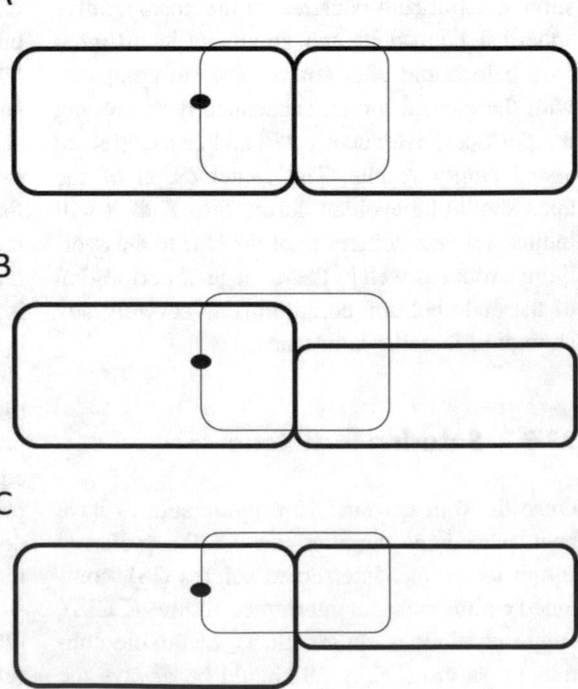

Fig. 23.2 Normal appearance of the graft–host junction with correct aligning of Bowman's layer of the donor and host corneas, with needle passed at a 90 % depth in both sides (**a**). If care is not taken in cases of a thin recipient cornea, steps will remain at the graft–host junction, leaving an irregular astigmatism and exposed sutures that need to be replaced (**b**). To avoid this, a partial thickness bite (50–70 % depth) should be performed at the donor side (**c**)

cases of previous keratoconus does not differ from other PK indications, with a complete suture removal generally recommended after 12–15 months.

23.3.3 Outcomes

Penetrating keratoplasty offers good long-term visual rehabilitation for keratoconus patients, and compared with other indications for PK there is a relatively low rate of graft failure and long mean graft survival. Rejection rate has been reported to be 5.8–41 % with a long-term follow-up, where most rejections occurred in the first 2 years [29–33]. Larger host trephine size, male donor gender, and nonwhite donor race have been associated with increased rejection hazard [29]. Despite this observed rejection rate, only a 4–6.3 % graft failure rate has been reported with a mean follow-up of 15 years, with an estimated 20-year probability of 12 % [29, 30, 34]. Fukoka et al. reported a cumulative probability of graft survival at 10, 20, and 25 years after PK of 98.8 %, 97.0 %, and 93.2 %, respectively, while Pramanik et al. estimated a graft survival rate of 85.4 % at 25 years after initial transplantation [30, 34]. Summarizing, the existing evidence shows that the graft survival rate gradually decreases after 20 years post-PK.

An average best-corrected visual acuity (BSCVA) in logarithm of the minimum angle of resolution (LogMAR) at preoperation, 10, 20, and 25 years after surgery of 1.54±0.68, 0.06±0.22, 0.03±0.17, and 0.14±0.42, respectively, has been reported [30]. Best spectacle-corrected visual acuity (BSCVA) of 0.14±0.11 LogMAR has been reported with a mean period of 33.5 months, while a BSCVA of 20/40 or better with a mean follow-up of 14 years was observed in 73.2 % of patients [33, 34].

An open angle glaucoma rate of 5.4 % with a mean follow-up of 14 years has been reported [34].

Claesson et al. reported a poorer survival and worse visual outcome of regrafts compared with first grafts in patients where the original indication was keratoconus: the failure rate was three times higher with regrafts and the observed visual acuity with preferred correction was ≥ 0.5 in 69 % of first grafts, while only 55 % of regrafts achieved that level [35].

23.4 Deep Lamellar Anterior Keratoplasty in Keratoconus

The goal of deep lamellar anterior keratoplasty in keratoconus is to achieve a depth of dissection as close as possible to the Descemet Membrane (DM). There are various ways to create a plane of separation between DM and the deep stromal layers, mainly variations of the two basic strategies: the Anwar big bubble method and the Melles manual dissection.

23.4.1 Surgical Techniques

23.4.1.1 The Big Bubble Method

Anwar based the big bubble method on a discovery in 1998 that intrastromal injection of balanced salt solution (BSS) was often effective at establishing cleavage plane just above the DM [36], taking advantage of the loose adhesion between DM and the posterior stroma. Anwar and Teichman described the current big bubble procedure in 2002 using air instead of BSS [9].

After a partial trephination of 70–80 % of the corneal stroma, pneumatic pressure is used to detach DM by injecting air into the deep stroma with a 30G needle. The air injected into the stroma produces a dome-shaped detachment of the DM that is seen under the surgical microscope as a ring meaning that the big bubble has been formed. The stromal tissue above the DM plane is removed with spatula and scissors, making first sure to exchange the air in the supradescemetic plane with viscoelastic to avoid inadvertent puncture of the DM. When all of the stromal tissue is successfully removed, the DME membrane exposed is characteristically smooth (Fig. 23.3).

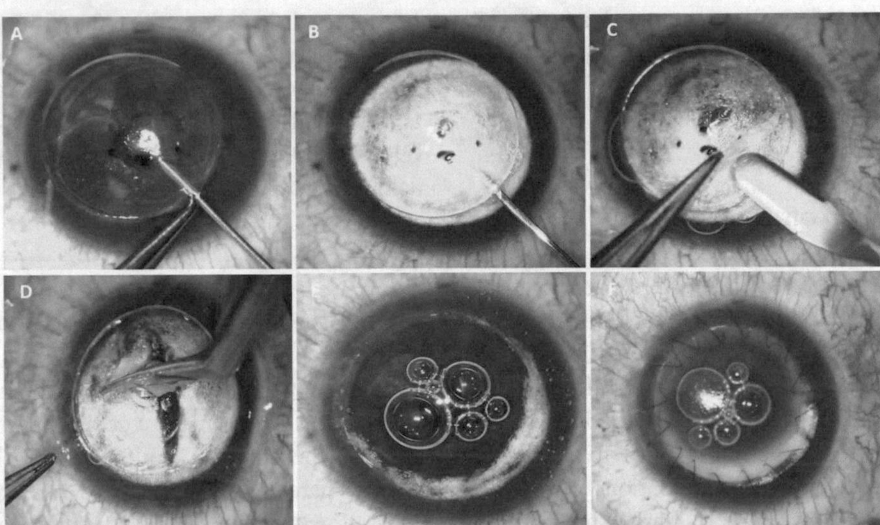

Fig. 23.3 DALK Big Bubble Technique: after a partial trephination of 70–80 % of the corneal stroma, pneumatic pressure is used to detach DM by injecting air into the deep stroma with a 27G needle (**a**). Once the air is injected it produces a dome-shaped detachment of the DM that is seen under the surgical microscope as a ring meaning that the big bubble has been formed (**b**). Then a lamellar dissection with a Crescent blade of the anterior stroma is performed (**c**) followed by the removal of the stromal tissue above the DM plane with spatula and scissors (**d**), making first sure to exchange the air in the supradescemetic plane with viscoelastic to avoid inadvertent puncture of the DM. When all of the stromal tissue is successfully removed, the DME membrane exposed is characteristically smooth (**e**), and the donor cornea without its DM and endothelium is then sutured with the preferred suture technique (**f**)

23.4.1.2 Melles Manual Method

This technique is based on the air–endothelium interface [8]. First the anterior chamber is filled with air. Then, using a series of curved spatulas through a scleral pocket, the stroma is carefully dissected away from the underlying DM. The difference in refractive index between the air and the corneal tissue creates a reflex in front of the surgical spatulas, and the distance between the instrument and the reflex is used to judge the amount of remaining tissue. Viscoelastic is injected through the scleral incision into the stromal pocket. Once the desired plane is reached, the superficial stroma is removed using trephine and lamellar dissection (Fig. 23.4).

Since the original descriptions, there have been many variations to the standard technique. Lamellar dissection can be made with diamond knife, nylon wire, microkeratome [37], or femtosecond laser. To help guiding the dissection plane trypan blue, ultrasound pachymetry [38] or real time optical coherence tomography [39] (OCT) has been tried. Partharsathy et al. describe the "small bubble" technique for confirming the presence of the big bubble [40].

For corneas with extreme peripheral thinning, a modified procedure has been proposed dubbed "tuck-in lamellar keratoplasty" [41, 42]. In this technique, the central anterior stromal disc is removed and a centrifugal lamellar dissection is performed using a knife to create a peripheral intrastromal pocket extending 0.5 mm beyond the limbus. The donor cornea is prepared in such a way that it has a central full thickness graft with a peripheral partial thickness flange. The edges of a large anterior lamellar graft are tucked in below to add extra thickness.

23.4.2 Outcomes

Most studies have found equivalent visual and refractive results between PK and DALK provided stromal dissection reaches the level or

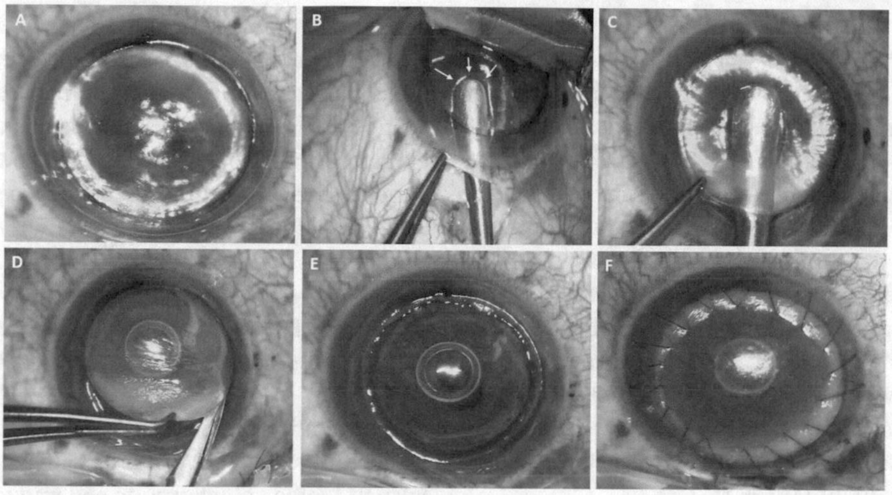

Fig. 23.4 DALK Melles Technique: first the anterior chamber is filled with air and a partial trephination of 70 % of the corneal stromais performed (**a**). Then, using a series of curved spatulas through a scleral pocket, the stroma is carefully dissected away from the underlying DM (**b**). The difference in refractive index between air and corneal tissue creates a reflex of the surgical spatulas, and the distance between the instrument and reflex is used to judge the amount of remaining underlying tissue (**b**, *arrows*). Viscoelastic is injected through the scleral incision into the stromal pocket and the dissection can be completed through the trephination edge (**c**). Once it is completed, the superficial stroma is removed (**d**), the DME membrane exposed, (**e**) and the donor cornea sutured (**f**)

close to the DM [12, 43–48], although 20/20 vision seems more likely after PK [12, 48]. For instance, in a recent study from Australian patients including 73 consecutive patients with keratoconus, the mean BCVA was not significantly different for DALK (0.14 logMAR, SD 0.2) versus PK (0.05 logMAR, SD 0.11) [12, 44]. A review of published literature that included 11 comparative studies on DALK and PK found that visual and refractive outcomes are comparable if the residual bed thickness in DALK cases is between 25 and 65 μm [14].

In those studies where the visual outcomes of DALK were inferior to PK [49], the dissection plane was "predescemetic" and the incomplete stromal dissection and the not fully baring of the DM had a negative impact in the results [49]. The problem seems to be related to the depth of the undissected stromal bed rather than to its smoothness as predescemetic DALKs performed by laser ablation did not outperform those dissected manually.

The recently published Australian graft registry data compared the outcomes of PKs and DALKs performed for KC over the same period of time and found that overall, both graft survival and visual outcomes were superior for PK. In a recent study from the UK, Jones et al. compared the outcomes after PKP and DALK for keratoconus [12]. The risk of graft failure for DALK was almost twice that for PKP. Probably, in the day-to-day clinical practice, visual outcomes with DALK, although comparable with PK, may be just slightly inferior or less predictable compared with PK, given surgical inexperience, and unpredictable issues regarding residual stromal thickness and DM folds. Nonetheless, elimination of risk of endothelial rejection compensates for this difference.

Lastly, one of the important advantages of DALK is a lower rate of endothelial loss compared with PK. The reported endothelial cell loss is as high as 34.6 % after PK, whereas it was 13.9 % after DALK [50].

23.4.3 Complications

Allograft reactions are less frequent in DALK than in PK and less likely to result in graft failure if correct treatment is initiated. Subepithelial and stromal rejection after DALK has been reported in the range of 3–14.3 % whereas in PKP ranges from 13 to 31 % in the first 3 years after surgery [11]. Endothelial rejection is not an issue in DALK.

Increases in IOP following DALK has been reported to be only 1.3 % of operated eyes, compared with 42 % of eyes after PK [50]. Development of glaucoma may also be up to 40 % less [51]. It is attributed to the lower steroid requirement of DALK [52].

Urrets–Zavalia Syndrome first reported following PK in KC and causing fixed, dilated pupil with iris atrophy is a rare entity following DALK [53].

There are also a few complications that are unique to DALK and the presence of a donor–host interface. One of the major problems with DALKs is intraoperative DM perforation, which may occur in 0–50 % of the eyes [11]. Surgeon's inexperience, corneal scarring near the DM, and advanced ectasias with corneal thickness less than 250 μm increase the risk [54, 55]. Depending on the size of the perforation, conversion to PK may be required to avoid double anterior chamber and persistent corneal edema, especially when the rupture leads to the collapse of the anterior chamber (macroperforation). Incidence of pseudoanterior chamber or double anterior chamber is in the range of 1 % [56]. It can occur because of retention of fluid secondary to breaks in the DM, or, because of incomplete removal of viscoelastic in the interface [57]. Large pseudo chambers must be managed surgically by drainage of the fluid and anterior chamber injection of air or gas [58]. The presence of DM folds caused by a mismatch between donor button and the recipient bed is usually transient and disappear over time, but interface wrinkling when central and persistent may affect quality of vision [59]. Occasionally an eye with anatomically correct DALK may require a reoperation secondary to interface haze and poor visual acuity, usually stemming from incomplete or predescemetic stromal dissection [11]. Interface keratitis is a serious complication of DALK and it is caused mainly by Candida [60] but Klebsiella pneumonia [61], and nontuberculous mycobacteria [62] have also been isolated in several cases. Conservative treatment is usually unsuccessful and most cases need a therapeutic PK [60]. Interface vascularization can occur because of inflammatory, infective, and traumatic episodes and can be treated with injection of bevacizumab [63].

23.5 Femtosecond Laser-Assisted Keratoplasty for Keratoconus

The capability of femtosecond laser energy to create different cutting patterns with a controlled level of biological interaction and minimal tissue trauma has provided a new possibility for corneal surgeons in both penetrating and nonpenetrating keratoplasty procedures. From case to case the cutting profile can be more convenient in one specific shape, what was impossible to be made before with the manual trephination techniques. The potential advantages of femtosecond laser-assisted keratoplasy are the following [64, 65]:

1. More precise and regular cuts
2. No risk of injury for intraocular structures
3. Perfect donor–recipient size matching
4. Less injury to donor endothelium
5. Customization of the cutting pattern
6. More donor–host tissue interaction promoting better wound healing
7. Potentially less induction of surgically induced astigmatism
8. Shorter visual rehabilitation time
9. Stronger and probably more stable wounds with earlier suture removal

23.5.1 Femtosecond-Assisted Keratoplasty Incision Profiles

Intralase (AMO) provides the more sophisticated and complex patterns when compared to the other technologies. The combination of simpler incisions (posterior side cut, anterior side cut, and lamellar cut) can be combined in limitless number of complex edge profile graft combinations [66] with a very high level of precision in dimensions and concentration which is not possible with other techniques [67].

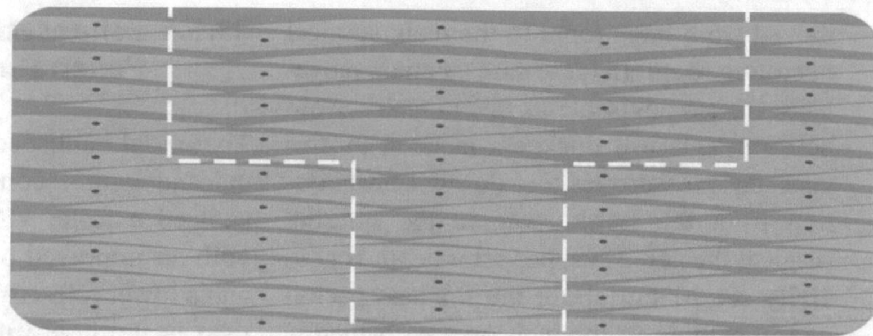

Fig. 23.5 Mushroom-based edge profile

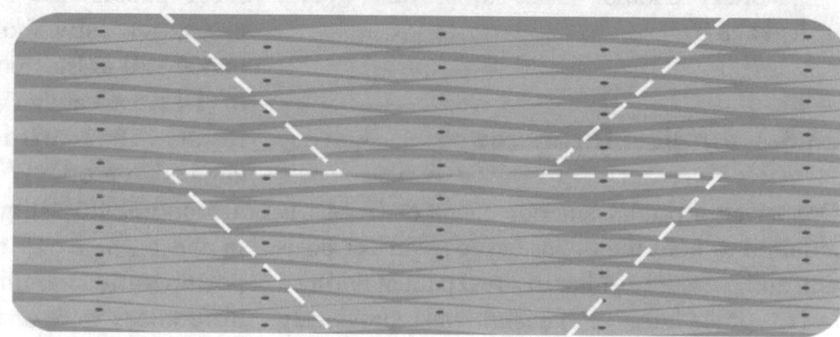

Fig. 23.6 Zigzag-based edge profile

- *Top-hat-based edge profile*
- This type of architecture maximizes the posterior tissue to be transplanted. Not suitable for keratoconus.
- *Mushroom-based edge profile*
- The inverted version of a top-hat is known as mushroom (Fig. 23.5) and is often used for anterior surface surgery, being composed of a narrower posterior side cut and a wider anterior side cut both intersected by the ring lamellar cut. The broader anterior section maximizes the anterior stroma area to be transplanted, what makes it suitable for keratoconus.
- *Zigzag-based edge profile*
- Zigzag profile (Fig. 23.6) is composed of a slanted anterior and posterior side cuts connected by the ring lamellar cut. It can be adapted to maximize either anterior or posterior surface, which makes it suitable to a wide variety of situations, including keratoconus.

23.5.2 Basics on Femtosecond Graft Architecture

Regardless of the profile being used, it is important to understand the basics of femtosecond incisions and stepped graft architecture [64].

- *Incision intersection*
  Femtosecond laser-assisted keratoplasty is formed by a combination of straight incisions that need to interact with each other in order to obtain a clear and continuous graft cutting profile that is easy to dissect, handle, and be later extracted. The overlapping degree is generally set between 10 and 30 μm.
- *Lamellar cut depth*
  As a thumb rule, lamellar cut depth is set at 50 % of average pachymetry in both donor and recipient corneas.
- *Oversizing*
  Femtosecond laser is able to create identical sized grafts in terms of diameter regardless of the keratometry readings, which has led to recommend using the exact same diameter in donor and recipient corneas [66, 68]. It is then up to the surgeon to decide oversizing primarily just in terms of postoperative spherical refraction needs.
- *Deepest posterior point*
  When designing the donor graft in PKP, posterior depth must be set below the maximum pachymetric reading in the incision area in order to assure a clean and full thickness incision. On the other hand, recipient might be

moved from laser room to the main surgical operating room. In these cases, patient movement makes advisable to intentionally avoid performing a full thickness incision to prevent any pressure leaking during transportation from the Lasik room to the suturing surgical theater. Thus, posterior depth is generally set 70 μm above the thinnest pachymetric reading in the incision area, which is generally enough tissue to prevent wound leakage [69].

23.5.3 Surgical Technique

Donor: an artificial anterior chamber (AAC) is required to hold the donor tissue in proper position and pressure similar to a real patient during a lasik procedure; *Recipient*: as previously described, it is necessary to leave a safety gap of posterior noncut tissue on the recipient cornea which prevents any aqueous humor leakage during transportation [69]; *Graft manipulation*: a Sinskey hook is used to dissect the different incisions being the procedure identical in both donor and recipient corneas. However, recipient cornea partial thickness cut will be completed with a diamond blade and curved scissors.

23.5.4 Femtosecond-Assisted Penetrating Keratoplasty

The initial published evidence comparing manual and femtosecond laser-assisted PK (f-PK) showed a faster visual rehabilitation together with an improved best corrected visual acuity, and a lower refractive and topographic astigmatism in the laser group [70–73]. Nevertheless, these papers had a limited follow-up of the cases, generally shorter than a year. Little evidence still exists about the long-term outcomes of f-PK: Chamberlain et al. published their results with 2-year follow-up and using a "zig-zag" edge profile [74]. They could demonstrate a topographic astigmatism significantly lower in the f-PK group but only during the first 6 postoperative months. Afterward no significant differences were observed regarding the refractive or topographic astigmatism and visual acuity. Only a few papers have been published comparing the different cutting edge profiles [75]. Our impression is that there are not significant differences in the visual or refractive outcomes regarding the preferred edge profile, although studies comparing the "zig-zag" and "mushroom" profiles in keratoconus are still required (Fig. 23.7).

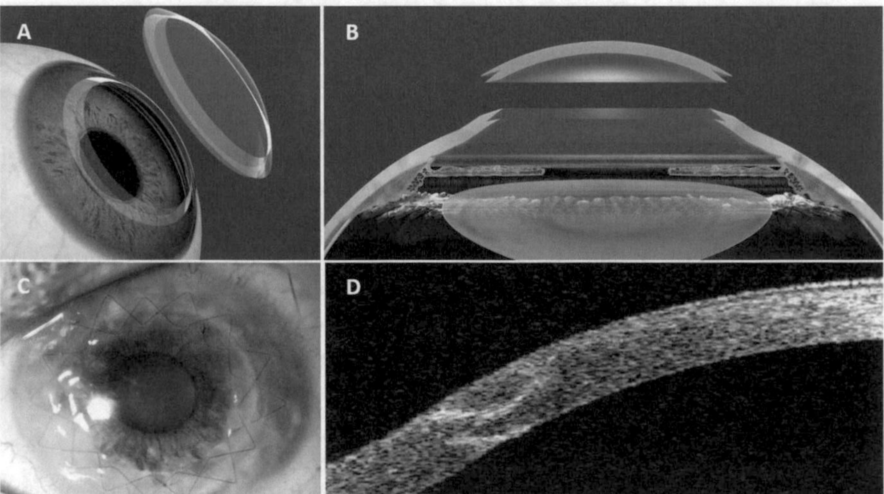

Fig. 23.7 Femtosecond laser-assisted penetrating keratoplasty with a "Zig-Zag" edge profile (**a**, **b**; courtesy of Abbott Medical Optics, USA). Postoperative clinical picture (**c**) and an anterior segment OCT capture (**d**) where it is possible to appreciate the zig-zag edge profile at the host–donor interface with a perfect coalescence of the edges

23.5.5 Femtosecond-Assisted Deep Anterior Lamellar Keratoplasty

The use of the femtosecond laser in DALK (f-DALK) avoids manual trephination and allows more precise identification of tissue depth and insertion of the air needle by following the plane between the lamellar and posterior laser side cuts. As variability in stromal thickness in eyes with advanced keratoconus, ectasia, or dense and deep stromal scars may limit the ability of the femtosecond laser to produce a uniform lamellar plane, we use the laser only to create the side cut both in donor and recipient cornea, while leaving a minimal amount of residual corneal tissue. With this we try to control the potential risk of creating a DM perforation with the femtosecond laser.

Femtosecond laser mushroom configuration is the preferred profile for DALK (Fig. 23.8). For the side cut a full thickness mushroom configuration cut is made on the donor cornea first and then a nonpenetrating mushroom configuration on the recipient. In the recipient cornea, the depth of the anterior side cut is about 60 % of the thinnest corneal pachymetry, the depth of the posterior side cut about 80 % of the thinnest corneal pachymetry, leaving a ring lamellar cut of 1 mm (Fig. 23.9). In the donor cornea, the Descemet's membrane (DM) and endothelium is debrided assisted by trypan blue dye.

Femtosecond laser-assisted DALK might have an advantage in keratoconus cases because it provides a larger amount of donor–recipient tissue to interact for the purpose of corneal wound healing consistency, and it has been demonstrated recently by our group that f-DALK shows a more active wound healing leading to leucomatous wounds [76]. We established a grading for the side cut corneal healing pattern as observed by slit lamp examination (Table 23.1), and we could observe that 52 % of f-DALK cases

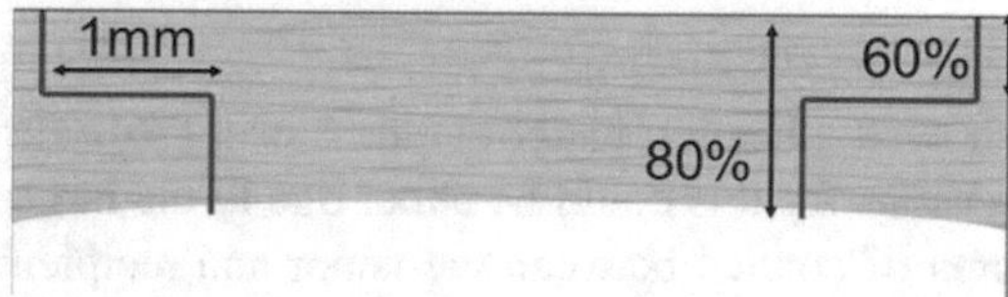

Fig. 23.9 Mushroom DALK configuration: the depth of the anterior side cut is about 60 % of the thinnest corneal pachymetry, the depth of the posterior side cut about 80 % of the thinnest corneal pachymetry, leaving a ring lamellar cut of 1 mm

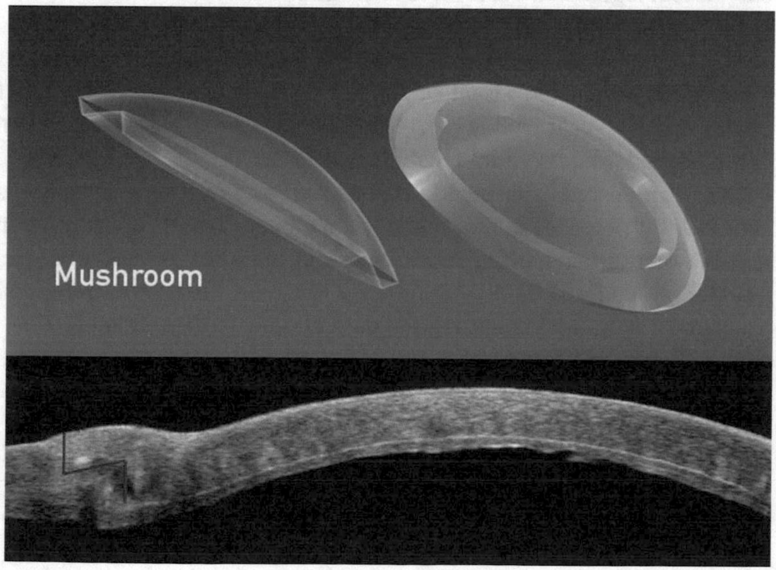

Fig. 23.8 Femtosecond laser-assisted DALK with a "Mushroom" edge profile (*up*: courtesy of Abbott Medical Optics, USA). Postoperative anterior segment OCT capture (*down*) where it is possible to appreciate the mushroom edge profile at the host–donor interface

Table 23.1 Analysis of femtosecond laser side cut corneal wound healing pattern

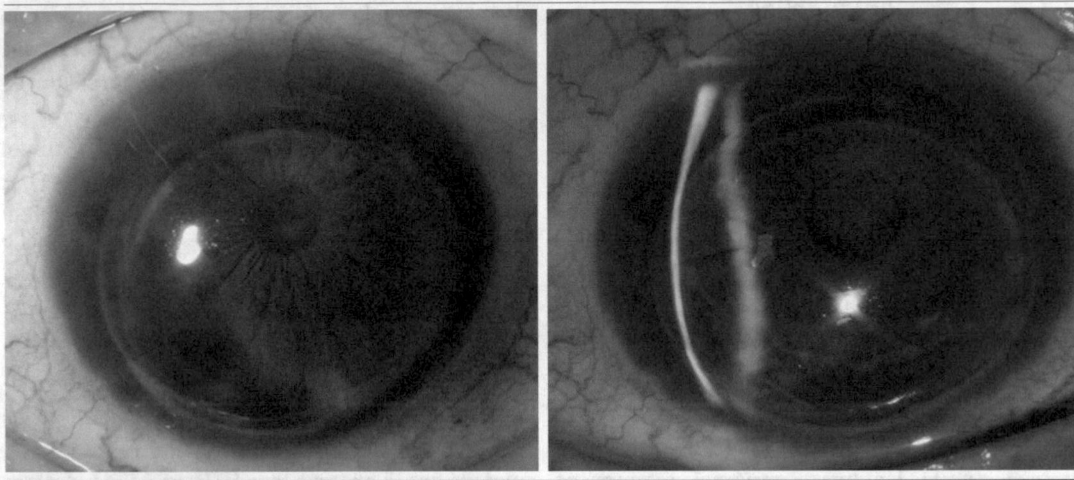

Keratoconus recurrence 17 years after a penetrating keratoplasty (*left*). Observe the severe thinning of the recipient stroma at the graft–host junction (*right*)

showed a healing pattern grade 3 or 4 [76]. The reasons for this could be either due to the larger area of contact between the donor and recipient tissues and/or to femtosecond laser-related biological activation of the corneal tissues, which should be related to the level of energy used for the creation of the side cut.

Equivalent to f-PK, f-DALK accelerates the visual rehabilitation, showing a better visual result during the immediate postoperative period, but without significant differences after the sixth postoperative month [77]. In a recent study of our group, we could not demonstrate significant differences regarding the visual or refractive outcomes after 1-year follow-up. However, we demonstrated a faster visual rehabilitation in the f-DALK group versus manual DALK as well as significant differences in the wound healing pattern between groups, being more intense in the f-DALK group [76].

Summarizing, and regarding the current evidence, femtosecond laser accelerates the visual rehabilitation after PK or DALK compared with the manual technique, obtaining better refractive and visual results along the immediate postoperative period; however, these benefits are lost later in the follow-up, not being able to improve the refractive or visual outcomes in the long term. Considering the high costs of this technology, these results do not justify its use as a gold standard for keratoplasty. Nevertheless, if available, femtosecond laser offers important intraoperative (easy wound closure) and perioperative (faster rehabilitation) advantages, together with a stronger surgical wound that allows a faster suture removal (depending on the wound healing pattern) and probably less risk of dehiscence against an ocular trauma in the long term.

23.6 Keratoconus Recurrence After Corneal Transplantation

We have already discussed the good long-term results of the different options of corneal grafting for keratoconus. Nevertheless, de Toledo et al. observed a progressive increase of keratometric astigmatism in 70 % of their cases from 10 years after suture removal, following an initial phase of refractive stability during the first 7 years after PK for keratoconus (4.05 ± 2.29 D 1 year after suture removal, 3.90 ± 2.28 D at year 3, 4.03 ± 2.49 D at year 5, 4.39 ± 2.48 D at year 7, 5.48 ± 3.11 D at year 10, 6.43 ± 4.11 D at year 15; 7.28 ± 4.21 D at year 20, and 7.25 ± 4.27 D at year

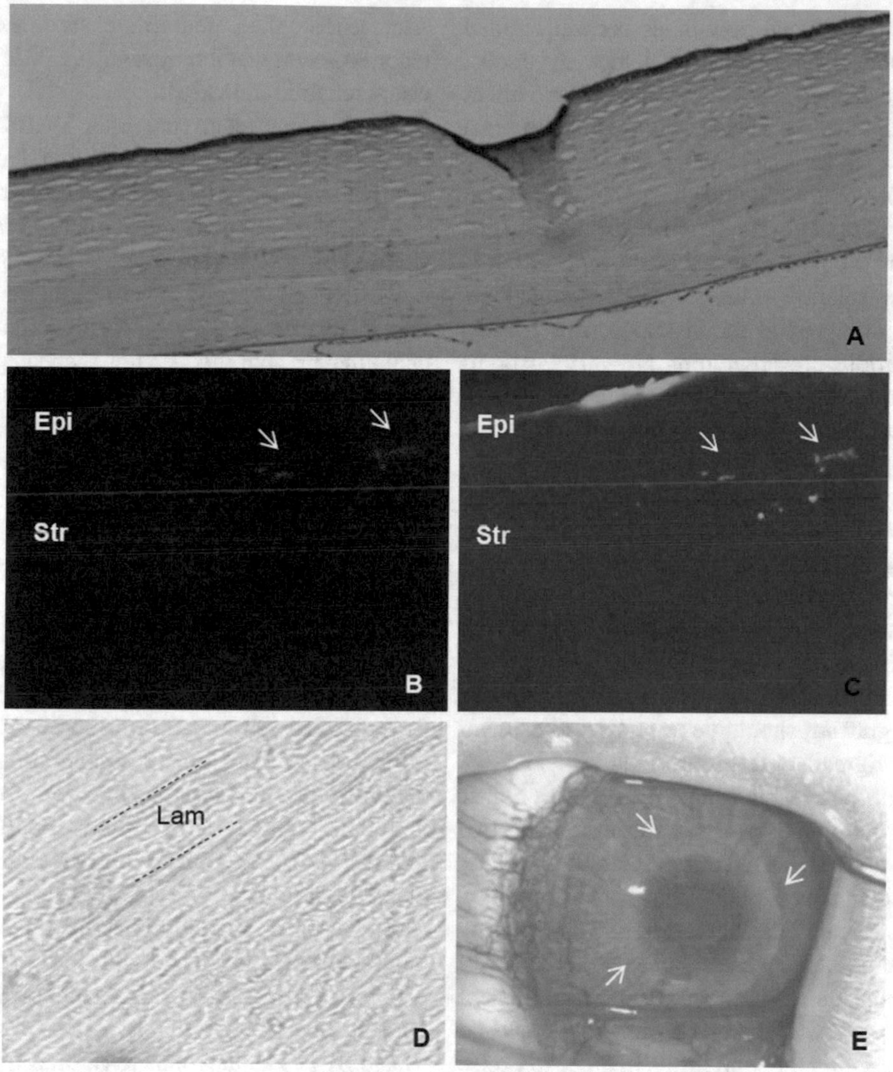

Fig. 23.10 Reconstruction of corneal stroma. (**a**) Hematoxylin–eosin staining of a rabbit cornea with an implanted graft of decellularized human corneal stroma with h-ADASC colonization: hypocellular band of ECM without vessels or any inflammatory sign (magnification ×200); (**b**) human cells labeled with CM-DiI around and inside the implant that express (**c**) human keratocan (human adult keratocyte specific marker; magnification ×400), confirming the presence of living human cells inside the corneal stroma and their differentiation into human keratocytes (*arrows*); (**d**) phase-contrast photomicrographs showing a morphologically unaltered corneal stroma (magnification ×400); (**e**) the graft remains totally transparent after 12 weeks of follow-up (magnification ×2) (*arrows* point to the slightly visible edge of the graft). *Epi* epithelium, *Str* stroma, *Lam* Lamina

25), so a late recurrence of the disease may occur with an increasing risk over time [16]. Actually, a 20 year post-PK probability of 10 % has been reported previously, with a mean time to recurrence of 17.9–21.9 years, so given the younger age at which keratoconus patients undergo corneal transplantation, these long-term findings should be explained to patients and incorporated into the preoperative counseling [29, 34, 78] (Fig. 23.10).

It is well known how other corneal stromal dystrophies, like granular or lattice dystrophy, tend to recur into the donor cornea, due to either colonization of the new stroma by the abnormal host keratocytes or epithelial secretion in early stages. In keratoconus this host keratocyte invasion has not been well stabilized as the main etiology for the post graft recurrent ectasia, but is likely in relation with the early keratoconic changes observed in the histology of explanted donor buttons after regrafting [78–80]. Postgraft ectasia is often preceded by thinning of the recipient stroma at the graft–host junction, so the disease progression at the host stroma is likely to be the underlying reason for these cases of recurrent ectasia and progressive astigmatism over time [16, 78]. In such cases, a mean keratometric sphere and cylinder increase of 4D and 3D, respectively, between final suture removal and diagnosis can be observed [78].

The management of recurrent ectasia after corneal grafting should be spectacle adjustment if low astigmatism levels are induced and rigid/hybrid gas permeable contact lenses with higher levels of astigmatism or significant anisometropia. For more advanced cases, scleral lenses may be considered before a surgical approach. If a second corneal transplant is required either a new full thickness PK versus lamellar keratoplasty can be considered. Large grafts are usually necessary as the whole area of thinning should be included within the graft limits in order to excise the whole cone to avoid a new recurrence and also to avoid suturing through a thin recipient cornea. As large grafts are associated with increased risk of rejection and glaucoma, lamellar techniques by manual dissection of the host and donor corneal stroma are always preferable as far as the donor endothelium presents healthy without signs of failure. If femtosecond dissection of the lamellar bed is chosen, gentian violet and cyanoacrylate glue can be used in the area of thinning as masking agents to minimize the risk of perforation [81]. Limbus may have to be recessed while suturing very large grafts that sit close to the limbus in order to avoid passing the suture through the conjunctiva at the host side. Recurrence after regrafting has also been reported, event that it may require a third graft for visual rehabilitation [78].

Keratoconus recurrence after DALK has not been described, being currently available very little evidence about its real incidence and impact. Feizi et al. reported a case where keratoconus recurred only 49 months after DALK [82]. They suggested that the time interval from transplantation to recurrence may be shorter after DALK than after PK, but this has not been supported or confirmed by other authors [83]. Further research analyzing the long-term outcomes after DALK for keratoconus is required in order to investigate its real incidence.

23.7 A Glance at the Future

Keratoconus is a corneal disease that affects primary the corneal stroma and Bowman layer. Current research and future therapeutic directions are focusing in the regeneration of corneal stroma by less or no invasive procedures that could avoid the common complications that we still see even with lamellar keratoplasty techniques.

Melles at al. recently described a new technique where an isolated Bowman layer is transplanted into a mid-stromal manually dissected corneal pocket in patients with an advanced (Stage III-IV) keratoconus [84]. They observed a modest improvement in the maximum keratometry and BSCVA but an unchanged best contact lens corrected visual acuity (BCLVA). This is a new interesting approach that it could have its indication for those advanced keratoconus non-suitable for corneal collagen crosslinking or intracorneal ring segments and intolerant to contact lenses but without visually significant corneal scars and therefore good BCLVA. In such cases Bowman's transplant could avoid or postpone the necessity of keratoplasty if the mild observed corneal flattening enables continued contact lens wear and the cone is stabilized (as it has been reported to happen but with only a sample of 20 eyes and a short mean follow-up of 21 months). Further research by alternative authors with a larger sample and longer follow-up is needed before introducing this technique into the routine clinical practice.

As discussed, Bowman's transplantation could have some benefits in cases of advanced keratoconus, but even if these results are finally confirmed by other authors, they offer a mild improvement to these patients without a significant functional/anatomical rehabilitation, so further techniques may focus on attempting the subtotal regeneration or substitution of the corneal stroma in order to achieve better results. Different types of stem cells have been used in various ways in several research projects in order to find the optimal procedure to regenerate the human corneal stroma: Corneal Stromal Stem Cells (CSSC), Bone Marrow Mesenchymal Stem Cells (BM-MSCs), Adipose Derived Adult Mesenchymal Stem Cells (ADASCs), Umbilical Cord Mesenchymal Stem Cells (UCMSCs), Embryonic Stem Cells (ESCs) [85]. These approaches can be classified into four techniques:

1. *Intrastromal injection of stem cells alone*

   Direct injection of stem cells inside the corneal stroma has been assayed in vivo in some studies, demonstrating the differentiation of the stem cells into adult keratocytes without signs of immune rejection. Our group demonstrated the production of human extracellular matrix when human ADASCs (h-ADASC) were transplanted inside the rabbit cornea [86]. Du et al. reported a restoration of the corneal transparency and thickness in lumican null mice (thin corneas, haze, and disruption of normal stromal organization) 3 months after the intrastromal transplant of human CSSCs. They also confirmed that human keratan sulfate was deposited in the mouse stroma and the host collagen lamellae were reorganized, concluding that delivery of h-CSSCs to scarred human stroma may alleviate corneal scars without requiring surgery [87]. Very similar findings were reported by Liu et al. using human UMSCs in the same animal model [88]. Recently, Thomas et al. found that, in a mice model for mucopolysaccharidosis, transplanted human UMSC participate both in extracellular glycosaminoglycans (GAG) turnover and enable host keratocytes to catabolize accumulated GAG products [89]. In our experience, the production of human extracellular matrix by implanted mesenchymal stem cells occurs, but not quantitatively enough to be able to restore the thickness of a diseased human cornea. However, the direct injection of stem cells may provide a promising treatment for corneal dystrophies including keratoconus, by regulating the abnormal host keratocyte collagen production, enabling collagen microstructure reorganization, and corneal scarring modulation.

2. *Intrastromal implantation of stem cells together with a biodegradable scaffold*

   In order to enhance the growth and development of the stem cells injected into the corneal stroma, transplantation together with biodegradable synthetic extracellular matrixes has been performed. Espandar et al. injected h-ADASCs with a semisolid hyaluronic acid hydrogel into rabbit corneal stroma, reporting better survival and keratocyte differentiation of the h-ADASCs when compared to their injection alone [90]. Ma et al. used rabbit ADSCs with a polylactic-co-glycolic (PLGA) biodegradable scaffold in a rabbit model of stromal injury, observing newly formed tissue with successful collagen remodeling and less stromal scarring [91]. Initial data show that these scaffolds could enhance stem cell effects over corneal stroma, although more research is required.

3. *Intrastromal implantation of stem cells with a nonbiodegradable scaffold*

   At the present time, no clinically viable human corneal equivalents have been produced by tissue engineering methods. The major obstacle to the production of a successfully engineered cornea is the difficulty with reproducing (or at least simulating) the stromal architecture. The majority of stromal analogs for tissue engineered corneas have been created by seeding human corneal stromal cells into collagen-based scaffoldings, which are apparently designed to be remodeled (see Ruberti et al. 2008 for a general review of corneal tissue engineering) [92]. The major drawback of these analogs is their lack of strength, thus unable to restore the normal mechanical properties of the cornea. New and improved biomaterials compatible with human corneas and with enhanced structural support have been developed leading to advanced scaffolds that can be used to engineer an artificial cornea (keratoprosthesis) [85]. The combination of these scaffolds with cells can generate promising corneal stroma equivalents, and some studies have already been published that use mainly corneal cell lines providing positive results regarding adhesion and cellular survival in vitro [93]. Our opinion is that stem cells do not differentiate properly into keratocytes in the presence of these synthetic biomaterials, losing their potential benefits and not resolving the major drawbacks with such substitutes: their relatively high extrusion rate and lack of complete transparency [94].

4. *Intrastromal implantation of stem cells with a decellularized corneal stromal scaffold*

   The complex structure of the corneal stroma has not been yet replicated, and there are well-known drawbacks to the use of synthetic scaffold-based designs. Recently, several corneal decellularization techniques have been described, which provide an acellular corneal extracellular matrix (ECM) [95]. These scaffolds have gained attention in the last few years as they provide a more natural environment for the growth and differentiation of cells when compared with synthetic scaffolds. In addition, components of the ECM are generally conserved among species and are tolerated well even by xenogeneic recipients. Keratocytes are essential for remodeling the corneal stroma and for normal epithelial physiology [96]. This highlights the importance of transplanting a cellular substitute together with the structural support (acellular ECM) to undertake these critical functions in corneal homeostasis. To the best of our knowledge, all attempts to repopulate decellularized corneal scaffolds have used corneal cells [97–99], but these cells have major drawbacks that preclude their autologous use in clinical practice (damage of the donor tissue, lack of cells, and inefficient cell subcultures), thus the efforts to find an extraocular source of autologous cells. In a recent study by our group, we showed the perfect biointegration of human decellularized corneal stromal sheets (100 μm thickness) with and without h-ADASC colonization inside the rabbit cornea in vivo (Fig. 23.10a,b), without observing any rejection response despite the graft being xenogeneic [100]. We also demonstrated the differentiation of h-ADASCs into functional keratocytes inside these implants in vivo, which then achieved their proper biofunctionalization (Fig. 23.10c). In our opinion the transplant of stem cells together with decellularized corneal ECM would be the best technique to effectively restore the thickness of a diseased human cornea, like in keratoconus. Through this technique, and using extraocular mesenchymal stem cells from patients, it is possible to transform allergenic grafts into functional autologous grafts, theoretically avoiding the risk of rejection.

23.8 Conclusion

Treatment of keratoconus has experienced great advances in the last two decades. From being limited only to rigid gas permeable contact lens wear and penetrating keratoplasty for the most advanced cases, to have nowadays different therapeutic alternatives to treat not only the cone and postpone/avoid the necessity of a corneal transplant, but also being able to halt the progression of the disease with a very high rate of efficacy and safety [101] (Figs. 23.11 and 23.12). Also the advances in refractive surgery including surface corneal ablation treatments and phakic intraocu-

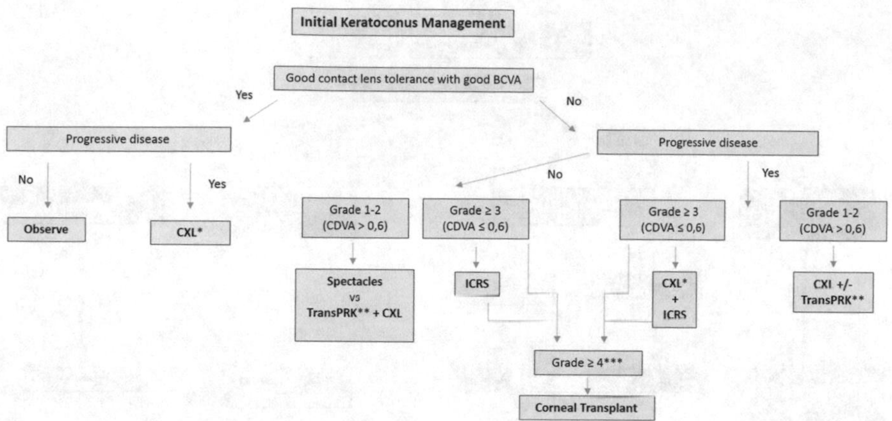

Fig. 23.11 Decision tree for intervention at presentation in keratoconus. Grading regarding the RETICS classification. *BCVA* best corrected visual acuity, *CDVA* corrected distance visual acuity, *CXL* corneal collagen crosslinking, *TransPRK* transepithelial photorefractive keratectomy, *ICRS* intracorneal ring segments (* if thinnest point>370 µm; ** wavefront guided transPRK (limited treatment) to reduce coma-like aberrations and increase CDVA; *** if corneal scarring, insufficient corneal thickness for ICRS implantation or ICRS failure with persistent contact/scleral lenses intolerance and poor CDVA)

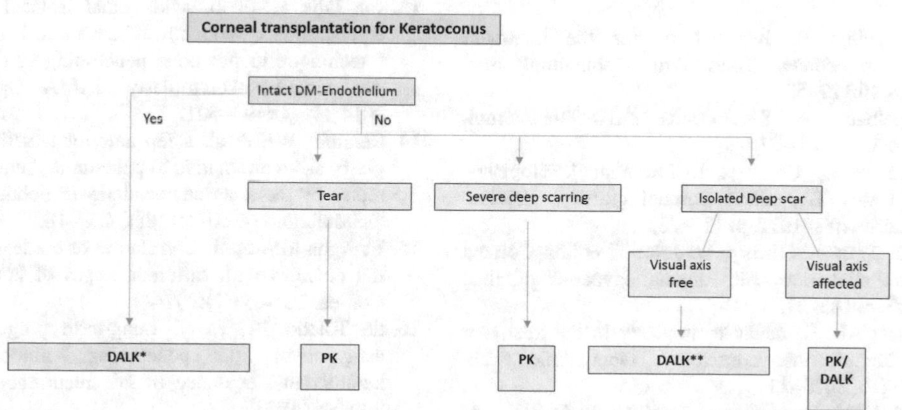

Fig. 23.12 Guideline for corneal transplant technique selection in cases of advanced keratoconus (*big bubble DALK as technique of choice due to its better visual performance; **assess manual DALK with "Melles" technique as big bubble technique will likely burst the Descemet membrane-endothelium layer)

lar lenses have allowed a better management and visual rehabilitation of these patients after a corneal transplant is required, being able to achieve, in many cases, a 20/20 unaided vision (Fig. 23.13). The future expected advances in transepithelial crosslinking, nanotechnology, and regenerative medicine predict an exciting future in this field and we will be looking forward to updating these guidelines.

Compliance with Ethical Requirements
Informed Consent: No human studies were carried out by the authors for this article.

Animal Studies: All institutional and national guidelines for the care and use of laboratory animals were followed.

Financial support or proprietary interest: None.
No conflicting relationship exists for any author.
No public or private support.

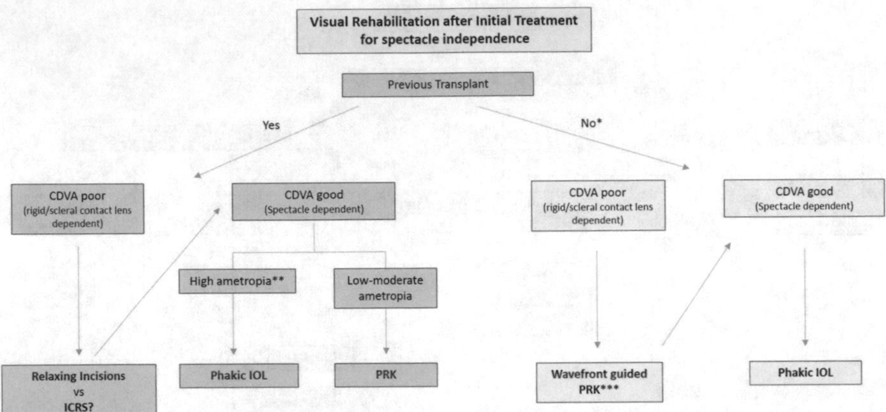

Fig. 23.13 Visual rehabilitation in order to achieve a spectacle independence for keratoconic eyes once the initial treatment has been completed and the stability of the disease has been confirmed (* gross shape correction with CXL±ICRS; ** mainly in cases of high cylinder or moderate-high hyperopia; *** if previous CXL has been done and stability is confirmed)

References

1. Castroviejo R. Keratoplasty for the treatment of keratoconus. Trans Am Ophthalmol Soc. 1948;46:127–53.
2. Appelbaum A. Keratoconus. Arch Ophthalmol. 1936;15(5):900–21.
3. Paufique L, Charleux J. Lamellar keratoplasty. In: Casey TA, editor. Corneal grafting. London: Butterworths; 1972. p. 121–76.
4. John T, et al. History. In: John T, editor. Corneal endothelial transplant. Panama: Jaypee-Highlights; 2010. p. 143–57.
5. Gasset AR. Lamellar keratoplasty in the treatment of keratoconus: conectomy. Ophthalmic Surg. 1979;10(2):26–33.
6. Archila EA. Deep lamellar keratoplasty dissection of host tissue with intrastromal air injection. Cornea. 1984;3(3):217–8.
7. Sugita J, Kondo J. Deep lamellar keratoplasty with complete removal of pathological stroma for vision improvement. Br J Ophthalmol. 1997;81(3):184–8.
8. Melles GR, et al. A new surgical technique for deep stromal, anterior lamellar keratoplasty. Br J Ophthalmol. 1999;83(3):327–33.
9. Anwar M, Teichmann KD. Big-bubble technique to bare Descemet's membrane in anterior lamellar keratoplasty. J Cataract Refract Surg. 2002;28(3):398–403.
10. Jhanji V, Sharma N, Vajpayee RB. Management of keratoconus: current scenario. Br J Ophthalmol. 2011;95(8):1044–50.
11. Parker JS, van Dijk K, Melles GR. Treatment options for advanced keratoconus: a review. Surv Ophthalmol. 2015;60(5):459–80.
12. Jones MN, et al. Penetrating and deep anterior lamellar keratoplasty for keratoconus: a comparison of graft outcomes in the United Kingdom. Invest Ophthalmol Vis Sci. 2009;50(12):5625–9.
13. van Dijk K, et al. Midstromal isolated Bowman layer graft for reduction of advanced keratoconus: a technique to postpone penetrating or deep anterior lamellar keratoplasty. JAMA Ophthalmol. 2014;132(4):495–501.
14. Reinhart WJ, et al. Deep anterior lamellar keratoplasty as an alternative to penetrating keratoplasty a report by the american academy of ophthalmology. Ophthalmology. 2011;118(1):209–18.
15. El-Agha MS, et al. Correlation of corneal endothelial changes with different stages of keratoconus. Cornea. 2014;33(7):707–11.
16. de Toledo JA, et al. Long-term progression of astigmatism after penetrating keratoplasty for keratoconus: evidence of late recurrence. Cornea. 2003;22(4):317–23.
17. Sharif KW, Casey TA. Penetrating keratoplasty for keratoconus: complications and long-term success. Br J Ophthalmol. 1991;75(3):142–6.
18. Tuft SJ, Gregory WM, Davison CR. Bilateral penetrating keratoplasty for keratoconus. Ophthalmology. 1995;102(3):462–8.
19. Olson RJ. Variation in corneal graft size related to trephine technique. Arch Ophthalmol. 1979;97(7):1323–5.
20. Wilson SE, Bourne WM. Effect of recipient-donor trephine size disparity on refractive error in keratoconus. Ophthalmology. 1989;96(3):299–305.
21. Javadi MA, et al. A comparison between donor-recipient corneal size and its effect on the ultimate refractive error induced in keratoconus. Cornea. 1993;12(5):401–5.
22. Kuryan J, Channa P. Refractive surgery after corneal transplant. Curr Opin Ophthalmol. 2010;21(4):259–64.

23. Lanier JD, Bullington Jr RH, Prager TC. Axial length in keratoconus. Cornea. 1992;11(3):250–4.
24. Tuft SJ, Fitzke FW, Buckey RJ. Myopia following penetrating keratoplasty for keratoconus. Br J Ophthalmol. 1992;76:642–5.
25. Busin M, et al. Intraoperative cauterization of the cornea can reduce postkeratoplasty refractive error in patients with keratoconus. Ophthalmology. 1998;105(8):1524–9.
26. Gasset AR, Kaufman HE. Thermokeratoplasty in the treatment of keratoconus. Am J Ophthalmol. 1975;79:226–32.
27. Javadi MA, et al. Comparison of the effect of three suturing techniques on postkeratoplasty astigmatism in keratoconus. Cornea. 2006;25(9):1029–33.
28. Solano JM, Hodge DO, Bourne WM. Keratometric astigmatism after suture removal in penetrating keratoplasty: double running versus single running suture techniques. Cornea. 2003;22(8):716–20.
29. Niziol LM, et al. Long-term outcomes in patients who received a corneal graft for keratoconus between 1980 and 1986. Am J Ophthalmol. 2013; 155(2):213–9.e3.
30. Fukuoka S, et al. Extended long-term results of penetrating keratoplasty for keratoconus. Cornea. 2010;29(5):528–30.
31. Choi JA, Lee MA, Kim MS. Long-term outcomes of penetrating keratoplasty in keratoconus: analysis of the factors associated with final visual acuities. Int J Ophthalmol. 2014;7(3):517–21.
32. Buzard KA, Fundingsland BR. Corneal transplant for keratoconus: results in early and late disease. J Cataract Refract Surg. 1997;23(3):398–406.
33. Javadi MA, et al. Outcomes of penetrating keratoplasty in keratoconus. Cornea. 2005;24(8):941–6.
34. Pramanik S, et al. Extended long-term outcomes of penetrating keratoplasty for keratoconus. Ophthalmology. 2006;113(9):1633–8.
35. Claesson M, Armitage WJ. Clinical outcome of repeat penetrating keratoplasty. Cornea. 2013;32(7):1026–30.
36. Amayem AF, Anwar M. Fluid lamellar keratoplasty in keratoconus. Ophthalmology. 2000;107(1):76–9; discussion 80.
37. Bilgihan K, et al. Microkeratome-assisted lamellar keratoplasty for keratoconus: stromal sandwich. J Cataract Refract Surg. 2003;29(7):1267–72.
38. Ghanem RC, Ghanem MA. Pachymetry-guided intrastromal air injection ("pachy-bubble") for deep anterior lamellar keratoplasty. Cornea. 2012;31(9): 1087–91.
39. De Benito-Llopis L, et al. Intraoperative anterior segment optical coherence tomography: a novel assessment tool during deep anterior lamellar keratoplasty. Am J Ophthalmol. 2014;157(2): 334–41.e3.
40. Parthasarathy A, Por YM, Tan DT. Use of a "small-bubble technique" to increase the success of Anwar's "big-bubble technique" for deep lamellar keratoplasty with complete baring of Descemet's membrane. Br J Ophthalmol. 2007;91(10):1369–73.
41. Vajpayee RB, Bhartiya P, Sharma N. Central lamellar keratoplasty with peripheral intralamellar tuck: a new surgical technique for keratoglobus. Cornea. 2002;21(7):657–60.
42. Kaushal S, et al. "Tuck In" Lamellar Keratoplasty (TILK) for corneal ectasias involving corneal periphery. Br J Ophthalmol. 2008;92(2):286–90.
43. Fontana L, et al. Influence of graft-host interface on the quality of vision after deep anterior lamellar keratoplasty in patients with keratoconus. Cornea. 2011;30(5):497–502.
44. Funnell CL, Ball J, Noble BA. Comparative cohort study of the outcomes of deep lamellar keratoplasty and penetrating keratoplasty for keratoconus. Eye (Lond). 2006;20(5):527–32.
45. Smadja D, et al. Outcomes of deep anterior lamellar keratoplasty for keratoconus: learning curve and advantages of the big bubble technique. Cornea. 2012;31(8):859–63.
46. Kim MH, Chung TY, Chung ES. A retrospective contralateral study comparing deep anterior lamellar keratoplasty with penetrating keratoplasty. Cornea. 2013;32(4):385–9.
47. Han DC, et al. Comparison of outcomes of lamellar keratoplasty and penetrating keratoplasty in keratoconus. Am J Ophthalmol. 2009;148(5):744–51.e1.
48. MacIntyre R, et al. Long-term outcomes of deep anterior lamellar keratoplasty versus penetrating keratoplasty in Australian keratoconus patients. Cornea. 2014;33(1):6–9.
49. Ardjomand N, et al. Quality of vision and graft thickness in deep anterior lamellar and penetrating corneal allografts. Am J Ophthalmol. 2007;143(2):228–35.
50. Zhang YM, Wu SQ, Yao YF. Long-term comparison of full-bed deep anterior lamellar keratoplasty and penetrating keratoplasty in treating keratoconus. J Zhejiang Univ Sci B. 2013;14(5):438–50.
51. Tan DT, et al. Visual acuity outcomes after deep anterior lamellar keratoplasty: a case-control study. Br J Ophthalmol. 2010;94(10):1295–9.
52. Musa FU, et al. Long-term risk of intraocular pressure elevation and glaucoma escalation after deep anterior lamellar keratoplasty. Clin Experiment Ophthalmol. 2012;40(8):780–5.
53. Niknam S, Rajabi MT. Fixed dilated pupil (Urrets-Zavalia syndrome) after deep anterior lamellar keratoplasty. Cornea. 2009;28(10):1187–90.
54. Michieletto P, et al. Factors predicting unsuccessful big bubble deep lamellar anterior keratoplasty. Ophthalmologica. 2006;220(6):379–82.
55. Baradaran-Rafii A, et al. Anwar versus Melles deep anterior lamellar keratoplasty for keratoconus: a prospective randomized clinical trial. Ophthalmology. 2013;120(2):252–9.
56. Sharma N, et al. Use of trypan blue dye during conversion of deep anterior lamellar keratoplasty to penetrating keratoplasty. J Cataract Refract Surg. 2008;34(8):1242–5.
57. Sarnicola V, et al. Descemetic DALK and predescemetic DALK: outcomes in 236 cases of keratoconus. Cornea. 2010;29(1):53–9.

58. Shimmura S, Tsubota K. Deep anterior lamellar keratoplasty. Curr Opin Ophthalmol. 2006;17(4):349–55.
59. Mohamed SR, et al. Non-resolving Descemet folds 2 years following deep anterior lamellar keratoplasty: the impact on visual outcome. Cont Lens Anterior Eye. 2009;32(6):300–2.
60. Kanavi MR, et al. Candida interface keratitis after deep anterior lamellar keratoplasty: clinical, microbiologic, histopathologic, and confocal microscopic reports. Cornea. 2007;26(8):913–6.
61. Zarei-Ghanavati S, Sedaghat MR, Ghavami-Shahri A. Acute Klebsiella pneumoniae interface keratitis after deep anterior lamellar keratoplasty. Jpn J Ophthalmol. 2011;55(1):74–6.
62. Murthy SI, et al. Recurrent non-tuberculous mycobacterial keratitis after deep anterior lamellar keratoplasty for keratoconus. BMJ Case Rep. 2013;2013. doi:10.1136/bcr-2013-200641.
63. Hashemian MN, et al. Deep intrastromal bevacizumab injection for management of corneal stromal vascularization after deep anterior lamellar keratoplasty, a novel technique. Cornea. 2011;30(2):215–8.
64. Alio JL, Vega-Estrada A, Soria F, editors. Femtosecond laser-assisted keratoplasty. 1st ed. New Delhi, India: Jaypee Brothers; 2013. p. 75–6.
65. Alió JL, Alió del Barrio JL, Abdelghany A, Vega-Estrada A. Láser de femtosegundo en la cirugía del trasplante corneal. Ponencia: Sociedad Española de Oftalmología; 2016 (in press).
66. Farid M, Kim M, Steinert RF. Results of penetrating keratoplasty performed with a femtosecond laser zigzag incision initial report. Ophthalmology. 2007;114:2208–12.
67. Sarayba MA, Maguen E, Salz J, et al. Femtosecond laser keratome creation of partial thickness donor corneal buttons for lamellar keratoplasty. J Refract Surg. 2007;23:58–65.
68. Price FW, Price MO. Femtosecond laser shaped penetrating keratoplasty: one-year results utilizing a top-hat configuration. Am J Ophthalmol. 2008;145:210–4.
69. McAllum P, Kaiserman I, Bahar I, et al. Femtosecond laser top hat penetrating keratoplasty: wound burst pressures of incomplete cuts. Ach Ophthalmol. 2008;126:822–5.
70. Farid M, Steinert RF, Gaster RN, et al. Comparison of penetrating keratoplasty performed with a femtosecond laser zig-zag incision versus conventional blade trephination. Ophthalmology. 2009; 116:1638–43.
71. Levinger E, Trivizki O, Levinger S, et al. Outcome of "mushroom" pattern femtosecond laser-assisted keratoplasty versus conventional penetrating keratoplasty in patients with keratoconus. Cornea. 2014;33:481–5.
72. Kamiya K, Kobashi H, Shimizu K, et al. Clinical outcomes of penetrating keratoplasty performed with the VisuMax femtosecond laser system and comparison with conventional penetrating keratoplasty. PLoS One. 2014;9:e105464.
73. Gaster RN, Dumitrascu O, Rabinowitz YS. Penetrating keratoplasty using femtosecond laser-enabled keratoplasty with zig-zag incisions versus a mechanical trephine in patients with keratoconus. Br J Ophthalmol. 2012;96:1195–9.
74. Chamberlain WD, Rush SW, Mathers WD, et al. Comparison of femtosecond laser-assisted keratoplasty versus conventional penetrating keratoplasty. Ophthalmology. 2011;118:486–91.
75. Shehadeh Mashor R, Bahar I, Rootman DB, et al. Zig Zag versus Top Hat configuration in IntraLase-enabled penetrating keratoplasty. Br J Ophthalmol. 2014;98:756–9.
76. Alio JL, Abdelghany A., Barraquer R, et al. Femtosecond laser assisted deep anterior lamellar keratoplasty outcomes and healing patterns compared to manual technique. BioMed Res Int. 2015; 2015, Article ID 397891. doi: 10.1155/2015/397891.
77. Shehadeh-Mashor R, Chan CC, Bahar I, et al. Comparison between femtosecond laser mushroom configuration and manual trephine straight-edge configuration deep anterior lamellar keratoplasty. Br J Ophthalmol. 2014;98:35–9.
78. Patel SV, et al. Recurrent ectasia in corneal grafts and outcomes of repeat keratoplasty for keratoconus. Br J Ophthalmol. 2009;93(2):191–7.
79. Bourges JL, et al. Recurrence of keratoconus characteristics: a clinical and histologic follow-up analysis of donor grafts. Ophthalmology. 2003;110(10):1920–5.
80. Brookes NH, et al. Recurrence of keratoconic pathology in penetrating keratoplasty buttons originally transplanted for keratoconus. Cornea. 2009;28(6):688–93.
81. Dang TQ, et al. Novel approach for the treatment of corneal ectasia in a graft. Cornea. 2014;33(3):310–2.
82. Feizi S, Javadi MA, Rezaei Kanavi M. Recurrent keratoconus in a corneal graft after deep anterior lamellar keratoplasty. J Ophthalmic Vis Res. 2012;7(4):328–31.
83. Romano V, et al. Long-term clinical outcomes of deep anterior lamellar keratoplasty in patients with keratoconus. Am J Ophthalmol. 2015;159(3):505–11.
84. van Dijk K, et al. Bowman layer transplantation to reduce and stabilize progressive, advanced keratoconus. Ophthalmology. 2015;122(5):909–17.
85. De Miguel MP, et al. Cornea and ocular surface treatment. Curr Stem Cell Res Ther. 2010;5(2): 195–204.
86. Arnalich-Montiel F, et al. Adipose-derived stem cells are a source for cell therapy of the corneal stroma. Stem Cells. 2008;26(2):570–9.
87. Du Y, et al. Stem cell therapy restores transparency to defective murine corneas. Stem Cells. 2009;27(7):1635–42.
88. Liu H, et al. Cell therapy of congenital corneal diseases with umbilical mesenchymal stem cells: lumican null mice. PLoS One. 2010;5(5):e10707.
89. Coulson-Thomas VJ, Caterson B, Kao WW. Transplantation of human umbilical mes-

enchymal stem cells cures the corneal defects of mucopolysaccharidosis VII mice. Stem Cells. 2013;31(10):2116–26.

90. Espandar L, et al. Adipose-derived stem cells on hyaluronic acid-derived scaffold: a new horizon in bioengineered cornea. Arch Ophthalmol. 2012;130(2):202–8.
91. Ma XY, et al. The graft of autologous adipose-derived stem cells in the corneal stromal after mechanic damage. PLoS One. 2013;8(10):e76103.
92. Ruberti JW, Zieske JD. Prelude to corneal tissue engineering – gaining control of collagen organization. Prog Retin Eye Res. 2008;27(5):549–77.
93. Hu X, et al. Tissue engineering of nearly transparent corneal stroma. Tissue Eng. 2005;11(11–12):1710–7.
94. Alio del Barrio JL, et al. Biointegration of corneal macroporous membranes based on poly(ethyl acrylate) copolymers in an experimental animal model. J Biomed Mater Res A. 2015,103(3):1106–18.
95. Lynch AP, Ahearne M. Strategies for developing decellularized corneal scaffolds. Exp Eye Res. 2013;108:42–7.
96. Wilson SE, Liu JJ, Mohan RR. Stromal-epithelial interactions in the cornea. Prog Retin Eye Res. 1999;18(3):293–309.
97. Choi JS, et al. Bioengineering endothelialized neo-corneas using donor-derived corneal endothelial cells and decellularized corneal stroma. Biomaterials. 2010;31(26):6738–45.
98. Shafiq MA, et al. Decellularized human cornea for reconstructing the corneal epithelium and anterior stroma. Tissue Eng Part C Methods. 2012;18(5):340–8.
99. Gonzalez-Andrades M, et al. Generation of bioengineered corneas with decellularized xenografts and human keratocytes. Invest Ophthalmol Vis Sci. 2011;52(1):215–22.
100. Alio del Barrio JL, et al. Acellular human corneal matrix sheets seeded with human adipose-derived mesenchymal stem cells integrate functionally in an experimental animal model. Exp Eye Res. 2015;132:91–100.
101. Alio JL, et al. Keratoconus management guidelines. Int J Keratoconus Ectatic Corneal Dis. 2015;4(1): 1–39.

The Use of Femtosecond Laser and Corneal Welding in the Surgery of Keratoconus

24

Luca Menabuoni, Alex Malandrini, Annalisa Canovetti, Ivo Lenzetti, Roberto Pini, and Francesca Rossi

24.1 Introduction

Since the beginning of the 2000s the femtosecond laser strongly entered the corneal surgery rooms. The major contribution of this technology is related to the enhanced cutting precision, speed of execution, and the ability to make a customized surgery in relation to specific patient's anatomy and pathology. All these characteristics effectively revolutionized the prognosis in corneal transplants surgery. The femtosecond laser is particularly suitable in the surgery of keratoconus patients, thanks to the opportunity to make customized intervention flaps, e.g., the femto DALK [1]. The technology evolution led to the development of high precision lasers, with increasing frequencies, so that surgeons have the ability to create accurate, reproducible incisions in a broad variety of shapes and patterns. The Prato Ophthalmic Department team, in collaboration with the researchers of the Institute of Applied Physics—Italian National Research Council of Florence designed and then realized the anvil profile in penetrating keratoplasty, showing self-sealing properties and mechanical resistance to external and internal loads [2]. Moreover, this profile is suitable to diode laser welding procedure. This original approach allows quick sealing of the surgical wounds and a rapid healing process. In the following paragraphs the characteristics of the anvil profile and of the laser welding processes are described. The results in clinical applications will be discussed in the final part of this chapter.

24.2 Femtosecond Laser Cutting Profile

The use of the femtosecond (FS) laser technology for corneal surgery has allowed great advances especially in penetrating keratoplasty (PK). Thanks to the FS laser, new variety of shapes and angulations in vertical and lamellar intrastromal incisions could be designed at a precise depth with minimal collateral tissue injury. Different incision patterns have been proposed in the past few years for the creation of a particular flap shape in PK, so that a watertight closuring effect of the surgical wound could be achieved together with a more biomechanically stable flap and an improved healing process. The best profile

L. Menabuoni, M.D. • A. Malandrini, M.D.
A. Canovetti, M.D. • I. Lenzetti, M.D.
U.O. Oculistica, Nuovo Ospedale S. Stefano,
Via Suor Niccolina Infermiera 20, Prato 59100, Italy
e-mail: luca.menabuoni@tin.it;
alexmalandrini@libero.it; canovetti.annalisa@gmail.it;
ilenzetti@usl4.toscana.it

R. Pini, Ph.D. • F. Rossi, Ph.D. (✉)
Institute of Applied Physics, Italian National
Research Council, Via Madonna del Piano 10,
Sesto Fiorentino 50019, Italy
e-mail: r.pini@ifac.cnr.it; f.rossi@ifac.cnr.it

J.L. Alió (ed.), *Keratoconus*, Essentials in Ophthalmology, DOI 10.1007/978-3-319-43881-8_24

would be the one ensuring a wider wound incision, improving the fit and stability of the graft–host junction.

Variations from a vertical wound in PK include top hat, mushroom, zigzag, Christmas tree, and the more recent anvil.

Every FS-designed pattern has the purpose to create a more structurally stable and predictable wound configuration with the aim of a faster recovery of vision and higher optical quality in comparison with the conventional blade trephination.

In patients with keratoconus, selected to PK, it is important to preserve the largest part of patient's endothelial cells, because they are generally quite young and they have a good endothelium. Moreover, having a key-hole wound effect is crucial to have a good suture apposition and to decrease the astigmatism after surgery. Therefore, the use of FS technology could find a wide application in these patients: the anterior diameter of the donor cornea should be wider than the posterior one; a good centration of the cut can be easily achieved than manual trephination. In addition, the cutting pattern can be customized on the pachimetry in order to avoid misalignment between host and donor tissue.

Between the different FS-laser proposed shapes, mushroom pattern has been widely used for PK in keratoconus patients [3–5].

Recently, a new anvil-shaped laser incision called "anvil" has been proposed (Fig. 24.1): it is particularly suitable in keratoconus corneas because this graft shape provides a large contact surface in between donor and recipient corneas, improving the donor tissue stabilization in the recipient bed. This original profile also enables a perfect match with the laser welding procedure.

24.3 Laser Welding

Laser welding of biological tissues is a technique used to join tissues by inducing a photothermal effect within the wound walls. It has been proposed in several surgical fields over the last 30 years. The first successful test was reported at the end of the 70s, when a neodymium:YAG laser was used to join small blood vessels [6]. Since then, several experiments have been performed using a variety of lasers for sealing many tissue types, including blood vessels, nerves, skin, urethra, stomach, and colon (see also previous reviews [7, 8]). Laser welding has progressively gained relevance in the clinical setting, where it now appears as a valid alternative to standard surgical techniques.

Laser welding technique holds the promise to provide instantaneous, watertight seals, which is important in many critical surgeries, such as in ophthalmology, without the introduction of foreign materials (sutures). Other advantages over conventional suturing include reduced operation times; fewer skill requirements; decreased foreign body reaction; and therefore reduced inflammatory response, increased ability to induce regeneration of the original tissue architecture, and an improved cosmetic appearance. The final aim of this procedure is to improve the quality of life of patients by reduction of healing times and the risk of postoperative complications.

The laser–tissue interaction occurring during a laser-mediated welding of biological tissues is considered to be photothermal [7, 8]. This interaction is distinguished by the absorption of the light emitted by the laser source, which generates heat through a target volume. The thermal changes induced within the tissue about the lesion result, in turn, in a bond between its adjoining edges. The heat is produced through the absorption of the laser energy by endogenous or exogenous chromophores.

In the laser welding approach, optimized by our research team, we proposed the application of a photo-enhancing dye in the tissue and the use of a laser emitting in the near infrared region. The corneal tissue, as well as most of biological tissues, is transparent to the light in this wavelength region, while the stained tissue presents the optical absorbance peak at the laser wavelength. This means that when irradiating the corneal wounds, only the stained tissue is absorbing the laser light and the induced photothermal effect is confined in the stained region.

The result is the selective fusion of wound walls at low irradiation power per target area,

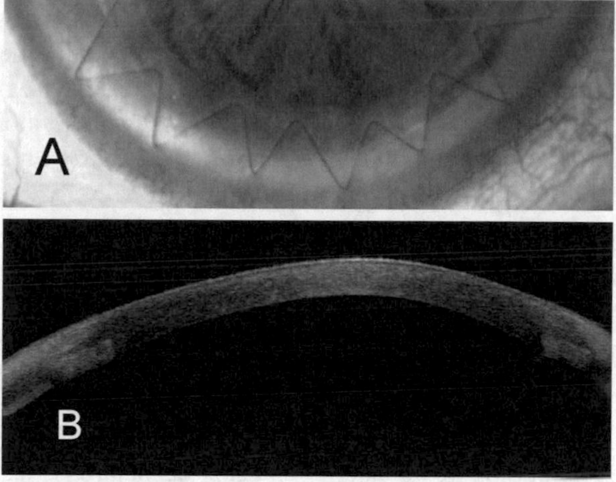

Fig. 24.1 The laser welded anvil profile at slit lamp (**a**) and OCT (**b**), 15 p.o. days

thus reducing the risk of thermal damage to surrounding tissues. The welding effect may be modulated in the depth of the transparent tissue, thus resulting in a more effective closure of the wound. Various chromophores have been employed as photo-enhancing dyes, including Indocyanine Green (ICG), fluorescein, basic fuchsin, and India ink [9]. A very popular setting of tissue laser welding includes the use of a near infrared laser, which is poorly absorbed by the biological tissue, in conjunction with the topical application of a chromophore absorbing in the same spectral region. Current examples of this modality are in the transplant of the cornea, in cataract surgery, in vascular tissue welding, in skin welding, and in laryngotracheal mucosa transplant [10, 11]. In all these cases, diode lasers emitting around 800 nm and the topical application of ICG have been used.

24.3.1 Surgical Applications of Thermal Laser Welding in Keratoplasty

To the best of our knowledge, the technique optimized and proposed by our research team is the only one laser welding application which has reached the preclinical and clinical phases. It is based on the use of a near infrared diode laser emitting at 810 nm and the topical application of the chromophore ICG, which shows high optical absorption at the laser wavelength emission [12–15]. The procedure consists in a preliminary staining phase with the chromophore, followed by an irradiation phase. ICG has been chosen because of its biocompatibility, which has already favored its exploitation in several biomedical applications. In practice, the chromophore is prepared in the form of an aqueous saturated solution of commercially available Indocyanine Green for biomedical applications (e.g., IC-GREEN Akorn, Buffalo Grove, IL or ICG-Pulsion Medical Systems AG, Germany). This solution is accurately positioned in the tissue area to be welded, using particular care to avoid the staining of surrounding tissues, and thus their accidental absorption of laser light. Then the wound edges are approximated and laser welding is performed under a surgical microscope.

The laser used in preclinical tests and in the clinical applications is typically an AlGaAs diode laser (e.g., Mod. WELD 800 by El.En. SpA, Italy) emitting at 810 nm and equipped with a fiber-optic delivery system.

We proposed two different protocols, to be used in penetrating keratoplasty [12, 13, 16] and in endothelial transplantation [17]. The first one is used in keratoconus patients, in combination with the femtosecond laser to cut donor and recipient tissues.

In penetrating keratoplasty, the technique has been named the continuous wave laser welding (CWLW). Noncontact, CW diode laser irradiation is used for the welding of corneal wounds, in substitution or in conjunction with traditional suturing procedures. The CWLW procedure developed to weld human corneal tissues in penetrating keratoplasty is as follows. The donor and recipient cornea are trephined by the use of a femtosecond laser. The donor cornea is then applied onto the patient's eye and secured by 8–16 interrupted stitches or continuous suturing. The ICG chromophore solution is prepared in sterile water (10 % w/w) in the surgery room, soon before its use. The surgeon places a small quantity of chromophore solution inside the corneal cut, using an anterior chamber cannula, in an attempt to stain the walls of the cut in depth. A bubble of air is injected into the anterior chamber prior to the application of the staining solution, so as to avoid perfusion of the dye. A few minutes after the application, the solution is washed out with abundant water. The stained walls of the cut appear greenish, indicating that ICG has been absorbed by the stroma. Lastly, the whole length of the cut is subjected to laser treatment. Laser energy is transferred to the tissue in a noncontact configuration, through a 300-μm core diameter fiber. The fiber is mounted in a handpiece and moved by the surgeon as a pencil. A typical value of the laser power density clinically used is around 10 W/cm^2, which results in a good welding effect. During irradiation, the fiber tip is kept at a working distance of about 1 mm, and at an angle of 20°–30° with respect to the corneal surface (side irradiation technique). This particular fiber position provides in-depth homogenous irradiation of the wound and prevents accidental irradiation of deeper ocular structures. The fiber tip is continuously moved over the tissue to be welded, with an overall laser irradiation time of about 120 s for a 360°. This procedure has been performed up to now on 300 patients with very satisfactory results [2, 12, 16]. The position of the apposed margins has been found to be stable over time, thus assuring optimal results in terms of postoperatively induced astigmatism after cataract and keratoplasty surgery. The lower number of stitches reduces the incidence of foreign body reactions, thus improving the healing process. Objective observations on treated patients have proved that the laser-welded tissues regain a good morphology (without scar formation) and pristine functionality (clarity and good mechanical load resistance, see Figs. 24.2 and 24.3).

In endothelium keratoplasty, the technique is called Pulsed Laser Welding (PLW). In this protocol, single laser spots (lasting tens of milliseconds) are delivered to the tissue, resulting in a photothermal effect localized within the spot dimension (a few hundreds of micrometers in diameter): the induced effect is a hard laser welding, consisting in a photocoagulation of the collagen confined at the donor/host interface. The result of the collagen denaturation at the welded site is a strong adhesion between the donor and host tissues, thus providing a suturing effect that is impossible to obtain with standard technique. The tissue regains his natural appearance in a short follow-up (1 month) and the adhesion between donor/host tissue is improved by the welding provided in the very early stage of the healing phase. However, this protocol is not used in keratoconus cases.

24.3.2 Mechanism of Thermal Laser Welding

The proposed approach has been characterized by the use of different experimental and theoretical studies, such as thermal modeling and microscopic analyses [11–15]. These include traditional methods as optical and fluorescence microscopy which allow for an investigation at the micron scale [18] and transmission and scanning electron microscopy (TEM and SEM, respectively) which are useful when studying nanometric structures [19–21]. Other used techniques are atomic force microscopy (AFM) and second-harmonic generation (SHG) microscopy which provide complementary information [22–24]. These studies have been helpful (although not exhaustive) in elucidating the different dynamics behind the sealing process.

The CWLW is based on the "soft" laser welding effect, as briefly described in this paragraph, while the PLW is based on "hard" laser welding.

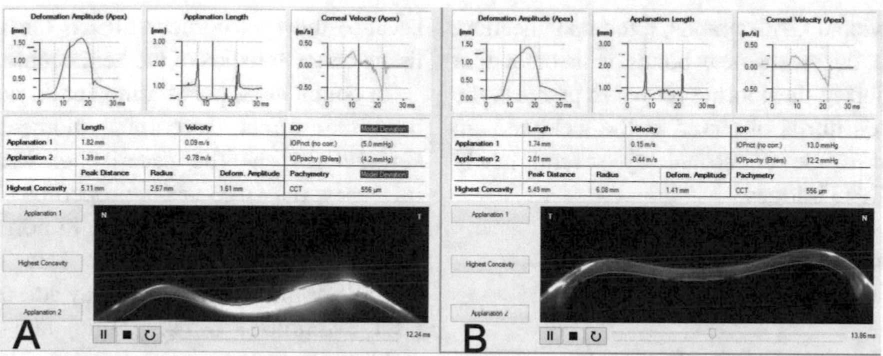

Fig. 24.2 Representative displays of the Corvis ST in a keratoconic eye (**a**) and in an eye of the same patient, following fs-penetrating keratoplasty (**b**). The deformation amplitude (DA) at the highest concavity in keratoconic eye (1.61 mm) is deeper than in fs-PK eye (1.41 mm)

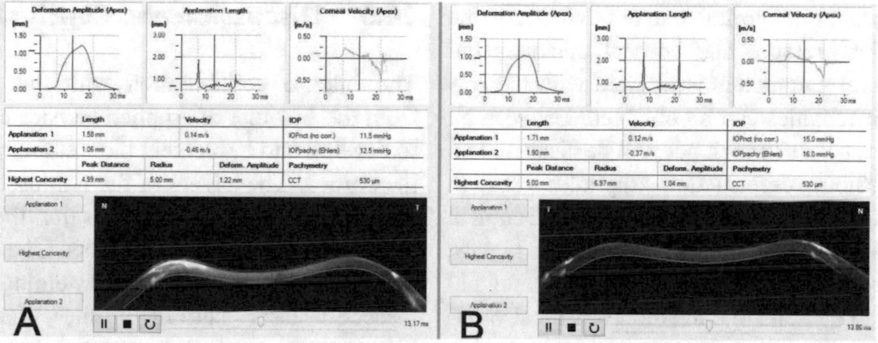

Fig. 24.3 Images from the Corvis ST at the highest concavity: simple femtosecond penetrating keratoplasty anvil profiled (**a**) versus laser welded fs-PK anvil profiled (**b**) of the same patient. Note the DA in laser welded fs-PK (1.04 mm) is smaller than in simple fs-PK (1.22 mm): this shows a greater biomechanical stability of the procedure. The anvil profile is evident in Scheimpflug image: a perfect synergy is remarkable at the host–graft junction

The main difference is the maximum induced temperature in the tissue and the treatment time duration, resulting in different biological effects. The "hard" photothermal effect results in the photocoagulation of the collagen content of the corneal stroma; the "moderate" effect consists in the "interdigitation" of collagen fibrils; and the "soft" effect results in the reorganization of the nonfibrillar components of the corneal stroma (mainly proteoglycans—PG- and glycosaminoglycans—GAGs).

As it has been pointed out, during hard laser welding the induced temperatures are higher than 70 °C. In these conditions there is a localized, strong loss of the regular appearance of the fibrillar collagen following laser welding. This is described as a full homogenization of the tissue (also called hyalinosis) [11, 25]; the appearance of fibrils fused together with a drastically altered morphology is the consequence of a complete denaturation of the collagen matrix occurring at high temperature values. Another frequently accompanying effect is the disruption of the cell membranes causing leakage of the cellular material in the extracellular space. In these cases, the wound sealing mechanism has been attributed to the photocoagulation of collagen and of other intracellular proteins, which act like micro-solders or endogenous glue on laser activation, thus forming new interactions between the tissue interfaces upon cooling [25].

In CWLW, it seems that the GAGs bridges connecting collagen fibrils in the native tissue are broken at the characteristic temperatures of diode laser welding (in the 50–65 °C range).

The individual GAG strands, freed upon heating, subsequently create new bonds with other free strands during the cooling phase. In practice, the interwoven fibrils observed at the weld site are supposed to be connected by several newly formed GAG bridges.

24.4 Clinical Results

A new dynamic Scheimpflug analyzer (Corvis ST, Oculus Optikgeräte, Wetzlar, Germany) has become available for clinical use. Because dynamic deformation of the cornea by a constant pressure air pulse is recorded through this ultra-high-speed Scheimpflug camera, not only the intraocular pressure and corneal thickness but also several parameters associated with the corneal biomechanics can be obtained. Between all these parameters (which not will be discussed on this occasion), deformation amplitude (DA; in mm) is defined as the displacement of the corneal apex from the original position at the highest concavity and it is significantly more useful and intuitive to demonstrate the biomechanical variations induced by transplant surgery.

In previous studies DA was found to be significantly greater in keratoconic eyes than in normal eyes and however, is widely accepted that the anterior segment surgery may change the biomechanical behavior of the cornea too.

Our findings showed that the DA in the keratoconic eyes underwent femtolaser penetrating keratoplasty (fs-PK) was significantly greater than in the control but not greater than in the fs-PK to which was applied the laser welding (see Figs. 24.2 and 24.3).

Some factors might have contributed to the changes in DA (and others parameters) after fs-PK: the biomechanical characteristics of the transplanted corneal button, the fibrotic wound healing of the host–graft junction site, and the application of laser welding have a positive recovering effect on DA, whereas the biomechanical characteristics of the corneoscleral rim of the residual recipient cornea may increase it, because the host cornea still has the weakened tissue characteristics of the keratoconic cornea.

In conclusion, penetrating keratoplasty has a beneficial effect on corneal biomechanics in keratoconus; as the severity of keratoconus increases, the viscoelastic properties of the cornea decrease but nearly return to normal levels with corneal transplantation. This beneficial effect is amplified when we may add the femtolaser technology (anvil profile) and the laser welding: both these elements are able to positively modulate the biomechanical behavior of the cornea [26–28].

24.5 Discussion and Conclusions

The intense collaboration with the physicists from the Institute of Applied Physics allowed us to develop and implement the welding process of the cornea. The advent of the femtosecond laser then has created new models for the surgical treatment of corneal transplants. The combination of these procedures, laser welding and femtosecond laser cutting profiles, has further increased the surgical success and the good quality of patient's life in postoperative treatment. Laser welding can definitely overcome the problems related to the restlessness of the incongruous surgical maneuvers, the risk of micro-traumas, and the possibility of reopening the wound walls at the time of stitches removal (even 16–18 months p.o.). The recovery of the work activities and sports is greatly encouraged by this procedure. The combination of these laser-based techniques can provide a quiet postoperative period for both the surgeon and the patient.

Compliance with Ethical Requirements Luca Menabuoni, Annalisa Canovetti, Alex Malandrini, Ivo Lenzetti, Roberto Pini, and Francesca Rossi declare that they have no conflict of interest.

All procedures followed were in accordance with the ethical standards of the responsible committee on human experimentation (institutional and national) and with the Helsinki Declaration of 1975, as revised in 2000. Informed consent was obtained from all patients for being included in the study.

References

1. Buzzonetti L, Petrocelli G, Valente P. Femtosecond laser and big-bubble deep anterior lamellar keratoplasty: a new chance. J Ophthalmol. 2012;2012: 264590. doi:10.1155/2012/264590.
2. Canovetti A, Malandrini A, Lenzetti I, Rossi F, Pini R, Menabuoni L. Laser-assisted penetrating keratoplasty: one year's results in patients, using a laser-welded "anvil"-profiled graft. Am J Ophthalmol. 2014. doi:10.1016/j.ajo.2014.07.010.
3. Levinger E, Trivizki O, Levinger S, Kremer I. Outcome of "mushroom" pattern femtosecond laser-assisted keratoplasty versus conventional penetrating keratoplasty in patients with keratoconus. Cornea. 2014;33(5):481–5. doi:10.1097/ICO.0000000000000080.
4. Shehadeh-Mashor R, Chan CC, Bahar I, Lichtinger A, Yeung SN, Rootman DS. Comparison between femtosecond laser mushroom configuration and manual trephine straight-edge configuration deep anterior lamellar keratoplasty. Br J Ophthalmol. 2014;98(1):35–9. doi:10.1136/bjophthalmol-2013-303737.
5. Shivanna Y, Nagaraja H, Kugar T, Shetty R. Femtosecond laser enabled keratoplasty for advanced keratoconus. Indian J Ophthalmol. 2013;61(8):469–72. doi:10.4103/0301-4738.116060.
6. Jain KK, Gorisch W. Repair of small blood vessels with the neodymium-YAG laser: a preliminary report. Surgery. 1979;85(6):684–8.
7. McNally KM. Chapter 39: Laser tissue welding. In: Vo-Dihn T, editor. Biomedical photonics handbook. Boca Raton: CRC Press; 2003. p. 1–45.
8. Pini R, Rossi F, Matteini P, Ratto F. Laser tissue welding in minimally invasive surgery and microsurgery. In: Pavesi L, Fauchet PM, editors. Biophotonics, Biological and medical physics, biomedical engineering. Berlin: Springer; 2008. p. 275–99.
9. Poppas DP, Scherr DS. Laser tissue welding: a urological surgeon's perspective. Haemophilia. 1998;4(4):456–62.
10. Ott B, Zuger BJ, Erni D, Banic A, Schaffner T, Weber HP, Frenz M. Comparative in vitro study of tissue welding using a 808 nm diode laser and a Ho:YAG laser. Lasers Med Sci. 2001;16(4):260–6.
11. Rossi F, Pini R, Menabuoni L, Mencucci R, Menchini U, Ambrosini S, Vannelli G. Experimental study on the healing process following laser welding of the cornea. J Biomed Opt. 2005;10(2):024004.
12. Buzzonetti L, Capozzi P, Petrocelli G, Valente P, Petroni S, Menabuoni L, Rossi F, Pini R. Laser welding in penetrating keratoplasty and cataract surgery in pediatric patients: early results. J Cataract Refract Surg. 2013;39(12):1829–34. doi:10.1016/j.jcrs.2013.05.046.
13. Menabuoni L, Pini R, Rossi F, Lenzetti I, Yoo SH, Parel J-M. Laser-assisted corneal welding in cataract surgery: a retrospective study. J Cataract Refract Surg. 2007;33:1608–12.
14. Rossi F, Pini R, Menabuoni L. Experimental and model analysis on the temperature dynamics during diode laser welding of the cornea. J Biomed Opt. 2007;12(1):014031.
15. Rossi F, Matteini P, Ratto F, Menabuoni L, Lenzetti I, Pini R. Laser tissue welding in ophthalmic surgery. J Biophotonics. 2008;1:331–42.
16. Menabuoni L, Canovetti A, Rossi F, Malandrini A, Lenzetti I, Pini R. The 'anvil' profile in femtosecond laser-assisted penetrating keratoplasty. Acta Ophthalmol. 2013;91:e494–5. doi:10.1111/aos.12144.
17. Rossi F, Canovetti A, Malandrini A, Lenzetti I, Pini R, Menabuoni L. An "All-laser" endothelial transplant. J Vis Exp. 2015;(101):e52939. doi:10.3791/52939.
18. Savage HE, Halder RK, Kartazayeu U, Rosen RB, Gayen T, McCormick SA, Patel NS, Katz A, Perry HD, Paul M, Alfano RR. A NIR laser tissue welding of in vitro porcine cornea and sclera tissue. Lasers Surg Med. 2004;35(4):293–303.
19. Matteini P, Rossi F, Menabuoni L, Pini R. Microscopic characterization of collagen modifications induced by low-temperature diode-laser welding of corneal tissue. Lasers Surg Med. 2007;39:597–604.
20. Menovsky T, Beek JF, van Gemert MJC. Laser tissue welding of dura mater and peripheral nerves: a scanning electron microscopy study. Lasers Surg Med. 1996;19(2):152–8.
21. Schober R, Ulrich F, Sander T, Durselen H, Hessel S. Laser-induced alteration of collagen substructure allows microsurgical tissue welding. Science. 1986;232(4756):1421–2.
22. Matteini P, Ratto F, Rossi F, Cicchi R, Stringari C, Kapsokalyvas D, Pavone FS, Pini R. Photothermally-induced disordered patterns of corneal collagen revealed by SHG imaging. Optics Exp. 2009;17:4868–78.
23. Matteini P, Sbrana F, Tiribilli B, Pini R. Atomic force microscopy and transmission electron microscopy analyses on low-temperature laser welding of the cornea. Lasers Med Sci. 2009;24:667–71.
24. Tan HY, Teng SW, Lo W, Lin WC, Lin SJ, Jee SH, Dong CY. Characterizing the thermally induced structural changes to intact porcine eye, part 1: second harmonic generation imaging of cornea stroma. J Biomed Opt. 2005;10:540191–5.
25. Murray LW, Su L, Kopchok GE, White RA. Crosslinking of extracellular matrix proteins: a preliminary report on a possible mechanism of argon laser welding. Lasers Surg Med. 1989;9(5):490–6.
26. Hon Y, Lam AK. Corneal deformation measurement using Scheimpflug non contact tonometry. Optom Vis Sci. 2013;90:e1-8.
27. Maeda N, Ueki R, Fuchilhata M, Fujimoto H, Koh S, Nishida K. Corneal biomechanical properties in 3 corneal transplantation techniques with a dynamic Scheimpflug analyzer. Jpn J Ophthalmol. 2014;58:483–9.
28. Yenerel NM, Kucumen RB, Gorgun E. Changes in corneal biomechanics in patients with keratoconus after penetrating keratoplasty. Cornea. 2010;29(11):1247–51.

Part VI

Refractive Surgery in Keratoconus

Refractive Surgery in Keratoconus 25

Pablo Sanz Díez, Alfredo Vega Estrada, and Jorge L. Alió

This chapter is a general introduction to summarize the current status of implementation of refractive surgery in keratoconus. In separate chapters to this, we will discuss in detail the excimer laser surgery and phakic lenses use in these cases, due to its current relevance. Keratoconus is an ectatic corneal disorder characterized by progressive corneal thinning that results in corneal protrusion, irregular astigmatism, and decreased vision. This corneal disorder induces myopia and astigmatism in both regular and irregular forms, often leading to marked visual impairment.

Keratoconus is probably one of the most common so-called rare diseases. Occurrence in the general population is low, between 4/1000 and 6/1000 [1]. Others have reported a lower incidence (between 1 and 2.3/1000) [2]. According to other authors, the current incidence is 1/2000 per year [2, 3] and depends on the geographic region; though there are also studies supporting the fact that the prevalence is higher in zones with higher UV exposure or with a combination of genetic and environmental factors [4]. Its prevalence is probably higher than that reported by the majority of studies if we take into account subclinical or forme fruste keratoconus.

The management of keratoconus depends on the stage and evolution of ectasia. In early cases, contact lenses are the main support treatment for keratoconus and one of the first treatments of choice due to corneal surface irregularity [5–7].

Nowadays, there are different and varied options for surgery in keratoconus:

- Lenticular refractive surgery.
  - Refractive lens exchange with toric intraocular lenses.
  - Toric phakic intraocular lenses
- Intracorneal ring segment insert.
- Corneal Cross-linking.
- Corneal transplantation.
  - Penetrating keratoplasty.
  - Deep anterior lamellar keratoplasty.
- Thermokeratoplasty.

From refractive surgery solution, the two primary lines of action are phakic lens (PIOL) implantation [8–13] and corneal tissue ablation using photorefractive keratectomy (PRK).

P. Sanz Díez, O.D., M.Sc.
J.L. Alió, M.D., Ph.D., F.E.B.O. (✉)
Keratoconus Unit, Department of Refractive Surgery, Vissum Alicante, Calle Cabañal, 1, Alicante, Spain

Division of Ophthalmology, Miguel Hernández University, Calle Cabañal, 1, Alicante 03016, Spain
e-mail: pablosanz9143@gmail.com; jlalio@vissum.com

A. Vega Estrada, Ph.D.
Keratoconus Unit, Vissum Alicante, Alicante, Spain
e-mail: alfredovega@vissum.com

J.L. Alió (ed.), *Keratoconus*, Essentials in Ophthalmology, DOI 10.1007/978-3-319-43881-8_25

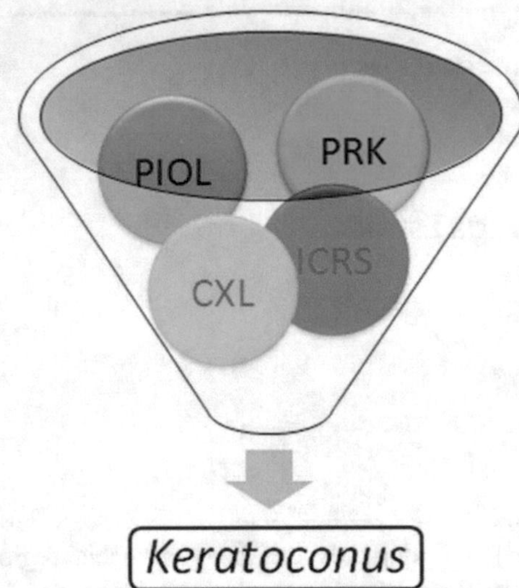

Fig. 25.1 Options of refractive surgery in keratoconus

These techniques have also been used in combination with cross-linking (CXL) [14–19] and intracorneal ring segment (ICRS) [20, 21] (Fig. 25.1).

These techniques are normally used in patients with forme fruste keratoconus or stable keratoconus [13] and are not choice in progressive keratoconus, although there are some studies along these lines [15, 19, 22].

We have always followed the same stability criteria in our work. If one (or several) of the circumstances described later occurs in an interval of less than 1 year, keratoconus is considered progressive and we consider it is not appropriate to apply some of these techniques:

- Increase in astigmatism of 1.0 D or more.
- Significant changes in the orientation of refractive axes.
- Increase of 1.0 D or more in the optical power of the steepest corneal meridian.
- Decrease of 25 μm or more in corneal thickness.

25.1 Phakic Intraocular Lenses (PIOL)

Several studies have reported significant visual improvements with good safety and efficacy indices for phakic intraocular lens insertion in keratoconus [23, 24].

The use of phakic lenses has advantages such as efficient and stable ametropia compensation, preservation of accommodation, centered and rotational stability not dependent on corneal morphology, retinal image magnification in patients with high myopia, and reversibility in the event of failure.

Negative effects of phakic lens implantation include accelerated endothelial cell loss, cataract formation, pupil ovalization, lens rotation or decentration, photic phenomena, and retinal detachment in isolated cases.

25.1.1 Implantation Criteria

Based on our experience and that described in medical literature, we believe the criteria in Table 25.1 should be met for phakic lens implantation in keratoconus:

According to a recent study by our group with the largest number of case studies on phakic lens implantation in keratoconus reported to date [13], the safety of this procedure in visual terms is high (post-CDVA/pre-CDVA = 1.19 ± 0.29). It is also an effective operation (post-UDVA/pre-CDVA = 0.90 ± 0.26). In fact, many patients stopped wearing glasses after phakic lens implantation. These results are roughly consistent with those reported by other authors [8–12].

It is also interesting to note that, based on the results of this study, implantation of a foldable lenses can be as safe and effective as implantation of a hard lens. The following models were studied: foldable Artiflex lens (Ophtec, Netherlands) and the ICL (implantable collamer lens, STAAR Surgical, United States). This result is particularly interesting, because flexible lenses can be inserted and removed through smaller incisions thanks to their flexibility.

We recommend that, whenever possible, implantation be performed using this type of microincision surgery (with incision of 1.8–2.00 mm) to ensure that the ectatic process is not affected as a result of the operation. It has been widely demonstrated that use of this type of incision causes minimal alternations in the cornea [25, 26].

Table 25.1 Criteria for phakic lens implantation in keratoconus

Indications	Relative indications	Contraindications
Corneal topography stable and age >35–40 years	Keratoconus, stable following CCL (topography and refraction)	Progressive keratoconus, unstable corneas
Good spectacle-corrected visual acuity (>0.6; 20/30)	Following DALK or PKP	Young patients (<25 years-old?)
Stable refraction for about 2 years. Spherical equivalent greater than −2.75 D	Moderately good vision but with poor tolerance to glasses or contact lenses	Highly aberrated eyes (total HOA >3 μm) with poor best spectacle corrected visual acuity (<0.5)
Absence of clinically significant irregular astigmatism. We consider irregular astigmatism to be clinically significant when there is a difference greater than one line of corrected vision between the vision obtained with glasses and the vision obtained with hard contact lenses	Anisometropia with adequate refractive anatomy and stable refraction	

25.2 Photorefractive Keratectomy (PRK)

This is a technique that ablates the stroma without performing the corneal flap. The cornea is reshaped using the excimer laser onto Bowman's layer and the anterior stroma. The epithelium can be removed mechanically (by brush, blade, or epikeratome), chemically (most often with approximately 20 % alcohol), or by laser.

PRK for the treatment of keratoconus has been discussed by several authors. While the precision obtained in ablating the corneal surface with laser ablation may be very high in normal corneas, it is unclear whether the same occurs with keratoconic patients due to preexisting corneal asymmetry and to the reduced reliability and repeatability of keratometry measurements in such patients [27]. In addition, ablating corneal tissue in patients whose corneal biomechanics are already altered is a risk factor to bear in mind. Obviously, unlike phakic lenses, this technique cannot be used to treat high levels of myopia (which are frequent in keratoconus), because the ablation is so deep in these cases. Furthermore, this technique is not reversible.

Exclusion Criteria

- Advanced or progressive keratoconus.
- Keratometry >56 D.
- Pachymetry less than 440 μm.
- Large displacement of the apex.
- Presence of scars or rupture of the Bowman membrane.

Our experience shows that it is a safe technique (1.03±0.08) with a high degree of efficacy (0.91±0.18), but we have only been able to confirm these results in the short term. Moreover, we detected some cases in which the ectasia became progressive. Hence the need for combined use with cross-linking and for more cases studied with longer follow-up.

Interestingly, regarding the use of this surgery on keratonic eyes, some authors like Vinciguerra et al. [28] suggest using corneal topography data before epithelial removal to avoid the masking effect over the stroma that may occur in keratoconus. This is obviously an inconvenient practice for the patient but a well-founded one in our opinion.

Lastly, in these cases, the ablation should not exceed 50 μm [29] and regarding the ablation profile to use, we think it is better to use wavefront-guided ablation as opposed to topography-guided ablation. This is because with the latter technique the operation is conducted based on the aberrometric profile of the anterior corneal surface. As has been widely reported in the literature, high internal astigmatism is common in keratoconic eyes due to large disparities between the anterior and posterior corneal surfaces [30]. For this reason, we believe it is better to use a customized wavefront profile.

In any case, as stated earlier, we do not consider PRK on its own to be the technique of choice in keratoconus, despite the high efficacy rates obtained (in a small series of only 21 eyes), due to doubts concerning long-term stability [31].

25.3 Combined Treatments

In recent years, refractive surgery of keratoconus has evolved combining different techniques to achieve the following objectives: improve visual quality and stop the progression of the disease. Currently, both PRK and PIOL are combined with CXL and ICRS.

In the combined treatment with CXL, the following principles must be taken into account:

- Indications:
  - Clinical manifestations of progressive keratoconus [32, 33].
  - Age: under 35 years [34].
  - Visual acuity less than 0.8 (20/25; LogMAR 0.1) [34].
  - Pachymetry over 400 μm [33, 35].
  - Keratometry readings less than 58 D [32, 34].
- Contraindications:
  - Pregnancy and breastfeeding [33, 36].
  - Age: can be a risk factor causing visual loss, but for the moment no limit has been established [37].
  - Visual acuity: as a visual loss risk factor, CVA ≥0.8 (20/25; LogMAR 0.1) [34].
  - Cornea with central opacity [38].
  - Serious dry eye syndrome [39].

Regarding combined treatments with ICRS, we must take a number of preoperative indications into account [40], in order to increase the likelihood of attaining the best possible postoperative outcomes for the patient:

- Corrected distance visual acuity (CDVA) <0.9.
- Stable cases. Patients with refractive and topographic stability, confirmed in the past 12 months.
- Aligning of refractive and keratometric axes. The least curved meridian of the cornea (K1) should be aligned with the refractive cylinder axis (expressed as a negative value). When the meridian and the axis form an angle of between 0° and 15° they are considered properly aligned.
- Internal astigmatism <3 D.
- Corneal pachymetry in tunnel area >300 μm (Ferrara); > 450 μm (Intacs); > 250 μm (Keraring), with these being minimum thicknesses depending on the thickness of each intracorneal segment.
- Absence of corneal leukoma.

25.3.1 Photorefractive Keratectomy

25.3.1.1 PRK and CXL

The rationale for this surgical approach is to halt the progression of keratoconus and to provide better refractive, topographic, and HOA results than with CXL treatment alone by reshaping the cornea and flattening and regularizing the anterior corneal surface, while ensuring stable outcomes over time in terms of nonprogression of the disease. It is very important to know that the CXL significantly increases corneal rigidity immediately after treatment, with a 71.9% increase of Young's modulus in pig corneas and a 328.9% increase in human corneas [41] and therefore, a cross-linked cornea may withstand low tissue ablations.

There are two possibilities for this combination:

- *Sequential treatment (PRK several months after CXL).*

Kanellopoulos and Binder [14] described a case with bilateral progressive keratoconus treated on one eye with topography-guided PRK and who had undergone CXL on both eyes 12 months before. PRK was attempted to improve the post-CXL refractive error; a significant clinical improvement and apparent stability was successfully achieved after two surgeries. At the 18 months follow-up visit, the uncorrected visual acuity (UCVA) and corrected distance visual acuity (CDVA) were improved from 20/100 to 20/20 and from 20/50 to 20/20, respectively, and there was no evidence of topographic progression.

- *Simultaneous treatment (PRK + CXL).*

  Kymionis et al. [16] reported promising results in study about customized topography-guided PRK followed by immediate CXL in 12 patients with keratoconus. The preoperative mean (logMAR) UCVA was 0.99±0.81, which increase postoperatively to 0.16±0.15.

  Other studies have also shown good results with simultaneous PRK and CXL [16, 18, 42]. It improved in SE, UDVA, CDVA, and KMAX and did not show evidence of topographic progression at 12 months follow-up visit.

- *Sequential vs. Simultaneous.*

  Kanellopoulos [17] compared these techniques. For this he used different sequence and timing which were evaluated in consecutive keratoconus cases. This study included a total of 325 eyes with keratoconus divided into two groups:

  - The sequential group had topo-guided PRK 6 months after the CXL procedure (127 eyes).
  - The simultaneous group had a CXL procedure immediately after the MMC topo-guided PRK (198 eyes).

  The simultaneous group demonstrated statistically superior results in CDVA, spherical equivalent (SE) reduction, maximum keratometry (Kmax) reduction, and corneal haze score. Furthermore, it was not observed progression of ectasia in either group after a mean follow-up of 36 months.

- *Concluding remarks.*
  - Low ablation of tissue seems to be safe and effective in keratoconic cross-linked corneas according to the current evidence.
  - Topo-guided PRK provides refractive error correction and HOAs decrease.
  - Simultaneous PRK+CXL has shown better outcomes than the sequential strategy.
  - Therefore, PRK+CXL is a promising tool in keratoconus that needs further investigation to assess its stability in the long term and to establish the indications.

25.3.1.2 PRK and CXL + ICRS

Not many research groups have studied about this type of multisurgery. Coskunseven et al. [43] performed a prospective case series (16 eyes with progressive keratoconus). All patients underwent topography-guided transepithelial PRK after Keraring ICRS implantation followed by CXL treatment. They applied a three-step sequence where the time interval between each of the three operations was 6 months. The results are promising: mean SE was significantly decreased from −5.66±5.63 to −0.98±2.21 D. Regarding visual results: the preoperative mean (LogMAR) UDVA and CDVA were significantly improved from 1.14±0.36 to 0.25±0.13 and 0.75±0.24 to 0.13±0.06, respectively. In other study [44], observed cases with moderate keratoconus who had previous Intacs ICRS implantation with the Intralase laser at least 6 months before PRK-CXL. They found that it satisfactorily changed the UDVA, CDVA, and central *K* values from 0.20±0.12 to 0.55±0.15, from 0.58±0.13 to 0.77±0.17, and from 50.91±5.50 to 46.61±4.52 D, respectively.

Two different studies have performed Intacs implantations followed by same-day PRK and CXL in patients with keratoconus. The results are satisfactory: UDVA, CDVA, and sphere and cylinder refractive measurements all significantly improved after surgery, with most eyes gaining two lines of CDVA or more [45, 46].

25.3.2 Phakic IOL

In progressive cases of keratoconus, surgical alternatives to corneal transplantation have been suggested. These include phakic IOL implantation, CXL, and ICRS. Once the keratoconus has stabilized, refractive solutions can be considered. A perfect power calculation of intraocular lens is essential to achieve good visual results, because we are in cases with high curvature and corneal irregularity.

25.3.2.1 PIOL and CXL

CXL is the only treatment that has proved effective in stabilizing the cone and PIOLs have been extensively used to correct a wide range of refractive errors in nonkeratoconic eyes and keratoconic eyes. The combination of these two methods has been reported as an effective and safe procedure [19, 47, 48]. Izquierdo et al. [47] performed a prospective comparative study (11 eyes with progressive keratoconus). They propose a minimal interval between CXL and Artiflex PIOL implantation of 6 months to allow consideration of the changes to refractive errors and *K* values produced by CXL because these changes can affect the calculation of PIOL power. They observed a reduction in the mean maximum keratometry value was 1.27 D at 6 months after CXL and 2.14 D at 6 months after Artiflex PIOL implantation (12 months after CXL). They also report a significant reduction in the mean spherical refractive error; however, the cylinder remained unchanged because the Artiflex toric PIOL model was not commercially available at the time of their study.

Güell et al. [19] reported a retrospective study (17 eyes with progressive keratoconus). This study evaluated the outcomes of CXL performed first to stabilize the cone followed by toric iris-claw PIOL implantation (Artiflex (15 eyes) and Artisan (two eyes)) to correct regular astigmatism in eyes with keratoconus. The median interval between CXL and PIOL implantation was 3.9±0.7 months. They showed the following results: 14 eyes were within±0.50 D of the attempted spherical equivalent correction and 13 eyes were within±1.00 D of the attempted cylinder correction. The mean difference in simulated keratometry between preoperatively and the last follow-up was 0.17±0.45 D. The postoperative uncorrected distance visual acuity was 20/40 or better in 16 eyes and no eye lost lines of corrected distance visual acuity.

Fadlallah et al. [48] published a retrospective study (16 eyes with keratoconus). In this study they combined CXL and Visian toric ICL implantation. The two procedures were done at an interval of 6 months. The postoperative follow-up was at 6 month after ICL implantation. They showed good results: mean UDVA improved from 1.67±0.49 to 0.17±0.06 logMAR and mean CDVA improved from 0.15±0.06 to 0.12±0.04 logMAR. Mean SE decreased from −7.24±3.53 to −0.89±0.76 D and mean cylinder decreased from 2.64±1.28 to 1.16±0.64 D.

25.3.2.2 PIOL and ICRS

Coskunseven et al. [49] evaluated three eyes of two patients who had undergone posterior chamber toric Implantable Collamer Lens (ICL) after Intacs implantation. This procedure was performed at intervals between 6 and 10 months after Intacs implantation. An improvement in uncorrected distance visual acuity and corrected distance visual acuity was found after the Intacs and toric ICL procedures in all eyes. The mean manifest refractive spherical equivalent refraction reduced from −18.50±2.61 D to 0.42 D.

Another study [50] evaluated the same PIOL, but combined with other type of ICRS, being in this case: Keraring ICRS. This study is composed of 40 eyes with keratoconus who had ICRS implantation followed 6 months later by PIOL implantation with corneal relaxing incisions. The mean UDVA was 0.11±0.05 preoperatively and 0.18±0.14 at 6 months after ICRS implantation, and 0.50±0.27 at 6 months after PIOL implantation. The mean CDVA was 0.56±0.23 before ICRS implantation, 0.68±0.25 at 6 months after ICRS implantation, and 0.71±0.19 at 1 month after PIOL implantation. The mean spherical equivalent after PIOL implantation was −1.19±1.33 D. Six months after PIOL implantation, the efficacy index was 0.88 and the safety index, 1.28.

Other studies also found promising results using this combined treatment (PIOL and ICRS) obtained an improvement in UDVA and CDVA and significant reduction in the mean SE after PIOL implantation [51, 52].

25.4 Conclusions

Usually, keratoconus has been traditionally considered a contraindication for refractive surgery, but performing a precise evaluation of each keratoconus patient (stage of disease, visual function, corneal topography, aberrometry, etc.) the refractive surgery can be, in some cases, a safe and effective option.

Today there is the possibility of combining different treatments to improve visual quality and stop the progression of the disease; however, we need more investigations to have a safer indication of each combination treatment.

Compliance with Ethical Requirements Pablo Sanz Díez, Alfredo Vega Estrada, and Jorge L. Alió declare that they have no conflict of interest. All procedures followed were in accordance with the ethical standards of the responsible committee on human experimentation (institutional and national) and with the Helsinki Declaration of 1975, as revised in 2000. Informed consent was obtained from all patients for being included in the study. No animal studies were carried out by the authors for this article.

This study has been supported in part by a grant from European Regional Development Fund (Fondo europeo de desarrollo regional FEDER) and the Spanish Ministry of Economy and Competitiviness, Instituto Carlos III, Red Temática de Investigación Cooperativa en Salud (RETICS) "Prevención, detección precoz y tratamiento de la patología ocular prevalente, degenerativa y crónica". Subprograma "dioptrio ocular y patologías frecuentes" (RD12/0034/0007).

References

1. Rabinowitz YS. Keratoconus. Surv Ophtalmol. 1998;42:297–319.
2. Barbara A, Rabinowitz YS. Chapter 6: Clinical signs and differential diagnosis of keratoconus. In: Kymionis GD, Plaka AD, Kontadakis GA, editors. Textbook on keratoconus. New insights. New Delhi: Jaypee Brothers Medical Publishers (P) Ltd; 2012.
3. Kennedy RH, Bourne WM, Dyer JA. A 48-year clinical and epidemiologic study of keratoconus. Am J Ophthalmol. 1986;101:267–73.
4. Barbara A, Rabinowitz YS. Chapter 1: Epidemiology of keratoconus. In: François M, Ancele E, Butterwoth J, editors. Textbook on keratoconus. New insights. New Delhi: Jaypee Brothers Medical Publishers (P) Ltd; 2012.
5. Rabinowitz YS, Garbus JJ, Garbus C, McDonnell PJ. Contact lens selection for keratoconus using a computer-assisted videophotokeratoscope. CLAO J. 1991;17:88–93.
6. Rosenthal P, Cotter JM. Clinical performance of a spline-based apical vaulting keratoconus corneal contact lens design. CLAO J. 1995;21:42–6.
7. Yeung K, Eghbali F, Weissman BA. Clinical experience with piggyback contact lens systems on keratoconic eyes. J Am Optom Assoc. 1995;66:539–43.
8. Sedaghat M, Ansari-Astaneh MR, Zarei-Ghanavati M, Davis SW, Sikder S. Artisan iris-supported phakic IOL implantation in patients with keratoconus: a review of 16 eyes. J Refract Surg. 2011;27:489–93.
9. Kamiya K, Shimizu K, Kobashi H, Komatsu M, Nakamura A, Nakamura T, Ichikawa K. Clinical outcomes of posterior chamber toricphakic intraocular lens implantation for the correction of high myopic astigmatism in eyes with keratoconus: 6-month follow-up. Graefes Arch Clin Exp Ophthalmol. 2011;249:1073–80.
10. Venter J. Artisan phakic intraocular lens in patients with keratoconus. J Refract Surg. 2009;25:759–64.
11. Kurian M, Nagappa S, Bhagali R, Shetty R, Shetty BK. Visual quality after posterior chamber phakic intraocular lens implantation in keratoconus. J Cataract Refract Surg. 2012;38:1050–7.
12. Leccisotti A, Fields SV. Angle-supported phakic intraocular lenses in eyes with keratoconus and myopia. J Cataract Refract Surg. 2003;29:1530–6.
13. Alió JL, Peña-García P, Abdulla F, Zein G, Abumustafa S. Phakic intraocular lenses in keratoconus; comparison between Artiflex (iris-claw) and posterior chamber implantable Collamer phakic intraocular lenses. J Cataract Refract Surg. 2014;40(3):383–94.
14. Kanellopoulos AJ, Binder PS. Collagen cross-linking (CCL) with sequential topography-guided PRK; a temporizing alternative for keratoconus to penetrating keratoplasty. Cornea. 2007;26:891–5.
15. Krueger RR, Kanellopoulos AJ. Stability of simultaneous topography-guided photorefractive keratectomy and riboflavin/ UVA cross-linking for progressive keratoconus: case reports. J Refract Surg. 2010;26: S827–32.
16. Kymionis GD, Kontadakis GA, Kounis GA, Portaliou DM, Karavitaki AE, Magarakis M, Yoo S, Pallikaris IG. Simultaneous topography-guided PRK followed by corneal collagen cross-linking for keratoconus. J Refract Surg. 2009;25(9):S807–S11.
17. Kanellopoulos AJ. Comparison of sequential vs same-day simultaneous collagen cross-linking and topography-guided PRK for treatment of keratoconus. J Refract Surg. 2009;25:S812–8.
18. Stojanovic A, Zhang J, Chen X, Nitter TA, Chen S, Wang Q. Topography-guided transepithelial surface ablation followed by corneal collagen cross-linking performed in a single combined procedure for the treatment of keratoconus and pellucid marginal degeneration. J Refract Surg. 2010;26:145–52.
19. Güell JL, Morral M, Malecaze F, Gris O, Elies D, Manero F. Collagen cross-linking and toric iris-claw phakic intraocular lens for myopic astigmatism in progressive mild to moderate keratoconus. J Cataract Refract Surg. 2012;38(3):475–84.
20. Navas A, Tapia-Herrera G, Jaimes M, Graue-Hernández EO, Gomez-Bastar A, Ramirez-Luquín T, Ramirez-Miranda A. Implantable collamer lenses after intracorneal ring segments for keratoconus. Int Ophthalmol. 2012;32(5):423–9.
21. Moshirfar M, Fenzl CR, Meyer JJ, Neuffer MC, Espandar L, Mifflin MD. Simultaneous and sequential implantation of intacs and verisyse phakic intraocular lens for refractive improvement in keratectasia. Cornea. 2011;30:158–63.
22. Alessio G, L'abbate M, Sborgia C, La Tegola MG. Photorefractive keratectomy followed by cross-linking versus cross-linking alone for management of

progressive keratoconus: two-year follow-up. Am J Ophthalmol. 2013;155(1):54–65.
23. Budo C, Bartels MC, van Rij G. Implantation of Artisan toric phakic intraocular lenses for the correction of astigmatism and spherical errors in patients with keratoconus. J Refract Surg. 2005;21(3):218–22.
24. Leccisotti A. Refractive lens exchange in keratoconus. J Cataract Refract Surg. 2006;32(5):742–6.
25. Denoyer A, Denoyer L, Marotte D, et al. Intraindividual comparative study of corneal and ocular wavefront aberrations after biaxial microincision versus coaxial small-incision cataract surgery. Br J Ophthalmol. 2008;92(12):1679–84.
26. Mojzis P, Piñero DP, Studeny P, et al. Comparative analysis of clinical outcomes obtained with a new diffractive multifocal toric intraocular lens implanted through two types of corneal incision. J Refract Surg. 2011;27(9):648–57.
27. McMahon TT, Anderson RJ, Roberts C, et al. CLEK Study Group. Repeatability of corneal topography measurement in keratoconus with the TMS-1. Optom Vis Sci. 2005;82(5):405–15.
28. Vinciguerra P, Muñoz MI, Camesasca FI, Grizzi F, Roberts C. Long-term follow-up of ultrathin corneas after surface retreatment with phototherapeutic keratectomy. J Cataract Refract Surg. 2005;31(1):82–7.
29. Ziaei M, et al. Reshaping procedures for the surgical management of corneal ectasia. J Cataract Refract Surg. 2015;41(4):842–72.
30. Alió JL, Piñero DP, Alesón A, Teus MA, Barraquer RI, Murta J, Maldonado MJ, Castro de Luna G, Gutiérrez R, Villa C, Uceda-Montanes A. Keratoconus-integrated characterisation considering anterior corneal aberrations, internal astigmatism, and corneal biomechanics. J Cataract Refract Surg. 2011;37(3):552–68.
31. Peña-García P. Vectorial analysis of astigmatic correction in stable keratoconus. PRK vs PIOLs. JCRS-2014-081 (Sent).
32. Meek KM, Hayes S. Corneal cross-linking—a review. Ophthalmic Physiol Opt. 2013;33(2):78–93.
33. Raiskup F, Spoerl E. Corneal cross-linking with riboflavin and ultraviolet A. Part II. Clinical indications and results. Ocul Surf. 2013;11:93–108.
34. Koller T, Mrochen M, Seiler T. Complication and failure rates after corneal cross-linking. J Cataract Refract Surg. 2009;35:1358–62.
35. Hafezi F, Mrochen M, Iseli H, Seiler T. Collagen cross-linking with ultraviolet A and hypo-osmolar riboflavin solution in thin corneas. J Cataract Refract Surg. 2009;35:621–4.
36. Hafezi F, Iseli HP. Pregnancy-related exacerbation of iatrogenic keratectasia despite corneal collagen cross-linking. J Cataract Refract Surg. 2008;34:1219–21.
37. NICE guidance on Photochemical corneal collagen cross-linkage using riboflavin and ultraviolet A for keratoconus. Issued November 2009; 27 Oct 2011.
38. Abad J, Panesso J. Corneal collagen cross-linking induced by UVA and riboflavin (CXL). Tech Ophthalmol. 2008;6:8–12.
39. Spoerl E, Mrochen M, Sliney D, et al. Safety of UVA-riboflavin cross-linking of the cornea. Cornea. 2007;26:385–9.
40. Peña-García P, Alió JL, Vega-Estrada A, Barraquer RI. Internal, corneal and refractive astigmatism as prognostic factor for ICRS implantation in mild to moderate keratoconus. J Cataract Refract Surg. 2014;40(10):1633–44.
41. Wollensak G, Spoerl E, Seiler T. Stress-strain measurements of human and porcine corneas after riboflavin-ultraviolet- A-induced cross-linking. J Cataract Refract Surg. 2003;29:1780–5.
42. Mukherjee AN, Selimis V, Aslanides I. Transepithelial photorefractive keratectomy with crosslinking for keratoconus. Open Ophthalmol J. 2013;7:63–8.
43. Coskunseven E, Jankov II MR, Grentzelos MA, Plaka AD, Limnopoulou AN, Kymionis GD. Topography-guided transepithelial PRK after intracorneal ring segments implantation and corneal collagen CXL in a three-step procedure for keratoconus. J Refract Surg. 2013;29(1):54–8.
44. Kremer I, Aizenman I, Lichter H, Shayer S, Levinger S. Simultaneous wavefront-guided photorefractive keratectomy and corneal collagen crosslinking after intrastromal corneal ring segment implantation for keratoconus. J Cataract Refract Surg. 2012;38(10):1802–7.
45. Al-Tuwairqi W, Sinjab MM. Intracorneal ring segments implantation followed by same-day topography-guided PRK and corneal collagen CXL in low to moderate keratoconus. J Refract Surg. 2013;29(1):59–63.
46. Iovieno A, Légaré ME, Rootman DB, Yeung SN, Kim P, Rootman DS. Intracorneal ring segments implantation followed by same-day photorefractive keratectomy and corneal collagen cross-linking in keratoconus. J Refract Surg. 2011;27(12):915–8.
47. Izquierdo Jr L, Henriquez MA, McCarthy M. Artiflex phakic intraocular lens implantation after corneal collagen cross-linking in keratoconic eyes. J Refract Surg. 2011;27(7):482–7.
48. Fadlallah A, Dirani A, El Rami H, Cherfane G, Jarade E. Safety and visual outcome of Visian toric ICL implantation after corneal collagen cross-linking in keratoconus. J Refract Surg. 2013;29(2):84–9.
49. Coskunseven E, Onder M, Kymionis GD, Diakonis VF, Arslan E, Tsiklis N, Bouzoukis DI, Ioannis PI. Combined Intacs and posterior chamber toric implantable Collamer lens implantation for keratoconic patients with extreme myopia. Am J Ophthalmol. 2007;144:387–9.
50. Alfonso JF, Lisa C, Fernández-Vega L, Madrid-Costa D, Poo-López A, Montés-Micó R. Intrastromal corneal ring segments and posterior chamber phakic intraocular lens implantation for keratoconus correction. J Cataract Refract Surg. 2011;37(4):706–13.
51. El-Raggal TM, Abdel Fattah AA. Sequential Intacs and Verisyse phakic intraocular lens for refractive improvement in keratoconic eyes. J Cataract Refract Surg. 2007;33:966–70.
52. Ferreira TB, Güell JL, Manero F. Combined intracorneal ring segments and iris-fixated phakic intraocular lens for keratoconus refractive and visual improvement. J Refract Surg. 2014;30(5):336–41.

26

Excimer Laser Ablation in Keratoconus Treatment: Sequential High Definition Wavefront-Guided PRK After CXL

Mohamed Shafik Shaheen and Ahmed Shalaby

26.1 Introduction

Laser refractive surgery in patients with such irregular corneas has long been contraindicated because of the risk of postoperative progression of the disease process. However, numerous studies claim the safety of surface ablation in suspected keratoconus or in "forme fruste keratoconus" as in photorefractive keratectomy (PRK). In patients with mild to moderate keratoconus, combined PRK and collagen cross-linking has been proven to be a safe and effective alternative to correct minor refractive error, stabilizing the remaining stromal bed and avoiding progression of ectatic disease [1, 2].

Kanellopoulos and Binder (2007) proposed a two-step procedure with corneal CXL and topography-guided PRK after a 1-year interval. They studied the effect of this two-step approach on keratoconus progression and concluded that there was significant clinical improvement and apparent stability for more than a year compared to the untreated mate eye that continued to progress over the same period [3].

Kanellopoulos and Asimellis also described the ATHENS protocol of simultaneous topography-guided PRK with same-day collagen CXL [4]. Kanellopoulos found superior results of this protocol compared to sequential CXL with later PRK after 6 months in his study that included 325 eyes with progressive keratoconus [5].

Thus, combination of laser surface ablation and CXL provides a potential treatment for keratoconus.

26.2 Higher Order Aberrations and Keratoconus

Keratoconus causes a reduction in the optical quality of the eye as a result of corneal distortion, corneal scarring, and higher order aberrations. The correction of these optical aberrations would significantly improve the visual performance of keratoconic eyes. However, the first step would be to measure the optical flaws in keratoconus accurately, which in itself presents a challenge. In keratoconus, corneal thinning causes marked shape changes which create large amounts of higher order optical aberrations, which differ significantly from the aberrations found in normal eyes [6].

Increased negative vertical coma, the major aberrometric finding in keratoconus, is caused by

M. Shafik Shaheen, M.D., Ph.D. (✉)
Department of Ophthalmology, University of Alexandria, Egypt, P.O. Box 27, Ibrahimia, Alexandria 21321, Egypt
e-mail: m.shafik@link.net

A. Shalaby, M.D.
Department of Ophthalmology, University of Alexandria Main Hospitals, Alexandria, Egypt
e-mail: dr_ahmadshalaby@yahoo.com

J.L. Alió (ed.), *Keratoconus*, Essentials in Ophthalmology, DOI 10.1007/978-3-319-43881-8_26

the relatively slower wavefront in the inferior part of the cornea; the relatively advanced wavefront in the superior part of the cornea is also an indicator of infero-superior asymmetry [7].

Measurement of the wavefront error of the eye provides an accurate method to assess the optical properties of the eye beyond sphere and cylinder, evaluate therapy (e.g., refractive surgery) designed to improve the optical properties of the eye, and provide the necessary information to design optical prescriptions for the eye to minimize all refractive errors.

Modern high-definition aberrometers that were introduced to the ophthalmic armamentarium could read the aberrations of such irregular corneas and generate a dependable ablation profile out of them for precise correction [8].

26.3 Wavefront vs. Topography-Guided Ablation

Attempts to treat irregular cornea by laser vision correction (LVC) started early by the work of Fernandez et al. (2000). They used a kind of primitive topography-guided ablation profile (contoured ablation pattern = Custom CAP) to treat irregular cornea cases including stable keratoconic patients. The results were disappointing, as the authors mentioned in their work, due to: The variability of refractive condition (sphere, cylinder, and irregular astigmatism) made it difficult to predict the precise spherical or regular cylindrical component that will remain, the ablation profile which was a primitive topo-guided one did not provide good tackling for the cause–effect relationship, the calculation and positioning of the laser beam lacked by that time the precision to address such irregularity with no compensation for cyclotorsion and no compensation for pupil centroid shift [9].

The use of wavefront-guided laser technology for the management of aberrated corneas has been shown to effectively reduce HOAs in corneas with residual refractive errors post keratorefractive surgeries [10]. Wavefront-guided technology has also shown efficacy in addressing irregularities in pathologic corneas once their biomechanical weakening has been addressed through the application of CXL [1]. However, limitations of wavefront-guided procedures have been described, mainly related to the technical limitations of aberrometers in measuring ocular aberrations [11].

After the introduction of the high-definition aberrometers, irregular astigmatism accompanying highly aberrated corneas could be handled [8, 10]. Modern aberrometers that were introduced to the ophthalmic armamentarium could read the aberrations of the irregular cornea and generate a dependable and reliable ablation profile out of them. Few years ago, a newer version of high-definition Hartmann-Shack aberrometer (iDesign system®) was introduced to the field of refractive surgery by Abbott Inc. with reports about their abilities to read and treat precisely the highly aberrated corneas [8].

26.4 Sequential vs. Simultaneous Treatment

The simultaneous approach is thought to be too invasive (two techniques at the same sitting), does not address emmetropia due to the prolonged flattening effect of CXL with uncontrolled refractive outcome [12].

Besides, the sequential protocol is, in fact, making use of the stable cornea provided by previous CXL. This stable corneal surface provides, in turn, a stable refractive surface (even still irregular) from which we can calculate a reliable and dependable ablation profile to correct the irregularity and avoid refractive surprises and changes that can potentially occur with the use of the simultaneous approach [8].

26.5 Wavefront-Guided PRK After CXL

We recommend Sequential wavefront-guided PRK using the ablation profile generated by the high-definition Hartmann-Shack aberrometer (iDesign system®, Abbott, USA) in cross-linked stable keratoconic eyes after at least 12 months of the cross-linking according to the data of a pilot study published recently by our team [8]. It is also recommended to have the cross-linking done by an epithelium-off approach to guarantee maximum corneal tissue compactness and stiffness before ablating a thin part of it.

The following selection criteria are recommended:

- Stage I, II keratoconus cases according to Amsler-Krumeich classification [13].
- Stable keratoconus after corneal collagen cross-linking as defined by stability of subjective refraction (± 0.5 diopters (D) change in spherical equivalent) in three consecutive monthly visits after 1 year of corneal CXL together with keratometric stability (no increase of the cone apex keratometry of ≥0.75 D) in the last 6 months of follow-up [14].
- Manifest refraction spherical equivalent ≤6 D.
- Corneal thickness at the thinnest location ≥400 μm.
- Clear cornea in the pupillary area.

26.6 Preoperative and Postoperative Examination

Preoperative ophthalmic examination should include manifest and cycloplegic refraction, UDVA and CDVA testing, pupil diameter measurement under mesopic conditions using the Colvard pupillometer (Oasis, Glendora, CA, USA), slit lamp anterior segment examination, corneal topography, and anterior segment imaging using the Pentacam-HR system (Oculus Inc., Wetzlar, Germany) or similar Scheimpflug imaging device, ocular aberrometry (iDesign aberrometer, Abbott Medical Optics, AMO, Santa Ana, CA), applanation tonometry, and funduscopy. With the Pentacam topography system, the following topographic and pachymetric parameters were recorded and evaluated: flattest and steepest keratometric readings (K1 and K2), maximum keratometry (K-max), corneal asphericity (*Q*) for an 8-mm diameter, central corneal thickness (CCT), minimum corneal thickness (MCT), maximum anterior corneal elevation (AE) for an 8-mm diameter, index of surface variation (ISV), index of vertical asymmetry (IVA), keratoconus index (KI), center keratoconus index (CKI), index of height asymmetry (IHA), index of height decentration (IHD), and minimal radius of curvature (R_{min}).

With the high-resolution aberrometer, the following parameters are recorded and evaluated for a 6-mm pupil: total root mean square (RMS), HOAs RMS, primary coma RMS $\left(Z_3^{\pm 1}\right)$, trefoil RMS $\left(Z_3^{\pm 3}\right)$, and the Zernike term corresponding to the primary spherical aberration (Z_4^0).

Postoperatively, patients should be examined the third day after surgery and at 1 week postoperatively to assess the status of the corneal epithelial healing and if a complete epithelialization is present, the therapeutic contact lens fitted has to be removed. Afterward, patients should be examined at 1, 3, 6, and 12 months after surgery. UDVA and CDVA testing, manifest refraction, corneal topography, ocular aberrometry, and biomicroscopic examination are performed in these four visits. In all postoperative visits, the level of corneal haze has to be evaluated on a scale from 0 to 4 (0 = clear cornea, 1 = mild haze, 2 = moderate haze, 3 = severe haze, and 4 = reticular haze obstructing iris details) [5].

26.7 Surgical Procedure

All surgical procedures are performed under topical anesthesia (benoxinate hydrochloride 0.4 % Sterile Ophthalmic Solution). In all cases, the corneal epithelium is removed using the 9.0-mm Amoils brush (Innovative Excimer Solutions, Inc., Toronto, Canada) and the laser ablation iw then applied. A WFG-PRK laser treatment is applied using the VISX Star S4IR excimer laser (Abbott Medical Optics, Santa Ana, California) and an ablation profile generated according to the measurements obtained with the iDesign system. An adjustment to the profile is applied as needed to reduce the maximum ablation depth to a maximum of 15 % of the corneal thickness at the thinnest location, reducing only the sphere component without changing the cylinder. The sphere adjustment is limited to 2.50 D, which is the maximum adjustment allowed by the manufacturer.

After laser ablation, a 6-mm cellulose disc soaked in Mitomycin C (MMC) 0.02 % solution is applied over the ablated tissue for 20 s followed by irrigation with 30 mL of chilled balanced salt solution. A bandage contact lens is then fitted, remaining in place until full reepithelialization. The postoperative treatment regimen consists of Topical Antibiotics/Corticosteroids, e.g., moxifloxacin hydrochloride 0.5 % (Vigamox, Alcon Laboratories) applied four times daily up to 2 weeks after complete reepithelialization, a combination of tobramycin 3 mg/mL with dexamethasone 1 mg/mL (Tobradex, Alcon Laboratories, UK) applied four times daily until complete reepithelialization and then gradual tapering over 2 weeks, preservative-free tear substitutes applied every 2 h for 2 weeks (e.g., Refresh plus, Allergan, Inc, USA), and oral analgesic nonsteroidal anti-inflammatory drug applied three times daily for 3 days (Catafast, Novartis, Switzerland).

26.8 Clinical Results

A study by Shafik Shaheen et al. was done on 34 eyes with stage I and II keratoconus meeting the above-mentioned criteria who had previous CXL at least 1 year before treatment to demonstrate the effect of this wavefront-guided laser surface correction on visual, refractive, corneal morphology, and aberrometric data (Recently published: Shafik Shaheen M, Bardan AS, Pinero D, Ezzeldin H, El-Kateb M, Helaly H, Khalifa M. Wave Front–Guided Photorefractive Keratectomy Using a High-Resolution Aberrometer After Corneal Collagen Cross-Linking in Keratoconus. Cornea 2016;35(7):946–953).).

It demonstrated a statistically significant improvement in the mean logMAR UDVA from 0.93 ± 0.33 (mean ± SD) preoperatively to 0.14 ± 0.11 (mean ± SD) at the last follow-up visit and the mean logMAR CDVA has been improved from 0.28 ± 0.24 (mean ± SD) preoperatively to 0.05 ± 0.06 (mean ± SD) at the last follow-up visit; (p-value <0.001) for both. The mean MRSE has been reduced from −3.22 preoperatively to −0.68 at the 12th month postoperatively. The magnitude of reduction is shown in Fig. 26.1. The study demonstrates a high safety and efficacy indices at the last follow-up visit. Efficacy index was 1.58 ± 1.11 (mean ± SD), $p < 0.001$, safety index was 1.96 ± 1.52 ($p < 0.001$) proving safety and efficacy regarding VA improvement.

About the predictability of the procedure, at the sixth month postoperatively, 76.5 % of eyes had a manifest refraction within ±1.00 D of emmetropia, 47.1 % were within ±0.50 D. At the last follow-up visit 62 % of the cases reached within ±0.50 D. Summary is shown in Fig. 26.1.

As shown in Fig. 26.2, 97.1 % of the study subjects reached ≥ 20/40 UDVA at the last follow-up visit compared to 73.5 % only reaching CDVA of ≥ 20/40 preoperatively. Hundred percent reached ≥ 20/50 UDVA at the last follow-up visit at 1 year postoperatively.

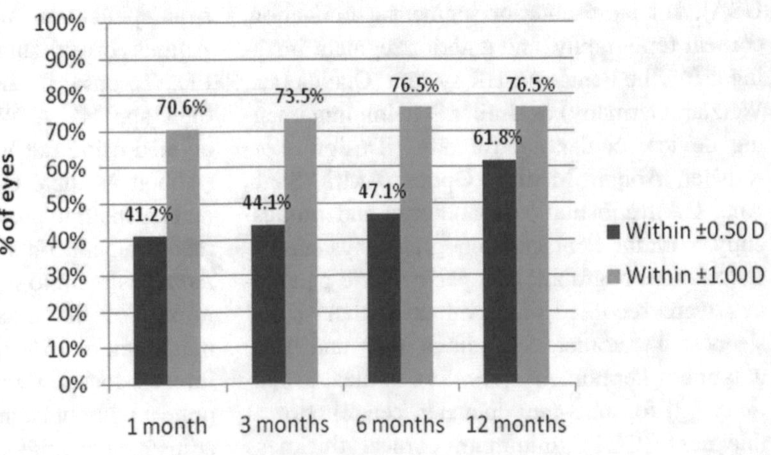

Fig. 26.1 Summary of the predictability outcomes after surgery in the analyzed sample

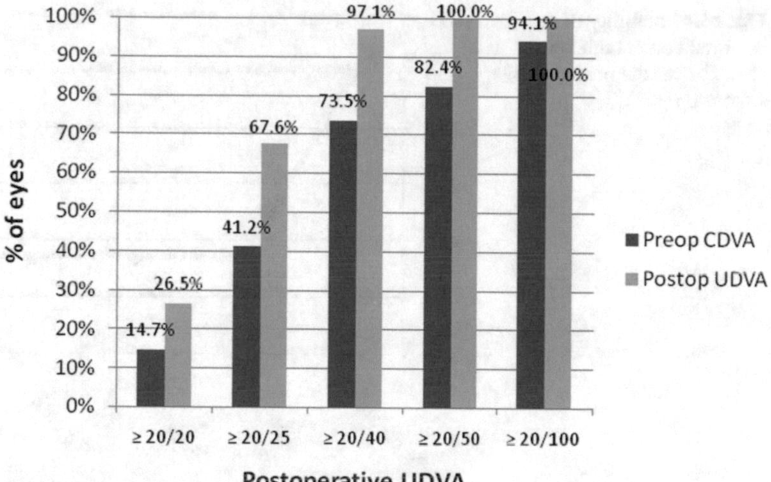

Fig. 26.2 Comparison of the distribution of the postoperative UDVA (after 1 year) and the preoperative CDVA outcomes

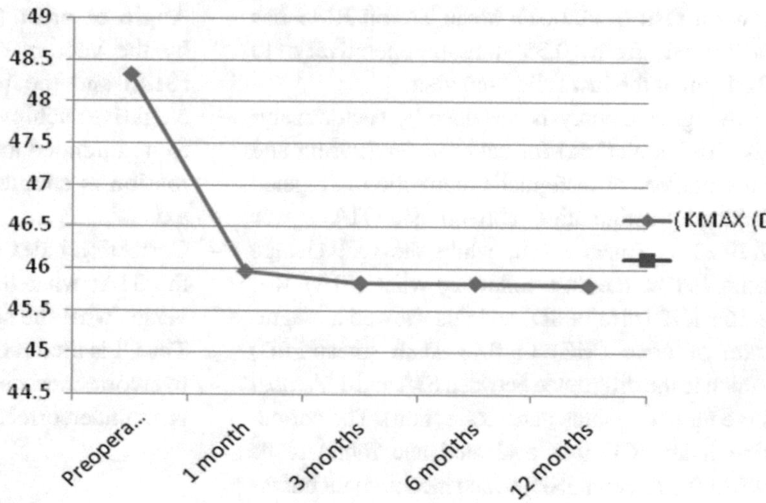

Fig. 26.3 Stability of the maximum keratometry (K-MAX) over the postoperative follow-up

The study demonstrated many changes in the corneal morphology. First of all the reduction of the maximum K reading from a mean of 48.32 D preoperatively to a mean of about 45.8 D at month 3 which remained in the same range over the first year postoperatively as shown in Fig. 26.3. Mean *Q*-value has decreased from −0.44 to −0.26. Central corneal thickness has decreased from 491.12 ± 39.19 μm (mean ± SD) preoperatively to 429.56 ± 61.81 μm at the last follow-up visit. Minimal corneal thickness decreased from 478.32 μm (mean) preoperatively to about 414 μm (mean) which remained stable over the period of follow-up as shown in Fig. 26.4. All the results are statistically significant ($p < 0.001$).

About the corneal indices, the results showed decrease in the values of the eight Pentacam indices studied. The reduction in IVA, IHA, IHD, and CKI was not statistically significant. While the reduction in ISV, R_{min}, and KI was statistically significant. The study showed also stability of the indices through the period of follow-up.

There was a statistically significant reduction in the higher order aberrations in general demonstrated by the significant reduction of total RMS; *p*-value <0.001, and the RMS HOA; ($p = 0.003$), and reduction of coma ($p = 0.001$) and trefoil ($p < 0.001$). The primary coma RMS has decreased from 0.60 ± 0.59 μm (mean ± SD) preoperatively to 0.37 ± 0.37 μm at the last fol-

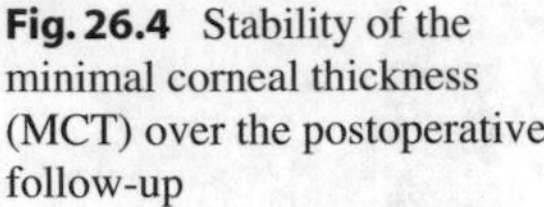

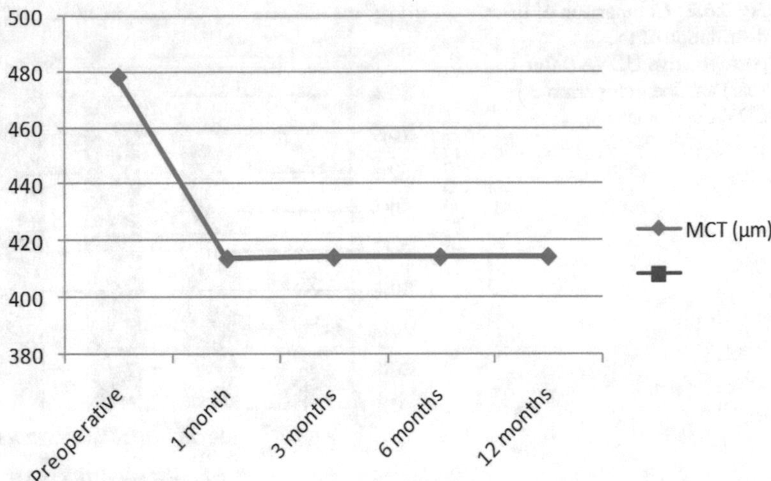

Fig. 26.4 Stability of the minimal corneal thickness (MCT) over the postoperative follow-up

low-up visit ($p=0.001$). Mean Trefoil RMS has decreased from 0.35 μm preoperatively to 0.21 μm at the last follow-up visit.

Astigmatic analysis was done by vector analysis (Alpins method) for better understanding and presentation of astigmatic correction. Targeted induced astigmatic correction (TIA) was 2.79 ± 1.82 (mean ± SD), while the real change achieved at the last follow-up visit (SIA) was 2.36 ± 1.72 (mean ± SD) and this showed a magnitude of error (ME) of 0.43 ± 0.86 (mean ± SD) which is the difference between SIA and TIA (positive number means undercorrection). The correction index (CI) was evaluated and found to be 0.88 ± 0.29 (mean ± SD) which means slight undercorrection. This is described in detail in Table 26.1.

The following vectors were determined and evaluated: targeted induced astigmatism (TIA) as the vector of intended change in cylinder for each treatment, surgically induced astigmatism (SIA) as the vector of the real change achieved, and difference vector (DV) as the additional astigmatic change that would enable the initial surgery to achieve its intended target. Additionally, the following parameters derived from the relationship between these vectors were calculated and analyzed in each postoperative visit:

- Magnitude of error (ME): the arithmetic difference between the magnitudes of the SIA and TIA. Positive: undercorrection; negative: overcorrection.
- Angle of error (AE): the angle described by the vectors of the achieved correction (SIA) and the intended correction (TIA): Negative: achieved correction is clockwise to its intended axis. Positive: achieved correction is counterclockwise to its intended axis
- Correction index (CI): The ratio of the SIA to the TIA; what the surgery actually induced versus what the surgery was meant to induce. The CI is preferably 1; it is greater than 1 if an overcorrection occurs and less than 1 if there is an undercorrection.

Case Example 1

A 25-year-old female patient. Wavefront-guided PRK was performed 2 years after corneal collagen cross-linking. Table 26.2 represents the preoperative clinical data, Pentacam and iDesign wavefront measurements compared to the findings at the final postoperative follow-up visit (12 months postop).

In this case there is a noticeable reduction in the total RMS value by (52 %), RMS HOA by (51.4 %), Coma reduction by (58.9 %), trefoil reduction by (40.2 %). This improvement was reflected on the patient's visual outcome (logMAR CDVA was improved from +0.50 to 0.00). Figures 26.5, 26.6, 26.7, 26.8, and 26.9 show the pre- and postoperative investigations and the ablation profile of this patient.

Table 26.1 Summary of the parameters derived from the vector analysis of ocular astigmatic changes at the end of the follow-up in the analyzed sample (Alpins method)

Vector parameters	Mean (SD) Median (range)
TIA (D)	2.79 (1.82)
	3.00 (0.00 to 7.00)
SIA (D)	2.36 (1.72)
	2.39 (0.00 to 7.95)
DV (D)	1.06 (0.92)
	0.75 (0.00 to 3.25)
ME	0.43 (0.86)
	0.28 (2.58 to −0.95)
CI	0.88 (0.29)
	0.83 (0.26 to 1.61)
AE (°)	2.57 (15.43)
	2.34 (48.76 to −44.86)

TIA targeted intended astigmatism, *SIA* surgically induced astigmatism, *DV* difference vector, *ME* magnitude of error, *AE* angle of error, *CI* correction index, *SD* standard deviation

Table 26.2 Summary of preoperative and postoperative data of case 1

Preoperative data		Final postoperative data
UDVA (logMAR)	+1.30	+0.10
CDVA (logMAR)	+0.50	0.00
Refraction	+0.75 − 4.00 × 110	−0.25 − 1.00 × 155
Pentacam corneal data		
Thinnest location	422 μm	374 μm
ISV	67	51
IVA	0.83	0.49
KI	1.19	1.17
CKI	1.03	1.05
R_{min}	6.78	6.98
IHA	9.8	15.3
IHD	0.061	0.057
iDesign data at 5 mm WFD		
RMS total	3.65 μm	1.75 μm
RMS HOA	2.72 μm	1.32 μm
Coma	1.16574	0.47882
Trefoil	0.67390	0.40287
Spherical aberrations	−0.00306	−0.21724

Case Example 2

A 30-year-old female patient. Wavefront-guided PRK was performed 3 years after corneal collagen cross-linking. Table 26.3 represents the preoperative clinical data, Pentacam and iDesign wavefront measurements compared to the findings at the final postoperative follow-up visit (12 months postop).

In this case there is a noticeable reduction in the total RMS value by (67.6 %), RMS HOA by (24.6 %), Coma reduction by (28.8 %). This improvement was reflected on the patient's visual outcome (logMAR UDVA was improved from +0.70 to 0.00). Figures 26.10, 26.11, 26.12, 26.13, and 26.14 show the pre- and postoperative investigations and the ablation profile of this patient.

26.9 Discussion

Keratoconus has a great impact on the visual performance which in turn affects the patient's quality of life owing to the highly aberrated irregular cornea that lead to image quality degradation. Retinal image quality is degraded by scatter, diffraction, and wavefront aberrations (better known as wavefront errors) [15].

In the modern era, a great breakthrough in the management of keratoconus was achieved by introducing the corneal collagen cross-linking that halts the disease progression and makes the cornea stiffer and more stable. Moreover, advances in laser vision correction changed the way of thinking and added a lot of options to the armamentarium of irregular cornea management [16–19].

Attempts to implement surface ablation to treat early to moderate keratoconus have evolved in the era of CXL. Some authors preferred the simultaneous approach [1, 2, 5] (same day PRK + CXL) while others preferred the sequential PRK after CXL [3, 8].

In his work, Kanellopoulos advised using topography-guided ablation to treat early and moderate keratoconus with simultaneous same day CXL. He stated that he was not able to use

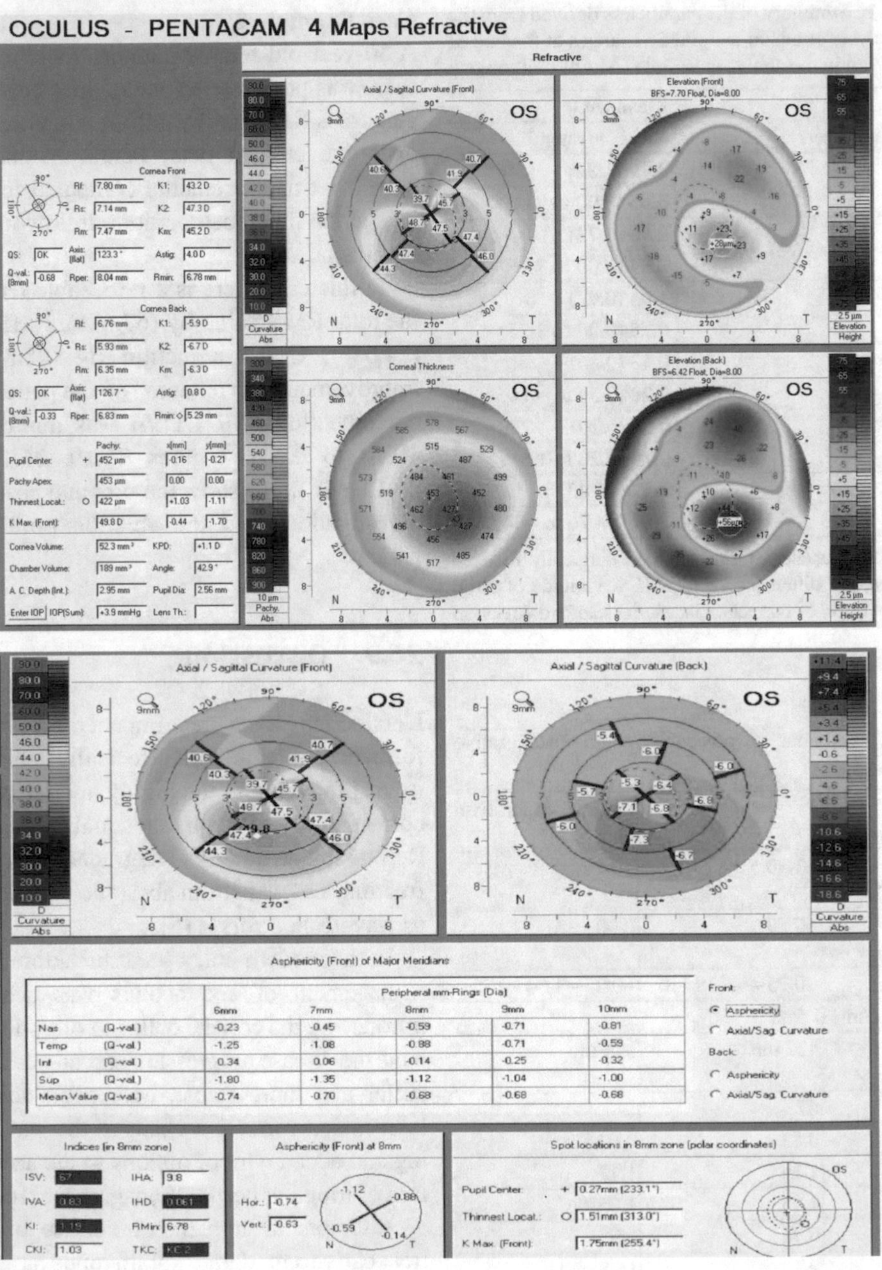

Fig. 26.5 Preoperative Pentacam of case 1

a wavefront-guided ablation profile because the highly irregular keratoconic eyes were beyond the limits of wavefront measuring devices making topo-guided approach more efficient in such cases. He also claimed superior results of the simultaneous over the sequential technique for three reasons: the combination reduces the patient's time away from work, performing both procedures at the same time with topography-guided PRK first appeared to minimize the potential superficial stromal scarring resulting from PRK, and when topography-guided PRK is performed after the CXL procedure, some of the cross-linked anterior cornea is removed, minimizing the potential benefit of CXL [5].

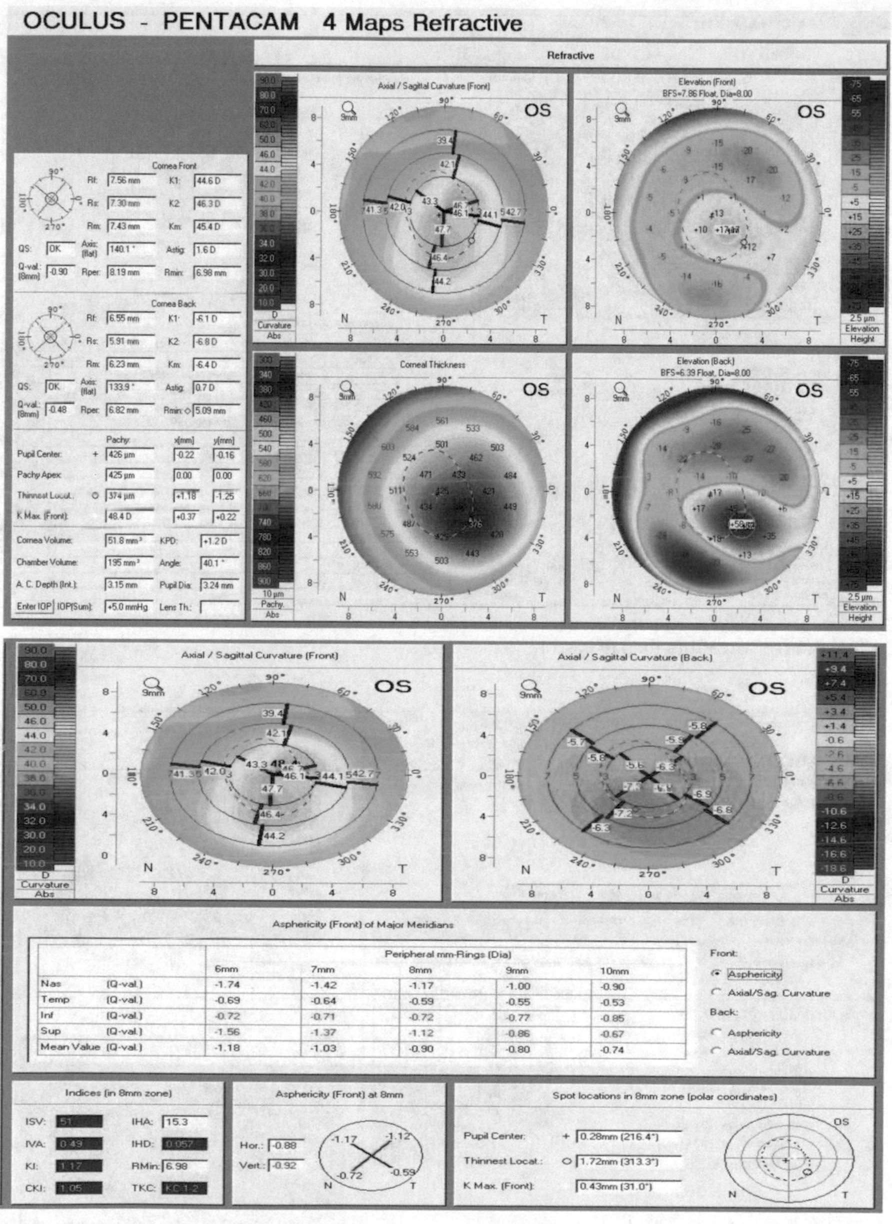

Fig. 26.6 Postoperative (final follow-up visit) Pentacam of case 1

Innovations in ablation profiles, excimer laser technology, and diagnostic equipments have allowed surgeons not only to correct LOAs but also to minimize HOAs, increasing the levels of postoperative efficacy, predictability, and visual quality [20]. Even so, the management of significantly irregular corneas remains as a challenge for refractive surgeons.

The use of wavefront-guided laser technology for the management of aberrated corneas has been shown to effectively reduce HOAs in corneas with residual refractive errors post keratorefractive surgeries [10, 21]. Wavefront-guided technology has also shown efficacy in addressing irregularities in pathologic corneas once their biomechanical weakening has been addressed

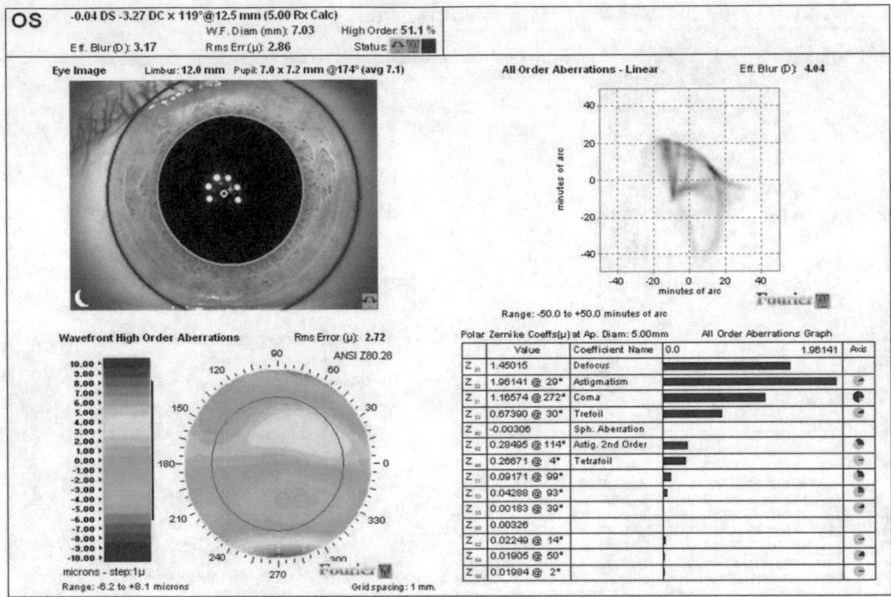

Fig. 26.7 Preoperative wavefront map of case 1

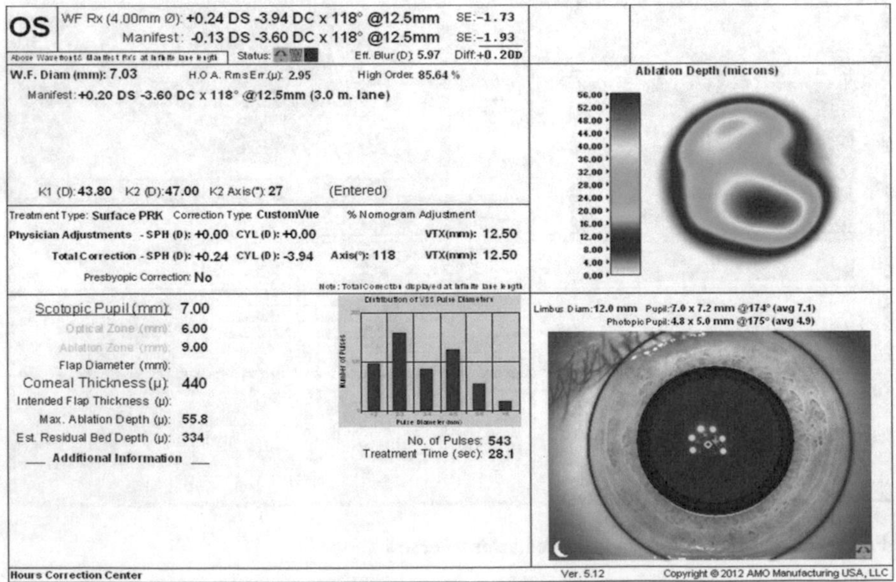

Fig. 26.8 Ablation profile generated by iDesign® for case 1

through the application of CXL [22]. However, limitations of wavefront-guided procedures have been described, mainly related to the technical limitations of aberrometers in measuring ocular aberrations [11].

Recently after the introduction of the high-definition aberrometers, irregular astigmatism accompanying highly aberrated corneas could be handled [8, 10]. Modern aberrometers that were introduced to the ophthalmic armamentarium could read the aberrations of the irregular cornea and generate a dependable and reliable ablation profile out of them. Few years ago, a newer version of high-definition Hartmann-Shack aberrometer

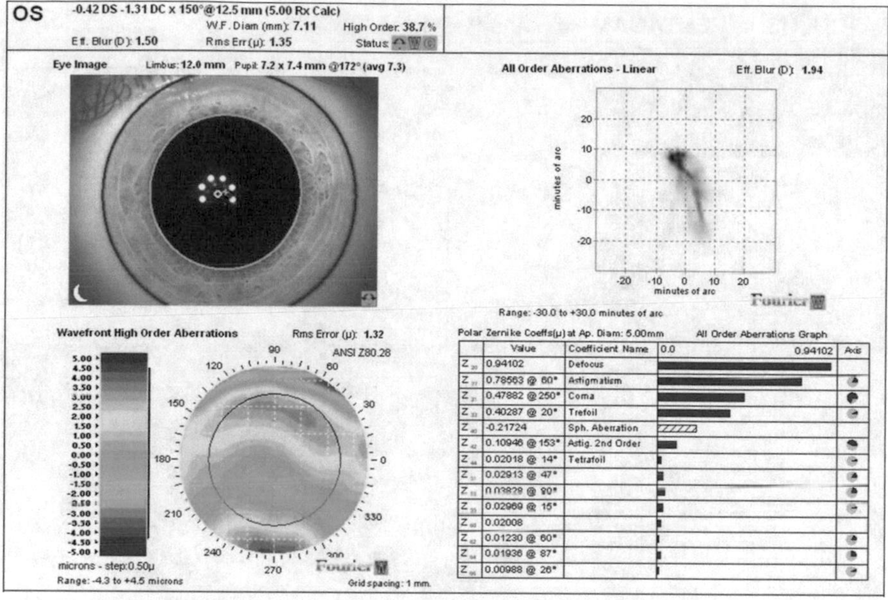

Fig. 26.9 Postoperative (final) wavefront map of case 1

Table 26.3 Summary of preoperative and postoperative data of case 2

Preoperative data		Final postoperative data
UDVA (logMAR)	+0.70	0.00
CDVA (logMAR)	+0.10	0.00
Refraction	−2.75−0.50×180	0.00−0.25×80
Pentacam corneal data		
Thinnest location	501 μm	468 μm
ISV	25	21
IVA	0.26	0.26
KI	1.06	1.04
CKI	1.01	1.00
R_{min}	7.22	7.52
IHA	14.3	22.1
IHD	0.033	0.032
iDesign data at 5 mm WFD		
RMS total	2.72 μm	0.88 μm
RMS HOA	0.69 μm	0.52 μm
Coma	0.23022	0.16375
Trefoil	0.07142	0.16481
Spherical aberrations	−0.01702	−0.08772

(iDesign system®) was introduced to the field of refractive surgery with reports about their abilities to read and treat precisely the highly aberrated corneas [8].

Our point of view in performing the sequential approach to treat keratoconic eyes after stabilizing them with CXL is due to the potential disadvantages of the simultaneous approach. The simultaneous approach is thought to be too invasive (two techniques at the same sitting) and does not address emmetropia due to the prolonged flattening effect of CXL with uncontrolled refractive outcome [12, 23].

The previously explained points were behind the philosophy of choosing the sequential wavefront-guided PRK after stabilizing the cornea with CXL.

Our study (under publication) demonstrated clearly in a statistically proved number of eyes ($n=34$) the safety and efficacy of a sequential high-definition aberrometer-guided PRK in providing a satisfactory visual outcome for the patients. The mean efficacy index (ratio of the postoperative UDVA to the preoperative CDVA)

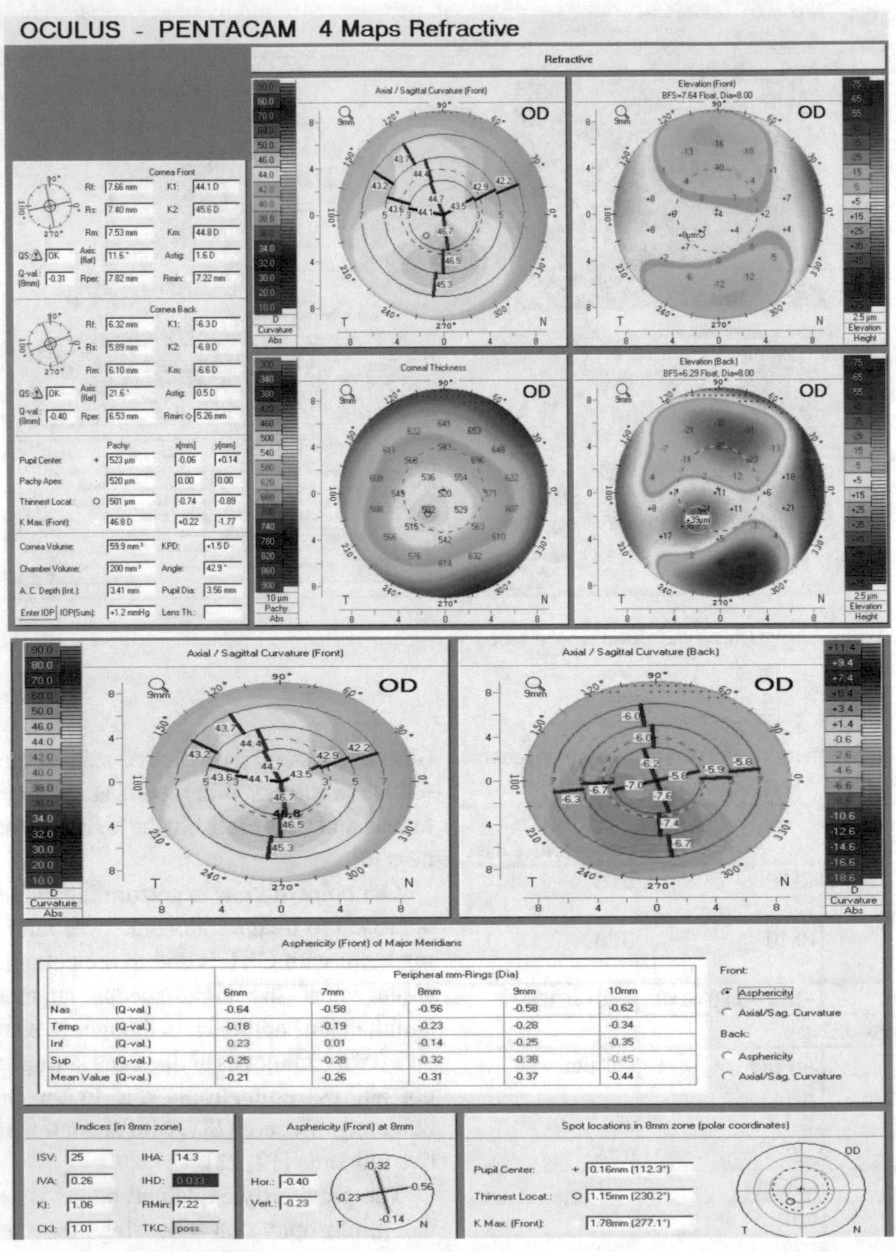

Fig. 26.10 Preoperative Pentacam of case 2

calculated after 1 year of follow-up was 1.58 ± 1.11 (mean ± SD); *p*-value <0.001. Whereas the safety index (ratio of the postoperative CDVA to the preoperative CDVA) calculated after 1 year of follow-up was 1.96 ± 1.52 (mean ± SD); *p*-value <0.001.

At the last follow-up visit, the preoperative logMAR UDVA of 0.93 ± 0.33 (mean ± SD) has been improved to 0.14 ± 0.11 postoperatively; *p*-value <0.001, and logMAR CDVA has been improved from 0.28 ± 0.24 preoperatively to 0.05 ± 0.06 (mean ± SD) postoperatively; *p*-value <0.001. Results also showed reduction in MRSE from −3.22 ± 1.32 D (mean ± SD) preoperatively to −0.68 ± 0.64 D at the last follow-up visit. About the predictability of the procedure, at the sixth month

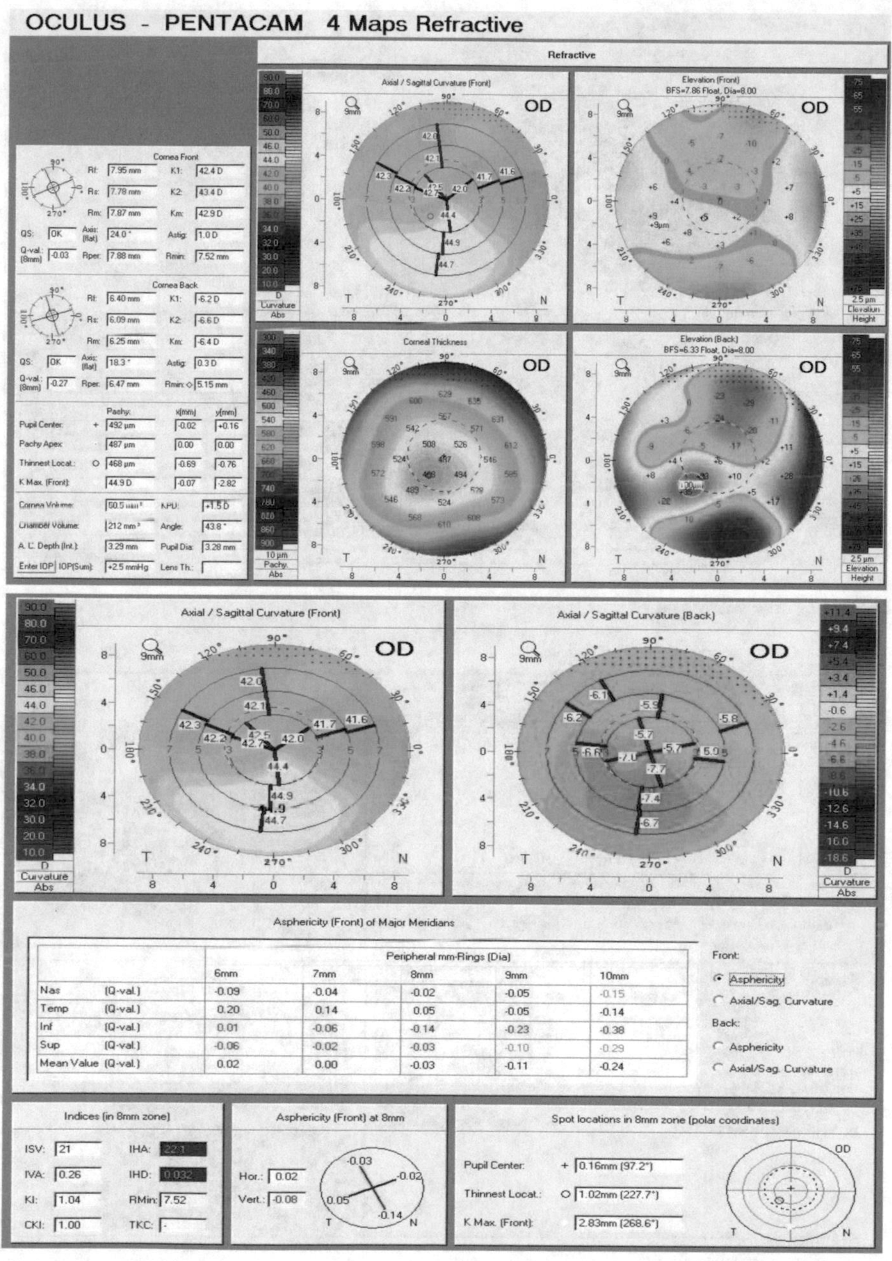

Fig. 26.11 Postoperative (final follow-up visit) Pentacam of case 2

postop, 76.5 % of eyes had a manifest refraction within ±1.00 D of emmetropia, 47.1 % were within ±0.50 D. At the last follow-up visit 62 % of the cases reached within ±0.50 D. A total of 97.1 % of our patients reached ≥20/40 UDVA at the last follow-up compared to 73.5 % only reaching CDVA of ≥20/40 preoperatively. Hundred percent of our patients reached ≥20/50 UDVA at the final follow-up. A total of 44.1 % of our patients gained two or more lines in the CDVA at month 12.

Our work also demonstrated a statistically significant reduction in the maximum keratometric reading from 48.32 ± 4.25 (mean ± SD) preoperatively to 45.81 ± 3.45 at the last follow-up visit. There was insignificant change in its value over the follow-up period.

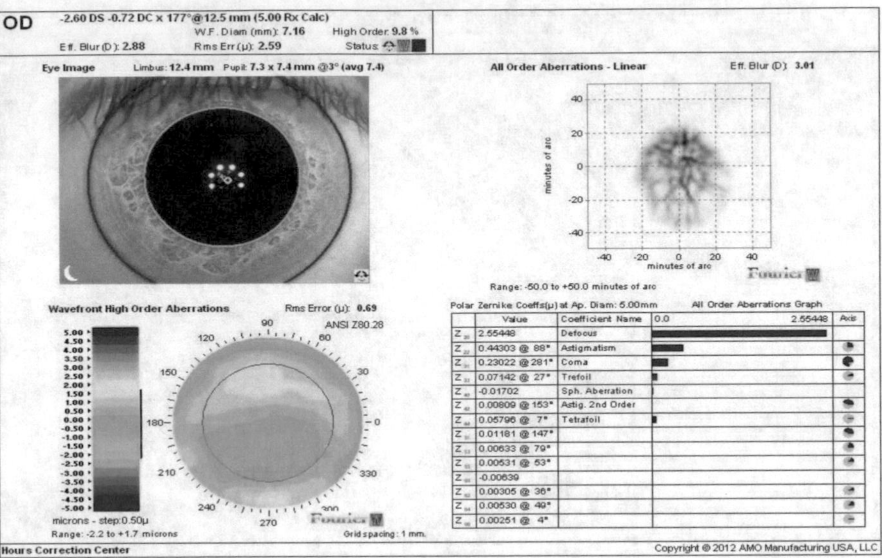

Fig. 26.12 Preoperative wavefront of case 2

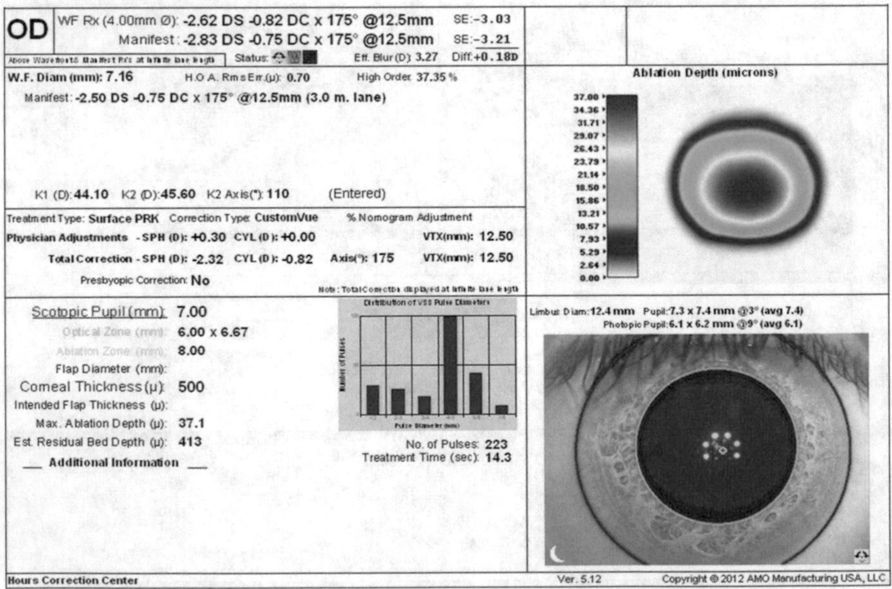

Fig. 26.13 Ablation profile generated by iDesign® for case 2

The mean starting central corneal thickness of the studied group was 491.12 ± 39.19 μm (mean ± SD) at the thinnest location that was reduced to 429.56 ± 61.81 μm at the last follow-up visit. It decreased as a result of excimer laser ablation and then remained stable through the follow-up period. The mean intended ablation depth for our patients was 54.53 ± 11.44 μm (mean ± SD). The ablation depth percentage calculated as (max. ablation depth in μm/corneal thinnest location thickness in μm) presented a mean of 11.4 % and a SD of 3.2 %. To some extent this exceeds the ablation depth in most of other reviewed studies. Many authors used a maximum ablation depth of 50 μm, this value was chosen arbitrarily by the authors based on

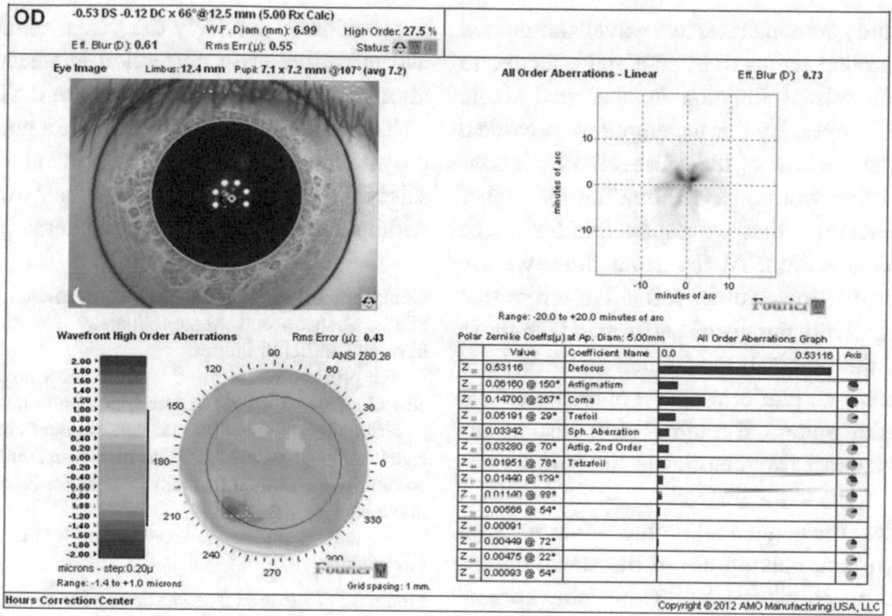

Fig. 26.14 Postoperative (final) wavefront of case 2

their own experience [5]. In our work, the maximum intended ablation depth did not exceed 15% of the corneal thinnest location thickness and the results showed stability of the cornea over the follow-up period (1 year).

There was a statistically significant reduction in the higher order aberrations in general demonstrated by the significant reduction of total RMS p-value <0.001 and the RMS HOA p-value 0.003, and reduction of coma, trefoil with p-value 0.001, <0.001, respectively. It is to be mentioned that the reduction of HOA in these eyes is considered number one reason behind the postoperative improvement in both UDVA and CDVA. From our point of view, this is a real addressing to what was named "Cause–Effect relationship" in Tamayo work [9].

In our study, vector analysis of ocular astigmatic changes was done (Alpins method) for better understanding and presentation of astigmatic correction. Targeted induced astigmatic correction (TIA) was 2.79 ± 1.82 (mean ± SD), while the real change achieved at the last follow-up visit (SIA) was 2.36 ± 1.72 (mean ± SD) and this showed a magnitude of error (ME) of 0.43 ± 0.86 (mean ± SD) which is the difference between SIA and TIA (positive number means undercorrection). The correction index (CI) was evaluated and found to be 0.88 ± 0.29 (mean ± SD) which means slight undercorrection.

There was insignificant corneal haze in the whole sample, six eyes had mild haze (grade 1) on the scale used and this was present from the start after CXL. The apparently insignificant postoperative haze could be attributed to the use of MMC in all of the cases after finalizing the laser ablation procedure.

The corneal indices were included in our study in an attempt to study the impact of corneal ablation by iDesign-guided profile on improving the corneal irregularities in these eyes; we noted reduction in values of the corneal indices. The reduction in IVA, IHA, IHD, and CKI was not statistically significant. While the reduction in ISV, R_{min}, and KI was statistically significant. The study shows also stability of the indices through the follow-up period. By studying these values, it is to be noted that the improvement of visual performance in these patients was achieved without increasing their corneal irregularities. On the contrary, all corneal regularity indices demonstrated a trend toward a more regular cornea although it was not statistically significant in some of the studied indices.

Our study demonstrates that wavefront-guided PRK treatment seems to be safe and effective to restore the visual function in aberrated stable keratoconic eyes. By this technique we provide a better management of the cause–effect relationship. In other words, we are treating the higher order aberrations that are responsible for image quality degradation. At the same time, we are correcting the lower order refractive errors that affect negatively the visual performance of those patients, the precisely positioned excimer laser beam using a platform that compensates for cyclotorsion and pupil centroid shift ensures targeting the exact irregularities in the corneal surface that degrade the image.

Besides, the sequential protocol that we suggest is, in fact, making use of the stable cornea provided by previous CXL. This stable corneal surface provides, in turn, a stable refractive surface (even still irregular) from which we can calculate a reliable and dependable ablation profile to correct the irregularity and avoid refractive surprises and changes that can potentially occur with the use of the simultaneous approach.

We strongly believe that the proposed protocol could be a very good modality to provide a useful glasses-independent vision for selected keratoconic eyes after CXL.

Of course, in the dilemma of keratoconus, the treating surgeon cannot promise perfection but at least can deliver to his patient, by the proposed protocol, a useful good vision using the patient's own cornea without the need for keratoplasty modalities with all their known complications.

26.10 Conclusions

High-definition aberrometers are able to read highly aberrated corneas (such as in stable keratoconus) and generate out of them a reliable ablation profile which can be used to reduce refractive error / HOAs in such eyes and provide better quality of vision for those patients.

Wavefront-guided ablation profile seems to be a good option to address visual rehabilitation in stable keratoconic eyes.

Sequential PRK for keratoconic eyes after doing corneal CXL seems to be a good option as it can address precisely the visual rehabilitation and refractive error correction in selected cases after having the maximum effect of CXL.

The proposed protocol could be a good tool to provide a useful glasses-independent vision for selected keratoconic eyes using their own cornea without the need for any type of keratoplasty.

Compliance with Ethical Requirements Mohamed Shafik Shaheen and Ahmed Shalaby declare that they have no conflict of interest.

All procedures followed were in accordance with the ethical standards of the responsible committe on human experimentation (institutional and national and with the Helsinki Declaration of 1975, as revised in 2000. Informed consent was obtained from all patients for being included in the study.

No animal studies were performed by the authors for this chapter.

Financial disclosure: The studies by the authors included in this chapter were supported in part by an unrestricted educational grant from Abbott Medical Optics Inc.

References

1. Kymionis GD, Portaliou DM, Kounis GA, Limnopoulou AN, Kontadakis GA, Grentzelos MA. Simultaneous topography-guided photorefractive keratectomy followed by corneal collagen cross-linking for keratoconus. Am J Ophthalmol. 2011;152(5):748–55.
2. Krueger RR, Kanellopoulos AJ. Stability of simultaneous topography-guided photorefractive keratectomy and riboflavin/UVA cross-linking for progressive keratoconus: case reports. J Refract Surg. 2010;26(10):S827–32.
3. Kanellopoulos AJ, Binder PS. Collagen cross-linking (CCL) with sequential topography-guided PRK: a temporizing alternative for keratoconus to penetrating keratoplasty. Cornea. 2007;26(7):891–5.
4. Kanellopoulos AJ, Asimellis G. Keratoconus management: long-term stability of topography-guided normalization combined with high-fluence CXL stabilization (the Athens Protocol). J Refract Surg. 2014;30(2):88–93.
5. Kanellopoulos AJ. Comparison of sequential vs same-day simultaneous collagen cross-linking and topography-guided PRK for treatment of keratoconus. J Refract Surg. 2009;25(9):S812.
6. Weed K, Macewen C, McGhee C. The Dundee University Scottish Keratoconus Study II: a prospective study of optical and surgical correction. Ophthalmic Physiol Opt. 2007;27(6):561–7.
7. Bühren J, Kühne C, Kohnen T. Defining subclinical keratoconus using corneal first-surface higher-order aberrations. Am J Ophthalmol. 2007;143(3):381–9.e2.

8. Shafik Shaheen M, El-Kateb M, Hafez TA, Piñero DP, Khalifa MA. Wavefront-guided laser treatment using a high-resolution aberrometer to measure irregular corneas: a pilot study. J Refract Surg. 2015;31(6):411–8.
9. Fernandez GET, Serrano MG. Early clinical experience using custom excimer laser ablations to treat irregular astigmatism. J Cataract Refract Surg. 2000;26(10):1442–50.
10. Alió JL, Piñero DP, Puche ABP. Corneal wavefront-guided photorefractive keratectomy in patients with irregular corneas after corneal refractive surgery. J Cataract Refract Surg. 2008;34(10):1727–35.
11. López-Miguel A, Maldonado MJ, Belzunce A, Barrio-Barrio J, Coco-Martín MB, Nieto JC. Precision of a commercial Hartmann-Shack aberrometer: limits of total wavefront laser vision correction. Am J Ophthalmol. 2012;154(5):799–807.e5.
12. Koller T, Pajic B, Vinciguerra P, Seiler T. Flattening of the cornea after collagen crosslinking for keratoconus. J Cataract Refract Surg. 2011;37(8):1488–92.
13. Alió JL, Shabayek MH. Corneal higher order aberrations: a method to grade keratoconus. J Refract Surg. 2006;22(6):539.
14. Chelala E, El Rami H, Dirani A, Fadlallah A, Fakhoury O, Warrak E. Photorefractive keratectomy in patients with mild to moderate stable keratoconus: a five-year prospective follow-up study. Clin Ophthalmol. 2013;7:1923.
15. Applegate RA, Marsack JD, Ramos R, Sarver EJ. Interaction between aberrations to improve or reduce visual performance. J Cataract Refract Surg. 2003;29(8):1487–95.
16. Wollensak G, Spoerl E, Seiler T. Riboflavin/ultraviolet-A-induced collagen cross-linking for the treatment of keratoconus. Am J Ophthalmol. 2003;135(5):620–7.
17. Wollensak G. Cross-linking treatment of progressive keratoconus: new hope. Curr Opin Ophthalmol. 2006;17(4):356–60.
18. Koller T, Seiler T. Therapeutic cross-linking of the cornea using riboflavin/UVA. Klin Monbl Augenheilkd. 2007;224(9):700–6.
19. Koller T, Mrochen M, Seiler T. Complication and failure rates after corneal cross-linking. J Cataract Refract Surg. 2009;35(8):1358–62.
20. Schallhorn SC, Tanzer DJ, Kaupp SE, Brown M, Malady SE. Comparison of night driving performance after wavefront-guided and conventional LASIK for moderate myopia. Ophthalmology. 2009;116(4):702–9.
21. Kanellopoulos AJ, Pe LH. Wavefront-guided enhancements using the wavelight excimer laser in symptomatic eyes previously treated with LASIK. J Refract Surg. 2006;22(4):345–9.
22. Kymionis GD, Kontadakis GA, Kounis GA, Portaliou DM, Karavitaki AE, Magarakis M, et al. Simultaneous topography-guided PRK followed by corneal collagen cross-linking for keratoconus. J Refract Surg. 2009;25(9):S807–11.
23. Mazzotta C, Caporossi T, Denaro R, Bovone C, Sparano C, Paradiso A, et al. Morphological and functional correlations in riboflavin/UVA corneal collagen cross-linking for keratoconus. Acta Ophthalmol. 2012;90(3):259–65.

Iris-Supported Phakic IOLs Implantation in Patients with Keratoconus

27

Pablo Sanz Díez, Alfredo Vega Estrada, Roberto Fernández Buenaga, and Jorge L. Alió

27.1 Introduction

Keratoconus is a corneal disorder in which the central or paracentral cornea undergoes progressive thinning and steepening, causing irregular astigmatism and corneal scarring. Keratoconus can lead to severe vision deterioration through the development of this irregular astigmatism. The general incidence has been estimated in 1:2000 of the general population, with a prevalence of 54:100,000 in the USA and 229:100,000 in Asian countries [1].

Nowadays, keratoconus treatment has become expanded and several techniques are now available. Keratoconus presents different treatment options: corneal stabilization or regularization (intrastromal corneal ring segment (ICRS) and corneal collagen crosslinking (CXL)) [2, 3], refractive treatment or a combination of these. In the treatment of visual impairment, the phakic intraocular lenses (pIOL) implantation has an important role.

Phakic IOLs can be classified into the following three categories based on their position in the eye or their mechanism of fixation: anterior chamber angle supported, *anterior chamber iris-fixated*, and posterior chamber. When there are no contraindications to implantation of phakic lenses, this refractive technique is the best choice for young patients with moderate to high refractive errors in which corneal refractive procedures are contraindicated. The advantages provided by these lenses, among others, are to maintain the accommodation and the reversibility of the process.

This chapter discusses the role of anterior chamber iris-fixated pIOLs (ARTIFLEX and ARTISAN (Ophtec BV, Groningen, The Netherlands)) in cases of keratoconus.

P. Sanz Díez, O.D., M.Sc.
J.L. Alió, M.D., Ph.D., F.E.B.O. (✉)
Keratoconus Unit, Department of Refractive Surgery, Vissum Alicante, Alicante, Spain

Division of Ophthalmology, Miguel Hernández University, Alicante, Spain
e-mail: pablosanz9143@gmail.com; jlalio@vissum.com

A. Vega Estrada, Ph.D.
Keratoconus Unit, Vissum Alicante, Alicante, Spain
e-mail: alfredovega@vissum.com

R. Fernández Buenaga, M.D., Ph.D.
Keratoconus Unit, Department of Refractive Surgery, Vissum Corporation, Avda de Denia s/n, Edificio Vissum, Alicante, 03016, Spain
e-mail: rfernandezbuenaga@gmail.com

J.L. Alió (ed.), *Keratoconus*, Essentials in Ophthalmology, DOI 10.1007/978-3-319-43881-8_27

27.2 Iris Fixated Phakic IOL

The first iris fixation IOLs were initially used in aphakic eyes after intraocular cataract extraction. In 1978, Jan G.F. Worst designed the iris-claw intraocular lenses [4]. These lenses began with the idea of being implemented after intracapsular cataract extraction. The one-piece PMMA lens was fixated to a fold on the middle periphery of the iris stroma (relatively stationary portion).

In 1986, Worst and Fechner developed an anterior chamber lens for the treatment of myopic phakic patients based on the original idea of a fixating iris-claw intraocular lens [5]. The follow-up showed a good predictability but a loss of endothelial cells around 7 % [6, 7].

In 1991, some modifications were incorporated into the phakic lens design, resulting in a convex–concave Artisan Myopia lens. The new design decreased the potential for complications, improved the optical performance, and facilitated the surgical implantation technique. In 2001, the Artisan toric lens was introduced into the market.

In 2005 and 2009, Artiflex Myopia lens and Artiflex Toric lens were introduced into the market, respectively.

In recent years, knowledge about these lenses has grown exponentially. These phakic lenses are based on the principle of iris fixation. This method of intraocular fixation allows relatively unrestricted constriction and dilation of the pupil; ensures stable fixation to the iris due to the two diametrically opposed haptics; permits centration of the lens over the pupil and is extremely versatile, permitting fixation horizontally, vertically, or obliquely.

Cases with keratoconus present topographic irregularity, so that toric versions of each of the mentioned phakic lenses. These lenses are ARTIFLEX toric® and ARTISAN toric® (Ophtec BV, Groningen, The Netherlands).

The *ARTIFLEX® toric* pIOL has a flexible optic of ultraviolet light-filtering silicone and two rigid polymethyl methacrylate haptics (Fig. 27.1). It has an anterior spherical surface and a posterior toric surface. The dioptric power range of ARTIFLEX Toric includes a spherical correction from −1.0 to −13.5 diopters in combination with a cylinder correction from −1.0 to −5.0 diopters.

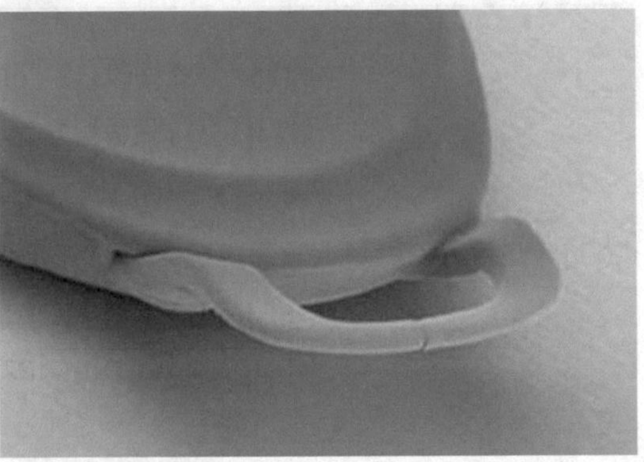

Fig. 27.1 Scanning electron microscopy (SEM) of ARTIFLEX pIOL

It has a flexible optic with a diameter of 6 mm. The total diameter of the lens is 8.5 mm and the maximum width of the haptics is 3 mm (Fig. 27.2 and Table 27.1), so that it can be inserted through a small incision (3.2 mm), with the benefits this entails.

This pIOL is available with a 0° or a 90° cylinder. This enables implantation of the Toric PIOL in a horizontal or slightly oblique position through a 12 o'clock incision, as well as in a more or less vertical position through a temporal incision. Essentially no change in the surgeon's implantation technique is required. The iris fixation method ensures exact positioning on the cylinder axis, without risk of lens rotation or decentration (Fig. 27.3).

Its concave–convex shape makes the distance between the peripheral margin of the optic and the corneal endothelium constant regardless of the dioptric power. In addition, this also enables a separation of 1.18 mm anterior to the iris plane, which facilitates normal aqueous flow, thus preventing a pupillary block (although it is advisable to perform iridotomy). Its insertion is done through a specially designed spatula.

The *ARTISAN® toric* pIOL is designed for the correction of astigmatism in combination with myopia or hyperopia. The asymmetric optic has two components: sphere and cylinder. All (spherical) ARTISAN lenses for myopia and hyperopia can be supplied with cylinders between 1 and 7.5 diopters. It is also possible to supply optics with only a cylindric correction (Table 27.2).

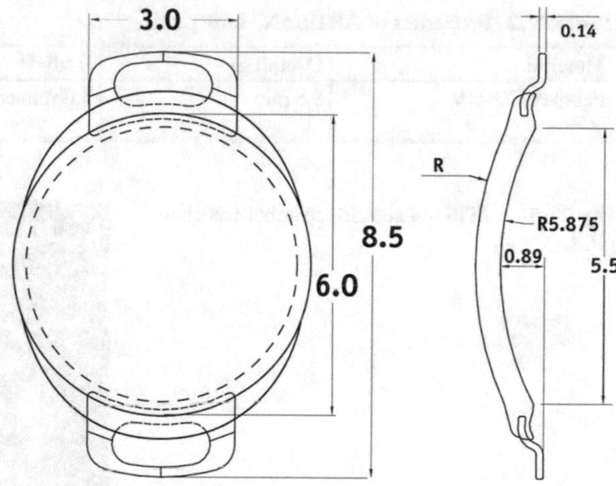

Fig. 27.2 Lens design

Table 27.1 Properties of ARTIFLEX toric pIOL

Optic material	Claw material	Overall Ø	Body Ø	Edge design	Refractive index
Hydrophobic Polysiloxane	PMMA CQ-UV	8.5 mm	6.0 mm	Polynomial	1.43

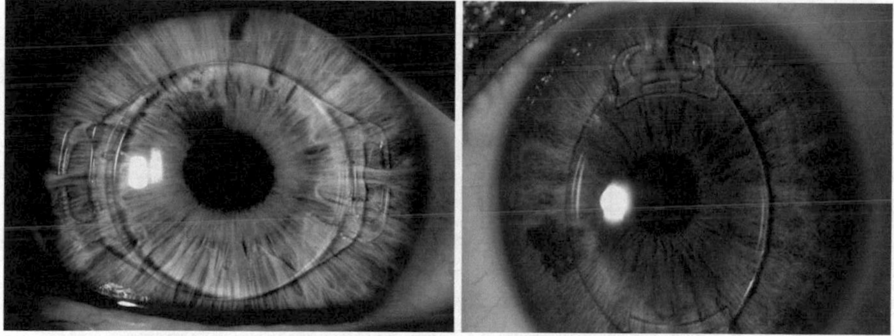

Fig. 27.3 ARTIFLEX anterior chamber iris claw pIOL

The ARTISAN pIOL shows in cross-section a low profile within the eye. The distance from the edge of the optic to the corneal endothelium is approximately >1.0 mm, depending on the anterior chamber depth and the dioptric power.

This lens is biconcave and made of poly (methyl methacrylate) with an ultraviolet-absorbing Perspex material. It has an overall 8.5 mm diameter, 5.0 mm lens width, 5.0 mm optic zone, 1.04 mm height, and a 0.93 mm thickness (Fig. 27.4).

The Artisan toric PIOL has two models. Model A has a 0° cylinder axis corresponding to the main lens axis, which runs through the claws. This model is implanted in cases where the cylinder axis to be corrected is between 0° and 45° or in cases with astigmatic meridians between 135° and 180° if the surgeon prefers a superior approach. Model B has its cylinder axis at 90°, perpendicular to the main lens axis, which runs through the claws. It is implanted when the cylinder axis to be corrected is between 45° and 135° if the surgeon prefers a superior approach. When performing a temporal approach, the previous two models could be used but in the reversed manner—model A for correction of astigmatism between 45° and 135° and model B for correction

Table 27.2 Properties of ARTISAN® toric pIOL

Material	Overall Ø	Body Ø	Availability
Perspex CQ-UV	8.5 mm	5.0 mmlconcave–convex	Can correct astigmatism from 1 to 7.5 diopters

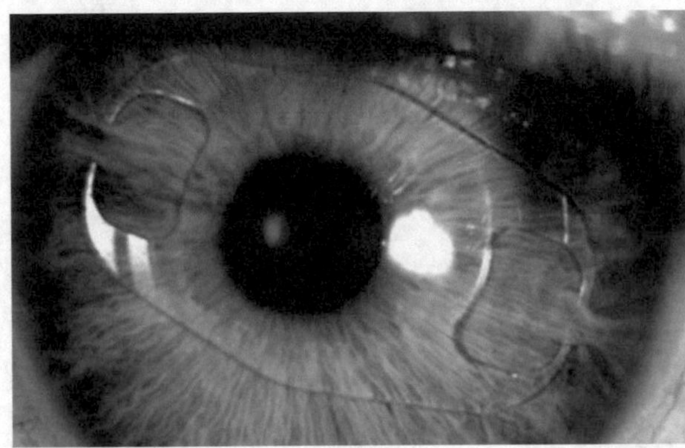

Fig. 27.4 ARTISAN anterior chamber iris claw pIOL

Table 27.3 Dioptric powers (positive cylinder range)

Positive cylinder range			
Cylinder power	Minimal sphere power	Maximal sphere power	Sphere power increments
1	−23.0	6.5	0.5
1.5	−23.0	6.5	0.5
2	−23.0	6.5	0.5
2.5	−23.0	6.5	0.5
3	−23.0	6.5	0.5
3.5	−23.0	6.5	0.5
4	−23.0	6.5	0.5
4.5	−23.0	6.5	0.5
5	−23.0	6.5	0.5
5.5	−23.0	6.5	0.5
6	−23.0	6.5	0.5
6.5	−23.0	6.5	0.5
7	−23.0	6.5	0.5
7.5	−23.0	6.5	0.5

Table 27.4 Dioptric powers (negative cylinder range)

Negative cylinder range			
Cylinder power	Minimal sphere power	Maximal sphere power	Sphere power increments
−1	−22	7.5	0.5
−1.5	−21.5	8	0.5
−2	−21	8.5	0.5
−2.5	−20.5	9	0.5
−3	−20	9.5	0.5
−3.5	−19.5	10	0.5
−4	−19	10.5	0.5
−4.5	−18.5	11	0.5
−5	−18	11.5	0.5
−5.5	−17.5	12	0.5
−6	−17	12.5	0.5
−6.5	−16.5	13	0.5
−7	−16	13.5	0.5
−7.5	−15.5	14	0.5

of astigmatism between 0° and 45° or in cases with astigmatic meridians between 135° and 180° (Tables 27.3 and 27.4).

27.3 Surgical Technique

The surgical technique is similar to the nontoric pIOLs, except for the need to fixate the lens on a precise axis. Preoperative determination and marking of the cylinder axis is therefore essential for an optimal refractive correction.

The incision width required for implantation of the lens is 5.5 mm for the ARTISAN toric lens, and 3.2 mm for the ARTIFLEX toric lens. This incision should be perpendicular to the enclavation axis.

Being cases of keratoconus, which are characterized by a destabilized corneal geometry, we propose to perform a tunneled scleral incision because an incision in the corneal area could lead

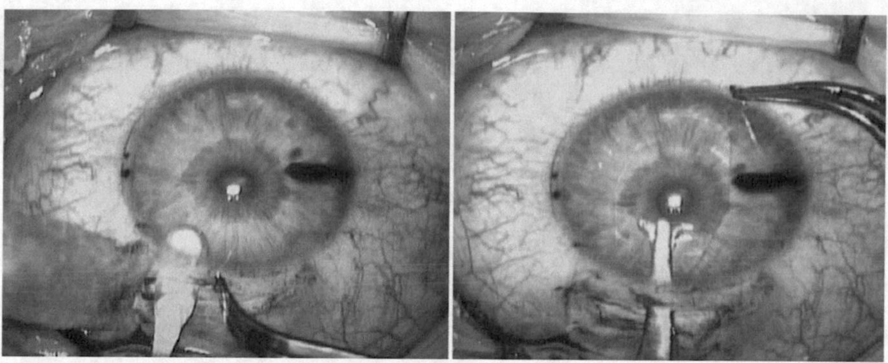

Fig. 27.5 Scleral incision to not affect the corneal structure and inserting the pIOL

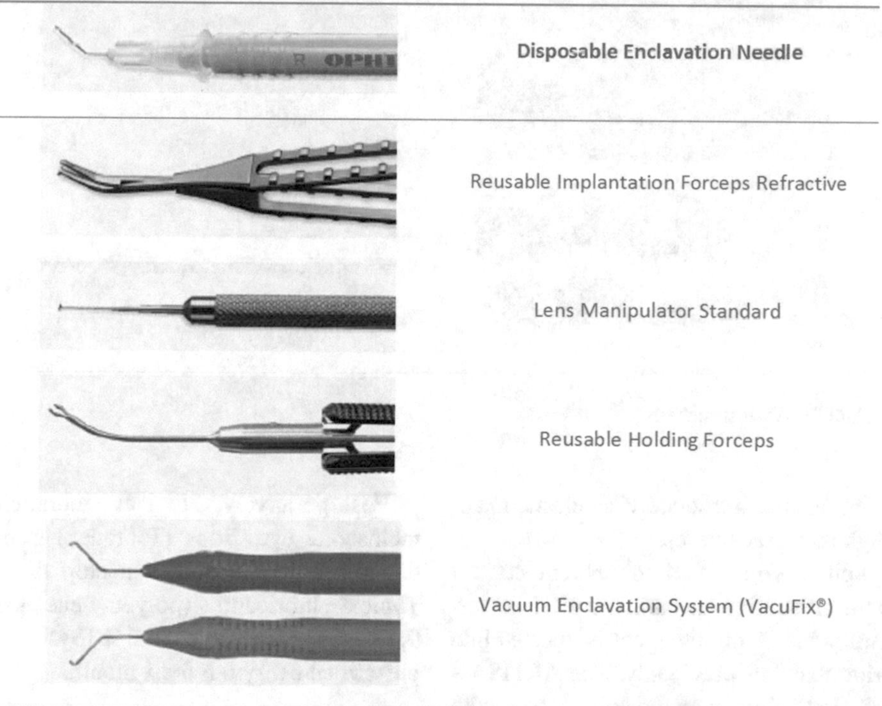

Fig. 27.6 ARTISAN instruments

to a weakening of the corneal tissue and unpredictable astigmatic change (Fig. 27.5) favoring even more the process of instability present in the irregular cornea.

At the time of surgical manipulation of each of the lenses, the ARTIFLEX pIOL is manipulated from haptic because these are PMMA CQ-UV, thus avoiding damage of the optic. In contrast, the ARTISAN pIOL is manipulated through the optic zone, because the lens as a whole is rigid (Perspex CQ-UV). We should note that each of these lenses has a specific instrumentation for proper implantation in the eye (Figs. 27.6 and 27.7).

Astigmatic marker is used to mark the astigmatic axis selected for lens implantation using slit-lamp microscopy, not in the supine position, to avoid any possible cyclotorsion or rotation movement of the eye.

Make two paracenteses of 1.2 mm at 10 and 2 o'clock, pointing downwards, oriented toward

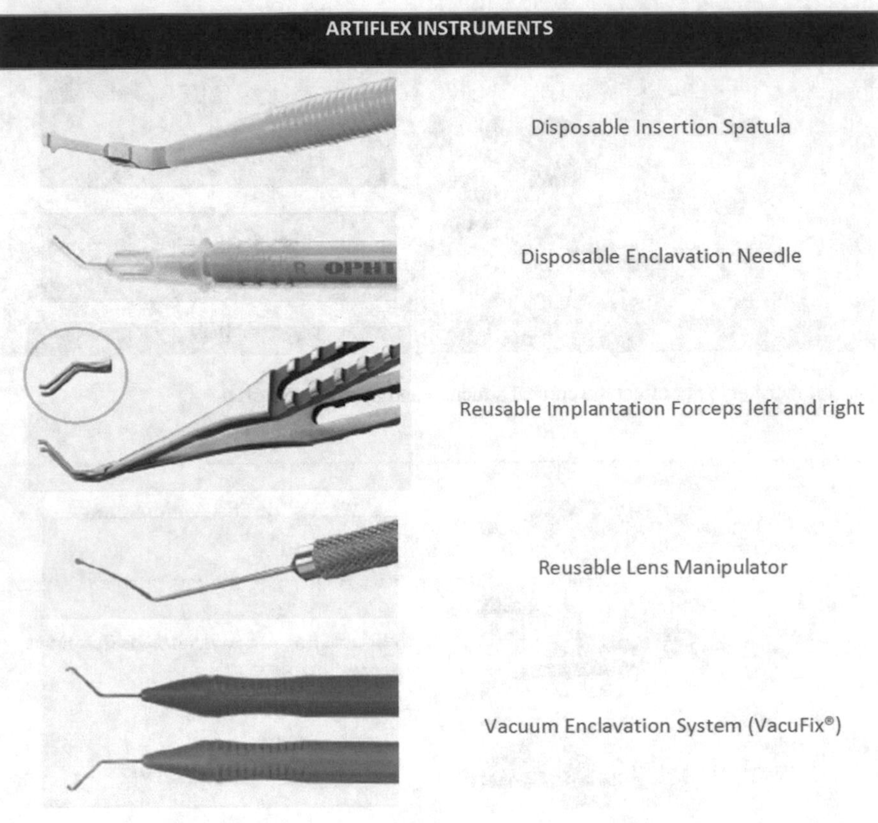

Fig. 27.7 ARTIFLEX instruments

the enclavation site. Introduce viscoelastic material through the paracenteses.

The pupil is constricted to prevent contact between the crystalline lens and the pIOL or surgical instruments. A miotic agent is injected into the anterior chamber previously. The ARTISAN pIOL is fixated using an enclavation needle with a bent shaft and a bent tip that pushes the iris into both claws. For insertion of the ARTIFLEX lens into the anterior chamber, a specific Disposable Insertion Spatula is used.

For both lenses, it is very useful to use the instrument VacuFix® because it helps the surgeon to grasp a fold of iris tissue, putting the toric pIOL in the correct orientation.

A surgical iridectomy (with vitrectome or laser) is important to allow for the normal flow of aqueous humor.

Topical anesthesia with preservative-free lidocaine 2.0 % is used with midazolam before the implantation of the pIOLs.

Postoperatively, topical tobramycin–dexamethasone eye drops (Tobradex) is used every 6 h for 2 weeks and then stop the treatment. Topical lubricants (polyethylene glycol 400 0.4 %–propylene glycol 0.3 % [Systane]) are also prescribed every 6 h for 1 month.

27.4 Results

The surgical correction of refractive errors in cases of keratoconus has been a continuous challenge in refractive surgery, with various surgical techniques having been attempted in these cases for the past years. The implantation of pIOLs has been showing very good results in these cases, as evidenced by the scientific literature [8, 9].

Regarding the use of toric phakic lenses in keratoconus, there are a number of published studies to allow sound conclusions on the safety and efficacy of this surgical technique in such cases with some complexity.

Budo et al. [10] implanted ARTISAN toric pIOLs in both eyes of three patients with keratoconus and high astigmatism with clear central corneas and contact lens intolerance. They reported good visual results in these six cases: best spectacle-corrected subjective visual acuity after lens implantation was unchanged in one eye and improved in five eyes. Spherical equivalent refraction was significantly reduced in all eyes ($p=0.03$) and the safety index was 1.49.

In the same way as the previous study, Sedaghat et al. [11] implanted 14 Artisan pIOLs and two toric ARTISAN pIOLs in 16 eyes with stable keratoconus who had contact lens intolerance. They obtained good visual and refractive outcomes: all patients had a final UDVA of 20/40 or better, and 84.6 % had final CDVA of 20/32 or better. A two-line improvement in CDVA was achieved in 50 % of eyes. The improvements in UDVA and CDVA were statistically significant ($p<0.0001$ and $p<0.002$, respectively). Mean final spherical and cylindrical refractions were −0.03 ± 1.81 D (range: +2.25 to −3.50 D) and 2.08 ± 1.04 D (range: 0.50–3.50 D), respectively. Mean final spherical equivalent refraction was −0.90 ± 1.90 D.

They contend that toric ARTISAN lenses can be considered for patients who show significant increases in CDVA with astigmatism correction (two lines). These patients have more regular astigmatism, and the axis of astigmatism can be approximated in subjective refraction.

Venter [12] performed a study on the use of Artisan pIOL for the correction of myopia and astigmatism in patients with stable keratoconus. He analyzed 18 eyes primarily for 6-month follow-up and finally, for 1-year follow-up. At 6 months postoperatively, all 18 eyes were available for follow-up. Nine eyes were available for follow-up at 9 months postoperatively and five eyes were available for follow-up at 1 year postoperatively. The majority of eyes were within 0.50 D of the intended correction 6 months postoperatively. At 6 months postoperatively, 22 % (4/18) of eyes saw 1.0 or better without correction. Six months after ARTISAN pIOL implantation, no eyes lost BSCVA and 33 % (6/18) of eyes gained two or more lines of BSCVA. Eighteen months postoperatively, keratoconus progressed in one eye, which required an exchange of the Artisan IOL. He concludes that the use of this lens in cases of stable keratoconus is safe, predictable and effective, with minimal complications.

Regarding ARTIFLEX pIOL, not many studies have been performed in eyes with keratoconus. Our group reported good results for this pIOL in cases with stable non-progressive keratoconus graded as mild to moderate on the Amsler-Krumeich scale. The iris-claw pIOL was implanted in 20 eyes. The UDVA, CDVA, and SE improved from preoperatively to postoperatively. The keratometric analysis showed: K1 changed from 44.46 ± 2.24 D (range 40.16–50.56 D) to 46.06 ± 3.82 D (range 42.17–50.47 D), K2 changed from 46.74 G 2.24 D (range 43.97–52.48 D) to 49.29 ± 2.43 D (range 45.88–51.84 D), and the mean K changed from 45.60 ± 2.04 D (range 43.29–51.52 D) to 47.65 ± 2.68 D (range 45.39–50.96 D). The mean efficacy index was 0.96 ± 0.22 and the safety index was 1.22 ± 0.33. The conclusion of our study is that the implantation of this lens can be considered a safe and effective procedure in the treatment of stable keratoconus over a wide range of ametropia (Table 27.5 and Fig. 27.8) [13].

Others studies have evaluated the possibility of a combined treatment [14–17]. These include phakic IOL implantation combined with cross-linking or intracorneal ring segments or both. The general idea is to first stop the progression of keratoconus and once the keratoconus has stabilized, refractive solutions can be considered. The combination of these methods has been reported as an effective and safe procedure [14–17].

27.5 Indications

Although keratoconus is not a currently accepted indication for pIOL implantation, some surgeons have performed such procedures and reported reasonable outcomes [9–18].

Based on our experience and that described in medical literature, we believe the following criteria should be met for phakic lens implantation in eyes with keratoconus:

Table 27.5 Comparisons in iris-claw pIOL group (20 eyes) [13]

Parameter	Preoperative	Postoperative	Difference	*p* Value
Decimal UDVA				
Mean ± SD	0.08 ± 0.06	0.72 ± 0.28	0.64	<0.001
Range	0.02, 0.3	0.03, 1.10		
Decimal CDVA				
Mean ± SD	0.75 ± 0.27	0.83 ± 0.24	0.08	0.004
Range	0.17, 1.00	0.03, 1.04		
LogMAR UDVA				
Mean ± SD	1.22 ± 0.38	0.14 ± 0.17	1.08	<0.001
Range	0.52, 1.77	−0.04, 0.52		
LogMAR CDVA				
Mean ± SD	0.12 ± 0.16	0.06 ± 0.10	0.06	0.003
Range	0.00, 0.47	−0.02, 0.32		
Sphere (D)				
Mean ± SD	−8.66 ± 5.51	0.13 ± 0.72	8.79	<0.001
Range	−21, −0.50	−1.75, 2.00		
Cylinder (D)				
Mean ± SD	−2.29 ± 1.90	−0.70 ± 0.80	1.59	<0.001
Range	−7.00, 0.25	−3.00, 0.00		
SE (D)				
Mean ± SD	−8.91 ± 4.57	−0.28 ± 0.81	8.63	<0.001
Range	−20.75, −2.75	−3.25, 1.00		
ECC (cells/mm²)				
Mean ± SD	2830 ± 590	2522 ± 282	308	0.012
Range	1992, 3937	1953, 2950		

CDVA corrected distance visual acuity, *ECC* endothelial cell count, *SE* spherical equivalent, *UDVA* uncorrected distance visual acuity

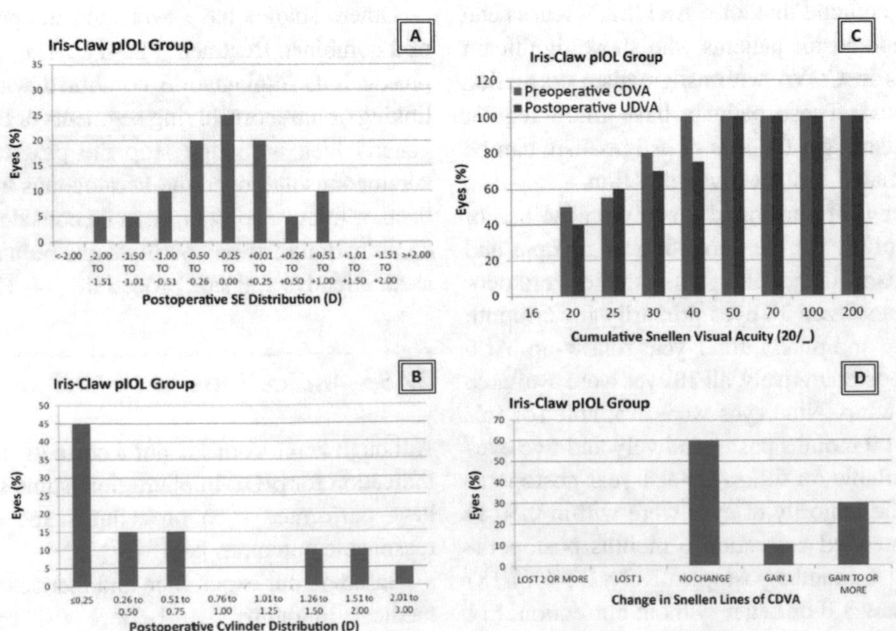

Fig. 27.8 (**a**) postoperative spherical equivalent (SE) distribution 2 months postoperatively. (**b**) Postoperative refractive cylinder distribution 2 months postoperatively. (**c**) Efficacy. (**d**) Safety

- Stable Refraction for 1 year and age of more than 21 years.
- Not a candidate for corneal refractive surgery.
- Anterior chamber depth ≥2.85 mm.
- Iridocorneal angle ≥35°.
- Crystalline lens elevation <200 μm.
- Flat iris configuration.
- Endothelial cell count:
  - ≥3000 cells if age <25 years.
  - ≥2500 cells if age 25–30 years.
  - ≥2200 cells if age >30 years.
- Toric: Refractive cylinder ≥1.25–1.5 D.

Contraindications

- Progressive keratoconus, unstable corneas.
- Highly aberrated eyes (total HOA >3 μm) with poor best spectacle corrected visual acuity (<0.5).
- Any condition that can compromise proper alignment of the IOL:
  - Zonular deficiencies.
  - Lens subluxation.

The clinician should always consider the complications that can be caused by this type of phakic intraocular lenses [19, 20]:

- Endothelial cell damage.
- Cataract formation.
- Glare.
- Disengagement of the haptics.
- Pigmentary dispersion.
- Large corneal incision.

27.6 Conclusions

The use of phakic lenses in selected cases of stable keratoconus with high refractive error seems to be a valid therapeutic alternative for the treatment of ametropia that accompanies this disease. In the vast majority of studies, it has shown a high degree of effectiveness and safety of treatment, along with a great satis faction of patients. More studies are needed to evaluate the best options for the intraocular management of refractive errors in patients with keratoconus.

Compliance with Ethical Requirements Pablo Sanz Díez, Alfredo Vega Estrada, Roberto Fernández Buenaga, and Jorge L. Alió declare that they have no conflicts of interest. All procedures were in accordance with the ethical standards of the responsible committee on human experimentation (institutional and national) and with the Helsinki Declaration of 1975, as revised in 2000. Informed consent was obtained from all patients for inclusion in the study. No animal studies were carried out by the authors of this chapter.

This study has been supported in part by a grant from the European Regional Development Fund (Fondo europeo de desarrollo regional FEDER) and the Spanish Ministry of Economy and Competitiviness, Instituto Carlos III, Red Temática de Investigación Cooperativa en Salud (RETICS) "Prevención, detección precoz y tratamiento de la patología ocular prevalente, degenerativa y crónica". Subprograma "dioptrio ocular y patologías frecuentes" (RD12/0034/0007).

References

1. Rabinowitz YS. Keratoconus. Surv Ophthalmol. 1998;42:297–319.
2. Raiskup F, Theuring A, Pillunat LE, Spoerl E. Corneal collagen crosslinking with riboflavin and ultraviolet-A light in progressive keratoconus: ten-year results. J Cataract Refract Surg. 2015;41(1):41–6.
3. Piñero DP, Alio JL, El Kady B, et al. Refractive and aberrometric outcomes of intracorneal ring segments for keratoconus: mechanical versus femtosecond-assisted procedures. Ophthalmology. 2009;116(9):1675–87.
4. Worst JG. Iris claw lens. J Am Intraocul Implant Soc. 1980;6:166–7.
5. Fechner PU, van der Heijde GL, Worst JG. Intraocular lens for the correction of myopia of the phakic eye. Klin Monbl Augenheilkd. 1988;193:29–34.
6. Fechner PU, Singh D, Wulff K. Iris-claw lens in phakic eyes to correct hyperopia: preliminary study. J Cataract Refract Surg. 1998;24:48–56.
7. Fechner PU, Haubitz I, Wichmann W, Wulff K. Worst-Fechner biconcave minus power phakic iris-claw lens. J Refract Surg. 1999;15:93–105.
8. Moshirfar M, Grégoire FJ, Mirzaian G, Whitehead GF, Kang PC. Use of Verisyse iris-supported phakic intraocular lens for myopia in keratoconic patients. J Cataract Refract Surg. 2006;32(7):1227–32.
9. Kamburoglu G, Ertan A, Bahadir M. Implantation of Artisan toric phakic intraocular lens following Intacs in a patient with keratoconus. J Cataract Refract Surg. 2007;33(3):528–30.
10. Budo C, Bartels MC, van Rij G. Implantation of Artisan toric phakic intraocular lenses for the correction of astigmatism and spherical errors in patients with keratoconus. J Refract Surg. 2005;21(3):218–22.
11. Sedaghat M, Ansari-Astaneh MR, Zarei-Ghanavati M, Davis SW, Sikder S. Artisan iris-supported phakic IOL

implantation in patients with keratoconus: a review of 16 eyes. J Refract Surg. 2011;27(7):489–93.
12. Venter J. Artisan phakic intraocular lens in patients with keratoconus. J Refract Surg. 2009;25(9):759–64.
13. Alió JL, Peña-García P, Abdulla F, Zein G, Abumustafa S. Phakic intraocular lenses in keratoconus; comparison between Artiflex (iris-claw) and posterior chamber implantable collamer phakic intraocular lenses. J Cataract Refract Surg. 2014;40(3):383–94.
14. Izquierdo Jr L, Henriquez MA, McCarthy M. Artiflex phakic intraocular lens implantation after corneal collagen cross-linking in keratoconic eyes. J Refract Surg. 2011;27(7):482–7.
15. Alfonso JF, Lisa C, Fernández-Vega L, Madrid-Costa D, Poo-López A, Montés-Micó R. Intrastromal corneal ring segments and posterior chamber phakic intraocular lens implantation for keratoconus correction. J Cataract Refract Surg. 2011;37(4):706–13.
16. Güell JL, Morral M, Malecaze F, Gris O, Elies D, Manero F. Collagen crosslinking and toric iris-claw phakic intraocular lens for myopic astigmatism in progressive mild to moderate keratoconus. J Cataract Refract Surg. 2012;38(3):475–84.
17. Coskunseven E, Onder M, Kymionis GD, Diakonis VF, Arslan E, Tsiklis N, Bouzoukis DI, Ioannis Pallikaris I. Combined Intacs and posterior chamber toric implantable collamer lens implantation for keratoconic patients with extreme myopia. Am J Ophthalmol. 2007;144:387–9.
18. Kamiya K, Shimizu K, Ando W, Asato Y, Fujisawa T. Phakic toric implantable collamer lens implantation for the correction of high myopic astigmatism in eyes with keratoconus. J Refract Surg. 2008;24(8):840–2.
19. Lovisolo CF, Reinstein DZ. Phakic intraocular lenses. Surv Ophthalmol. 2005;50(6):549–87.
20. Benedetti S, Casamenti V, Marcaccio L, Brogioni C, Assetto V. Correction of myopia of 7 to 24 diopters with the Artisan phakic intraocular lens: two-year follow-up. J Refract Surg. 2005;21:116–26.

28 Toric Implantable Collamer Lens for Correction of Myopia and Astigmatism in Keratoconus

Mohamed Shafik Shaheen and Hussam Zaghloul

28.1 Introduction

Phakic refractive IOLs are becoming more and more popular because of the ease of implantation and the predictability of refractive and visual results.

Myopia and astigmatism are often associated with keratoconus, and patients with keratoconus often ask for refractive surgery. In such eyes, when corneal topography shows a keratoconic aspect or suggests a keratoconus fruste, implantation of a refractive IOL may be considered to avoid a postoperative fragile cornea. Moreover, the indication is easily considered because the anterior chamber depth is usually greater than 3.00 mm in such cases [1].

Phakic IOLs (PIOLs) allow correction outside the limits of the corneal refractive surgery [1]. The insertion of an implant in a phakic eye preserves accommodation and is reversible. Current IOL choices include AC PIOLs; angle-supported or iris-fixated models; and PC PIOLs, sulcus-fixated or free-floating models.

Historically, the idea of curing refractive problems by means of built-in or integrated additional optics (built-in glasses or contact lenses) sounds logical; however, even the great surgeons of our time failed initially with this approach that dates back to the late 1950s.

Despite the well-known setbacks of Strambelli [2–4], individual scientists never allowed the idea of PIOL implantation to die. Three different scientists pursued three different anatomic concepts for PIOLs at roughly the same time: Baikoff saw a solution in the angle-supported anterior chamber lens [5].

Fechner developed another solution in the modification of Worst's iris fixated lobster claw IOL and Fyodorov implanted a silicon lens into the posterior chamber [6].

The Baikoff design, angle-supported PIOLs evolved from 4-point fixation polymethyl methacrylate (PMMA) versions [5] to three-point PMMA versions, and then to foldable IOLs to decrease induced astigmatism. The PMMA versions failed basically due to endothelial cell loss, pupil ovalization, and induced astigmatism. To overcome these problems, the material was changed from PMMA to hydrophilic acrylate or hydrophobic acrylate. However, severe complications such as

M. Shafik Shaheen, M.D., Ph.D. (✉)
Department of Ophthalmology, University of Alexandria, Egypt, P.O. Box 27 Ibrahimia, Alexandria 21321, Egypt, Alexandria 21321, Egypt
e-mail: m.shafik@link.net

H. Zaghloul, M.D.
Department of Ophthalmology, Alexandria Armed Forces Hospital, 19 Ibrahim Elattar St. Zezinia, Alexandria, Egypt
e-mail: hussamhamed@gmail.com

J.L. Alió (ed.), *Keratoconus*, Essentials in Ophthalmology, DOI 10.1007/978-3-319-43881-8_28

endothelial decompensation [7] and pupil ovalization [8] after implantation of an anterior PIOL have resulted in several European countries having recalled these lenses for the correction of refractive errors [9].

The iris-fixated PIOL for the correction of myopia was introduced in 1986 as a rigid single-piece PMMA model with a 5.0- or 6.0-mm optic. The iris-fixated PIOL has been implanted for more than 20 years through a 5.0- to 6.0-mm incision. The goal of reducing surgically induced astigmatism was achieved with the development of the foldable iris-fixated model with silicone optic and PMMA haptics introduced in 2003.

The foldable design makes implantation possible through a 3.2-mm incision. However, this PIOL may be associated occasionally with recurrent intraocular inflammation, enhanced iris dispersion with posterior synechiae [10], and lenticular glistering [11].

The posterior chamber PIOLs to correct myopia was introduced first by Fyodorov in 1986 [6]. The first-generation Fyodorov PC PIOL was a one-piece silicon lens fixated by a haptic in the PC. In 1990, this lens was replaced by a second-generation model. Using knowledge of the early model of silicon posterior PIOL designs as a basis, two manufacturers, i.e., Medennium Inc., Irvine, CA, USA and STAAR Surgical Co., Monrovia, CA, USA, currently are researching and marketing posterior PIOL designs.

28.2 The Implantable Collamer Lens (ICL) (STAAR Surgical Co.)

The ICL has undergone many modifications in design since 1993. The latest model, V 4c, developed in 2011, made significant improvement in the amount of vaulting over the anterior lens capsule from the previous model [1]. The lens has a one-piece plate design with a rectangular shape, 7.5–8.0 mm wide, available in four standard overall lengths: 11.5–13.5 mm for myopic lenses and 11.0–13.0 mm for hyperopic lenses to adapt to eyes of different sizes.

The diameter of the optic zone is 4.65–5.5 mm in the myopic lenses, based on the desired dioptric power, and 5.5 mm for hyperopic ICLs.

Available powers for myopic lenses range from −3.0 to −22.0 D and from +3.0 to +20.0 D for hyperopic lenses [12].

The lens is introduced by means of a STAAR microinjector.

The proximity of the ICL to the crystalline lens, a dynamic phenomenon, has been postulated to be a risk factor for cataract development, which has been the main concern with this lens, and a greater vault would be expected to decrease ICL–crystalline lens contact [1, 12]. However, it is also possible that interference with lens nutrition instead of IOL contact of the crystalline lens may be the cause of cataract [13].

The main differences between the ICL and the phakic refractive lens (PRL) are the lens material and lens dynamics. The ICL is made of a collamer, which is hydrophilic acrylic with some cross-linked porcine collagen [13].

The PRL is made of hydrophobic silicone and rests on the zonulas and floats in the PC, whereas the ICL is fixated and supported in the ciliary sulcus. Cataract formation has been reported less frequently with the PRL [14]. However, rotation of the PRL in the PC excludes the possibility for cylinder compound whereas the ICL has the toric alternative for myopic eyes with astigmatism [15].

28.2.1 Device Description

The STAAR Surgical Visian ICL (Implantable Collamer Lens) is an intraocular implant manufactured from a proprietary hydroxyethyl methacrylate (HEMA)/porcine-collagen based biocompatible polymer material. The Visian ICL contains a UV absorber made from a UV absorbing material. The Visian ICL features a plate-haptic design with a central convex/concave optical zone and incorporates a forward vault to minimize contact of the Visian ICL with the central anterior capsule.

The Visian ICL features an optic diameter with an overall diameter that varies with the dioptric power; the smallest optic/overall diameter being 4.9 mm/12.1 mm and the largest 5.8 mm/13.7 mm. The lenses are capable of being folded and inserted into the posterior chamber through an incision of 3.2 mm or less.

The Visian ICL is intended to be placed entirely within the posterior chamber directly behind the iris and in front of the anterior capsule of the human crystalline lens when correctly positioned, the lens functions as a refractive element to optically reduce moderate to high myopia.

28.2.2 Material

Collagen—Copolymer (Collamer™) Biocompatible, Refractive index 1.45 at 35 °C, optically clear, UV Absorbing (10 % transmission).

28.2.3 Manufacture

Lathe cut, Laser engraved, Hydrated, Steam Sterilized, Single—Piece Design.

28.2.4 Different Versions of the Toric ICL

The development of the toric ICL has passed by many modifications since the first version in 1993 with appearance of the V family of the lens in 2007 which was stored in NaCl container and has no holes which necessitates making a peripheral iridotomy to help prevent pupillary block, in 2010 the improved version V4b came with two perioptic holes to facilitate removal of viscoelastic material behind the lens and the lens was stored in BSS not NaCl as before, in 2013 the newer version V4c was introduced with a central hole which allowed for the implantation of the lens without the need for the peripheral iridotomy (see Figs. 28.1, 28.2, and 28.3).

28.2.5 Recommended Criteria for the Toric ICL Implantation in KC Patients

- Normal systemic history and normal physical examination results.
- Absence of any history or physical signs of ocular disease with the exception of keratoconus and myopia.
- Age between 20 and 45 years.
- Best Spectacle Corrected visual acuity of 0.3 (20/60) or better in the eye to be treated.
- Stable refraction for at least 12 months after corneal collagen cross-linking.
- Clear central cornea.
- Normal anterior segment with an anterior chamber depth of at least 2.80 mm.
- Normal intraocular pressure.

28.2.6 Preoperative Assessment of Patients

- Manifest (Subjective) and Cycloplegic (Objective) refraction.
- Best spectacle corrected visual acuity:

Every single measure should be used to verify the subjective refraction before the calculation of the ICL power. The accurate subjective refraction in these cases is defined as the lowest sphere and cylinder values that give the best spectacle corrected visual acuity. These values together with the exact axis of the cylinder should be properly determined using all the available optometric tricks. The subjective refraction that gives the best spectacle corrected visual acuity should be checked in three consecutive monthly visits after at least 9 months of the CXL to get sure of the stability of refraction. The stability of the subjective refraction over the monthly visits is one of the most important parameters before planning to implant a toric ICL (TICL) for those patients. It indicates the stability of the keratoconic state after the CXL, hence the stability of the visual outcome after the TICL implantation. One of the

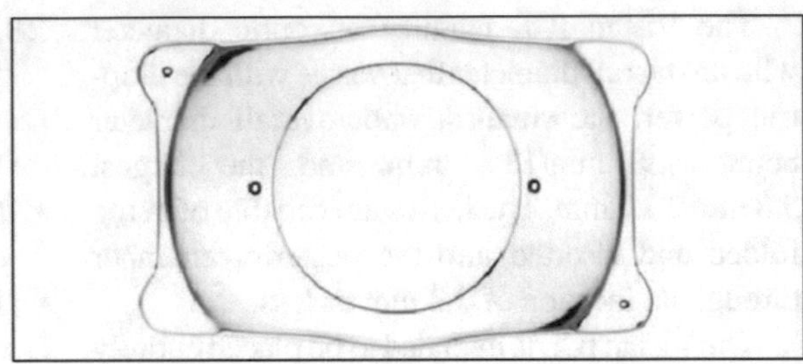

Fig. 28.1 Different periods of vaulting of the implanted toric ICL

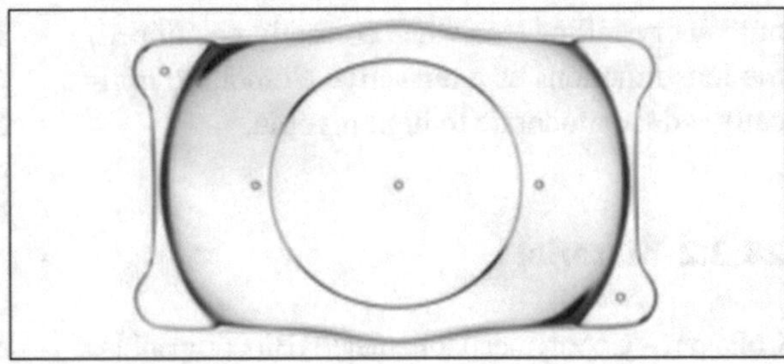

Fig. 28.2 The ICL V4b IOL

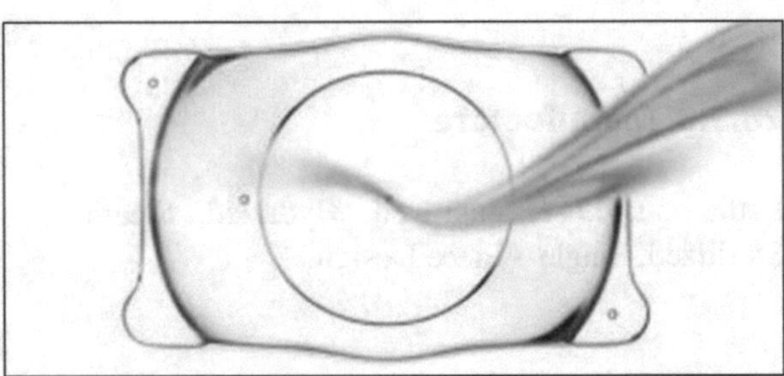

Fig. 28.3 The ICL V4c iol

useful clinical tricks is to prescribe glasses for those patients and encourage them to wear their glasses for at least 2 weeks before ordering the ICL. Patient's satisfaction and fair visual performance with the glasses before the TICL implantation are very good indicators of a good postoperative visual performance. Again, it is to be noted that there is usually a discrepancy between the value of the subjective and cycloplegic refraction in keratoconic eyes as a result of the corneal multifocality induced by the keratoconus [16].

Verification of the power of the sphere together with the power and exact axis of the cylinder give the best subjective spectacle corrected visual acuity is the key point of the success of the TICL implantation to give visual performance satisfaction for those patients.

- Anterior chamber depth using IOL Master (Carl Zeiss, Jena, Germany), a Scheimpflug anterior segment imaging (e.g., Pentacam), or anterior segment OCT.
- Corneal Curvature information (*K* readings).
- White-to-white measurement using a Caliper and/or IOL Master (Carl Zeiss, Jena, Germany).
- Assessment of anterior, posterior corneal surfaces and Anterior Chamber using a Scheimpflug camera system (e.g., Pentacam, Oculus Inc).
- The ICL power can be calculated using the software ICL POWER CHOICE OF STAAR SURGICAL. The verified stable subjective refraction, as described earlier, is the one that is used to calculate the TICL power.

28.3 Surgical Technique

- In order to dilate the pupil of the eye to be operated, 1 h before surgery, a Tropicamide 1 % (Mydriacyl, Alcon laboratories, Inc. Fort Worth, USA) and phenylephrine® ophthalmic solution 2.5 % (Alcon laboratories, Inc. Fort Worth, USA) are instilled every 15 min.
- Marking the exact horizontal and vertical axes of the cornea at the slit lamp with a pen marker.
- Checking and confirming that the pupil is fully dilated.
- Confirmation of the received TICL power and diameter.
- Reviewing the orientation diagram supplied by the manufacturer and establishing the implantation direction.
- Cleaning of the operative site with Povidone Iodine (Betadine®).
- Draping the patient and the operative site with sterile towels.
- Preparing the TCL for loading into the injector cartridge:
  - Open the lens container
  - Hydrate the micro-Staar foam tip (STAAR Surgical) inside the ICL container
  - Wet the inside of the micro-Staar injector with BSS.
  - Lubricate the inside of the cartridge with viscoelastic Healon® (10 mg/mL Sodium hyaluronate; Abbott).
  - Getting the ICL from its container using the foam tip
  - Loading the ICL inside the cartridge under the microscope on the side table using the foam tip and the coaxial forceps (Janach, J3864.1, sold by STAAR)
  - Insertion of the foam tip inside the micro-Staar injector.
  - Finally load the cartridge inside the injector.
- Cutting of the drape and exposing the operative eye with a self-retaining speculum.
- Bores and Mendez tool is used to determine the proper axis for the lens position as indicated by the implantation diagram.
- Marking the axis on the limbus using a surgical pen marker.
- Performing two sideport incisions (paracentesis) one at 12:00 o'clock and one at 6:00 o'clock.
- Temporal clear corneal tunnel of 3.00–3.2 mm with a disposable keratome after fixing the globe with 0.12 fixation forceps.
- Injection of viscoelastic in the anterior chamber.
- Insertion of the ICL using the injector.
- Injection of viscoelastic on top of the lens in the anterior chamber.
- Manipulating the distal haptic under the edge of the iris through the side port using an ICL special manipulator.
- Manipulation of the proximal haptic under the iris edge through the main 3.2 mm incision.
- ICL centration and rotation as necessary referring to the implantation guide.
- Removal of the viscoelastic using Simcoe irrigation/Aspiration cannula.
- Constriction of the pupil using Miochol-E (acetylcholine chloride intraocular solution) 1:100 with Electrolyte Diluent (Novartis, Switzerland).
- Surgical iridectomy after pupil constriction is achieved using Vitrectomy cutter in case of implanting the V4b version of the ICL (not necessary in the new version of V4c ICL as it has a central hole).
- Checking for wound leakage.
- Instillation of antibiotic eye drops.
- Removal of the drapes.
- Antibiotic and corticosteroid drops four times daily for 10 days.
- In cases of bilateral implantation, the second eye can be operated upon within the first postoperative week of the fellow eye.
- Postoperative follow up should include; uncorrected visual acuity (UCVA), CDVA, slit-lamp examination, Manifest and Cycloplegic refraction, funduscopy, and IOP measurements.
- Assessment of the postooerative ICL vaulting should be done using the slit lamp, the anterior segmant OCT and/or a Scheimpflug camera system (Pentacam, Oculus Inc.).

28.4 Clinical Results

In a study that was conducted by our team [16] to assess the use of the toric ICL to correct the ametropia in the stable keratoconus patients after corneal collagen cross-linking, a prospective interventional clinical study included 16 eyes that we followed for more than 3 years which is considered the longest follow-up period for this technique in published data.

The results demonstrate the efficacy of the technique in restoring a good visual acuity for those patients having residual high sphere and cylinder after corneal collagen cross-linking.

28.4.1 Visual Acuity

- Table 28.1 presents the different periods of the CDVA after the corneal cross-inking and ICL implantation, as noticed, the mean CDVA improved from 0.56 before cross-linking to >0.8 after 1 week of the ICL implantation, and this improvement was maintained throughout the follow-up period. The beta type 2 error was 0.0987.
- Table 28.2 presents the difference between the CDVA before the surgery and the postoperative UDVA demonstrating a significant improvement in the visual acuity as the mean for the preoperative CDVA was 0.63±0.14 and the mean of the postoperative UDVA was about 0.8 at 1 week and maintained throughout the rest of the follow-up or even got slightly better. The beta type 2 error was 0.0842.

28.4.2 Refraction

Considering the sphere, the preoperative mean was about −6.00±4.00 D, which improved to almost undetectable levels postoperatively. Preoperatively, the mean cylinder was about −5:00±1.50 D, and this improved to 0.0 D postoperatively; the spherical equivalent preoperatively was −8.50±4.00 D, and this improved postoperatively to less than −0.25 D. The beta type 2 error was 0.0835.

Table 28.1 Different periods of the CDVA after the corneal cross-linking and ICL implantation

CDVA	Before cross-linking	Before ICL	After 7 days	After 1 month	After 6 months	After 1 year	After 3 years
Range	0.40–0.80	0.40–0.80	0.60–1.20	0.60–1.20	0.60–1.20	0.60–1.20	
Mean±SD	0.56±0.13	0.63±0.14	0.82±0.16	0.87±0.15	0.89±0.17	0.89±0.17	0.89±0.17
Median	0.60	0.60	0.85	0.85	0.90	0.90	0.90
F (*p*)							
Mean difference (p_1)		0.063* (0.002)	0.256* (<0.001)	0.306* (0.028)	0.325* (<0.001)	0.325* (<0.001)	0.325* (<0.001)
Mean difference (p_2)			0.194* (0.002)	0.244* (<0.001)	0.263* (<0.001)	0.263* (<0.001)	0.263 (<0.001)
Mean difference (p_3)				0.050* (0.032)	0.069 (0.139)	0.069 (0.139)	0.069 (0.139)
Mean difference (p_4)					0.019 (1.000)	0.019 (1.000)	0.019 (1.000)
Mean difference (p_5)						0.0 (–)	0.0 (–)
Mean difference (p_6)							0.0 (–)

p_1, Bonferroni-adjusted *P* value for comparison between pre-cross-linking with each other period; p_2, Bonferroni-adjusted *P* value for comparison between pre-ICL with each other period; p_3, Bonferroni-adjusted *P* value for comparison between after 7 days with each other period; p_4, Bonferroni-adjusted *P* value for comparison between after 1 month with each other period; p_5, Bonferroni-adjusted *P* value for comparison between after 6 months with each other period; p_6, Bonferroni-adjusted *P* value for comparison between after 1 year and after 3 years

*Statistically significant at $P \leq 0.05$

Table 28.2 Difference between the CDVA before the surgery and the postoperative UDVA

UCVA	CDVA before ICL	After 7 days	After 1 month	After 6 months	After 1 year	After 3 years
Range	0.40–0.80	0.60–1.20	0.60–1.20	0.60–1.20	0.60–1.20	0.60–1.20
Mean ± SD	0.63 ± 0.14	0.79 ± 0.16	0.83 ± 0.16	0.85 ± 0.15	0.88 ± 0.18	0.88 ± 0.18
Median	0.60	0.80	0.80	0.80	0.85	0.85
F (*p*)			43.022* (<0.001)			
Mean difference (p_1)		0.169* (0.002)	0.206* (<0.001)	0.250* (<0.001)	0.250* (<0.001)	0.250* (<0.001)
Mean difference (p_2)			0.038 (0.135)	0.081* (0.042)	0.081* (0.042)	0.081* (0.042)
Mean difference (p_3)				0.044 (0.210)	0.044 (0.210)	0.044 (0.210)
Mean difference (p_4)					0.0 (–)	0.0 (–)
Mean difference (p_5)						0.0 (–)

p_1, Bonferroni-adjusted *P* value for comparison between pre-ICL with each other period; p_2, Bonferroni-adjusted *P* value for comparison between after 7 days with each other period; p_3, Bonferroni-adjusted *P* value for comparison between after 1 month with each other period; p_4, Bonferroni-adjusted *P* value for comparison between after 6 months with each other period; p_5, Bonferroni-adjusted *P* value for comparison between after 1 year and after 3 years; UCVA, uncorrected distant visual acuity
*Statistically significant at $P \leq 0.05$

The preoperative manifest refraction is used to calculate the TICL power. The beta type 2 error was 0.0762.

28.4.3 Vaulting of the TICL

The mean values were 539.13 ± 161.94 μm, 524.88 ± 151.61 mm, 509.12 ± 121.7 mm, 508.75 ± 132.4 μm, 508.90 ± 111.6 μm, and 507.12 ± 117.3 μm for the 1-week; 1-, 3-, 6-, 12-month; and 3-year postoperative periods of the follow-up, respectively (see Fig. 28.4).

28.4.4 Intraocular Pressure

The mean values were 12.0 ± 1.03 mmHg, 14.38 ± 2.45 mmHg, 13.0 ± 1.51 mmHg, 12.19 ± 1.33 mmHg, 11.94 ± 1.12 mmHg, and 11.94 ± 1.12 mmHg for the 1-week; 1-, 3-, 6-, 12-month; and 3-year postoperative periods of the follow-up, respectively.

28.4.5 Endothelial Cell Count

The mean preoperative endothelial cell count was 2850 cells per square millimeter; after 1 year, it was 2705 cells per square millimeter (−5.08 % cell loss). After 2 years, it was 2650 cells per square millimeter (−7.01 % cell loss), and after 3 years, it was 2594 cells per square millimeter (−8.89 % cell loss).

No complications occurred during the surgical procedures.

No eye needed explantation or repositioning of the TICL. Decentration of the TICL optic was not observed, and no case of pupillary block was detected.

28.5 Discussion

Refractive surgical correction of ametropia in patients with keratoconus remains challenging.

Progressive thinning and subsequent anterior bulging of the cornea can lead to high astigmatism

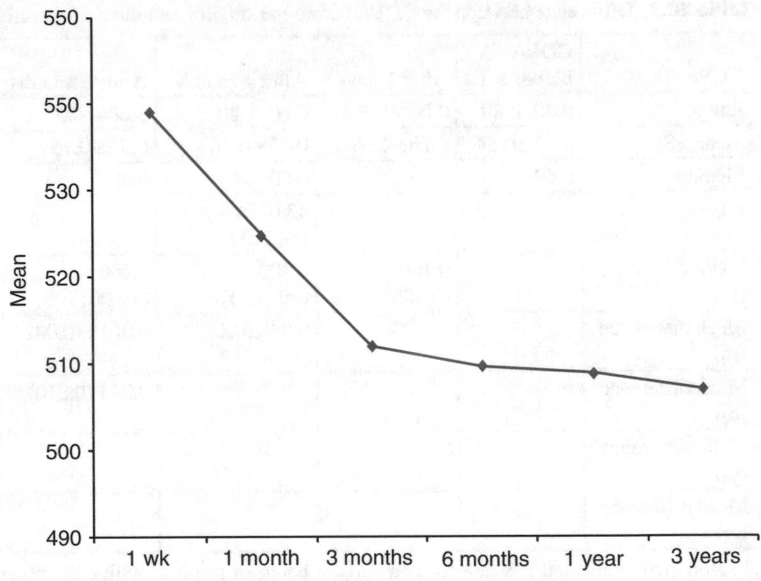

Fig. 28.4 The ICL V4c IOL. The KS-Aquaport is designed to restore a more natural aqueous flow and eliminate the need for an iridotomy

that is often accompanied by myopia and sometimes central scarring, resulting in mild-to-marked impairment in the quantity and quality of vision [17, 18].

Spectacles and contact lenses are the usual optical treatment options in the early stages of keratoconus [19].

In more advanced cases with severe corneal astigmatism and stromal opacity, patients may not tolerate contact lenses or there may be no improvement in visual acuity on using contact lenses. In these cases, a penetrating keratoplasty (PKP) or a deep anterior lamellar keratoplasty is necessary to restore visual function [20].

Collagen cross-linking using riboflavin and UV light was lately introduced [21]; however, cross-linking alone stabilizes and stiffens the cornea by inducing more corneal collagen cross-links of keratoconus, and the remaining refractive errors will still need to be corrected.

Our prospective nonrandomized clinical interventional study of 16 eyes, aimed to determine whether the implantation of a TICL in corneas that had been cross-linked and showed refractive stability for at least 12 months is safe, predictable, and effective in correcting different ranges of myopia and astigmatism in eyes with early stage keratoconus [16].

We obtained very satisfactory refractive outcomes in predictability with all the eyes being within 0.5 D of the intended spherical equivalent; the mean spherical equivalent was <0.25 D 3 years after the surgery. In addition, the astigmatism decreased significantly to nearly clinically insignificant values. Regarding visual outcomes, the efficacy was good with >81 % of the eyes having a postoperative UDVA of ≥0.8 and all the operated eyes maintaining a CDVA or gaining multiple lines of CDVA [16]. All the studied cases demonstrated line(s) gain in their postoperative BCVA. The improvement of the postoperative visual performance of these patients is attributed to many optical factors: The effect of the CXL on regularization of the corneal surface and relative recentering of the cone and then the correction of the remaining refractive error by the ICL which provides a magnification of image and improvement of the image details by correcting the refractive error at a level near to the nodal point. We think that the above-mentioned factors are responsible for the superior visual performance of the cross-linked keratoconic eyes after implantation of Toric ICL to correct their ametropia.

The efficacy and predictability of posterior chamber phakic toric IOLs in the treatment of different degrees of myopia combined with low to high astigmatism in virgin ametropic eyes are supported by many reports [15, 22–25]. Some studies demonstrated the efficacy and predictability of these lenses to treat similar refractive errors in stable keratoconic eyes [26]. Their long-term stability was also reported in our study [16].

The most commonly reported postoperative complications of the ICL implantation are anterior subcapsular cataract [27–29] and increased IOP [30, 31].

Sanders [32] reported that anterior subcapsular opacities and cataract occurred 5 years after surgery in the Food and Drug Administration trial.

Although approximately 6–7 % of eyes developed anterior subcapsular opacities ≥7 years after phakic IOL implantation, the opacity progressed to a clinically significant cataract in only 1–2 % during the same period, with most cases being observed in older patients and in eyes with very high myopia.

There were no cases of chronic increased postoperative IOP or anterior subcapsular cataract in our study.

Another concern is the degree of vaulting of the implanted ICL and how it changes over time; a study performed by Kojima et al. [33] 1 year after ICL implantation in 36 eyes showed that the mean vault was 0.53 ± 0.25 mm. A result consistent with the results in our study, which showed a mean vault of 0.509 ± 0.141 mm at 1 year postoperatively.

We also demonstrated that a high vault gradually decreases over time. The reason for the decrease in the initial vaulting measures especially from the 1-week to 1-month period of the postoperative follow-up may be related to the residual viscoelastic material that was present between the ICL and the crystalline lens, although meticulous irrigation/aspiration was performed.

A complete irrigation is often difficult because of the presence of a narrow space between the crystalline lens and the ICL.

It is preferable that TICL implantation not be performed until refraction and keratometry are stable after corneal collagen cross-linking. We prefer to wait for a least 1 year of the CXL to insure the stability of the refraction in those eyes.

The recommended indications for TICL implantation in keratoconus are as follows:

CDVA ≥20/60, clear central cornea, stable refraction at least 12 months after cross-linking and those patients who are satisfied with their spectacles prescription after CXL. Of course all measures should be exhausted to provide the best subjective spectacle corrected visual acuity before ordering the spectacles after stabilizing the cornea. If these criteria were not met, TICL is not considered as a good tool for ametropia correction and visual rehabilitation in keratoconic eyes a kind of keratoplasty would probably provide better visual outcomes.

In other words, TICL implantation should not be considered a true alternative to keratoplasty but rather an alternative treatment in cases of early-to-moderate stages of keratoconus with a relatively low irregular/regular astigmatism. The key point of success with this modality is to base the TICL power calculation on the subjective best spectacle correction refraction. This value should be meticulously verified and approved by both the patient and surgeon prior to TICL calculation, ordering, and implantation. A keratoconus patient who is happy with his glasses after CXL will be almost sure after TICL implantation as a result of the optical correction of his refractive error on a plane nearer to the nodal point by the ICL. We advise waiting for at least 1 year after the CXL to implant the TICL to get sure of the stability of the refraction and corneal state.

Refraction stability could be verified by 3 monthly consecutive visits in which the subjective refraction value that guarantees the best spectacle corrected visual performance is revised each time to insure stability before ordering and implanting the TICL.

All intraocular procedures entail some degree of endothelial cell loss, and insertion of a phakic IOL induces between 2.1 and 7.6 % [34]. Postoperative endothelial loss is also an important issue. For the ICL, the 1-year endothelial cell loss rate was 5.17 % in one study [35] and, in another, a cumulative decrease of 7.7 % was seen in the endothelial cell density over 5 years [36].

The reason for the discrepancy is possibly because of chronic low-grade inflammation [37].

28.6 Conclusion

Correction of spherical and cylindrical refractive errors in keratoconic eyes by TICL implantation after cross-linking seems to have significantly good outcomes, particularly in the astigmatic component of refraction. The significant visual improvement after this procedure could be attributed to two factors: the effect of the cross-linking on flattening/regularizing the cornea and the correcting effect of the TICL on a plane near the nodal point of the line of sight.

It is recommended to meticulously repeat the refraction of these eyes to obtain the subjective refraction that provides the best spectacle corrected visual performance and to calculate the ICL power using it to target postoperative emmetropia.

28.7 Example of a Clinical Case from Our Study

A 26-year-old female patient with progressing keratoconus who had corneal collagen cross-linking of her both eyes and showed refractive stability after 12 months. (Fig. 28.5 shows Pentacam study before CXL and 12 months after CXL.) The refractive stability was verified over the last 3 monthly visits of the patient. The patient had a BCVA of 0.4 (OD) and 0.8 (OS) with the subjective refraction of −9.50 −4.00 × 46 and −4.50 −3.50 × 138, respectively. The patient was given glasses to wear them over 2 months and she was very satisfied with them. A pair of toric ICLs was ordered for her based on the subjective refraction. The IOL Master (Zeiss, Germany) was used to provide values of the *K* readings, anterior chamber depth, and white-to-white measurements of both eyes (Fig. 28.6). Bilateral toric ICL implantation was performed 14 months after the CXL according to the provided data and the implantation forms provided by the manufacturer (Figs. 28.7 and 28.8). One month after the surgery the UCVA was 0.7 (OD) and 1.2 (OS) with a quite bilateral anterior segment, normal bilateral IOP, and an ICL central vault of 600 μm bilaterally as

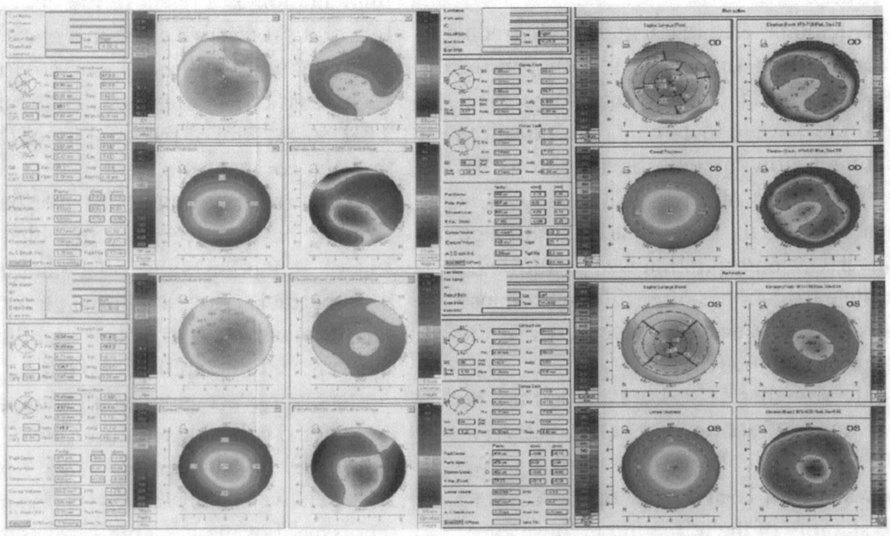

Fig. 28.5 Bilateral Scheimpflug images pre and 12 months postcorneal collagen cross-linking

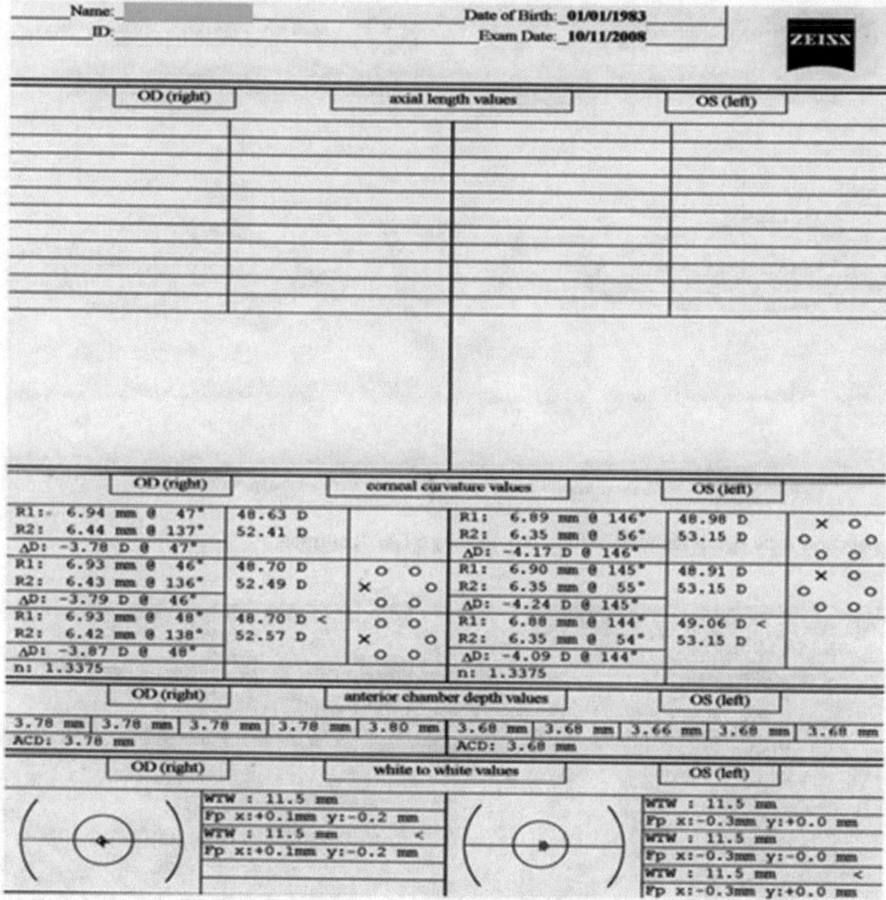

Name:
ID:
Date of Birth: 01/01/1983
Exam Date: 10/11/2008
ZEISS

OD (right) | axial length values | OS (left)

OD (right) | corneal curvature values | OS (left)

OD (right)		OS (left)	
R1: 6.94 mm @ 47°	48.63 D	R1: 6.89 mm @ 146°	48.98 D
R2: 6.44 mm @ 137°	52.41 D	R2: 6.35 mm @ 56°	53.15 D
ΔD: -3.78 D @ 47°		ΔD: -4.17 D @ 146°	
R1: 6.93 mm @ 46°	48.70 D	R1: 6.90 mm @ 145°	48.91 D
R2: 6.43 mm @ 136°	52.49 D	R2: 6.35 mm @ 55°	53.15 D
ΔD: -3.79 D @ 46°		ΔD: -4.24 D @ 145°	
R1: 6.93 mm @ 48°	48.70 D <	R1: 6.88 mm @ 144°	49.06 D <
R2: 6.42 mm @ 138°	52.57 D	R2: 6.35 mm @ 54°	53.15 D
ΔD: -3.87 D @ 48°		ΔD: -4.09 D @ 144°	
n: 1.3375		n: 1.3375	

OD (right) | anterior chamber depth values | OS (left)

OD (right)					OS (left)				
3.78 mm	3.78 mm	3.78 mm	3.78 mm	3.80 mm	3.68 mm	3.68 mm	3.66 mm	3.68 mm	3.68 mm
ACD: 3.78 mm					ACD: 3.68 mm				

OD (right) | white to white values | OS (left)

OD (right)	OS (left)
WTW : 11.5 mm	WTW : 11.5 mm
Fp x:+0.1mm y:-0.2 mm	Fp x:-0.3mm y:+0.0 mm
WTW : 11.5 mm <	WTW : 11.5 mm
Fp x:+0.1mm y:-0.2 mm	Fp x:-0.3mm y:-0.0 mm
	WTW : 11.5 mm <
	Fp x:-0.3mm y:+0.0 mm

Fig. 28.6 Bilateral corneal curvature data, anterior chamber depth, and white-to-white measurements as measured using the IOL Master® (Zeiss, Germany))

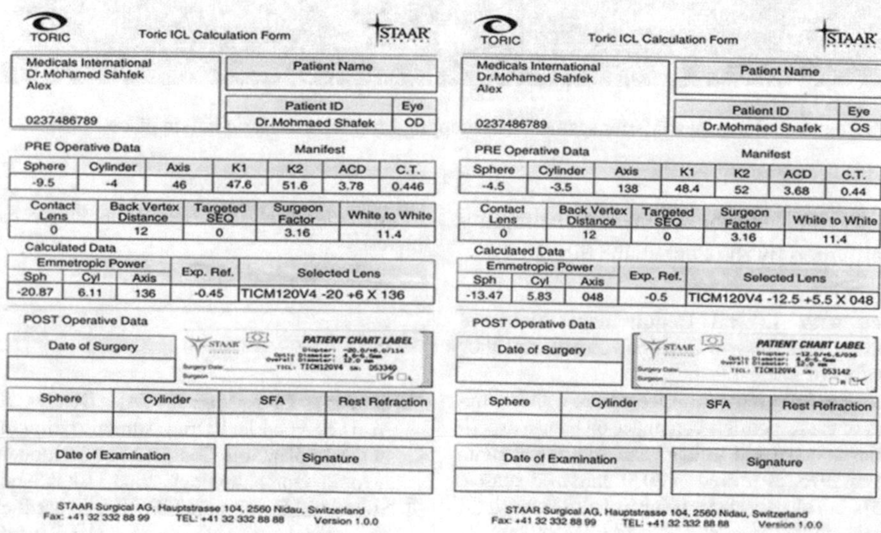

TORIC — Toric ICL Calculation Form — STAAR (OD)

Medicals International
Dr.Mohamed Sahfek
Alex
0237486789

Patient Name	
Patient ID	Eye
Dr.Mohmaed Shafek	OD

PRE Operative Data — Manifest

Sphere	Cylinder	Axis	K1	K2	ACD	C.T.
-9.5	-4	46	47.6	51.6	3.78	0.446

Contact Lens	Back Vertex Distance	Targeted SEQ	Surgeon Factor	White to White
0	12	0	3.16	11.4

Calculated Data

Emmetropic Power Sph	Cyl	Axis	Exp. Ref.	Selected Lens
-20.87	6.11	136	-0.45	TICM120V4 -20 +6 X 136

POST Operative Data

Date of Surgery — PATIENT CHART LABEL

Sphere	Cylinder	SFA	Rest Refraction

Date of Examination	Signature

STAAR Surgical AG, Hauptstrasse 104, 2560 Nidau, Switzerland
Fax: +41 32 332 88 99 TEL: +41 32 332 88 88 Version 1.0.0

TORIC — Toric ICL Calculation Form — STAAR (OS)

Medicals International
Dr.Mohamed Sahfek
Alex
0237486789

Patient Name	
Patient ID	Eye
Dr.Mohmaed Shafek	OS

PRE Operative Data — Manifest

Sphere	Cylinder	Axis	K1	K2	ACD	C.T.
-4.5	-3.5	138	48.4	52	3.68	0.44

Contact Lens	Back Vertex Distance	Targeted SEQ	Surgeon Factor	White to White
0	12	0	3.16	11.4

Calculated Data

Emmetropic Power Sph	Cyl	Axis	Exp. Ref.	Selected Lens
-13.47	5.83	048	-0.5	TICM120V4 -12.5 +5.5 X 048

POST Operative Data

Date of Surgery — PATIENT CHART LABEL

Sphere	Cylinder	SFA	Rest Refraction

Date of Examination	Signature

STAAR Surgical AG, Hauptstrasse 104, 2560 Nidau, Switzerland
Fax: +41 32 332 88 99 TEL: +41 32 332 88 88 Version 1.0.0

Fig. 28.7 Bilateral toric ICL calculation form provided by STAAR surgical

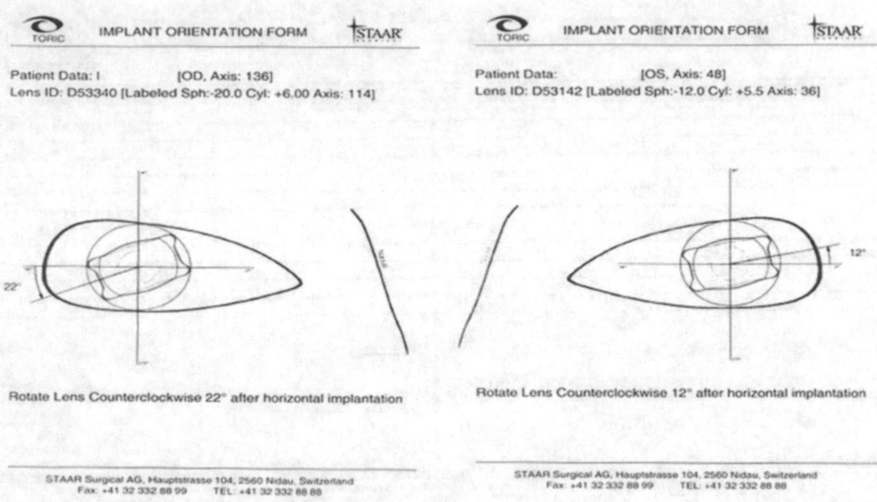

Fig. 28.8 Bilateral toric ICL implantation form provided by STAAR surgical

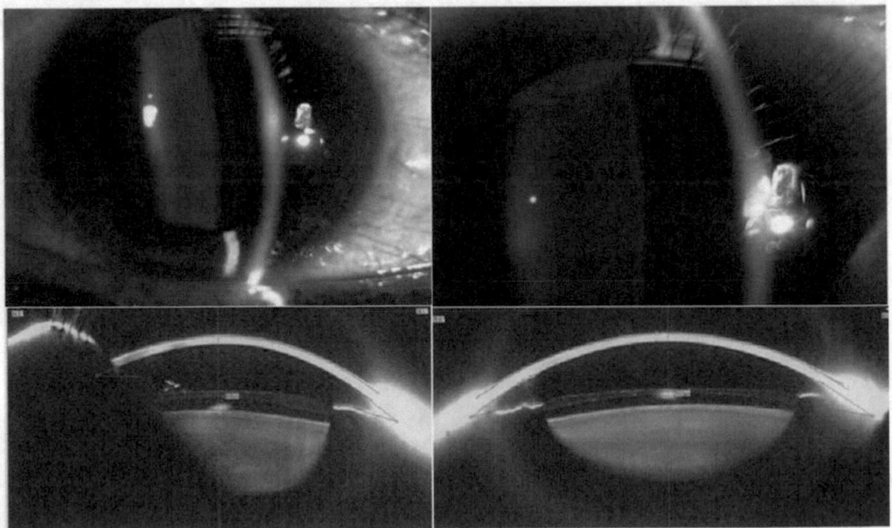

Fig. 28.9 Bilateral slit lamp and anterior segment Scheimpflug images of the toric ICL in place

measured by the anterior segment Scheimpflug imaging provided by the Pentacam (Fig. 28.9).

Compliance with Ethical Requirements Mohamed Shafik Shaheen and Hussam Zaghloul declare that they have no conflict of interest.

All procedures followed were in accordance with the ethical standards of the responsible committee on human experimentation (institutional and national and with the Helsinki Declaration of 1975, as revised in 2000. Informed consent was obtained from all patients for being included in the study.

No animal studies were performed by the authors for this chapter.

Financial disclosure: None of the authors has financial interest.

References

1. Sanders DR, Vukich JA, Doney K, Gaston M. U.S. Food and Drug Administration clinical trial of the Implantable Contact Lens for moderate to high myopia. Ophthalmology. 2003;110:255–66.
2. Strambelli B. Sopportabilitádi lenti acrilliche in camera anteriore nella afachia e nei vizi di refrazione. Ann Ottamol Clin Oculist. 1954;80:75–82.

3. Barraquer J. Anterior chamber plastic lenses. Results of and conclusions from five years' experience. Trans Ophthalmol Soc UK. 1959;79:393–424.
4. Choyce DP. Intra-cameral and intra-corneal implants. A decade of personal experience. Trans Ophthalmol Soc UK. 1966;86:507–25.
5. Baikoff G, Joly P. Comparison of minus power anterior chamber intraocular lenses and myopic epikeratoplasty in phakic eyes. Refract Corneal Surg. 1990;6:252–60.
6. Fyodorov S, Zuev V, Aznabayev B. Intraocular correction of high myopia with negative posterior chamber lens. Ophthalmosurgery. 1991;3:57–8.
7. Coullet J, Mahieu L, Malecaze F, Fournie P, Leparmentier A, Moalic S, Arne JL. Severe endothelial cell loss following uneventful angle-supported phakic intraocular lens implantation for high myopia. J Cataract Refract Surg. 2007;33:1477–81.
8. Leccisotti A. Angle-supported phakic intraocular lenses in hyperopia. J Cataract Refract Surg. 2005;31:1598–602.
9. Kohnen T. Evaluation of new phakic intraocular lenses and materials. J Cataract Refract Surg. 2007;33:1347.
10. Koss MJ, Cichocki M, Kohnen T. Posterior synechias following implantation of a foldable silicone iris-fixated phakic intraocular lens for the correction of myopia. J Cataract Refract Surg. 2007;33:905–9.
11. Cisneros-Lanuza A, Hurtado-Sarrio M, Duch-Samper A, Gallego-Pinazo R, Menezo-Rozalen JL. Glistenings in the Artiflex phakic intraocular lens. J Cataract Refract Surg. 2007;33:1405–8.
12. Lackner B, Pieh S, Schmidinger G, Hanselmayer G, Dejaco-Ruhswurm I, Funovics MA, Skorpik C. Outcome after treatment of ametropia with implantable contact lenses. Ophthalmology. 2003;110:2153–61.
13. Olson RJ, Werner L, Mamalis N, Cionni R. New intraocular lens technology. Am J Ophthalmol. 2005;140:709–16.
14. Pallikaris IG, Kalyvianaki MI, Kymionis GD, Panagopoulou SI. Phakic refractive lens implantation in high myopic patients: one-year results. J Cataract Refract Surg. 2004;30:1190–7.
15. Sanders DR, Schneider D, Martin R, Brown D, Dulaney D, Vukich J, Slade S, Schallhorn S. Toric implantable collamer lens for moderate to high myopic astigmatism. Ophthalmology. 2007;114:54–61.
16. Shafik Shaheen M, El-Kateb M, El-Samadouny M, Zaghloul H. Evaluation of a toric implantable collamer lens after corneal collagen crosslinking in treatment of early-stage keratoconus: 3-year follow-up. Cornea. 2014;33:475–80.
17. Davis LJ, Schechtman KB, Wilson BS, et al. Longitudinal changes in visual acuity in keratoconus. Invest Ophthalmol Vis Sci. 2006;47:489–500.
18. Zadnik K, Barr JT, Edrington TB, et al. Corneal scarring and vision in keratoconus: a baseline report from the collaborative longitudinal evaluation of keratoconus (CLEK) study; the CLEK study group. Cornea. 2000;19:804–12.
19. Mahadevan R, Arumugam AO, Arunachalam V, et al. Keratoconus—a review from a tertiary eye-care center. J Optom. 2009;2:166–72.
20. Gordon MO, Steger-May K, Szczotka-Flynn L, et al. Baseline factors predictive of incident penetrating keratoplasty in keratoconus. Am J Ophthalmol. 2006;142:923–30.
21. Wollensak G, Spoerl E, Seiler T. Riboflavin/ultraviolet-a-induced collagen crosslinking for the treatment of keratoconus. Am J Ophthalmol. 2003;135:620–7.
22. Kamiya K, Shimizu K, Igarashi A, et al. Comparison of collamer toric [corrected] contact lens implantation and wavefront-guided laser in situ keratomileusis for high myopic astigmatism. J Cataract Refract Surg. 2008;34:1687–93; erratum, 2011.
23. Sanders DR, Sanders ML. Comparison of the toric implantable collamer lens and custom ablation LASIK for myopic astigmatism. J Refract Surg. 2008;24:773–8.
24. Alfonso JF, Fernández-Vega L, Fernandes P, et al. Collagen copolymer toric posterior chamber phakic intraocular lens for myopic astigmatism: one-year follow-up. J Cataract Refract Surg. 2010;36:568–76.
25. Alfonso JF, Baamonde B, Madrid-Costa D, et al. Toric phakic intraocular collamer posterior chamber lenses to correct high degrees of myopic astigmatism. J Cataract Refract Surg. 2010;36:577–86.
26. Kamiya K, Shimizu K, Ando W, et al. Phakic toric implantable collamer lens implantation for the correction of high myopic astigmatism in eyes with keratoconus. J Refract Surg. 2008;24:840–2.
27. Gonvers M, Bornet C, Othenin-Girard P. Implantable contact lens for moderate to high myopia; relationship of vaulting to cataract formation. J Cataract Refract Surg. 2003;29:918–24.
28. Sanders DR, Vukich JA. Incidence of lens opacities and clinically significant cataracts with the implantable contact lens: comparison of two lens designs; the ICL in treatment of myopia (ITM) study group. J Refract Surg. 2002;18:673–82.
29. Jiménez-Alfaro I, Benítez del Castillo JM, García-Feijoó J, et al. Safety of posterior chamber phakic intraocular lenses for the correction of high myopia; anterior segment changes after posterior chamber phakic intraocular lens implantation. Ophthalmology. 2001;108:90–9; discussion by SM MacRay, 99.
30. Chung TY, Park SC, Lee MO, et al. Changes in iridocorneal angle structure and trabecular pigmentation with STAAR implantable collamer lens during 2 years. J Refract Surg. 2009;25:251–8.
31. Chun YS, Park IK, Lee HI, et al. Iris and trabecular meshwork pigment changes after posterior chamber phakic intraocular lens implantation. J Cataract Refract Surg. 2006;32:1452–8.

32. Sanders DR. Anterior subcapsular opacities and cataracts 5 years after surgery in the visian implantable collamer lens FDA trial. J Refract Surg. 2008;24:566–70.
33. Kojima T, Maeda M, Yoshida Y, et al. Posterior chamber phakic implantable collamer lens: changes in vault during 1 year. J Refract Surg. 2010;26:327–32.
34. Lovisolo CF, Reinstein DZ. Phakic intraocular lenses. Surv Ophthalmol. 2005;50:549–87.
35. Jiminez-Alfaro I, Benitez del Castillo JM, Garcia-Feijoo J, et al. Safety of posterior chamber phakic intraocular lenses for the correction of high myopia: anterior segment changes after posterior chamber phakic intraocular lens implantation. Ophthalmology. 2001;108:90–9.
36. Alfonso JF, Baamonde B, Fernández-Vega L, et al. Posterior chamber collagen copolymer phakic intraocular lenses to correct myopia: five-year follow up. J Cataract Refract Surg. 2011;37:873–80.
37. Bozkurt E, Yazici AT, Yildirim Y, et al. Long-term follow-up of first generation posterior chamber phakic intraocular lens. J Cataract Refract Surg. 2010;36:1602–4.

29 Cataract Surgery in the Patient with Keratoconus

Roberto Fernández Buenaga and Jorge L. Alió

29.1 Introduction

It has been reported that keratoconus patients are more likely to develop cataract compared with nonkeratoconus patients [1, 2]. Keratoconus is a progressive noninflammatory disease characterized by thinning and protrusion of the cornea. This results in high irregular astigmatism and myopia and a reduced visual acuity. Therefore, toric pseudophakic intraocular lenses (IOLs) are a very attractive option in these cases. Modern toric pseudophakic IOLs have shown excellent efficacy, predictability, and safety in correcting astigmatism at time of cataract surgery in eyes with normal corneas and regular astigmatism [3]. Clinical studies have shown significantly better UDVA and refractive astigmatism outcomes following toric IOL implantation compared with spherical IOL implantation in eyes with a cylinder power of 1.50 D or higher [4–6]. However, there are very few publications about toric pseudophakic lenses performance in keratoconic eyes [1, 2, 7–10]. In this chapter, we will review the patient selection, limitations of toric IOLs in keratoconic eyes, IOL power calculation, considerations during the cataract surgery, and the results published of cataract surgery in kerataconus.

29.2 Preoperative Examination

Preoperatively, a full ophthalmological examination is mandatory. It should include uncorrected distance visual acuity (UDVA) and corrected distance visual acuity (CDVA), manifest refraction, slit-lamp evaluation, Goldmann applanation tonometry, corneal topography and measurement of corneal aberrations, biometry, endothelial cell count, and funduscopy.

A topographer that analyzes both anterior and posterior corneal surfaces is preferred. Regarding the biometry, axial length and anterior chamber depth measured by partial coherence interferometry is desirable.

29.3 Patient Selection

There are two main limiting factors regarding cataract surgery in a keratoconic eye:

R. Fernández Buenaga, M.D., Ph.D.
Keratoconus Unit, Department of Refractive Surgery, Vissum Corporation, Avda de Denia s/n, Edificio Vissum, Alicante 03016, Spain
e-mail: rfernandezbuenaga@gmail.com

J.L. Alió, M.D., Ph.D., F.E.B.O. (✉)
Keratoconus Unit, Department of Refractive Surgery, Vissum Alicante, Alicante, Spain

Division of Ophthalmology, Miguel Hernández University, Alicante, Spain
e-mail: jlalio@vissum.com

J.L. Alió (ed.), *Keratoconus*, Essentials in Ophthalmology, DOI 10.1007/978-3-319-43881-8_29

- First, the decision of whether to perform the surgery or not is not easy. The difficulty for the clinician to evaluate the influence of the cataract on the visual acuity is probably one of the reasons why surgeons do not decide to operate in many of these cases. In other words, the clinician cannot measure separately the effect on one hand of the ectasia and on the other of the cataract on the visual limitation and cannot decide which the most influential factor is and therefore it is difficult to be sure if the surgery is really needed.
- Second, formulas for the calculation of the IOLs used are the same as those applied in nonkeratoconic patients. Measurement of high keratometry values in keratoconic eyes is not reliable and results vary depending on where the measurement is taken on the cornea. Additionally, keratoconic eyes are multifocal and the visual axis is not at the apex of the cornea but on the slope of the cone [11]. Thus, keratometry readings may be artificially high for the purposes of IOL calculation. Software used for toric IOL calculation by various companies is calibrated and validated on nonkeratoconic eyes with regular astigmatism where the apex of the cornea often roughly coincides with the visual axis [8].

Inclusion criteria for toric pseudophakic IOL implantation [2, 8–10]

- Mild-to-moderate keratoconus (usually grade I–II in Amsler-Krumeich classification)
- Nonprogressive disease. Cataract surgery is usually performed in patients older than 40 years old and keratoconus is usually stable at that age. In any case, progressive keratoconus is a contraindication for toric IOL implantation as the achieved effect will not be stable over time.
- Patients that were not rigid contact lens dependent to achieve good visual acuity.
- Good historical corrected (with spectacles) visual acuity (better than 20/40).
- Not very irregular astigmatism in the central 4 mm of the cornea.

We advocate using a keratoconus classification defined by our research group (called RETICS classification). This classification is mainly based on the CDVA but also in some aberrometric parameters such us the coma like [12]. The interest of this grading system is that it is a functional classification. Grade I is for those cases with decimal CDVA better than 0.9. Grade 2 eyes with CDVA >0.6 and ≤0.9. Grade 3: 0.4<CDVA ≤0.6, Grade 4: CDVA ≤0.4, and Grade plus: CDVA <0.2. According to this grading system, cataract surgery with toric IOL could be performed in Grade I and in selected Grade 2 cases. In the rest of the eyes, a reshaping procedure like intracorneal ring segments (ICRS) implantation should be attempted before the cataract surgery.

Figure 29.1 shows an example of a good candidate for cataract surgery with toric IOL implantation. Right eye refraction is +2.50 − 5 × 35° with a historical CDVA of 0.9 (decimal scale). Left eye refraction is +1.75 − 2.25 × 145° with a historical CDVA of 1.0. Topographies and aberrometric analysis of both eyes are shown earlier.

Figure 29.2 shows an example of patient with cataract and keratoconus. The right eye refraction is +2.50 − 6.50 × 30° (CDVA: 0.5) and the left eye: +1.25 − 5.50 × 145° (CDVA: 0.4). However, in this case, the optical aberrations in both eyes are high and a combined procedure of ICRS to improve the corneal regularity and decrease the coma aberration followed by cataract surgery with toric IOL implantation might be considered.

29.4 IOL Calculation

This is obviously the main issue when planning cataract surgery in keratoconic eyes. In a series of refractive lens exchange with toric IOL in keratoconus, the authors used Pentacam or Orbscan II keratometry and interferometry IOL calculation. The SRK II formula was used for the IOL power calculation [9]. Other authors also chose the *K*-values obtained with the Pentacam for the IOL calculation; however in this case, manual keratometry (Javal-Schiotz; Rodenstock, Dusseldorf, Germany) was used to obtain accurate determination of the axis of corneal astigmatism and the

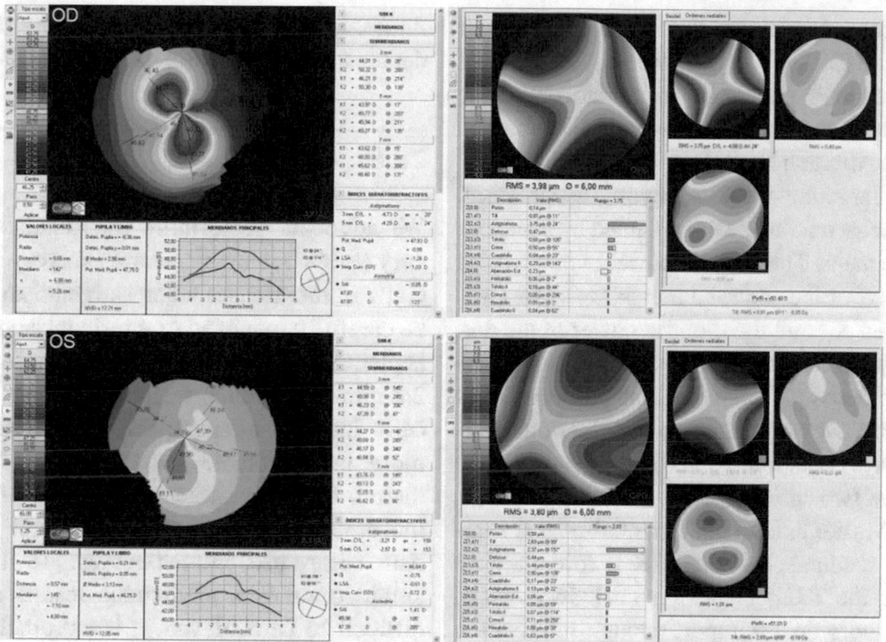

Fig. 29.1 An example of a good candidate for cataract surgery with toric IOL implantation. Right eye refraction is +2.50 − 5 × 35° with a historical CDVA of 0.9 (decimal scale). Left eye refraction is +1.75 − 2.25 × 145° with a historical CDVA of 1.0. Topographies and aberrometric analysis of both eyes are shown earlier

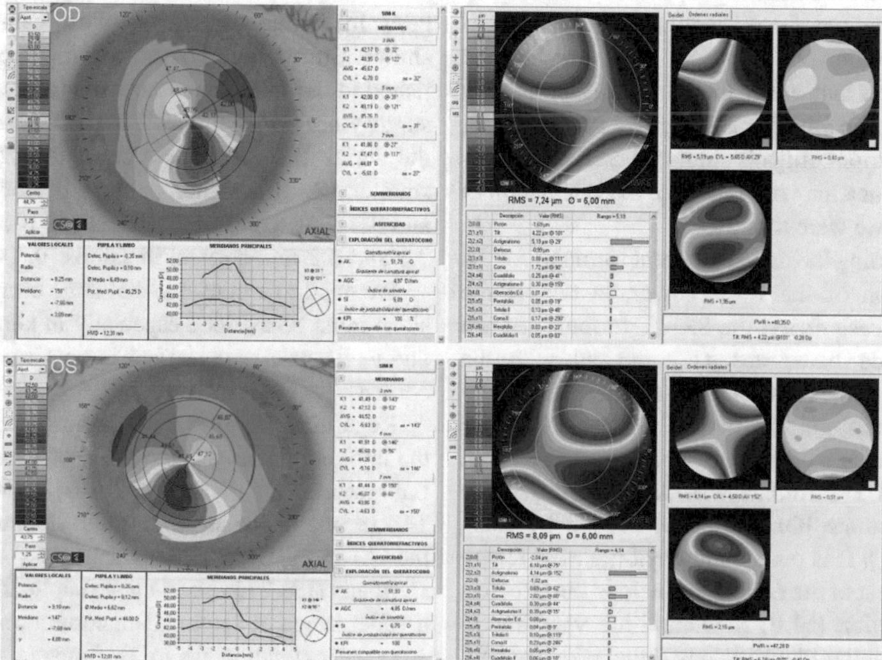

Fig. 29.2 This an example of patient with cataract and keratoconus. The right eye refraction is +2.50 − 6.50 × 30° (CDVA: 0.5) and the left eye is +1.25 − 5.50 × 145° (CDVA: 0.4). However, in this case, the optical aberrations in both eyes are high and a combined procedure of ICRS to improve the corneal regularity and decrease the coma aberration followed by cataract surgery with toric IOL implantation might be considered

elected formula was the Sanders–Retzlaff–Kraff theoretical (SRK/T) [2]. In the largest series of refractive lens exchange in keratoconus, the author calculated the IOL power by US biometry using the Allergan Humphrey 820 and Holladay 2 formula, targeting a residual myopic astigmatism. Keratometry readings were obtained by axial topographic maps. The dioptric power of the steepest meridian over the central 3 mm of the cornea was considered K_1, and the dioptric power of the flattest meridian over the central 3 mm of the cornea was considered K_2. Each meridian power was calculated by averaging its two semimeridian values, always considering the central 3 mm [13]. In a series of two cases of forme fruste keratoconus, the IOLMaster axial length, the Orbscan II keratometric readings, and the SRK II formula were used for the IOL calculation [14]. In contrast, other authors do not report enough information about how the IOL calculation was performed [8]. It is evident that there is big disparity among authors regarding the best method for IOL calculation in keratoconus patients. In any case, axial length measurement by optical interferometry and *K* readings from topographers are the preferred options. In our study [10], we had the impression that when the corneal shape is very altered, probably the deformity of the anterior and posterior cornea is similar, therefore the posterior cornea may not influence the calculation as much as we were thinking.

Regarding the use of different formulas for the calculation of the IOLs power, in one of the reported case series, the SRK/T formula seemed to provide better results compared with the Hoffer Q [10]. In contrast, in a different publication, the difference between the ideal IOL power and the calculated IOL power from SRK, SRK II, and SRK/T formulas was determined and the most accurate IOL power was found by using SRKII [1]. It is our opinion that the axial length and the rest of the factors that help in the effective lens position (ELP) prediction are very important. Formulas like Holladay II that take into consideration all these factors should be more accurate. We have also the hope that with the new ray tracing formulas we will be able to improve the predictability of these difficult cases in the future. In any case, greater series are needed to demonstrate which formula performs the best.

29.5 Surgery

We advocate performing microincisional surgery (MICS) in every cataract surgery but especially in those cases when astigmatism needs to be carefully managed or a toric intraocular lens is planned to be implanted. Incisions larger than 2.2 mm may induce variable amounts of surgically induced astigmatism (SIA) leading to a more unpredictable outcome [15–17]. Other factors that may affect the amount of SIA are the amount of preoperative corneal astigmatism, suture use, and patient age [18, 19]. As in keratoconus eyes predictable results are more difficult to be achieved, it is extremely important to avoid all the possible sources of error and uncontrolled surgically induced astigmatism due to a too large incision may be an important one. In a recent paper from our research group [10], the results of MICS surgery in keratoconus eyes with cataract are shown. Surprisingly, in most of the papers published to date, the incisions used to perform the surgery are larger than 2.2 mm. Only in two of the series the incisions size were 2.2 mm or smaller [2, 10]. Other authors performed 2.7 and 3.2 mm sclera tunnel incisions [8, 12], and 2.8 and 3.2 mm corneal incisions [9, 14].

We need to emphasize that large corneal incisions must be avoided especially in keratoconus due to its weakening effect in an already weak cornea.

Regarding the toric IOL, in most of the series the implanted IOL was the AcrySof Toric (Alcon Laboratories Inc. Ft Worth, Texas) [2, 9, 10, 13, 14]. In one of the series the IOL implanted was the AT TORBI 709M (Carl Zeiss Meditec, Germany) [8]. This bitoric plate haptic IOL offers a wider range of astigmatism correction than the AcrySof extending up to 12 diopters and even higher levels can be manufactured to order. At this moment it is necessary to remind that some manufactured toric IOL calculators consider the relation between cylinder power at the IOL plane and at the corneal plane as a fixed amount [20, 21]. This is an important error because the effective cylinder power of the IOL at the corneal plane is a function of the effective lens position and the spheroequivalent power of the IOL. The IOL cylindrical and spherical powers must first be converted into the two principal lens powers, after which both lens powers are calculated to the corneal plane using a standard vertex formula. The difference between both lens powers at the corneal plane should be used to select the most appropriate IOL cylinder power [3].

29.6 Results

Overall, outcomes after cataract surgery with toric IOL implantation in keratoconus are good. Nanavaty et al. [8] reported excellent outcomes with a UDVA of 20/40 or better in 75 % of the eyes and a reduction in the preoperative cylinder from 3.00 ± 1.00 D to 0.70 ± 0.80 D. Leccisotti [13] reported worse outcomes in his series of clear lens extraction and toric IOL implantation. IOL exchange surgery was needed in 11 cases (32 %) because the IOL power was not accurate due to the ultrasound biometry limitations. However, at 12 months, mean spherical equivalent (SE) was −1.31 ± 1.08 D and mean defocus equivalent was 1.94 ± 1.57 D. Twenty-two eyes (65 %) were within ±2 D of defocus equivalent, 16 eyes (47 %) were within ±1 D, and three eyes (9 %) were within ±0.5 D. The safety index was 1.38, and the efficacy index was 0.87.

Jaimes et al. [9], in their refractive lens exchange series in 19 keratoconus eyes showed that the mean preoperative sphere decreased from −5.25 ± 6.40 D to 0.22 ± 1.01 D postoperatively ($p < 0.001$). Mean preoperative cylinder and SE were 3.95 ± 1.30 and −7.10 ± 6.42, respectively, and improved to 1.36 ± 1.17 and −0.46 ± 1.12 after the surgery ($p < 0.001$). Preoperative mean UDVA was 1.35 ± 0.36 and changed to 0.29 ± 0.23 after the surgery ($p < 0.001$).

Thebpatiphat et al. [1] found a mean improvement in CDVA of four lines and a slight improvement in UDVA from 0.71 ± 0.41 to 0.63 ± 0.47; most of these patients were rigid contact lenses users before and after the surgery.

Our research group recently published the largest series of cataract surgery in keratoconic eyes [10]. Refractive outcomes before and after the surgery are presented in Table 29.1.

As it can be seen in the table, statistically significant improvements were found in the cylinder, defocus equivalent, UDVA, and CDVA. Meanwhile, the keratometry remained completely stable due to the neutral effect of the MICS incisions.

The safety index was 1.38 ± 0.58. Nine eyes (60 %) achieved postoperative UDVA ≥20/30. The efficacy index was 1.17 ± 0.66.

In Fig. 29.3a, b, the change in Snellen lines of corrected distance visual acuity versus percentage of eyes and the results for visual efficacy are shown.

In Fig. 29.4a, b, the postoperative spherical equivalent distribution and the attempted versus the achieved refraction can be seen. The black line corresponds to the fit line of the complete group.

It should be noticed in the graph earlier, that the refractive predictability of this surgery was very good for those patients with myopic astigmatism ($N = 10$), but not for patients with hyperopic astigmatism. However, the application of different formulas for the calculation of the IOL power (depending on the axial length) could influence the result.

There are also two more publications of cataract surgery in keratoconic eyes, they show good results but these papers are case report of only two cases each [2, 14].

According to the above-mentioned literature, toric IOL implantation in keratoconus at the time of cataract surgery reduces preoperative cylinder and overall improves patient's refraction. However, the predictability achieved is worse and not comparable with the predictability reported in eyes with normal corneas [3, 4, 6, 22–28].

29.7 Combined Procedures

In our clinical practice, we will also find cases with cataract and advanced keratoconus. In these patients, we usually need to combine several procedures. We may find two different situations:

Table 29.1 Changes in refractive, visual, and keratometric parameters for keratoconus stable patients operated of cataract using micro-inclusion cataract surgery

	Preoperative	Postoperative	Comparison (*p* value)
Sphere (D)	−1.77 ± 6.57 (−11.00 to 7.00)	0.08 ± 0.79 (−1.25 to 1.75)	0.211
Cylinder (D)	−2.95 ± 1.71 (−7.00 to −0.75)	−1.40 ± 1.13 (−3.25 to 0.00)	0.016*
Spherical equivalent (D)	−3.24 ± 6.14 (−11.75 to 5.63)	−0.62 ± 0.97 (−2.50 to 0.50)	0.158
Defocus equivalent (D)	5.73 ± 3.40 (0.25 to 11.75)	0.78 ± 0.84 (0.00 to 2.50)	0.001*
UDVA (logMAR)	1.33 ± 0.95 (0.40 to 2.77)	0.32 ± 0.38 (0.00 to 1.30)	0.008*
CDVA (logMAR)	0.32 ± 0.45 (0.01 to 1.77)	0.20 ± 0.36 (−0.03 to 1.30)	0.013*
K_1	43.93 ± 1.78 (42.05 to 46.32)	44.83 ± 2.38 (42.50 to 47.25)	0.593
K_2	46.95 ± 2.75 (44.35 to 50.05)	47.75 ± 2.29 (45.75 to 50.25)	0.580
K_M	45.44 ± 2.24 (43.70 to 48.19)	46.29 ± 2.14 (44.55 to 48.75)	0.625

CDVA corrected distance visual acuity, *UDVA* uncorrected distance visual acuity
The level of significance was $p = 0.05$
*Statistically significant difference

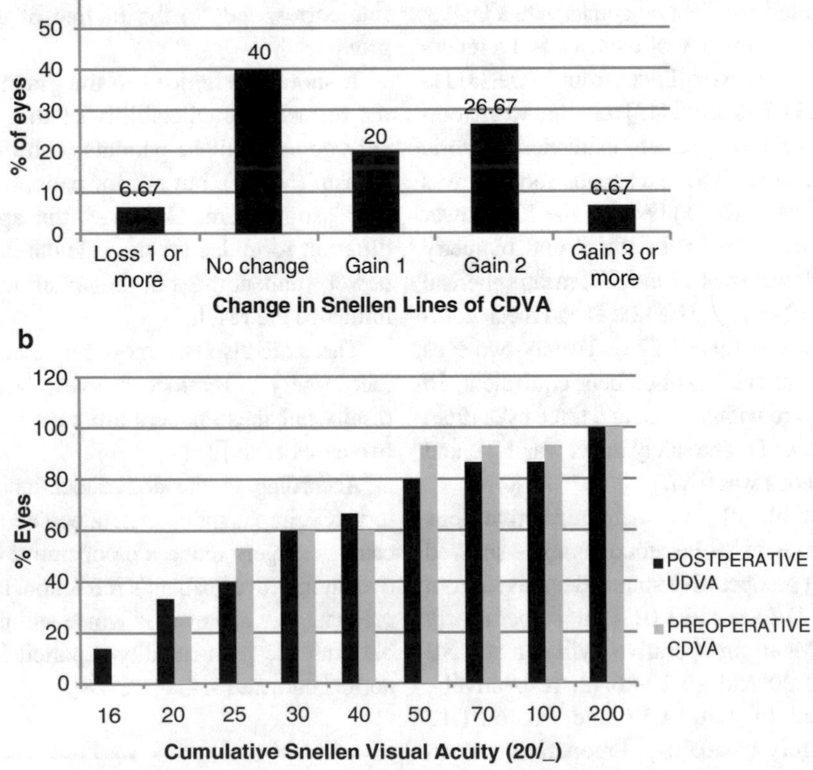

Fig. 29.3 (**a**, **b**) The change in Snellen lines of corrected distance visual acuity versus percentage of eyes and the results for visual efficacy are shown

1. Eyes with high irregular astigmatism and aberrations but with clear corneas and with the thinnest point at 6 mm of 400 µm or more. In these cases, we recommend to implant intracorneal ring segment/s to improve the corneal shape prior to the cataract surgery.

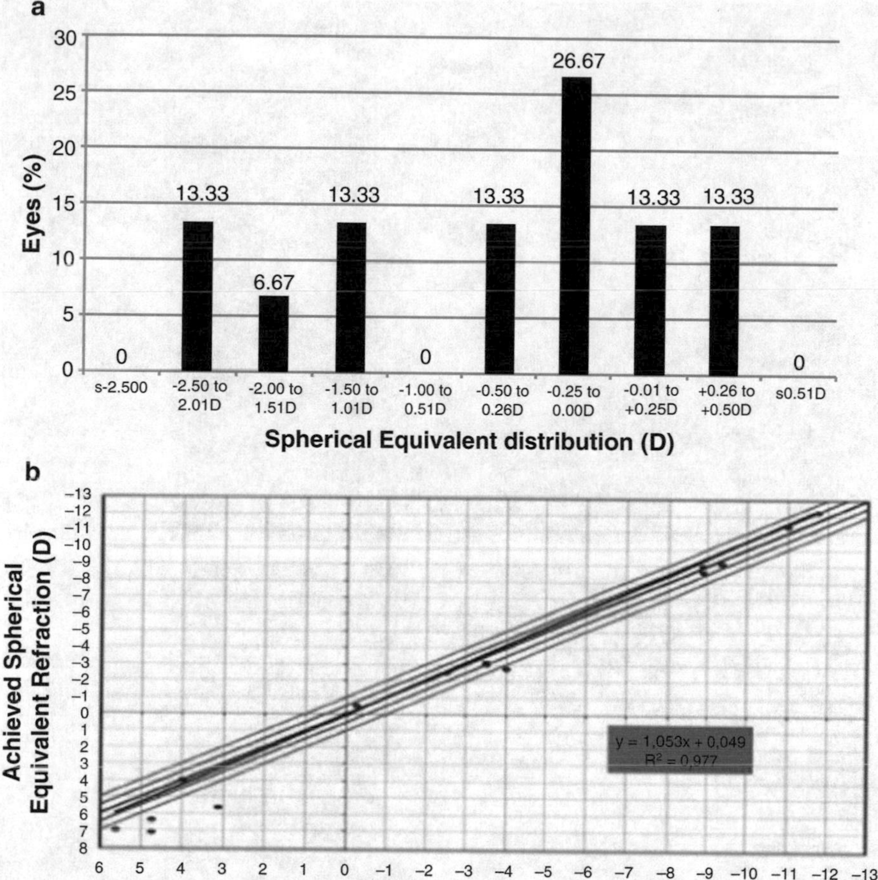

Fig. 29.4 (**a, b**) The postoperative spherical equivalent distribution and the attempted versus the achieved refraction can be seen. The *black line* corresponds to the fit line of the complete group

Once the corneal regularity is improved, we can proceed with the cataract surgery. A toric IOL may be implanted only in cases with low aberrations and low irregular astigmatism after the ICRS implantation.

2. Eyes with high irregular astigmatism and aberrations but with corneal scars (due to a previous hydrops) or too thin corneas for the ICRS implantation purpose. These are obviously the more extreme keratoconus cases and in these cases we need to combine corneal transplantation, preferably deep anterior lamellar keratoplasty (DALK), and cataract surgery. However, once again, we need to distinguish two different situations:
   (a) When the cataract is very dense or it is mild but penetrating keratoplasty (PK) is needed, it is better to perform the cataract surgery and the corneal transplantation at the same time.

   The endothelial cell number is always decreased after PK, thus the risk of corneal decompensation with cataract surgery is higher in eyes with previous PK.
   (b) When the cataract is not very dense and a DALK is planned, an interesting strategy is to first perform the DALK. Once the sutures are removed a cataract surgery is planned to improve the patient visual acuity but also with a refractive purpose, even implanting a toric IOL when the corneal regularity allows it (Fig. 29.5).

In a recent publication [29], toric IOL implantation results after corneal transplantation are analyzed in 21 cases. The authors show

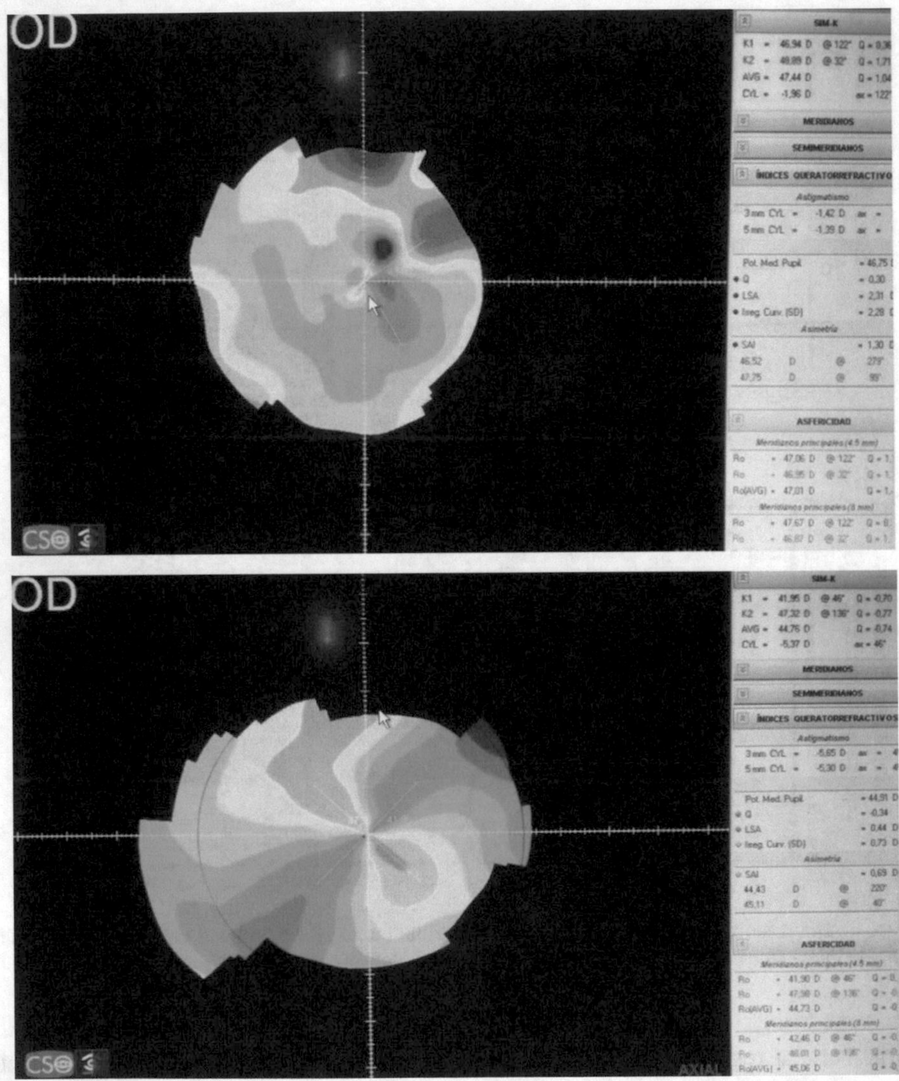

Fig. 29.5 This figure shows a case of sequential DALK and cataract surgery. This patient had advanced keratoconus and mild cataract. DALK was successfully performed and 1 year later, once the double running sutures were removed, cataract surgery with a toric IOL was performed to adjust the refractive outcomes. The first picture (*on top*) shows very low astigmatism (1.96 D) prior to the sutures removal. The second picture (*below*) shows increased astigmatism (5.37 D) after the suture removal. However, this is a nicely regular astigmatism

significant improvement in UDVA (logMAR, 0.90 ± 0.48 to 0.23 ± 0.25; $p = 0.0001$) and CDVA (logMAR, 0.31 ± 0.14 to 0.08 ± 0.13; $p = 0.0001$). A total of 14 of 21 eyes (67 %) and 17 of 21 eyes (81 %) had UDVA and CDVA of 20/30, respectively. Preoperative topographic astigmatism was 4.57 ± 2.05 D. Postoperative manifest refraction astigmatism was 1.58 ± 1.25 D.

Figure 29.5 shows a case of sequential DALK and cataract surgery. This patient had advanced keratoconus and mild cataract. DALK was successfully performed and 1 year later, once the double running sutures were removed, cataract surgery with a toric IOL was performed to adjust the refractive outcomes. The first picture (on top) shows very low astigmatism (1.96 D) prior to the sutures removal. The second picture (below) shows increased astigmatism (5.37 D) after the suture removal. However, this is a nicely regular astigmatism.

29.8 Conclusion

Cataract surgery in the keratoconic eye with the current technology improves the refraction and the quality of life of these patients. To achieve this satisfactory outcome, proper patient selection, IOL calculation with topography and optical biometry, microincisional cataract surgery, and toric IOL implantation in selected cases are mandatory.

Compliance with Ethical Requirements Roberto Fernández-Buenaga and Jorge L. Alió declare that they have no conflict of interest. "·"All procedures followed were in accordance with the ethical standards of the responsible committee on human experimentation (institutional and national) and with the Helsinki Declaration of 1975, as revised in 2000. Informed consent was obtained from all patients for being included in the study.

No animal studies were carried out by the authors for this chapter.

References

1. Thebpatiphat N, Hammersmith KM, Rapuano CJ, et al. Cataract surgery in keratoconus. Eye Contact Lens. 2007;33:244–6.
2. Visser N, Gast ST, Bauer NJ, et al. Cataract surgery with toric intraocular lens implantation in keratoconus: a case report. Cornea. 2011;30:720–3.
3. Visser N, Bauer N, Nuijts R. Toric intraocular lenses: historical overview, patient selection, IOL calculation, surgical techniques, clinical outcomes and complications. J Cataract Refract Surg. 2013;39:624–37.
4. Holland E, Lane S, Horn JD, Ernest P, Arleo R, Miller KM. The AcrySof toric intraocular lens in subjects with cataracts and corneal astigmatism; a randomized, subject-masked, parallel group, 1-year study. Ophthalmology. 2010;117:2104–11.
5. Statham M, Apel A, Stephensen D. Comparison of the AcrySof SA60 spherical intraocular lens and the AcrySof Toric SN60T3 intraocular lens outcomes in patients with low amounts of corneal astigmatism. Clin Exp Ophthalmol. 2009;37:775–9.
6. Ernest P, Potvin R. Effects of preoperative corneal astigmatism orientation on results with a low-cylinder-power toric intraocular lens. J Cataract Refract Surg. 2011;37:727–32.
7. Lee SJ, Kwon HS, Koh IH. Sequential intrastromal corneal ring implantation and cataract surgery in a severe keratoconus patient with cataract. Korean J Ophthalmol. 2012;26:226–9.
8. Nanavaty MA, Lake DB, Daya SM. Outcomes of pseudophakic toric intraocular lens implantation in keratoconic eyes with cataract. J Refract Surg. 2012;28:884–9.
9. Jaimes M, Xacur-Garcia F, Alvarez-Melloni D, et al. Refractive lens exchange with toric intraocular lenses in keratoconus. J Refract Surg. 2011;27:658–64.
10. Alió JL, Peña-García P, Abdulla Guliyeva F, Soria FA, Zein G, Abu-Mustafa SK. MICS with toric intraocular lenses in keratoconus: outcomes and predictability analysis of postoperative refraction. Br J Opthalmol. 2014;98(3):365–70.
11. Tan B, Baker K, Chen YL, et al. How keratoconus influences optical performance of the eye. J Vis. 2008;8(2):13.1–10.
12. Vega-Estrada A, Alio JL, Brenner LF, Javaloy J, Plaza-Puche AB, Barraquer RI, Teus MA, Murta J, Henriques J, Uceda-Montanes A. Outcome analysis of intracorneal ring segments for the treatment of keratoconus based on visual, refractive, and aberrometric impairment. Am J Ophthalmol. 2013;155:575–84.
13. Leccisotti A. Refractive lens exchange in keratoconus. J Cataract Refract Surg. 2006;32:742–6.
14. Navas A, Suárez R. One-year follow-up of toric intraocular lens implantation in forme fruste keratoconus. J Cataract Refract Surg. 2009;35:2024–7.
15. Kohnen T, Dick B, Jacobi KW. Comparison of the induced astigmatism after temporal clear corneal tunnel incisions of different sizes. J Cataract Refract Surg. 1995;21:417–24.
16. Oshika T, Nagahara K, Yaguchi S, Emi K, Takenaka H, Tsuboi S, Yoshitomi F, Nagamoto T, Kurosaka D. Three year prospective, randomized evaluation of intraocular lens implantation through 3.2 and 5.5 mm incisions. J Cataract Refract Surg. 1998;24:509–14.
17. Masket S, Wang L, Belani S. Induced astigmatism with 2.2- and 3.0-mm coaxial phacoemulsification incisions. J Refract Surg. 2009;25:21–4.
18. Lyhne N, Corydon L. Two year follow-up of astigmatism after phacoemulsification with adjusted and unadjusted sutured versus sutureless 5.2 mm superior scleral incisions. J Cataract Refract Surg. 1998;24:1647–51.
19. Storr-Paulsen A, Madsen H, Perriard A. Possible factors modifying the surgically induced astigmatism in cataract surgery. Acta Ophthalmol Scand. 1999;77:548–51.
20. Goggin M, Moore S, Esterman A. Outcome of toric intraocular lens implantation after adjusting for anterior chamber depth and intraocular lens sphere equivalent power effects. Arch Ophthalmol. 2011;129:998–1003.
21. Holladay JT. Exact toric intraocular lens calculations using currently available lens constants [letter]. Arch Ophthalmol. 2012;130:946–7.
22. Kim MH, Chung T-Y, Chung E-S. Long-term efficacy and rotational stability of AcrySof toric intraocular

lens implantation in cataract surgery. Korean J Ophthalmol. 2010;24:207–12.
23. Mingo D, Muñoz-Negrete FJ, Kim HRW, Morcillo R, Rebolleda G, Oblanca N. Comparison of toric intraocular lenses and peripheral corneal relaxing incisions to treat astigmatism during cataract surgery. J Cataract Refract Surg. 2010;36:1700–8.
24. Cervantes G, Garcia L, Mendoza E, Velasco C. High-cylinder acrylic toric intraocular lenses: a case series of eyes with cataracts and large amounts of corneal astigmatism. J Refract Surg. 2012;28:302–4.
25. Alió JL, Piñero DP, Tomás J, Alesón A. Vector analysis of astigmatic changes after cataract surgery with toric intraocular lens implantation. J Cataract Refract Surg. 2011;37:1038–49.
26. Tassignon M-J, Gobin L, Mathysen D, Van Looveren J. Clinical results after spherotoric intraocular lens implantation using the bag-in-the-lens technique. J Cataract Refract Surg. 2011;37:830–4.
27. Alió JL, Agdeppa MCC, Pongo VC, El Kady B. Microincision cataract surgery with toric intraocular lens implantation for correcting moderate and high astigmatism: pilot study. J Cataract Refract Surg. 2010;36:44–52.
28. Ahmed IIK, Rocha G, Slomovic AR, Climenhaga H, Gohill J, Grégoire A, Ma J, Canadian Toric Study Group. Visual function and patient experience after bilateral implantation of toric intraocular lenses. J Cataract Refract Surg. 2010;36:609–16.
29. Wade M, et al. Results of toric intraocular lenses for post-penetrating keratoplasty astigmatism. Ophthalmology. 2014;121:771–7.

30 Adjourn: A Glance at the Future of Keratoconus

Jorge L. Alió

The reader who has gone through the different chapters of this book has been able to confirm how improvements in genomics, proteomics, etiopathology, epidemiology, diagnostics, and therapy have improved our knowledge about keratoconus, jointly with a capability for early diagnosis which has indeed made keratoconus a more frequent disease because we can diagnose it properly. Most probably, this is just the beginning of a scientific and technical trend that will be further developed for a better understanding and treatment of keratoconus.

Looking at the future, we may guess that the computerized volumetric analysis of keratoconus will display not only the disease but also its capability to progress into different stages with different severities. The eye in keratoconus, for sure, is not only affected at the cornea but also at the scleral level. Further investigations will probably confirm early studies that are indicating that the sulcus and the anterior part of the sclera are indeed affected in keratoconus, which is something that seems to be just logical [1].

The advances in corneal surgery as applied in keratoconus today are clear but still with important limitations. Among the main ones are the unpredictable refractive and visual outcomes of corneal graft surgery in its different modalities. In spite of the recent advances with the use of femtosecond laser, deep anterior lamellar grafts and other sophistications, still the use of sutures that have to join a normal donor tissue to an abnormal tissue in harmonic shape and thickness make the outcomes unpredictable. Modern techniques based on the use of adhesives or diode laser welding most probably will eliminate the need for sutures or will make the use of sutures more adequate, useful, and predictable.

Invasive pharmacological therapy of the cornea initiated by the use of riboflavin and ultraviolet: the so-called corneal collagen cross linking therapy has just started. Ultraviolet is not the only radiation capable of crosslinking the cornea and riboflavin is not the only photosensitizer able to be stimulated and to make the oxidative changes that make the corneal collagen crosslinking in keratoconus possible. Most probably, the future use of nanotechnology and other methods that will be able to strengthen the corneal tissue collagen creating a different standard in treating keratoconus and perhaps even other diseases associated to the weakening of the ocular surface structure such as happens in high myopia.

We may forecast that the future knowledge and treatment is going to be completely different and better. Keratoconus, now treatable, will be in a

J.L. Alió, M.D., Ph.D., F.E.B.O. (✉)
Keratoconus Unit, Department of Refractive Surgery, Vissum Alicante, Alicante, Spain

Division of Ophthalmology, Miguel Hernández University, Alicante, Spain
e-mail: jlalio@vissum.com

J.L. Alió (ed.), *Keratoconus*, Essentials in Ophthalmology, DOI 10.1007/978-3-319-43881-8_30

given moment preventable, thanks to the help of genomics and proteomic diagnosis. The early application of invasive pharmacological therapy of the cornea will change the progression of the disease to stages in which surgery is today necessary. When necessary, surgery will be transformed to one with more predictable outcomes, using minimally invasive technology assisted by lasers and probably without the sutures used today.

The currently available and future developments that will happen in keratoconus treatment make this otherwise rare and frustrating corneal disease one of the most important issues that we have in cornea and basic and clinical research studies today.

Keratoconus is a model for the future understanding of the cornea and it is a model as well for future treatment of other corneal diseases. Let us participate in this most interesting and creative moment in the history of ophthalmology related to the technological and therapeutical development of the diseases of the cornea by the opportunity offered by keratoconus. The future of our patients and probably our understanding about today's partially known corneal diseases will improve and progress to a new and far better level of knowledge and ophthalmological practice.

Compliance with Ethical Requirements Jorge L. Alió declares that he has no conflict of interest. No human or animal studies were carried out by the author for this chapter.

Reference

1. Sorbara L, Maramb J, Mueller K. Use of the Visante™ OCT to measure the sagittal depth and scleral shape of keratoconus compared to normal corneae: Pilot study. J Optom. 2013;6:141–6.

Index

J.L. Alió (ed.), *Keratoconus*, Essentials in Ophthalmology, DOI 10.1007/978-3-319-43881-8

F

K

Printed in the United States
By Bookmasters